MW00654218

THERAPY FOR
MUCUS-CLEARANCE
DISORDERS

Property of Apollo College

LUNG BIOLOGY IN HEALTH AND DISEASE

Executive Editor

Claude Lenfant
Former Director, National Heart, Lung, and Blood Institute
National Institutes of Health
Bethesda, Maryland

ADDITIONAL VOLUMES IN PREPARATION

The opinions expressed in these volumes do not necessarily represent the views of the National Institutes of Health.

THERAPY FOR MUCUS-CLEARANCE DISORDERS

Edited by

Bruce K. Rubin
Wake Forest University School of Medicine
Winston-Salem, North Carolina, U.S.A.

Cees P. van der Schans
University for Professional Education "Hanzehogeschool"
Groningen, The Netherlands

MARCEL DEKKER, INC.   NEW YORK · BASEL

Although great care has been taken to provide accurate and current information, neither the author(s) nor the publisher, nor anyone else associated with this publication, shall be liable for any loss, damage, or liability directly or indirectly caused or alleged to be caused by this book. The material contained herein is not intended to provide specific advice or recommendations for any specific situation.

Trademark notice: Product or corporate names may be trademarks or registered trademarks and are used only for identification and explanation without intent to infringe.

Library of Congress Cataloging-in-Publication Data
A catalog record for this book is available from the Library of Congress.

ISBN: 0-8247-0716-8

This book is printed on acid-free paper.

Headquarters
Marcel Dekker, Inc., 270 Madison Avenue, New York, NY 10016, U.S.A.
tel: 212–696-9000; fax: 212–685-4540

Distribution and Customer Service
Marcel Dekker, Inc., Cimarron Road, Monticello, New York 12701, U.S.A.
tel: 800–228-1160; fax: 845–796-1772

Eastern Hemisphere Distribution
Marcel Dekker AG, Hutgasse 4, Postfach 812, CH-4001 Basel, Switzerland
tel: 41–61-260–6300; fax: 41–61-260–6333

World Wide Web
http://www.dekker.com

The publisher offers discounts on this book when ordered in bulk quantities. For more information, write to Special Sales/Professional Marketing at the headquarters address above.

Copyright © 2004 by Marcel Dekker, Inc. All Rights Reserved.

Neither this book nor any part may be reproduced or transmitted in any form or by any means, electronic or mechanical, including photocopying, microfilming, and recording, or by any information storage and retrieval system, without permission in writing from the publisher.

Current printing (last digit):

10 9 8 7 6 5 4 3 2 1

PRINTED IN THE UNITED STATES OF AMERICA

Introduction

As noted in the editors' preface to this monograph, in previous times airways mucus clearance was viewed as "disgusting" by members of the bourgeoisie, whereas the common people considered spitting a normal function consistent with well-being. Old-time physicians called it lung discharge, while today we refer to it as expectoration!

Irrespective of these perceptions and conventions, mucus and mucus clearnace have had a long and interesting history. Early Greek and Roman physicians thought that nasal discharge served to free the brain of excess fluid. This theory was eventually discarded, but nobody took mucus seriously until the late nineteenth century. Indeed, in 1888 F. H. Bosworth published a seminal paper on the physiology of the nose in which he ignored, if not belittled, mucus. It is noteworthy that this paper did not even mention a very fundamental publication that had appeared 100 years earlier! Its author was Charles Darwin—not the one famed for his work on the evolution of species, but a member of the same family. His publication, "Experiments Establishing the Criterion Between Mucoginous and Purulent Matter," provided the first demonstration that mucus clearance could be a vehicle for the discharge of pathogenic material.

Since that time, of course, much progress has been made. However, the turning point in this long journey of discovery was the relatively recent recognition that mucus clearance is a lung defense mechanism, but that if it does not function properly, it will cause respiratory function failure.

Since its beginning, the Lung Biology in Health and Disease series of monographs has addressed mucus and mucus clearance, but always to complement a discussion of another focus. Thus, only chapters—or even paragraphs—on mucus clearance have been presented. This volume provides a new and comprehensive perspective on mucus and mucus clearance. It is made up of three sections that lead the reader to what is important, that is, helping patients to feel better, if not to be cured of their illness. In developing the table of contents and selecting the contributors, the editors were cognizant of the objective, and they have developed a monograph that practicing physicians undoubtedly will value. The perspective, not to say guidance, reflects the experience of the best experts from many countries, a fact that makes this volume even more valuable.

All the authors, and the editors, Drs. Bruce Rubin and Cees van der Schans, have made an important and timely contribution. I am grateful for it, and for the opportunity to present it in the Lung Biology in Health and Disease series.

Claude Lenfant, M.D.
Bethesda, Maryland

Preface

The thought of mucus disturbs many people. Mucus is beneficial as the first defense of the airways. The mucus lining traps inhaled particles and allows them to be cleared from the airway by cilia and cough. The mucus layer also prevents dehydration and desiccation of the airway surface and provides a nutrient milieu for the ciliated epithelium. Mucus can also be quite bad. Airway mucus retention due to hypersecretion or poor mucus clearance is a characteristic of many airway diseases including cystic fibrosis, chronic bronchitis, bronchiectasis, and asthma. Mucus retention is thought to lead to airway obstruction, atelectasis, and tissue destruction by entrapping inflammatory mediators. It promotes microbial retention and growth. The Copenhagen longitudinal study showed that chronic mucus expectoration is associated with a poor prognosis in patients with chronic bronchitis. Mucus is also disgusting, and expectoration of sputum is often associated with lack of refinement and the spread of disease. It has even been postulated that, because of the social stigma associated with expectorating, persons who voluntary suppress cough and sputum expectoration are more likely to develop airway damage; this is called Lady Windemere's syndrome.

It is far to say that mucus is complex. Neither an ideal liquid nor a solid, mucus is a viscoelastic gel secreted by several different cell types and cleared from the airway by different mechanisms. Mucus is difficult to collect and a challenge to analyze. Because of this, mucus has proven fascinating to physicians, physical therapists, and physiologists, to pharmaceutical and biotechnology companies, and to epidemiologists and 8-year-old boys. There is now a critical group of investigators around the world studying many aspects of mucus secretion and clearance, and we are fortunate that many of these "phlegmish masters" have contributed their knowledge to this art book.

The book opens with an overview of airway mucus clearance by Duncan Rogers. This is an important review of the physiology and pharmacology of mucus secretion and clearance. Malcolm King then discusses methods for measuring mucus viscoelasticity and gives a practical underpinning for the use of mucolytic agents. Dr. King also explains the complex polymer chemistry involved in the biophysical evaluation of mucus properties. Dr. Jonathan Widdicombe follows this with a chapter on the regulation of mucus secretion describing how mucus secretion and clearance are coordinately regulated. He explains the mechanisms of mucus hypersecretion in persons with chronic airway inflammation and briefly discusses interventions that may reduce hypersecretion.

Medications to promote sputum clearance are sold without prescription around the world and represent a large share of the over-the-counter drug market, but proof of efficacy is very limited. One of the challenges facing those who develop, evaluate, and market mucus-clearance therapies is deciding on appropriate and meaningful outcome variables for clinical trials. In Chapter 4, the various efficacy measures that have been used are critically reviewed and specific recommendations given for choosing outcomes that are appropriate for the medication or device and for the patient population being studied. Because airway-clearance techniques can be effort- and time-intensive—especially when used several times daily for months and years, Dr. Webb and colleagues describe the results of studies evaluating adherance with common airway-clearance techniques, offering suggestions for improving adherance to therapy. These two chapters along with the final chapter in Part Two, by Dr. Babatunde Otulana and colleagues, provide useful guidelines for those interested in drug and devices development and clinical evaluation. Dr. Otulana has spent many years at the U.S. Food and Drug Administration and in industry. From this perspective he gives clear guidance on regulatory issues related to the development of drugs and airway-clearance devices.

Part Two discusses mucoactive medications. Many classification systems have been used to describe mucoactive medications. Chapter 6 provides a classification based on their putative mechanism of action. This chapter is also an overview of subsequent chapters discussing these different medications. Because mucoactive medications can be delivered orally, parenterally, or by therapeutic aerosol, Drs. Amirav and Newhouse review the advantages and disadvantages of each of these routes and discuss techniques for aerosol delivery in detail.

Expectorant medications increase the volume and water content of airway secretions. This is the class of mucoactive medication that has been in longest use, going back to ancient therapies for pulmonary diseases. Dr. Ziment reviews this fascinating history and provides an evidence-based assessment of the potential effectiveness of these medications.

Mucolytics are medications that specifically reduce the viscosity of mucus secretions by disrupting or disentangling the polymer structure of mucus. Classic mucolytics do this by virtue of effects on mucin polymers while peptide mucolytics disrupt the pathological DNA and actin polymers in sputum. Dr. King presents the molecular basis for mucolytic therapy.

Mucus is first cleared by coordinated ciliary activity. Drs. Rutland, Morgan, and de Iongh explain the physiology of mucociliary clearance and the contribution of ciliary beat force, beat frequency, and beat coordination (metachronicity) in this process. They describe primary and secondary disorders of ciliary activity and structure and how medications can affect mucociliary clearance.

Mucokinetic medications increase the cough transportability of sputum, usually by increasing expiratory air flow or by reducing the adhesion of mucus to epithelium. Surfactant phospholipids are the best described of the mucokinetic agents. Drs. Anzueto and Rubin describe the balanced processes of mucus-epithelium adhesion and abhesion and how abhesive medications like surfactant can improve mucus and sputum clearance in persons with chronic hypersecretory airway diseases associated with epithelial damage.

Mucoregulation is the process of decreasing chronic mucus hypersecretion that can obstruct and damage the airway. Dr. Tamaoki and colleagues explain the presumed mechanism of action of these agents and describe the clinical use of each of these types of medication, with special emphasis on the glucocorticosteroids and the macrolide antibiotics.

Hyperosmolar aerosol inhalation has been used both for sputum induction and to promote sputum clearance in persons with cystic fibrosis or bronchiectasis. Like ion-channel modifiers that increase the transport of ions (primarily sodium and chloride) and water into the airway lumen, hyperosmolar aerosols have been shown to increase mucus secretion, decrease sputum adhesion to the epithelium, and perhaps "thin" mucus by increasing airway water transport. Dr. Kishioka describes the physiology of ion and water transport in the airway and reviews the clinical use of this class of mucoactive medications.

Although mucoactive medications have primarily been used to treat pulmonary disease, the upper airway, including the paranasal sinuses and the eustachian tubes, are also mucus secretion ciliated epithelia. Otolaryngologists, allergists, and rhinologists have long recognized that sinus mucostasis can lead to recurrent bacterial infection and chronic sinusitis and otitis media. Professors Sakakura and his colleagues explore the use of mucoactive therapy for upper-airway disorders and give practical suggestions for using and assessing these therapies.

Chapters 16 and 17 then review the application of chest physical therapy and breathing techniques as physical means to enhance mucus clearance. The various airway-clearance device modalities are described in detail, as well as the physiology of mucus clearance by the application of physical therapy, with specific recommendations given for both. The term chest physical therapy usually suggests the application of various breathing techniques, hand clapping on the chest, and vibration and postural draining, all to promote more effective cough and sputum expectoration. Dr. Olséni and colleagues discuss the proposed mechanism of action for these maneuvers, the evidence for their effectiveness, and their common use to promote mucus clearance.

A variety of devices have been developed and tested that are meant to improve mucus clearance by altering the physical interaction of the secretions with the epithelium. High-frequency oscillation, positive expiratory pressure, and Flutter are thought to help secure airway patency and enhance expiratory airflow while helping to detach secretions bound to the airway wall. Mr. Fink and Dr. King differentiate these techniques and give evidence-based suggestions for their clinical application.

Chapter 18–20 describe special consideration related to airway-clearance techniques and medications for children, patients in the perioperative period, and those with neuromuscular disease. These are patient populations with special needs and requirements that are well described by the authors.

The child with acute or chronic difficulty with mucus clearance presents a special set of problems for the therapist. Children can have difficulty with the independent performace of physical therapy or breathing techniques and the youngest children (generally those less than 5 years of age) will rarely expectorate sputum even when coughing. Professor Zach and Dr Oberwaldner review the theraputic considerations in treating children and how these can be modified to be most effective at different ages.

Postoperative patients are at greater risk for mucostasis, atelectasis, and pneumonia because of immobility, pain, weakness, and any residual effects of anesthesia. Chapter 19 discusses the special risk posed by surgery and how to best prevent and treat mucostasis in the perioperative period.

Patients with neuromuscular diseases such as spinal motor atrophy, amyotrophic lateral sclerosis, or muscular dystrophy frequently develop chest infections from secretion aspiration and from poor cough due to muscle weakness. Dr. Bach cares for a large number of patients with neuromuscular disease and he has developed and tested specific and effective protocols and procedures to enhance mucus clearance and prevent atelectasis and infection.

The study of mucus secretions and clearance in health and disease is a rapidly evolving field. This has been one of the most difficult-to-treat components of asthma, cystic fibrosis, chronic bronchitis, and other chronic inflammatory airway disease, but appropriate therapies promises some of the greatest benefits in these diseases. This book gives an in-depth evaluation of the physiology of airway mucus secretion and clearance as well as medications and devices used to clear mucus from the lungs. It also provides specific guidelines for development and testing of new therapies.

Bruce K. Rubin
Cees van der Schans

Contributors

Janice Abbott, Ph.D. Professor of Health Physiology, Faculty of Health, University of Central Lancashire, Preston, England

Israel Amirav, M.D. Pediatric Department, R. Sieff Hospital, Kfar Hanassi, Israel

Antonio Anzueto, M.D. Associate Professor, Division of Pulmonary and Critical Care, University of Texas Health Science Center, San Antonio, Texas, U.S.A.

John R. Bach, M.D. Professor, Department of Physical Medicine and Rehabilitation and Department of Neurosciences, UMDNJ–The New Jersey Medical School, Newark, New Jersey, U.S.A.

Robb de Iongh Ph.D.* Concord Repatriation General Hospital, Concord, New South Wales, Australia

Linda Denehy, Ph.D. School of Physiotherapy, University of Melbourne, Parkville, Victoria, Australia

Mary E. Dodd, F.C.S.P. Consultant Physiotherapist Clinician, Adult Cystic Fibrosis Unit, Wythenshawe Hospital, Manchester, England

---

Current affiliation: Anatomy and Cell Biology, University of Melbourne, Parkville, Victoria, Australia

James B. Fink, M.S., R.R.T.   Aerogen, Inc., Mountain View, California, U.S.A.

John W. Georgitis, M.D.   Department of Pediatrics, Wake Forest University School of Medicine, Winston-Salem, North Carolina, U.S.A.

Donald J. Kellerman   Inspire Pharmaceuticals, Durham, North Carolina, U.S.A.

Malcolm King, Ph.D.   Pulmonary Research Group, University of Alberta, Edmonton, Alberta, Canada

Chikako Kishioka, M.D.   Department of Otorhinolaryngology, Mie University School of Medicine, Mie, Japan

Mitsuko Kondo   Tokyo Women's Medical University School of Medicine, Tokyo, Japan

Louise Lannefors   Department of Lung Medicine, University Hospital, Lund, Sweden

Yuichi Majima, M.D.   Department of Otorhinolaryngology, Mie University School of Medicine, Mie, Japan

Lucy Morgan   Concord Repatriation General Hospital, Concord, New South Wales, Australia

Richard J. Morishige   Aradigm Corporation, Hayward, California, U.S.A.

Atsushi Nagai   Tokyo Women's Medical University School of Medicine, Tokyo, Japan

Michael T. Newhouse, M.D.   Nektar Therapeutics, San Carlos, California, U.S.A.

Beatrice Oberwaldner, P.T.   Abteilung für Pulmonologie/Allergologie, Univeritatsklinik für Kinder- und Jugendheilkunde, University of Graz, Graz, Austria

Kosuke Okamoto, M.D.   Department of Otorhinolaryngology, Mie University School of Medicine, Mie, Japan

Lone Olséni, Med. Sci. R.P.T.   Department of Lung Medicine, University Hospital, Lund, Sweden

Babatunde A. Otulana, M.D. Aradigm Corporation, Hayward, California, U.S.A.

Duncan F. Rogers Thoracic Medicine, National Heart & Lung Institute, Imperial College, London, England

Bruce K. Rubin, M. Engr., M.D., F.R.C.P.C., F.C.C.P. Professor and Vice-Chair, Department of Pediatrics, and Professor of Biomedical Engineering, Physiology, and Pharmacology, Wake Forest University School of Medicine, Winston-Salem, North Carolina, U.S.A.

Jonathan Rutland Concord Repatriation General Hospital, Concord, New South Wales, Australia

Yasuo Sakakura, M.D. Professor and Chairman, Department of Otorhinolaryngology, Mie University School of Medicine, Mie, Japan

Jun Tamaoki First Department of Medicine, Tokyo Women's Medical University School of Medicine, Tokyo, Japan

Jodi Thomas, M.D. Department of Physical Medicine and Rehabilitation, UMDNJ–The New Jersey Medical School, Newark, New Jersey, U.S.A.

J. P. van de Leur, B.Sc. Department of Rehabilitation, University Hospital Groningen, Groningen, The Netherlands

Cees P. van der Schans, P.T., Ph.D. Professor of Nursing and Allied Health, University for Professional Education "Hanzehogeschool", Groningen, The Netherlands

A. Kevin Webb, F.R.C.P. Professor of Respiratory Medicine, Adult Cystic Fibrosis Unit, Wythenshawe Hospital, Manchester, England

J. H. Widdicombe, Ph.D. Department of Human Physiology, University of California–Davis, and Cardiovascular Research Institute, University of California–San Francisco, San Francisco, California, U.S.A.

Maximilian S. Zach, M.D. Abteilung für Pulmonologie/Allergologie, Univeritatsklinik für Kinder- und Jugendheilkunde, University of Graz, Graz, Austraia

Irwin Ziment, M.D. Professor and Chief of Medicine, Olive View–UCLA Medical Center, Sylmar, California

Contents

THERAPY FOR
MUCUS-CLEARANCE
DISORDERS

1

Overview of Airway Mucus Clearance

DUNCAN F. ROGERS

National Heart & Lung Institute
Imperial College
London, England

It goes up, mucus.
It goes down, mucus.
It comes out!
Eduardo Saurez

I. Introduction

Mucus clearance from the respiratory tract is a housekeeping job second to none. Inhalation of ~500 L of air per hour delivers up to 600 million particles to the lungs on a daily basis (1). Cigarette smoking could easily double the lung burden (2,3). This onslaught of soot, microbes, allergens, and irritants is prevented from impinging upon and penetrating the airway epithelium by a thin layer of slimy liquid, termed mucus. The coordinated beating of cilia wafts the mucus and flotsam to the throat, where they are unwittingly swallowed (Fig. 1) (4). Consequently, mucus clearance represents the first-line defense of the respiratory tract (5). If clearance falters, mucus accumulates and obstructs the airways (Fig. 2). Other mechanisms can be enlisted to help shift mucus, including two-phase gas-liquid flow (whereby energy is transferred from airflow to

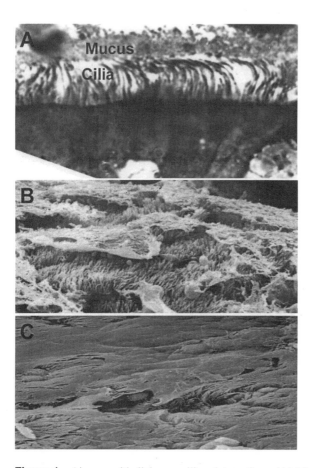

Figure 1 Airway epithelial mucociliary interactions. (A) Mucus movement on cilia in bovine trachea. Note differences in bending of the cilia at different stages of the beat cycle. (Courtesy of K. Pritchard.) (B) Scanning electron micrograph of mucus "flakes" or "rafts" resting on top of cilia in human bronchus. (Courtesy of P. K. Jeffery.) (C) Scanning electron micrograph of "sheets" of mucus in rat trachea. (Courtesy of P. K. Jeffery.)

mucus transport), airway "peristalsis," and cough (6). Cough and expectoration can invariably dislodge and remove excess mucus from larger diameter airways (7). However, patients with advanced airflow obstruction may be incapable of generating sufficiently forceful expiratory flows. Under these circumstances, cough becomes ineffective, leading to disparate mucociliary transport and markedly reduced clearance from central airways (8).

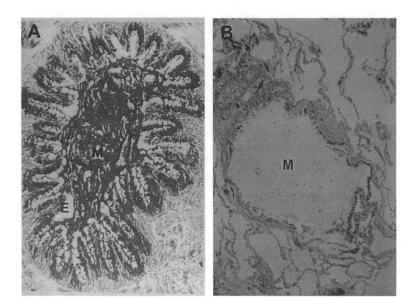

Figure 2 Mucus obstruction of the airways in asthma and COPD. (A) Fatal interaction between bronchoconstriction and lumenal mucus. Intrapulmonary airway of a patient who died of an acute severe asthma attack showing airway epithelium (E) thrown into folds by smooth muscle contraction, and occlusion of remaining lumen by mucus (M). (B) Mucus obstruction (M) in an intrapulmonary airway of a cigarette smoker.

Long-term impairment of mucus clearance can lead to significant airflow limitation in a number of severe respiratory conditions, including asthma (9), chronic obstructive pulmonary disease (COPD) (10,11), and cystic fibrosis (CF) (12). It should be noted, however, that subjects with primary ciliary dyskinesia (PCD) (also termed immotile cilia syndrome), a condition predisposing to respiratory disease, in most cases lead normal active lives by utilizing cough and "hawking" to dislodge and clear airway mucus (13,14). PCD apart, impaired airflow due to impaired mucus clearance is usually associated with increased morbidity and mortality in asthma (15), COPD (16), and CF (17,18). However, it should be noted that the impact of impaired mucus clearance on morbidity and mortality is not unequivocal or pertinent to all patients. Nevertheless, there are certain groups of patients, for example, those with COPD who have mucous hypersecretion and are prone to chest infections (19), in which a causal association has been demonstrated. Consequently, there is the perception that improving mucus clearance should have clinical benefit in hypersecretory conditions of the airways, and numerous pharmaceutical and other treatments are available or in development that are aimed, either directly or indirectly, at aiding clearance. However, although asthma, COPD, and CF share mucus obstruction as a clinical feature, the pathophysiological mechanisms underlying the impairment in mucus clearance may be different, to a greater or lesser extent, for each condition. For example, there are real and theoretical differences in the patho-physiology of airway mucous hypersecretion between asthma, COPD, and CF (Fig. 3). In addition, the structure and movement of individual cilia (defective in PCD) and the coordination of their beating, the amount, composition, and rheological properties of the mucus layer, whether or not there is defective trans-

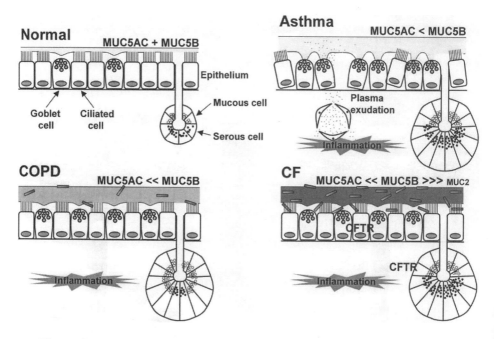

Figure 3 Putative differences in pathophysiology of airway mucus obstruction in asthma, COPD, and CF. Compared with normal, in asthma there is airway inflammation, increased luminal mucus, with an increased ratio of MUC5B to MUC5AC, epithelial "fragility" with loss of ciliated cells, marked goblet cell hyperplasia, submucosal gland hypertrophy (although without a marked increase in mucous-to-serous ratio), "tethering" of mucus to goblet cells, and plasma exudation. In COPD there is airway inflammation, increased luminal mucus, goblet cell hyperplasia, submucosal gland hypertrophy (with an increased proportion of mucous to serous acini), an increased ratio of mucin MUC5B to MUC5AC compared to that in asthma, and a susceptibility to infection. In CF there is airway inflammation, increased luminal mucus, goblet cell hyperplasia, submucosal gland hypertrophy, an increased ratio of MUC5B to MUC5AC, small amounts of MUC2 present in the mucus, and a marked susceptibility to infection. Many of these differences require confirmation (or otherwise) by data from greater numbers of subjects.

epithelial electrolyte flux (as in CF) (20,21), and the features of airway inflammation and remodeling that uniquely characterize different respiratory diseases are all factors that influence the efficiency of mucus clearance. Consequently, no one therapy is likely to be effective across the spectrum of mucus-obstructive conditions of the respiratory tract. It is possible that disease-specific therapy will be more successful.

This chapter gives an overview of airway mucus clearance, using asthma and COPD as examples of respiratory conditions that share impaired clearance as a clinical feature, but with specific differences in mucus pathophysiology. CF will be mentioned where appropriate for comparative purposes as a third respiratory condition with its own pathophysiology and mucus problems. Factors involved in the rational design of pharmacotherapeutic compounds to facilitate clearance will also be considered. A brief description of respiratory tract cilia, airway mucus, and cough is given first.

II. Airway Cilia and Ciliary Beat

Human lower airways are carpeted by half a square meter of ciliated epithelium comprising up to three thousand billion cilia (13). Each ciliated cell (Fig. 4) has ~200 cilia on its apical surface. The length of the cilia decreases with airway generation, from 5–7 µm in the trachea to 2–3 µm in the intrapulmonary bronchi (22). This is shorter than water-propelling cilia and is presumed to afford more rigidity for movement of mucus. The length is also related to the depth of the periciliary liquid layer (Sec. III) in which the cilia beat. Only the tips of the cilia engage with mucus, whereas longer cilia would pass through the mucus without imparting movement.

The mechanism of ciliary beat is based on the "9 + 2" architectural design that is evolutionarily conserved from protozoans through to humans (Fig. 5) (10,23). Each cilium contains nine outer interconnected doublet microtubules cross-linked to a sheath that surrounds two central microtubules. This arrangement is termed the axoneme. Each doublet comprises a complete microtubule, termed the A-subfiber, and a partial microtubule, termed the B-subfiber. The central microtubules terminate at the base of the cilium, while the doublets continue into the cytoplasm to form a basal body that is stabilized by a basal foot, a striated rootlet, and interconnections with the apical cytoskeleton. The doublets support a variety of attachments, the most important of which are paired adenosine triphosphatase (ATPase) or dynein arms that project from the A-subfiber. The dynein arms undergo a mechanochemical cycle of alternating sliding that generates ciliary motility (24,25). One ciliary abnormality in PCD is absence of the outer dynein arms (Fig. 6), which leads to impaired beating and reduced ability to move mucus.

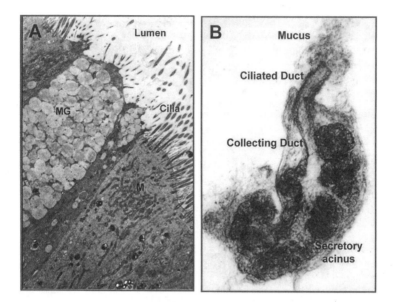

Figure 4 Mucociliary elements in the airways: goblet cell, ciliated cell, and submucosal gland. (A) Electron micrograph of human bronchus showing a goblet cell packed with intracellular mucin granules (MG), a ciliated cell with numerous cilia, and prominent mitochondria (M), the latter consistent with its high metabolic activity. (B) Isolated submucosal gland from dog trachea. Mucins secreted by mucous cells in mucous acini mix in the collecting duct with antibacterial agents secreted by serous cells in serous acini. Ciliary action in the ciliated duct helps deliver the mucus onto the airway surface.

FACING PAGE

Figure 5 Structure of airway cilia. (A) Longitudinal sectional view of the structure of a cilium. A ciliary membrane derived from the cell membrane surrounds the ciliary shaft. At the tip, hair-like claws attach internally to a dense cap at the top of the microtubules of the axoneme. At the base of the cilium is the basal body (BB) with a number of attachments including a striated rootlet (SR) and a basal foot (BF) with microfilament (MF) and microtubule (MT) tethers. (B) Electron micrograph of a cross section through a human nasal cilium. (C) Schematic representation of B. Nine outer doublet microtubules, each comprising a complete A-subfiber and an incomplete B-subfiber, surround two central microtubules. Inner and outer dynein arms (ID and OD) project from the A-subfiber towards the next doublet. The outer doublets are connected to each other via nexin links and to structures associated with the central tubules via radial spokes (RS) with dilated heads. (D) Schematic cross section through the basal body showing arrangement of the nine triplet microtubules, nexin links, and radial spokes. (Adapted from Refs. 10 and 23.)

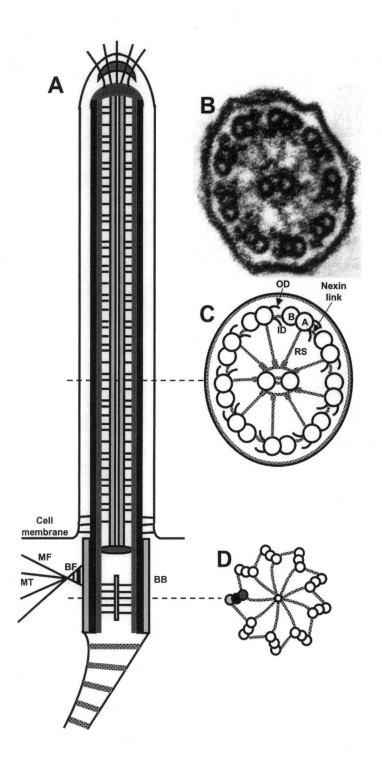

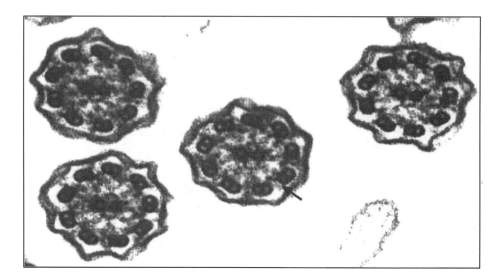

Figure 6 Airway ciliary ultrastructure in a patient with primary ciliary dyskinesia. Note absent or shortened (arrow) outer dynein arms. (Courtesy of K. Pritchard.)

Mucus is moved by an effective stroke whereby the cilia move in a plane perpendicular to the cell surface. A crown of short hair-like "claws" at the tips of the cilia engage with the mucus to aid traction (26). These claws are a feature of airway cilia and are not found in water-propelling cilia. Another feature of airway cilia is that the tips of the axoneme microtubules are embedded in the ciliary apical cap and are not completely free to slide. This causes the axoneme to twist as it bends, possibly enhancing the force of the effective stroke to aid movement of mucus (27). In addition, in contrast to water-propelling cilia, airway cilia incorporate a brief rest phase at the end of the effective stroke whereby the cilia lie with their tips pointing in the direction of mucus transport (28). This arrangement would tend to oppose retrograde mucus movement. The effective stroke occupies a quarter of the ciliary cycle. The other three quarters is for the recovery stroke whereby the cilia return to the rest position by curving back and to the side through the periciliary liquid layer (see Sec. III), near to the cell surface, to limit retrograde mucus movement. Ciliary beat frequency in the respiratory tract of healthy humans is 12–15 Hz (29).

For effective mucus movement, airway ciliary beat is coordinated into waves (23). In order to execute unhindered beat cycles, cilia move to a metachronal rhythm whereby each cilium is slightly out of phase with its neighbor. Hydrodynamic coupling between cilia facilitates metachronic coordination. However, airway metachrony is not as well coordinated as that of water-propelling cilia (28) and is presumably related to the specifics of movement of viscoelastic mucus; as each cilium progresses through its effective stroke in the periciliary layer, the tip eventually encounters mucus, which rapidly slows its velocity and upsets metachrony with the next cilium in sequence. The recovery phase, during which the cilia pass through low-viscosity periciliary liquid, is therefore utilized to recoordinate ciliary movement for each full cycle. However, metachronal sequences initiated by recovery strokes are not wide-ranging, which limits airway ciliary wave propagation to short distances (23). This creates numerous localized areas of ciliary activity. Ciliary beat within each area is coordinated, but not the beat between areas. This discontinuous metachronal activity facilitates airway mucus transport by compensating for elastic recoil; some areas of cilia are engaging with and moving mucus, while others are disengaging, ready to reengage and inch the mucus forward when other areas become disengaged.

From the above discussion it may be seen that airway cilia are optimized for transporting mucus by adaptation of their length, internal structure (causing axoneme twisting), external features such as apical claws, beat cycle (incorporating a rest phase), and metachronal rhythm (development of wave discontinuity). However, for effective mucociliary transport, airway mucus needs adaptations that complement those of the cilia.

III. Airway Mucus, Secretory Cells, and Mucins

Airway lumenal mucus is a complex dilute aqueous solution of lipids, glycoconjugates, and proteins. It comprises salts, enzymes and antienzymes, oxidants and antioxidants, exogenous bacterial products, endogenous antibacterial agents, cell-derived mediators and proteins, plasma-derived mediators and proteins, and cell debris such as DNA. Airway mucus is considered to form a liquid bi-layer whereby an upper gel layer floats above a lower, more watery sol, or periciliary liquid, layer (5). The gel layer traps particles and is moved on the tips of the cilia. The functions of the sol layer are debated, but are presumed to include "lubrication" of the beating cilia. Respiratory tract mucus requires the correct combination of viscosity and elasticity for optimal efficiency of ciliary interaction. Viscosity is a liquid-like characteristic and is the resistance to flow and the capacity to absorb energy when moving. Elasticity is a solid-like property and is the capacity to store the energy used to move or deform it. Viscoelasticity confers a number of properties upon the mucus that allow effective interaction with cilia. These properties have been variously described in terms of spinnability, adhesiveness, and wettability (10). An important characteristic of mucus is that it is non-Newtonian, whereby its viscosity decreases as the applied force increases (30). Consequently, the ratio of stress to rate of strain is nonlinear, with the result that the more forcefully the cilia beat, the more easily the mucus moves.

Viscoelasticity is conferred on the mucus primarily by high molecular weight mucous glycoproteins, termed mucins, that comprise up to 2% by weight of the mucus (31). In the airways, mucins are produced by goblet cells in the epithelium (32) and sero-mucous glands in the submucosa (33) (Fig. 4). Mucins are thread-like molecules comprising a linear peptide sequence (the latter termed apomucin), often with tandemly repeated regions, that is highly glycosylated, predominantly via *O*-linkages but also with additional *N*-linked glycans (Fig. 7). The glycosylation pattern is complex and extremely diverse (34) and is associated with complementary motifs on bacterial cell walls, thereby facilitating broad-spectrum bacterial attachment and subsequent clearance (35,36). Apomucins are encoded by specific mucin (MUC) genes, with 17 human MUC genes recognized to date, namely MUC1, 2, 3A, 3B, 4, 5AC, 5B, 6–9, 11–13, 16 (37, 38), 17 (39), and 18 (40). In general, the MUC gene products are poorly characterized biochemically and biophysically (31). The predicted sequences of the MUC1, 3, 4, 8, 11, and 13 gene products suggest they are membrane-bound, with an extracellular mucin domain and a hydrophobic membrane-spanning domain. In contrast, MUC2, 5AC, 5B, 6, and 7 gene products are secreted mucins.

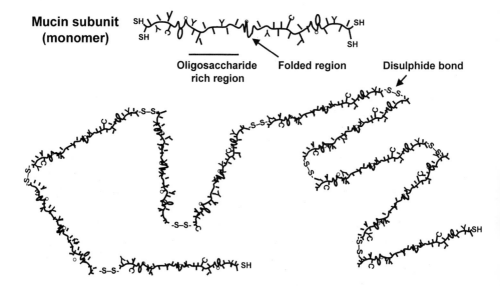

Figure 7 Schematic representation of a gel-forming mucin molecule. The mucin subunit (~500 nm in length) comprises an amino acid backbone with highly glycosylated areas and folded regions, stabilized via disulfide bonds, with little or no glycosylation. Glycosylation is via *O*-linkages and is highly diverse. In secretions, the subunits are joined end-to-end by disulfide bonds (S-S) into long thread-like molecules.

The technology for studying the contribution to physiology and pathophysiology of the individual MUC gene products lags well behind that of investigation of gene expression. Nine MUC genes are expressed in the normal human adult respiratory tract, namely MUC1, 2, 4, 5AC, 5B, 7, 8, 11, and 13 (41). MUC1, 2, and 8 genes are expressed in both the epithelium and submucosal glands, whereas MUC4, 5AC, and 13 are expressed primarily in the epithelium. In contrast, MUC5B and MUC7 genes are expressed primarily in the glands. Use of currently available antibodies confirms that the MUC5AC gene product is a goblet cell mucin, while MUC5B predominates in the glands, albeit that some MUC5AC and MUC7 is also usually present (31). Interestingly, MUC4 mucin localizes to the ciliated cells. MUC5AC and MUC5B are the major gel-forming mucins in respiratory secretions from normal subjects. The mucin content of secretions from patients with hypersecretory respiratory diseases may differ from normal (see Sec. VII).

From the above discussion it can be seen that the biochemical and biophysical characteristics of airway mucins and mucus are becoming increasingly better delineated. These features of mucus allow optimal interaction with cilia, making mucociliary interaction an effective mechanism for clearing airway mucus. When this interaction fails, other mechanisms, for example, cough, can clear airway mucus.

IV. Cough

Cough comprises an inhalation of air followed by closure of the glottis and a vigorous expiratory effort that, when coordinated with opening of the glottis, produces an expiratory blast. Cough is initiated via activation of sensory receptors in the epithelium and submucosa of the larynx, trachea, and bronchi (42,43). These receptors are described as being polymodal in that they respond to a wide variety of stimuli, usually adverse or noxious, including chemical and mechanical irritants and inflammatory mediators. Activation of the receptors sends nerve impulses along their respective nerve fibers to the brainstem to trigger cough. The receptors responsible mainly for initiating cough are the rapidly adapting receptors (RARs) in the airway epithelium (44,45). Airway C-fibers also contribute to initiation of cough (46–48). Aδ fibers with neuronal bodies in the jugular ganglia may also be involved in producing cough, although their precise contribution is currently unclear (49). These neuronal pathways interact and exhibit plasticity at the level of the periphery, the ganglia, and the central nervous system (CNS) (42,49,50). Although research into the complex nature of cough is beginning to delineate mechanisms underlying sensory initiation, neural propagation, and CNS integration, there remain few, if any, effective treatments that suppress cough (51,52). Most patients are usually treated for their respiratory disease, for example, asthma or COPD, rather than specifically for cough. Consequently, cough is controlled as the disease becomes managed. In addition, cough suppression may not necessarily be beneficial, considering its effectiveness at clearing airway mucus.

V.   Mucus Obstruction in Asthma and COPD

Asthma and COPD are chronic, severe inflammatory conditions of the airways in which mucous hypersecretion is a pathophysiological feature. This overproduction of mucus contributes to airway obstruction. The increase in airway lumenal mucus is associated with increases in amount of mucus-secreting tissue. In addition, there are pathological changes in the airway ciliated cells in both conditions that would further contribute to impaired mucociliary clearance.

A.   Asthma

Asthma is a chronic inflammatory condition of the airways characterized by variable airflow limitation that is at least partially reversible, either spontaneously or with treatment (53,54). It has specific clinical and pathophysiological features (55), including mucus obstruction of the airways (15). The latter is particularly evident in a proportion of patients who die in *status asthmaticus*, where many airways are occluded by mucus plugs (56–58). The plugs are highly viscous and comprise plasma proteins, DNA, cells, proteoglycans (59), and mucins (57,59,60). Incomplete plugs are found in the airways of asthmatic subjects who have died from causes other than asthma (61), which indicates that plug formation is a chronic, progressive process. There is also more mucus in the central and peripheral airways of both chronic and severe asthmatics compared with control subjects (62). Analysis of asthmatic sputum indicates that the mucus comprises DNA, lactoferrin, eosinophil cationic protein, and plasma proteins such as albumin and fibrinogen (63–65), as well as mucins (64,66,67). The increased amount of lumenal mucus reflects an increase in amount of airway secretory tissue, due to both goblet cell hyperplasia (62,67) and submucosal gland hypertrophy (57), although the latter is not characteristic of all patients with asthma (62).

Airway epithelial fragility, with epithelial shedding in extreme cases, is a significant feature of asthma (68). Shedding includes loss of ciliated cells, with presumably a concomitant reduction in mucus-clearing capacity. The ciliated cells themselves may also be damaged, with loss of cilia, vacuolization of the endoplasmic reticulum and mitochondria, and microtubule damage (69–71). These abnormalities could be caused by some of the inflammatory mediators generated in the airways of asthmatic patients, for example, eosinophil major basic protein (72). A variety of other ciliostatic and ciliotoxic compounds are also present in asthmatic airway secretions (9).

The combination of an increased amount of mucus-secreting tissue, with associated mucous hypersecretion, the production of viscid mucus, and abnormal ciliary function lead to reduced mucus clearance and the development of airway mucus obstruction in asthma.

B. COPD

COPD comprises three overlapping conditions: chronic bronchitis (airway mucus hypersecretion), chronic bronchiolitis (small airways disease), and emphysema (airspace enlargement due to alveolar destruction) (73). The following discussion considers the "bronchitic" component of COPD. The airways of patients with COPD contain excessive amounts of mucus (74), which is markedly increased in comparison to control subjects (75,76). The excessive lumenal mucus is associated with increased amounts of mucus secreting tissue. Goblet cell hyperplasia is a cardinal feature of chronic bronchitis (74), with increased numbers of goblet cells in the airways of cigarette smokers either with chronic bronchitis and chronic airflow limitation (77) or with or without productive cough (78). Submucosal gland hypertrophy also characterizes chronic bronchitis (74, 75,79,80), and the amount of gland correlates with the amount of lumenal mucus (75).

As in asthma, abnormalities in airway ciliated cells and cilia have been described in COPD. The number of ciliated cells and the length of individual cilia is decreased in patients with chronic bronchitis (81). Ciliary aberrations include compound cilia, cilia with an abnormal axoneme or intracytoplasmic microtubule doublets, and cilia enclosed within periciliary sheaths (82). These abnormalities coupled with mucous hypersecretion are presumably associated with reduced mucus clearance and airway mucus obstruction in the bronchitic component of COPD.

VI. Mucus Clearance in Asthma and COPD

Clearance of mucus from the airways is impaired in patients with a variety of respiratory diseases, including asthma and COPD (83). However, it should be noted that there are often discrepancies in results between studies that are invariably due to differences in methodology (84,85), but may also be due to observations made at different stages of disease.

A. Asthma

Airway mucociliary clearance is well documented as being impaired in asthma (9). Clearance is impaired even in patients in remission (86) and in those with mild stable disease (87). Mucus clearance is proportionally reduced in symptomatic asthmatics (88) and during exacerbations (89). In addition, the normal slowing of mucus clearance during sleep is more pronounced in asthmatic patients (90,91), and this could be a contributory factor in nocturnal asthma. The mechanisms underlying the reduced mucus clearance in asthma are not clearly defined, although airway inflammation is considered to be a major contributor (9).

B. COPD

Mucus clearance is generally considered to be impaired in patients with COPD (83). However, the validity of these studies is dependent upon patient selection and the exclusion of patients with asthma. For example, patients classified as having obstructive chronic bronchitis and with a bronchial reversibility of less than 15% had slower lung mucus clearance than patients with reversibility greater than 15% and who, therefore, were likely to be asthmatic (92). Nevertheless, mucus clearance is significantly reduced in heavy smokers (93) and in patients with chronic bronchitis (94). Lung mucus clearance differs between patients with chronic airway obstruction, with or without emphysema (95). Both groups of patients were smokers or ex-smokers and had productive cough, but lung elastic recoil pressure was reduced in the emphysema group. Mucus clearance from central airways was similar. In contrast, clearance from the peripheral lung was faster in the emphysema group than in the patients without emphysema. Importantly, forced expirations and cough markedly increased peripheral clearance in the nonemphysema group but not in the emphysema group. Comparable findings in a subsequent study led to the suggestion that cough compensates relatively effectively for decreased mucus clearance in patients with chronic bronchitis (96). Conversely, cough is not as effective in COPD patients with impaired lung elastic recoil.

VII. Differences in Pathophysiology Relating to Mucus Obstruction in Asthma and COPD

In order to develop appropriate models of airway mucus obstruction and develop drugs to aid mucus clearance, it is necessary to understand the similarities and differences in the features of mucus obstruction for different hypersecretory conditions. There are a number of differences in the pathophysiology of impaired mucus clearance between asthma and COPD (Fig. 3). First, although the underlying pulmonary inflammation of asthma and COPD shares many common features, there are specific characteristics unique to each condition (97–99). Asthma is invariably an allergic disease that affects the airways, rather than the lung parenchyma, and is characterized by Th2-lymphocyte orchestration of pulmonary eosinophilia. The reticular layer beneath the basement membrane is markedly thickened and the airway epithelium is fragile, features not usually associated with COPD. The bronchial inflammatory infiltrate comprises activated T cells (predominatly CD4+ cells) and eosinophils. Neutrophils are generally sparse in stable disease. In contrast, COPD is currently perceived as predominantly a neutrophilic disorder governed largely by macrophages and epithelial cells. It is associated primarily with cigarette smoking. Three conditions comprise COPD, namely mucous hypersecretion, bronchiolitis, and emphysema. The latter two features are not associated with asthma. In addition, and in contrast to asthma, CD8+ T lymphocytes predominate, and pulmonary eosinophilia is generally associated with exacerbations.

Both asthma and COPD have a characteristic "portfolio" of inflammatory mediators and enzymes, many of which differ (100,101). At a simplified level, histamine, interleukin (IL)-4, and eotaxin are associated with asthma, while IL-8, neutrophil elastase, and matrix metalloproteinases are associated with COPD. Thus, there are specific differences between asthma and COPD in their airway inflammation and remodeling. These differences may in turn exert different influences on the development of airway mucus obstruction in the two conditions (Fig. 2).

Airway mucus in asthma is more viscous than in COPD or CF, with the airways of asthmatic patients tending to develop, and subsequently become blocked by, gelatinous "mucus" plugs (15). Whether or not mucus in asthma has an intrinsic biochemical abnormality is unclear. In general terms, sputum from patients with asthma is more viscous than that from patients with chronic bronchitis or bronchiectasis (63,102,103). Mucus plugs in asthma differ from airway mucus gels in chronic bronchitis or CF in that they are stabilized by noncovalent interactions between extremely large mucins assembled from conventional sized subunits (60). This suggests an intrinsic abnormality in the mucus due to a defect in assembly of the mucin molecules and could account for the increased viscosity of the mucus plugs in asthma. Plug formation may also be due, at least in part, to increased airway plasma exudation in asthma compared with COPD (104). In addition, in direct contrast to COPD, exocytosed mucins in asthma are not released fully from the goblet cells, leading to "tethering" of luminal mucins to the airway epithelium (105). This tethering may also contribute to plug formation. One explanation of mucus tethering is that neutrophil proteinases, the predominant inflammatory cell in COPD (73), cleave goblet cell–attached mucins. In asthma, the inflammatory cell profile, predominantly airway eosinophilia (55), does not generate the appropriate proteinases to facilitate mucin release.

Different MUC gene products may be present in respiratory secretions in asthma and COPD. MUC5AC and a low-charge glycoform of MUC5B are the major mucin species in airway secretions from patients with asthma, COPD, or CF (106–110). There is significantly more of the low-charge glycoform of MUC5B in the respiratory diseases than in normal control secretions (110). An interesting difference between the disease conditions is that there is a proportional increase in the MUC5B mucin over the MUC5AC mucin in airway secretions from patients with CF or COPD compared with secretions from patients with asthma (106). These data require confirmation in more samples. The significance to bacterial colonization of the change in MUC5B glycoforms between the different diseases in unclear, although it is interesting that it is COPD and CF, both diseases in which patients are prone to infection (17,73), that share the same proportional difference, rather than asthma, a condition in which patients are not so notably prone to bacterial infection.

In contrast to normal airways, goblet cells in the airways from patients with COPD contain not only MUC5AC but also MUC5B (108,111) and MUC2 (31,112). This distribution is different from that in the airways of patients with asthma or CF, where MUC5AC and MUC5B show a similar histological pattern to normal controls (113,114). It is noteworthy that although MUC2 is located in goblet cells in irritated airways and MUC2 mRNA is found in the airways of smokers (76), MUC2 mucin is either not found in airway secretions from normal subjects or patients with chronic bronchitis (107) or is found only in very small amounts in asthma, COPD, or CF (110,115). The significance of the above combined observations is unclear, but suggests that there are differences in goblet cell phenotype between asthma, COPD, and CF.

Another notable difference between asthma and COPD is in the bronchial submucosal glands (116). In asthma, although hypertrophied, the glands are morphologically normal with an even distribution of mucous and serous cells. In contrast, in chronic bronchitis gland hypertrophy is characterized by an increased number of mucous cells relative to serous cells, particularly in severe bronchitis.

Finally, it is not clear whether or not there are differences in the airway ciliary abnormalities between asthma and COPD (Sec. V.A and B). However, epithelial fragility and shedding are features of asthma rather than COPD (97), which suggests that there may be greater loss of, and damage to, the ciliated cells in asthma.

From the above, it may be seen that there are theoretical and actual differences in the nature of airway mucus obstruction between asthma and COPD. How these relate to pathophysiology and clinical symptoms in the two conditions is, for the most part, unclear. However, these dissimilarities indicate that different treatments are required for effective treatment of airway mucus obstruction in asthma and COPD.

VIII. Considerations for Effective Treatment of Airway Mucus Obstruction

The prevalence of patient presentation with cough and expectoration of sputum and the perceived importance of mucus in the pathophysiology of many severe lung conditions, including asthma and COPD, have led to development of drugs intended to treat airway mucus obstruction (117). Numerous naturally occurring and synthetic compounds are available worldwide that are perceived to have potentially beneficial actions on some aspect of mucus or its secretion (118). These "mucoactive" compounds can be divided into mucolytics, peptide mucolytics, nondestructive mucolytics, expectorants, mucokinetic agents, abhesives, and mucoregulators (119). Mucolytics are compounds containing free sulfhydryl groups that dissociate disulfide bonds and directly thin mucus. Peptide mucolytics dissociate filaments of cell (predominantly neutrophil)-derived DNA and actin in airway mucus. Nondestructive mucolytics comprise compounds that disperse mucus by means of charge shielding. The mechanism of action of expectorants is varied, but in general they increase the volume and/or hydration of airway mucus. They may also stimulate cough. Mucokinetic agents increase mucociliary efficiency or cough efficiency, or both. Abhesives include surfactant and decrease mucus attachment to the cilia and epithelium, thereby facilitating cough and, possibly, mucociliary clearance. Mucoregulators inhibit airway mucus secretion and include indomethacin, glucocorticosteroids, anticholinergics, and certain macrolide antibiotics such as erythromycin (16). At least 15 drugs with mucoactive properties are listed in international pharmacopoeias for treatment of respiratory conditions associated with airway mucous hypersecretion (Table 1) (118). However, the characteristics of airway mucus obstruction in asthma and COPD (Sec. V) and the differences in pathophysiology of the obstruction (Sec. VII) demonstrate that therapy of mucus obstruction in these two diseases is likely to entail more than just "thinning" of mucus and could be different for each condition.

There are two objectives for treatment of airway mucus obstruction, namely, short-term relief of symptoms and long-term benefit (Table 2). Short-term benefit can be achieved by facilitating mucus clearance. In both asthma and COPD, this entails reducing the viscosity of mucus (and possibly increasing

Table 1 Internationally Listed Mucoactive Agents[a]

Mucolytics
  N-Acetylcysteine, L-ethylcysteine, sodium 2-mercaptoethane sulfonate (MESNA), methylcysteine hydrochloride, stepronine, thiopronine
Mucoregulators
  Carbocysteine, eprazinon hydrochloride, erdosteine, letosteine
Expectorants
  Ambroxol, bromhexine, guaifenesin, sobrerol
Peptide mucolytic
  Recombinant human DNase I (Dornase-alfa: degrades DNA)

[a]The 15 most frequently listed drugs in pharmacopoeias worldwide (118). Definitions: mucolytic = thins mucus; mucoregulatory = does not thin mucus (precise mechanism of action, if any, unknown); expectorant = increases cough and expectoration (may induce mucus secretion).

Table 2 Objectives for Effective Pharmacotherapy of Mucus Pathophysiology
in Asthma, COPD, and Cystic Fibrosis

Overall objective	Component objective
Facilitate mucus clearance (short-term relief of symptoms)	Reduce viscosity (?increase elasticity)
	Increase ciliary function
	Induce cough
	Facilitate release of "tethered" goblet cell mucin (asthma)
	Treat pulmonary infection (COPD and CF)
Reverse hypersecretory phenotype (long-term benefit)	Treat airway/pulmonary inflammation
	Reduce goblet cell number
	Reduce submucosal gland size
	Correct increased gland mucous:serous cell ratio (COPD)
	Reverse increased MUC5B:MUC5AC ratio (especially in COPD and CF)
	Inhibit plasma exudation (asthma)
	Inhibit production of MUC2 (CF)
	Inhibit development of epithelial "fragility" (asthma)

elasticity) to an optimal level, increasing ciliary function, and, possibly, encouraging cough. In addition, in asthmatic patients, facilitating release of the tethered goblet cell mucin should improve airflow. Long-term benefit entails reversal of the hypersecretory phenotype. For both asthma and COPD, reducing the number of goblet cells and the size of the submucosal glands might be a primary goal. In addition, in asthma it could be useful to inhibit plasma exudation. In COPD, correction of the increased submucosal gland mucous cell–to–serous cell ratio and any increased MUC5B-to-MUC5AC ratio may be of benefit.

The activity of current compounds intended to treat airway mucus obstruction, as well as those in development, on the above parameters of mucus pathophysiology is not clearly defined. Despite the abundance of mucoactive drugs available, few are recommended for use in respiratory diseases with mucus obstruction. For example, mucolytic drugs are not generally included in guidelines for management of asthma or COPD (53,54,73,120,121). For COPD, both the American Thoracic Society (122) and the Thoracic Society of Australia and New Zealand (123) suggest that mucolytic agents be considered as an adjunct to bronchodilators where there is an increase in symptoms or in severe exacerbations with highly viscous sputum. Interestingly, the latter suggestion preceded, and now concurs with, a recent review (118) and meta-analysis (124) that concluded that although maintenance treatment with mucolytic drugs is not beneficial in asthma or COPD, treatment of COPD patients with certain mucolytic drugs is associated with a reduction in exacerbations and days of illness. The effect is particularly pertinent to treatment with N-acetylcysteine (125,126).

The effectiveness of N-acetylcysteine in alleviating exacerbations of COPD makes an important point in that its mechanism of action is unknown. For example, it is a mucolytic compound in that it breaks disulfide bonds in mucus molecules (127), but is also an antioxidant (128) and hinders adherence of bacteria to airway epithelial cells (129). Any or all of these properties, or even properties as yet undiscovered, may contribute to its effectiveness. And this is true of virtually all of the other compounds that are currently available for treatment of airway mucus obstruction. Consequently, it should be remembered that any beneficial clinical effects of these compounds are not necessarily due to beneficial effects on mucus or mucus clearance. In contrast, the mechanism of action of Lomucin (MSI-1995), currently undergoing clinical trial for asthma and trials still ongoing/not published, is highly defined: it is a selective inhibitor of the human calcium activated chloride channel (hCLCA1) (130). This channel is upregulated in goblet cells in the airways of patients with asthma (131,132). Inhibition of this channel in experimentally induced animal models of asthma inhibits mucous metaplasia. It is suggested that similar inhibition in humans is an attractive therapeutic strategy to control mucus obstruction in respiratory diseases. The results of the clinical trials are awaited with great interest because they will indicate whether inhibition of a single pathophysiological target for mucus is a feasible therapeutic strategy for alleviating airway mucus obstruction, thereby aiding disease management.

IX. Conclusions

Clearance of mucus from the airways is a vital homeostatic mechanism that protects the respiratory tract from a barrage of inhaled insult. Precise interaction between cilia, the periciliary layer, and mucus is required for optimal clearance. However, abnormal or impaired ciliary activity and production of mucus can contribute to respiratory disease. Airway obstruction by mucus is a common feature of a number of severe respiratory conditions, including asthma, COPD and CF. These diseases share pulmonary inflammation and remodeling as a pathophysiological characteristic. Each also has a number of unique features that characterize its airway mucus obstruction. For example, plasma exudation, mucus plug formation, and mucus tethering are features of asthma, whereas submucosal gland hypertrophy with a disproportionate increase in the ratio of mucous to serous cells is a significant feature in COPD. Understanding of the relative importance of the differences and similarities in the pathophysiology of mucus obstruction between different respiratory diseases should lead to rational development of therapeutic interventions. However, it will require clinical trials of a range of classes of drug to determine whether intervention at a single, rationally determined pathophysiological mucus target will have therapeutic benefit over broader spectrum interventions, or even over interventions not specifically targeted at mucus, including generalized anti-inflammatory therapy, for example, the effective use of glucorticosteroids in management of asthma.

References

1. Seaton A, MacNee W, Donaldson K, Godden D. Particulate air pollution and acute health effects. Lancet 1995; 345:176–178.
2. Lippmann M, Yeates DB, Albert RE. Deposition, retention, and clearance of inhaled particles. Br J Ind Med 1980; 37:337–362.
3. Hollander W, Stober W. Aerosols of smoke, respiratory physiology and deposition. Arch Toxicol Suppl 1986; 9:74–87.
4. Rubin BK. Physiology of airway mucus clearance. Respir Care 2002; 47:761–768.
5. Knowles MR, Boucher RC. Mucus clearance as a primary innate defense mechanism for mammalian airways. J Clin Invest 2002; 109:571–577.
6. Pavia D, Agnew JE, Lopez-Vidriero MT, Clarke SW. General review of tracheobronchial clearance. Eur J Respir Dis Suppl 1987; 153:123–129.
7. Widdicombe JG. Advances in understanding and treatment of cough. Monaldi Arch Chest Dis 1999; 54:275–279.
8. Foster WM. Mucociliary transport and cough in humans. Pulm Pharmacol Ther 2002; 15:277–282.
9. Del Donno M, Bittesnich D, Chetta A, Olivieri D, Lopez-Vidriero MT. The effect of inflammation on mucociliary clearance in asthma: an overview. Chest 2000; 118:1142–1149.
10. Houtmeyers E, Gosselink R, Gayan-Ramirez G, Decramer M. Regulation of mucociliary clearance in health and disease. Eur Respir J 1999; 13:1177–1188.
11. Maestrelli P, Saetta M, Mapp CE, Fabbri LM. Remodeling in response to infection and injury. Airway inflammation and hypersecretion of mucus in smoking subjects with chronic obstructive pulmonary disease. Am J Respir Crit Care Med 2001; 164:S76–S80.
12. Robinson M, Bye PT. Mucociliary clearance in cystic fibrosis. Pediatr Pulmonol 2002; 33:293–306.
13. Afzelius BA. Role of cilia in human health. Cell Motil Cytoskeleton 1995; 32: 95–97.
14. Noone PG, Bennett WD, Regnis JA, Zeman KL, Carson JL, King M, et al. Effect of aerosolized uridine-5′-triphosphate on airway clearance with cough in patients with primary ciliary dyskinesia. Am J Respir Crit Care Med 1999; 160:144–149.
15. Liu YC, Khawaja AM, Rogers DF. Pathophysiogy of airway mucus secretion in asthma. In: Barnes PJ, Rodger IW, Thomson NC, eds. Asthma. Basic Mechanisms and Clinical Management. London: Academic Press, 1998:205–227.

16. Rogers DF. Mucus pathophysiology in COPD: differences to asthma, and pharmacotherapy. Monaldi Arch Chest Dis 2000; 55:324–332.
17. Davis PB. Cystic fibrosis. Pediatr Rev 2001; 22:257–264.
18. Quinton PM. Physiological basis of cystic fibrosis: a historical perspective. Physiol Rev 1999; 79(1 suppl):S3–S22.
19. Prescott E, Lange P, Vestbo J. Chronic mucus hypersecretion in COPD and death from pulmonary infection. Eur Respir J 1995; 8:1333–1338.
20. Kunzelmann K, Mall M. Pharmacotherapy of the ion transport defect in cystic fibrosis. Clin Exp Pharmacol Physiol 2001; 28:857–867.
21. Reddy MM, Quinton PM. Selective activation of cystic fibrosis transmembrane conductance regulator Cl– and HCO3– conductances. JOP 2001; 2(4 suppl):212–218.
22. Serafini SM, Michaelson ED. Length and distribution of cilia in human and canine airways. Bull Eur Physiopathol Respir 1977; 13:551–559.
23. Sanderson MJ. Mechanisms controlling airway ciliary activity. In: Rogers DF, Lethem MI, eds. Airway Mucus: Basic Mechanisms and Clinical Perspectives. Basel: Birkhäuser Verlag, 1997:91–116.
24. Afzelius BA. Ultrastructural basis for ciliary motility. Eur J Respir Dis Suppl 1983; 128:280–286.
25. Clarke SW. Rationale of airway clearance. Eur Respir J Suppl 1989; 7:599s–603s.
26. Foliguet B, Puchelle E. Apical structure of human respiratory cilia. Bull Eur Physiopathol Respir 1986; 22:43–47.
27. Dentler WL, LeCluyse EL. Microtubule capping structures at the tips of tracheal cilia: evidence for their firm attachment during ciliary bend formation and the restriction of microtubule sliding. Cell Motil 1982; 2:549–572.
28. Sanderson MJ, Sleigh MA. Ciliary activity of cultured rabbit tracheal epithelium: beat pattern and metachrony. J Cell Sci 1981; 47:331–347.
29. Helleday R, Huberman D, Blomberg A, Stjernberg N, Sandstrom T. Nitrogen dioxide exposure impairs the frequency of the mucociliary activity in healthy subjects. Eur Respir J 1995; 8:1664–1668.
30. Sleigh MA, Blake JR, Liron N. The propulsion of mucus by cilia. Am Rev Respir Dis 1988; 137:726–741.
31. Davies JR, Herrmann A, Russell W, Svitacheva N, Wickström C, Carlstedt I. Respiratory tract mucins: structure and expression patterns. In: Mucus Hypersecretion in Respiratory Disease. Chichester, UK: John Wiley and Sons, 2002: 76–88.
32. Rogers DF. The airway goblet cell. Int J Biochem Cell Biol 2003; 35:1–6.
33. Finkbeiner WE. Physiology and pathology of tracheobronchial glands. Respir Physiol 1999; 118:77–83.
34. Hanisch FG. O-Glycosylation of the mucin type. Biol Chem 2001; 382:143–149.
35. Dell A, Morris HR. Glycoprotein structure determination by mass spectrometry. Science 2001; 291:2351–2356.
36. Moniaux N, Escande F, Porchet N, Aubert JP, Batra SK. Structural organization and classification of the human mucin genes. Front Biosci 2001; 6:D1192–D1206.
37. Dekker J, Rossen JW, Buller HA, Einerhand AW. The MUC family: an obituary. Trends Biochem Sci 2002; 27:126–131.

38. Lapensee L, Paquette Y, Bleau G. Allelic polymorphism and chromosomal localization of the human oviductin gene (MUC9). Fertil Steril 1997; 68:702–708.

39. Gum JR Jr, Crawley SC, Hicks JW, Szymkowski DE, Kim YS. MUC17, a novel membrane-tethered mucin. Biochem Biophys Res Commun 2002; 291:466–475.

40. Wu GJ, Wu MW, Wang SW, Liu Z, Qu P, Peng Q, et al. Isolation and characterization of the major form of human MUC18 cDNA gene and correlation of MUC18 over-expression in prostate cancer cell lines and tissues with malignant progression. Gene 2001; 279:17–31.

41. Copin MC, Buisine MP, Devisme L, Leroy X, Escande F, Gosselin B, et al. Normal respiratory mucosa, precursor lesions and lung carcinomas: differential expression of human mucin genes. Front Biosci 2001; 6:D1264–D1275.

42. Widdicombe J. Neuroregulation of cough: implications for drug therapy. Curr Opin Pharmacol 2002; 2:256–263.

43. Morice AH, Widdicombe J, Dicpinigaitis P, Groenke L. Understanding cough. Eur Respir J 2002; 19:6–7.

44. Sant'Ambrogio G, Widdicombe J. Reflexes from airway rapidly adapting receptors. Respir Physiol 2001; 125:33–45.

45. Canning BJ. Interactions between vagal afferent nerve subtypes mediating cough. Pulm Pharmacol Ther 2002; 15:187–192.

46. Karlsson JA, Fuller RW. Pharmacological regulation of the cough reflex—from experimental models to antitussive effects in man. Pulm Pharmacol Ther 1999; 12:215–228.

47. Lee LY, Pisarri TE. Afferent properties and reflex functions of bronchopulmonary C-fibers. Respir Physiol 2001; 125:47–65.

48. Lee LY, Kwong K, Lin YS, Gu Q. Hypersensitivity of bronchopulmonary C-fibers induced by airway mucosal inflammation: cellular mechanisms. Pulm Pharmacol Ther 2002; 15:199–204.

49. Undem BJ, Carr MJ, Kollarik M. Physiology and plasticity of putative cough fibres in the guinea pig. Pulm Pharmacol Ther 2002; 15:193–198.

50. Pantaleo T, Bongianni F, Mutolo D. Central nervous mechanisms of cough. Pulm Pharmacol Ther 2002; 15:227–233.

51. Schroeder K, Fahey T. Systematic review of randomised controlled trials of over the counter cough medicines for acute cough in adults. BMJ 2002; 324:329–331.

52. Widdicombe J, Morice A. Over the counter cough medicines for acute cough. Good quality research is needed. BMJ 2002; 324:1158.

53. American Thoracic Society. Standards for the diagnosis and care of patients with chronic obstructive pulmonary disease (COPD) and asthma. Am Rev Respir Dis 1987; 136:225–244.

54. British Thoracic Society. The British guidelines on asthma management. Thorax 1997; 52(suppl 1):S1–S21.

55. Eapen SS, Busse WW. Asthma. Clin Allergy Immunol 2002; 16:325–353.

56. Houston JC, De Navasquez S, Trounce JR. A clinical and pathological study of fatal cases of status asthmaticus. Thorax 1953; 8:207–213.

57. Dunnill MS. The pathology of asthma with special reference to changes in the bronchial mucosa. J Clin Pathol 1960; 13:27–33.

58. Saetta M, Di Stefano A, Rosina C, Thiene G, Fabbri LM. Quantitative structural analysis of peripheral airways and arteries in sudden fatal asthma. Am Rev Respir Dis 1991; 143:138–143.

59. Bhaskar KR, O'Sullivan DD, Coles SJ, Kozakewich H, Vawter GP, Reid LM. Characterization of airway mucus from a fatal case of status asthmaticus. Pediatr Pulmonol 1988; 5:176–182.

60. Sheehan JK, Richardson PS, Fung DC, Howard M, Thornton DJ. Analysis of respiratory mucus glycoproteins in asthma: a detailed study from a patient who died in status asthmaticus. Am J Respir Cell Mol Biol 1995; 13:748–756.

61. Dunnill MS. The morphology of the airways in bronchial asthma. In: Stein M, ed. New Directions in Asthma. Park Ridge, IL: American College of Physicians, 1975:213–221.

62. Aikawa T, Shimura S, Sasaki H, Ebina M, Takishima T. Marked goblet cell hyperplasia with mucus accumulation in the airways of patients who died of severe acute asthma attack. Chest 1992; 101:916–921.

63. Lopez-Vidriero MT, Reid L. Chemical markers of mucous and serum glycoproteins and their relation to viscosity in mucoid and purulent sputum from various hypersecretory diseases. Am Rev Respir Dis 1978; 117:465–477.

64. Fahy JV, Steiger DJ, Liu J, Basbaum CB, Finkbeiner WE, Boushey HA. Markers of mucus secretion and DNA levels in induced sputum from asthmatic and from healthy subjects. Am Rev Respir Dis 1993; 147:1132–1137.

65. Fahy JV, Liu J, Wong H, Boushey HA. Cellular and biochemical analysis of induced sputum from asthmatic and from healthy subjects. Am Rev Respir Dis 1993; 147:1126–1131.

66. Lopez-Vidriero MT, Reid L. Bronchial mucus in health and disease. Br Med Bull 1978; 34:63–74.

67. Ordonez CL, Khashayar R, Wong HH, Ferrando R, Wu R, Hyde DM, et al. Mild and moderate asthma is associated with airway goblet cell hyperplasia and abnormalities in mucin gene expression. Am J Respir Crit Care Med 2001; 163:517–523.

68. Bousquet J, Jeffery PK, Busse WW, Johnson M, Vignola AM. Asthma. From bronchoconstriction to airways inflammation and remodeling. Am J Respir Crit Care Med 2000; 161:1720–1745.

69. Laitinen LA, Heino M, Laitinen A, Kava T, Haahtela T. Damage of the airway epithelium and bronchial reactivity in patients with asthma. Am Rev Respir Dis 1985; 131:599–606.

70. Beasley R, Roche WR, Roberts JA, Holgate ST. Cellular events in the bronchi in mild asthma and after bronchial provocation. Am Rev Respir Dis 1989; 139:806–817.

71. Carson JL, Collier AM, Fernald GW, Hu SC. Microtubular discontinuities as acquired ciliary defects in airway epithelium of patients with chronic respiratory diseases. Ultrastruct Pathol 1994; 18:327–332.

72. Gleich GJ, Loegering DA, Frigas E, Filley WV. The eosinophil granule major basic protein: biological activities and relationship to bronchial asthma. Monogr Allergy 1983; 18:277–283.

73. National Heart Lung, and Blood Institute/WHO. Global Initiative for Chronic Obstructive Lung Disease. Bethesda, MD: National Institutes of Health, 2001. Pub. No. 2701.

74. Reid L. Pathology of chronic bronchitis. Lancet 1954; i:275–278.

75. Aikawa T, Shimura S, Sasaki H, Takishima T, Yaegashi H, Takahashi T. Morphometric analysis of intraluminal mucus in airways in chronic obstructive pulmonary disease. Am Rev Respir Dis 1989; 140:477–482.

76. Steiger D, Fahy J, Boushey H, Finkbeiner WE, Basbaum C. Use of mucin antibodies and cDNA probes to quantify hypersecretion in vivo in human airways. Am J Respir Cell Mol Biol 1994; 10:538–545.

77. Saetta M, Turato G, Baraldo S, Zanin A, Braccioni F, Mapp CE, et al. Goblet cell hyperplasia and epithelial inflammation in peripheral airways of smokers with both symptoms of chronic bronchitis and chronic airflow limitation. Am J Respir Crit Care Med 2000; 161:1016–1021.

78. Mullen JB, Wright JL, Wiggs BR, Pare PD, Hogg JC. Structure of central airways in current smokers and ex-smokers with and without mucus hypersecretion: relationship to lung function. Thorax 1987; 42:843–848.

79. Reid L. Measurement of the bronchial mucous gland layer: a diagnostic yardstick in chronic bronchitis. Thorax 1960; 15:132–141.

80. Restrepo G, Heard BE. The size of the bronchial glands in chronic bronchitis. J Pathol Bacteriol 1963; 85:305–310.

81. Wanner A. Clinical aspects of mucociliary transport. Am Rev Respir Dis 1977; 116:73–125.

82. McDowell EM, Barrett LA, Harris CC, Trump BF. Abnormal cilia in human bronchial epithelium. Arch Pathol Lab Med 1976; 100:429–436.

83. Wanner A, Salathe M, O'Riordan TG. Mucociliary clearance in the airways. Am J Respir Crit Care Med 1996; 154:1868–1902.

84. Clarke SW, Pavia D. Lung mucus production and mucociliary clearance: methods of assessment. Br J Clin Pharmacol 1980; 9:537–546.

85. Pavia D, Sutton PP, Agnew JE, Lopez-Vidriero MT, Newman SP, Clarke SW. Measurement of bronchial mucociliary clearance. Eur J Respir Dis Suppl 1983; 127:41–56.

86. Pavia D, Bateman JR, Sheahan NF, Agnew JE, Clarke SW. Tracheobronchial mucociliary clearance in asthma: impairment during remission. Thorax 1985; 40: 171–175.

87. Bateman JR, Pavia D, Sheahan NF, Agnew JE, Clarke SW. Impaired tracheobronchial clearance in patients with mild stable asthma. Thorax 1983; 38:463–467.

88. Foster WM, Langenback EG, Bergofsky EH. Lung mucociliary function in man: interdependence of bronchial and tracheal mucus transport velocities with lung clearance in bronchial asthma and healthy subjects. Ann Occup Hyg 1982; 26: 227–244.

89. Messina MS, O'Riordan TG, Smaldone GC. Changes in mucociliary clearance during acute exacerbations of asthma. Am Rev Respir Dis 1991; 143:993–997.

90. Bateman JR, Pavia D, Clarke SW. The retention of lung secretions during the night in normal subjects. Clin Sci Mol Med Suppl 1978; 55:523–527.

91. Pavia D, Lopez-Vidriero MT, Clarke SW. Mediators and mucociliary clearance in asthma. Bull Eur Physiopathol Respir 1987; 23(suppl 10):89s–94s.
92. Moretti M, Lopez-Vidriero MT, Pavia D, Clarke SW. Relationship between bronchial reversibility and tracheobronchial clearance in patients with chronic bronchitis. Thorax 1997; 52:176–180.
93. Goodman RM, Yergin BM, Landa JF, Golivanux MH, Sackner MA. Relationship of smoking history and pulmonary function tests to tracheal mucous velocity in nonsmokers, young smokers, ex-smokers, and patients with chronic bronchitis. Am Rev Respir Dis 1978; 117:205–214.
94. Agnew JE, Little F, Pavia D, Clarke SW. Mucus clearance from the airways in chronic bronchitis—smokers and ex-smokers. Bull Eur Physiopathol Respir 1982; 18:473–484.
95. van der Schans CP, Piers DA, Beekhuis H, Koeter GH, van der Mark TW, Postma DS. Effect of forced expirations on mucus clearance in patients with chronic airflow obstruction: effect of lung recoil pressure. Thorax 1990; 45:623–627.
96. Ericsson CH, Svartengren K, Svartengren M, Mossberg B, Philipson K, Blomquist M, et al. Repeatability of airway deposition and tracheobronchial clearance rate over three days in chronic bronchitis. Eur Respir J 1995; 8:1886–1893.
97. Jeffery PK. Differences and similarities between chronic obstructive pulmonary disease and asthma. Clin Exp Allergy 1999; 29(suppl 2):14–26.
98. Saetta M, Turato G, Maestrelli P, Mapp CE, Fabbri LM. Cellular and structural bases of chronic obstructive pulmonary disease. Am J Respir Crit Care Med 2001; 163:1304–1309.
99. Djukanovic R. Airway inflammation in asthma and its consequences: implications for treatment in children and adults. J Allergy Clin Immunol 2002; 109(6 suppl): S539-S548.
100. Barnes PJ, Chung KF, Page CP. Inflammatory mediators of asthma: an update. Pharmacol Rev 1998; 50:515–596.
101. Barnes PJ. New treatments for COPD. Nat Rev Drug Discov 2002; 1:437–446.
102. Charman J, Reid L. Sputum viscosity in chronic bronchitis, bronchiectasis, asthma and cystic fibrosis. Biorheology 1972; 9:185–199.
103. Shimura S, Sasaki T, Sasaki H, Takishima T, Umeya K. Viscoelastic properties of bronchorrhoea sputum in bronchial asthmatics. Biorheology 1988; 25:173–179.
104. Rogers DF, Evans TW. Plasma exudation and oedema in asthma. Br Med Bull 1992; 48:120–134.
105. Shimura S, Andoh Y, Haraguchi M, Shirato K. Continuity of airway goblet cells and intraluminal mucus in the airways of patients with bronchial asthma. Eur Respir J 1996; 9:1395–1401.
106. Thornton DJ, Carlstedt I, Howard M, Devine PL, Price MR, Sheehan JK. Respiratory mucins: identification of core proteins and glycoforms. Biochem J 1996; 316: 967–975.
107. Hovenberg HW, Davies JR, Herrmann A, Linden CJ, Carlstedt I. MUC5AC, but not MUC2, is a prominent mucin in respiratory secretions. Glycoconj J 1996; 13: 839–847.
108. Wickstrom C, Davies JR, Eriksen GV, Veerman EC, Carlstedt I. MUC5B is a

major gel-forming, oligomeric mucin from human salivary gland, respiratory tract and endocervix: identification of glycoforms and C-terminal cleavage. Biochem J 1998; 334:685–693.

109. Sheehan JK, Howard M, Richardson PS, Longwill T, Thornton DJ. Physical characterization of a low-charge glycoform of the MUC5B mucin comprising the gel-phase of an asthmatic respiratory mucous plug. Biochem J 1999; 338:507–513.

110. Kirkham S, Sheehan JK, Knight D, Richardson PS, Thornton DJ. Heterogeneity of airways mucus: variations in the amounts and glycoforms of the major oligomeric mucins MUC5AC and MUC5B. Biochem J 2002; 361:537–546.

111. Chen Y, Zhao YH, Di YP, Wu R. Characterization of human mucin 5B gene expression in airway epithelium and the genomic clone of the amino-terminal and 5′-flanking region. Am J Respir Cell Mol Biol 2001; 25:542–553.

112. Davies JR, Carlstedt I. Respiratory tract mucins. In: Salthe M, ed. Cilia and Mucus: from Development to Respiratory Defense. New York: Marcel Dekker, 2001: 167–178.

113. Groneberg DA, Eynott PR, Lim S, Oates T, Wu R, Carlstedt I, et al. Expression of respiratory mucins in fatal status asthmaticus and mild asthma. Histopathology 2002; 40:367–373.

114. Groneberg DA, Eynott PR, Oates T, Lim S, Wu R, Carlstedt I, et al. Expression of MUC5AC and MUC5B mucins in normal and cystic fibrosis lung. Respir Med 2002; 96:81–86.

115. Davies JR, Svitacheva N, Lannefors L, Kornfalt R, Carlstedt I. Identification of MUC5B, MUC5AC and small amounts of MUC2 mucins in cystic fibrosis airway secretions. Biochem J 1999; 344:321–330.

116. Glynn AA, Michaels L. Bronchial biopsy in chronic bronchitis and asthma. Thorax 1960; 15:142–153.

117. Houtmeyers E, Gosselink R, Gayan-Ramirez G, Decramer M. Effects of drugs on mucus clearance. Eur Respir J 1999; 14:452–467.

118. Rogers DF. Mucoactive drugs for asthma and COPD: any place in therapy? Expert Opin Investig Drugs 2002; 11:15–35.

119. Rubin BK. The pharmacologic approach to airway clearance: mucoactive agents. Respir Care 2002; 47:818–822.

120. British Thoracic Society. BTS guidelines for the management of chronic obstructive pulmonary disease. Thorax 1997; 52 (suppl 5):S1–S28.

121. Siafakas NM, Vermeire P, Pride NB, Paoletti P, Gibson J, Howard P, et al. Optimal assessment and management of chronic obstructive pulmonary disease (COPD). The European Respiratory Society Task Force. Eur Respir J 1995; 8:1398–1420.

122. American Thoracic Society. Standards for the diagnosis and care of patients with chronic obstructive pulmonary disease. Am J Respir Crit Care Med 1995; 152 (suppl):S77–S120.

123. Jenkins C, Mitchell C, Irving L, Frith P, Young I. Guidelines for the management of chronic obstructive disease. Mod Med Australia 1995; 38:132–146.

124. Poole PJ, Black PN. Oral mucolytic drugs for exacerbations of chronic obstructive pulmonary disease: systematic review. BMJ 2001; 322:1271–1274.

125. Grandjean EM, Berthet P, Ruffmann R, Leuenberger P. Efficacy of oral long-term N-acetylcysteine in chronic bronchopulmonary disease: a meta-analysis of

published double-blind, placebo-controlled clinical trials. Clin Ther 2000; 22: 209–221.

126. Grandjean EM, Berthet PH, Ruffmann R, Leuenberger P. Cost-effectiveness analysis of oral N-acetylcysteine as a preventive treatment in chronic bronchitis. Pharmacol Res 2000; 42:39–50.

127. Sheffner AL, Medler EM, Jacobs LW, Sarett HP. The in vitro reduction in viscosity of human tracheobronchial secretions by acetylcysteine. Am Rev Respir Dis 1964; 90:721–729.

128. Ziment I. Acetylcysteine: a drug with an interesting past and a fascinating future. Respiration 1986; 50(suppl 1):26–30.

129. Riise GC, Qvarfordt I, Larsson S, Eliasson V, Andersson BA. Inhibitory effect of N-acetylcysteine on adherence of Streptococcus pneumoniae and Haemophilus influenzae to human oropharyngeal epithelial cells in vitro. Respiration 2000; 67: 552–558.

130. Zhou Y, Shapiro M, Dong Q, Louahed J, Weiss C, Wan S, et al. A calcium-activated chloride channel blocker inhibits goblet cell metaplasia and mucus overproduction. In: Mucus Hypersecretion in Respiratory Disease. Chichester, UK: John Wiley and Sons, 2002: 150–165.

131. Toda M, Tulic MK, Levitt RC, Hamid Q. A calcium-activated chloride channel (HCLCA1) is strongly related to IL-9 expression and mucus production in bronchial epithelium of patients with asthma. J Allergy Clin Immunol 2002; 109:246–250.

132. Hoshino M, Morita S, Iwashita H, Sagiya Y, Nagi T, Nakanishi A, et al. Increased expression of the human Ca2+-activated Cl⁻ channel 1 (CaCC1) gene in the asthmatic airway. Am J Respir Crit Care Med 2002; 165:1132–1136.

2

The Biophysical Properties of Mucus

MALCOLM KING

University of Alberta
Edmonton, Alberta, Canada

I. Introduction

The *rheology* of mucus is its capacity to undergo flow and deformation in response to the forces applied to it. The proper evaluation of mucus rheology is
essential for a complete understanding of mucociliary and cough clearance, for
monitoring the action of medications that might affect its behavior, and for
fitting the role of mucus into the context of epithelial function. However, since
the biophysical properties of mucus are complex, useful parameters that characterize its viscoelastic behavior are not easy to define in mathematical terms or
to measure experimentally. Indeed, many researchers believe that mucus is one
of the most difficult biological materials to analyze.

Airway mucus is a viscoelastic gel consisting of water and high-molecular-
weight glycoproteins, mixed with serum and cellular proteins (albumin, immunoglobulins, enzymes) and lipids. Normal mucus contains variable amounts of
cell debris and particulate matter.

Respiratory mucus is usually cleared by airflow and ciliary interactions.
Sputum—which is mucus mixed with inflammatory cells, cellular debris, and
bacteria—is generally cleared by cough. The clearance of airway mucus depends

on the biophysical or rheological properties of the mucus gel. These include its internal cohesive properties—viscosity and elasticity—as well as its surface and adhesive characteristics. In addition, mucus clearance depends on ciliary function, the nature of the serous fluid, and the interactions between mucus and airflow. This chapter focuses on the present status of and future prospects for research into the interrelationships between the driving forces for mucus clearance in the central airways and the viscoelastic properties of mucus.

II. Mucus Viscoelasticity

Many factors contribute to the viscoelasticity of mucus, including the type of mucus glycoprotein (mucin), the hydration of the secretions, and the degree of entanglement and crosslinking in the mucus gel. In turn, mucus gel formation is influenced by the pH and ion content of the secretions, as well as the presence of inflammatory mediators and enzymes. Disruption of the gel network (the process known as *mucolysis*) causes breakage or reduction of the bonds within the mucus gel. If carried out to the right extent, this process optimizes the ability of ciliary and airflow mechanisms to clear mucus. Mucolysis occurs through either physical intervention such as high-frequency oscillation (1) or biochemical or pharmacological agents (also referred to as *mucotropic* agents) such as *N*-acetylcysteine or dornase alfa (2). Mucolysis, by breaking macromolecular bonds or disrupting secondary bonding in the mucus gel structure, reduces the viscoelasticity of the mucus gel.

   Since mucus rheological behavior involves the crosslinking and entanglement of glycoproteins, it is described as "viscoelastic." In other words, it has the characteristics of both a liquid and a solid (3,4). *Viscosity* is resistance to flow, reflecting the absorption of energy from an object such as a solid particle, moving through a substance. In ideal fluids, viscosity is independent of the applied stress. *Elasticity* (elastic modulus) is the capacity of the material to transmit recoil energy back to the object. The elasticity of a mucus gel is a measure of the density of crosslink points within a given timeframe. At high-measurement frequencies or within short times, the effective number of crosslinks is greater than for longer times, when the gel network has more opportunity to rearrange in response to the applied stress.

   The viscosity of viscoelastic liquids such as mucus decreases with increasing stress or rate of strain (shear rate). Mucus responds to stress with an initial solid-like deformation followed by a viscoelastic deformation and finally by a period of steady flow with a constant rate of deformation. After the stress is removed, there is only partial recovery of the strain. This indicates that there has been a permanent deformation of the gel structure. This type of viscoelastic behavior is illustrated in Figure 1.

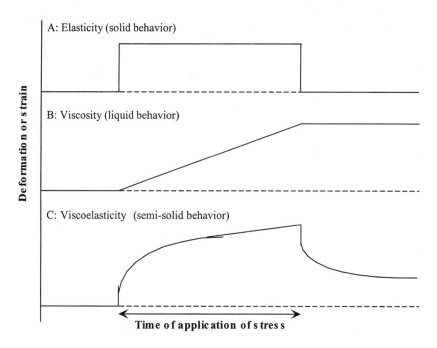

Figure 1 Diagram showing the viscoelastic behavior of a mucus gel. The first two panels illustrate stress–strain relationships in idealized materials, namely, an elastic solid, in which the displacement or strain is proportional to the applied force or stress, and a viscous liquid, in which the rate of strain (displacement/time) is proportional to the stress. Mucus is a viscoelastic semisolid. It responds instantaneously as a solid, with a very rapid displacement in response to an applied force. This is followed by a transition to a liquid-like response, where the rate of strain is constant with time. Finally a zone of viscous response is reached, where the rate of displacement is constant with time. After release of the applied force, the mucus gel only partially recoils to its initial position.

Mucus exhibits *shear thinning*; i.e., following exposure to high shear forces, mucus shows a decreased viscosity when retested at low shear rates. Some shear thinning may be permanent (that is, the viscosity is permanently reduced through an altered molecular structure) while some shear thinning may be reversible. Reversible shear thinning is known as *thixotropy*. When sputum is obtained by aspiration under pressure, shear thinning occurs, along with dilution by irrigation fluids, and the incorporation of air bubbles.

Water can influence viscosity by binding to mucus glycoprotein macromolecules. Dehydration of the mucus can increase viscosity, as can mucus–epithelium adhesion. In purulent sputum, there is a poor correlation between viscosity and the dry weight of solids. This may explain why mucus glycopro-

tein content is a poor index of viscoelasticity in chronic bronchitis, bronchiectasis, and cystic fibrosis (5). Because mucus viscosity and elasticity increase with
acidic pH (6), this is a predictor of reduced mucociliary clearability. Mucus
viscoelasticity is also dependent on the content of low-molecular-weight electro-
lytes. These properties reflect the polyelectrolyte nature of mucins (1,7,8).

Changes in mucus viscosity and elasticity are generally interrelated (6,9),
although interventions that break or add crosslinks can alter the close relationship (10,11). The low end of the normal range of viscoelasticity (3,12,13) promotes optimal mucociliary clearance of airway mucus, and a decrease in the
clearance rate (*transport*) occurs with increasing mucus elasticity and increasing
viscosity. Increasing viscosity at constant elasticity causes a pronounced decrease in the mucociliary transport rate (14). Decreasing mucus viscosity alone
results in increased cough transportability (3), which may explain the improvement in sputum mobilization following hydration or mucolytic drug therapy.

Another measure of elasticity is *spinnability*—the thread-forming ability
of mucus under the influence of large-amplitude elastic deformation. In model
studies, spinnability has been correlated positively with mucociliary clearance
(15) and negatively with cough clearance (16). Mucus spinnability and low-
amplitude viscoelasticity show no simple or consistent relationship; these two
variables should therefore be considered independent parameters describing the
biophysical properties of mucus.

Spinnability can be considered a measure of the cohesiveness of the mucus gel, or its resistance to rupture with applied tension. Mucus spinnability is
much more sensitive to mucolytic treatments involving molecular-weight reduction than to low-amplitude viscoelasticity (17).

True mucolytic treatments involve the rupture of polymer backbone elements such as disulfide bridges linking mucin subunits or the breakdown of
high-molecular-weight DNA. Having only a few ruptured linkages greatly reduces the resistance of the network to rupture at high strain, even though there
is relatively little change in the concentration of crosslinks (which determines
low-amplitude viscoelasticity). *Indirect mucolysis*, which involves rearrange-
ments of the macromolecular configuration (e.g., swelling of the network by
increasing water content or altering mucin polymer size by changes in ion content), may greatly alter the distance between crosslinks (crosslink density) and
yet do little to alter the cohesiveness or rupturability of the gel.

III. Surface Properties of Mucus

The surface properties of mucus have only recently been recognized as being
separate and distinct from bulk viscoelasticity. The surface properties are believed to be critically important for most aspects of mucus function, such as its

clearance by airflow and ciliary mechanisms, as well as its cytoprotective function. *Adhesiveness*, the ability of mucus to bond to a solid surface, is measured as the force of separation between one or more solid surfaces and the adhesive material: The degree of adhesion depends on the surface tension, hydration, wettability, and contact (dwell) time of the mucus.

The surface properties of mucus are important determinants of cough clearability (16,18–20). Surface-active phospholipids probably also play an important role in mucociliary clearance. A bronchial surfactant layer has been demonstrated between the mucus and periciliary fluid layers (21). This bronchial surfactant may help the mucus layer to spread evenly across the periciliary layer surface and maintain the integrity of these layers. It probably also acts as a lubricant and so increases the efficiency of the mucociliary apparatus. Allegra and colleagues (22) added surfactant to the excised frog palate and showed that this maneuver markedly increased the rate of mucociliary transport on this ciliated surface. In my laboratory, we demonstrated that the administration of exogenous surfactant to premature babies with neonatal respiratory distress syndrome dramatically improves the mucociliary clearability of their airway secretions (23). Finally, we also demonstrated that an artificial surfactant preparation instilled intrabronchially enhances the in vivo rate of mucociliary clearance in anesthetized dogs (24).

IV. Current Methods for Mucus Viscoelasticity

A. Controlled Shear Rate Rheometer

These classic instruments for measuring the bulk viscoelastic properties of biofluids are generally based on deformation in the cone-and-plate geometry or between double concentric cylinders. In both setups the shear rate in the testing fluid (i.e., the mucus) is definable and uniform. Since the viscoelastic properties of mucus are highly dependent on the rate of shear applied to the sample, this is a clear advantage. Testing can be dynamic (oscillatory motion) (25) and/or transient (steady rotation and recoil) (26). Both modes yield equivalent information in principle, that is, separate measures of viscosity and elasticity at different rates of shear or at different oscillatory frequencies. The main disadvantage of these instruments is that, because of edge or end effects, their use is limited to volumes of about 0.5 mL or more. This is not a serious limitation for sputum samples, but other rheological testing methods must be used for samples of mucus from humans without hypersecretion or from experimental animals.

B. Double-Capillary Method

When fluid is pulled from a reservoir through a simple capillary tube under vacuum pressure, the further it enters the tube the more the rate of progression decreases. Thus, no steady flow rate is reached, and no single value of viscosity (proportional to driving pressure over flow rate) can be defined. A smaller capillary tube segment within the larger tube can be used to overcome this problem. Because the pressure drop in a tube is inversely proportional to the fourth power of the radius, the smaller tube will account for most of the pressure drop and act essentially as a flow-limiting segment. The viscosity of mucus is then determined directly from the ratio of the pressure drop and the flow rate across the flow-limiting segment. The researcher can determine measurements of viscosity at different shear rates by varying the driving pressure, and determine a measure of the elastic modulus by observing the recoil after the pressure is released.

The double-capillary method is well suited to the study of mucus because it can easily be miniaturized down to the range of 20 μL sample volumes (27). Beyond that, the measurement of elasticity is limited by the fact that the meniscus changes shape during the recoil. Further miniaturization (down to the 100 nL range) has been achieved by converting to a plug flow setup (28), in which the changes in the shape of the two menisci tend to balance each other. However, with capillary flow, the shear rate within the mucus is not constant. It varies from a maximum at the wall to zero along the midline of the tube. It is also essential to ensure that the no-slip condition is met, i.e., that the mucus adheres firmly to the capillary surface. This could be problematic for mucus that is mixed with saliva or that contains surfactant or lipidic components. This consideration also applies to the macroscopic, controlled shear rate viscoelastometers discussed above.

C. Magnetic Microrheometers

Magnetic microrheometers are also designed to measure the viscoelastic properties of very small quantities of mucus. A steel ball is positioned in a 1–5 μL sample of mucus and oscillated by an electromagnet at different driving frequencies. The researcher can use the magnitude of displacement of the ball and its phase lag with respect to the driving force to calculate the viscoelasticity of the mucus (29). See Figure 2.

Because the magnetic rheometer depends on an optical detection system and mucus is semiopaque, this instrument works better with microliter quantities of mucus than with larger quantities. Although it is not size-limited in principle, miniaturization much beyond the magnetic rheometer's present microliter range would require the development of a stronger magnet and a more potent light source or a better optical detection system. The shear rate in the mucus is also not well defined, and it is difficult to work with samples that are too watery because the steel ball becomes nonbouyant and sinks to the bottom of the container. To overcome this latter problem an investigator has turned the rheometer on its side and applied a bias current to the magnet to balance the pull of gravity on the ball (30).

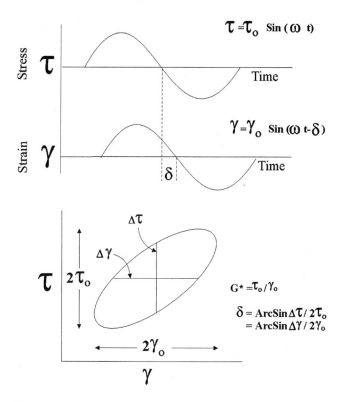

Figure 2 Stress–strain relationships in oscillatory rheological testing. In a viscoelastic material, strain lags behind the applied stress. The in-phase strain gives the elasticity, the out-of-phase component the viscosity.

The magnetic rheometer is probably insensitive to the presence of surfactants, since the rheological probe lies completely within the mucus and "sees" only the bulk properties, assuming no slippage between the ball and the mucus through which it moves. As with all microrheological methods, one must be aware that mucus is inherently heterogeneous in its rheological properties, and it is generally necessary to test multiple aliquots. A computer-assisted, automated magnetic rheometer has been developed, and this instrument has demonstrated improvements in accuracy and speed of analysis (31).

D. Filancemeter

Spinnability (*filance*, *Spinnbarkeit*) is the thread-forming capacity of mucus under the influence of large-amplitude elastic deformation. By conducting an electric signal through the mucus sample, the filancemeter measures spinnability as thread formation in millimeters. This measurement is performed with a 10–20 µL mucus sample at a retraction velocity of 10 mm/sec. To measure spinnability, the electric signal is interrupted at the point where the stretched mucus thread is broken (32). Spinnability has been correlated positively with mucociliary clearance on the frog palate (15), but negatively with cough clearability using a simulated cough machine (16). One of the major problems with the measurement of spinnability is the fact that it does not correlate well with other more basic measures of viscoelasticity.

V. Role of Mucus in Mucociliary Clearance

There are two major mechanisms for clearing airway mucus: mucociliary clearance and airflow interaction. The latter becomes important as lung disease develops (5). According to model studies, mucociliary clearance is critically dependent on maintaining the depth of periciliary fluid (33,34). The depth of mucus does not appear to vary a great deal within the bronchi, but the mucus layer may become discontinuous in the smaller airways (35,36). The normal daily volume of respiratory secretion arriving at the larynx is estimated to be approximately 10 mL/day. Although the total production of airway surface fluid throughout the airway system is not known, it is probably much higher than the volume actually reaching the larynx. This reduction in airway fluid volume is believed to be due to absorption of water through the lower bronchi via active ion transport mechanisms (37–39).

Mucociliary clearance rate (MCR) is affected by ciliary, serous fluid, and mucus factors. The ciliary factors that affect MCR are mainly ciliary amplitude and beat frequency, which together determine the maximal velocity at the tips of the cilia, and hence the maximal forward velocity of the mucus layer. There is little supporting evidence in the literature but it is a generally accepted principle that the faster the cilia beat, the higher the MCR. Also, longer cilia should be able to clear mucus faster because they can generate greater forward velocities, and the greater the distance between the cilia, the more energy will be dissipated in the mucus, thus reducing the net forward velocity. Cilia are generally shorter in smaller airways than in the large bronchi, and even though ciliary beat frequency may be comparable, the rate of momentum transfer to the mucus will be proportionately reduced.

Serous factors that affect MCR include viscosity and depth of serous fluid. If the serous fluid is too viscous, the cilia will not be able to move very well within it and the decreased ciliary tip velocity will lead to a reduction of MCR. This principle is well established for water-propelling cilia, but the serous fluid viscosity is unknown for the periciliary fluid in the two-layer mucociliary system. Active ion transport and its associated transepithelial water flux (38) are likely of critical importance in modulating serous fluid viscosity. Transepithelial protein fluxes may also reasonably be expected to contribute to serous fluid viscosity (40). The efficient transfer of momentum between the cilia and the mucus layer requires that the cilia firmly contact the mucus during their forward stroke while minimally interacting with it during the return. If the serous fluid is too deep or too shallow, MCR will decrease (34). The cilia must be also able to penetrate and pull through the mucus in the zone of contact. This might be aided by a surfactant layer, as suggested in experiments involving administration of exogenous surfactants (24).

Mucus factors affecting MCR are the depth and viscoelastic properties of mucus (3,4). Mucus that is deep is better suited to clearance by coughing (41) than to clearance by cilia. The elasticity of mucus is important for clearance by cilia because it efficiently transmits energy without energy loss. The viscosity of mucus results in energy loss, but it is necessary so that mucus can be extruded from submucosal glands and displaced and either expectorated or swallowed. A balance between these factors must be maintained for optimal MCR.

The transport velocity of mucus simulant gels is directly related to mucus elasticity and the depth of the periciliary fluid, and it is inversely related to mucus viscosity (3). An ideal viscoelastic ratio may exist for optimal mucociliary interaction. If so, an increase in viscosity and/or a decrease in elasticity would result in a reduced transport rate. Transport by cough or airflow interaction depends inversely on viscosity, elasticity (spinnability), and adhesivity (16). Mucus that is elastic rather than viscous is transported well by ciliary action, but less well by coughing (4).

VI. Mucus and Cough Clearance

In various lung diseases characterized by mucus hypersecretion and impaired airway clearance, elimination of the excess mucus by coughing becomes of paramount importance. Cough clearance derives from the high-velocity interaction between airflow and the mucus, leading to wave formation in the mucus layer, temporary reduction in crosslinking within the mucus gel, and ultimately to shearing and forward propulsion of portions of the mucus layer. The depth of mucus and the airflow linear velocity, are of course, critical determinants of cough clearance (42). Mucus properties that are important to cough clearance are the viscosity or internal cohesion of the mucus; the elastic component, which impedes forward motion and results in recoil after the cough event; and the surface properties, both at the air–mucus interface and at the interface with the periciliary layer (16). Adhesivity or surface tension inhibits cough clearance by suppressing mucus–airflow interaction, which manifests itself as wave formation in the mucus layer during the cough.

Viscosity

Viscosity is the primary variable governing cough clearance. For purely viscous materials, the mucus velocity profiles follow Newton's law.

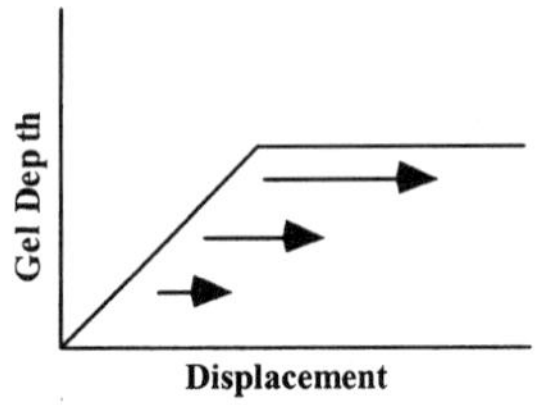

Gel Depth

Displacement

Spinnability

Spinnability or thread formation is a measure of large deformation elasticity. A high degree of spinnability inhibits viscous deformation by creating recoil in the mucus.

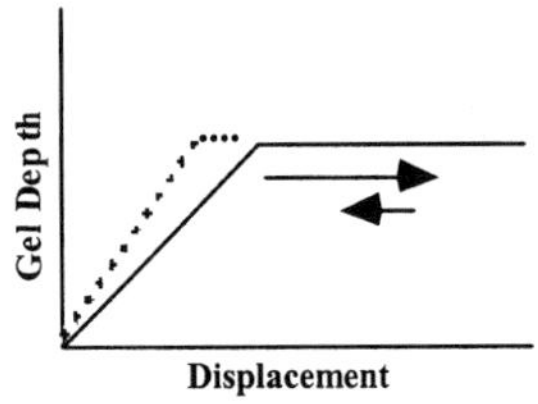

Gel Depth

Displacement

Adhesivity

High surface tension increases the work of adhesion of the mucus to the underlying surface, and inhibits wave formation in the mucus layer, reducing air-mucus interaction.

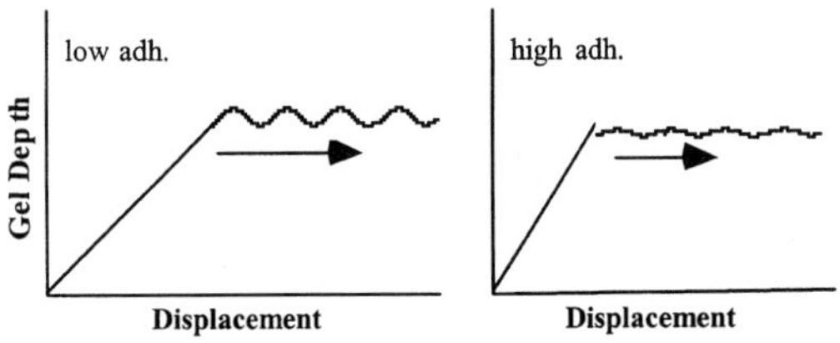

low adh.   high adh.

Gel Depth

Displacement   Displacement

Figure 3 Cough clearance, based on the results of studies involving the simulated cough machine (16), depends on three primary biophysical variables: 1) viscosity, 2) elasticity, and 3) adhesivity.

The dependence of cough clearance on mucus viscosity, elasticity, and adhesivity is illustrated in Figure 3. In addition, Zahm et al. (43) demonstrated that mucus thixotropy and shear-thinning were important in describing the movement of mucus in multiple rapid coughs and, by extension, high-frequency oscillation.

There is an optimal range of viscoelastic properties, and in some cases both mucociliary and cough clearance should be optimized. These findings suggest that therapeutic measures designed to modify the rheology of secretions should consider the initial state of the mucus, and that the monitoring of the viscoelastic properties of the mucus should be an essential part of any potential mucotropic therapy.

References

1. Dasgupta B, King M. Molecular basis for mucolytic therapy. Can Respir J 1995; 2:223–230.

2. Rubin BK, Tomkiewicz RP, King M. Mucoactive agents: old and new. In: Wilmott RW, ed. The Pediatric Lung. Basel, Switzerland: Birkhäuser, 1997:155–179.

3. King M. Mucus, mucociliary clearance and coughing. In: Bates DV, ed. Respiratory Function in Disease. 3rd ed. Philadelphia: Saunders, 1989:69–78.

4. King M, Rubin BK. Rheology of airway mucus: relationship with clearance function. In: Takishima T, Shimura S, eds. Airway Secretion: Physiological Bases for the Control of Mucous Hypersecretion. New York: Marcel Dekker, 1994:283–314.

5. King M, Rubin BK. Mucus physiology and pathophysiology: therapeutic aspects. In: Derenne JP, Whitelaw WA, Similowski T, eds. Acute Respiratory Failure in COPD. New York: Marcel Dekker, 1996:391–411.

6. Lutz RJ, Litt M, Chakrin LW. Physical-chemical factors in mucus rheology. In: Gabelnick HL, Litt M, eds. Rheology of Biological Systems. Springfield, IL: Charles C Thomas, 1973:158–194.

7. Lamblin G, Aubert JP, Perini JM, Klein N, Porchet N, Degand P, Roussel P. Human respiratory mucins. Eur Respir J 1992; 5:247–256.

8. Bansil R, Stanley E, LaMont JT. Mucin biophysics. Annu Rev Physiol 1995; 57: 635–657.

9. King M, Macklem PT. Rheological properties of microliter quantities of normal mucus. J Appl Physiol 1977; 42:797–802.

10. Meyer FA, Gelman RA. Mucociliary transference rate and mucus viscoelasticity: dependence on dynamic storage and loss modulus. Am Rev Respir Dis 1979; 120: 553–557.

11. Dasgupta B, Tomkiewicz RP, De Sanctis GT, Boyd WA, King M. Rheological properties in cystic fibrosis airway secretions with combined rhDNase and gelsolin treatment. In: Singh M, Saxena VP, eds. Advances in Physiological Fluid Dynamics. New Delhi, India: Narosa, 1996:74–78.

12. Dulfano MJ, Adler KB. Physical properties of sputum. VII. Rheologic properties and mucociliary transport. Am Rev Respir Dis 1975; 112:341–347.

13. Shih CK, Litt M, Khan MA, Wolf DP. Effect of nondialyzable solids concentration and viscoelasticity on ciliary transport of tracheal mucus. Am Rev Respir Dis 1975; 115:89–995.

14. King M. Relationship between mucus viscoelasticity and ciliary transport in guaran gel/frog palate model system. Biorheology 1980; 17:249–254.

15. Puchelle E, Zahm JM, Duvivier C. Spinability of bronchial mucus: relationship with viscoelasticity and mucus transport properties. Biorheology 1983; 20:239–249.

16. King M, Zahm JM, Pierrot D, Vaquez-Girod S, Puchelle E. The role of mucus gel viscosity, spinnability, and adhesive properties in clearance by simulated cough. Biorheology 1989; 26:737–745.

17. King M, Dasgupta B, Tomkiewicz RP, Brown NE. Rheology of cystic fibrosis sputum after in vitro treatment with hypertonic saline alone and in combination with rhDNase. Am J Respir Crit Care Med 1997; 156:173–177.

18. Agarwal M, King M, Rubin BK, Shukla JB. Mucus transport in a miniaturized simulated cough machine: effect of constriction and serous layer simulant. Biorheology 1989; 26:977–988.

19. Zahm JM, Pierrot D, Vaquez-Girod S, Duvivier C, King M, Puchelle E. The role of mucus sol phase in clearance by simulated cough. Biorheology 1989; 26:747–752.

20. Girod S, Galabert C, Pierrot D, Boissonade MM, Zahm JM, Baszkin A, Puchelle E. Role of phospholipid lining on respiratory mucus clearance by cough. J Appl Physiol 1991; 71:2262–2266.
21. Schürch S, Gehr P, Im Hof V, Geiser M, Green F. Surfactant displaces particles toward the epithelium in airways and alveoli. Respir Physiol 1990; 80:17–32.
22. Allegra L, Bossi R, Braga PC. Influence of surfactant on mucociliary transport. Eur J Respir Dis 1985; 67(suppl 142):71–76.
23. Rubin BK, Ramirez O, King M. The role of mucus rheology and transport in neonatal respiratory distress syndrome and the effect of surfactant therapy. Chest 1992; 101:1080–1085.
24. De Sanctis GT, Tomkiewicz RP, Rubin BK, Schürch S, King M. Exogenous surfactant enhances mucociliary clearance in the anesthetized dog. Eur Respir J 1994; 7: 1616–1621.
25. Braga PC. Sinusoidal oscillations method. In: Braga PC, Allegra L, eds. Methods in Bronchial Mucology. New York: Raven Press, 1988:63–71.
26. Davis SS. Practical applications of viscoelasticity measurement. Eur J Respir Dis 1980; 61(suppl 110):141–156.
27. Kim CS. Capillary type viscometer. In: Braga PC, Allegra L, eds. Methods in Bronchial Mucology. New York: Raven Press, 1988:93–103.
28. Leikauf GD, Ueki IF, Nadel JA. Autonomic regulation of viscoelasticity of cat tracheal gland secretion. J Appl Physiol 1984; 56:426–430.
29. King M. Magnetic microrheometer. In: Braga PC, Allegra L, eds. Methods in Bronchial Mucology. New York: Raven Press, 1988:3–83.
30. Majima Y, Hirata K, Takeuchi K, Hattori M, Sakakura Y. Effects of orally administered drugs on dynamic viscoelasticity of human nasal mucus. Am Rev Respir Dis 1990; 141:79–83.
31. Silveira PSP, Böhm GM, Yang HM, Wen CL, Guimar{{atilde}}es ET, Parada MAC, King M, Saldiva PHN. Computer-assisted rheological evaluation of microsamples of mucus. Comput Methods Programs Biomed 1992; 39:51–60.
32. Zahm JM, Puchelle E, Duvivier C, Didelon J. Spinability of respiratory mucus. Validation of a new apparatus: the Filancemeter. Bull Eur Physiopathol Respir 1986; 22:609–613.
33. Blake JR, Winet H. On the mechanics of mucociliary transport. Biorheology 1980; 17:125–134.
34. King M, Agarwal M, Shukla JB. A planar model for mucociliary transport: effect of mucus viscoelasticity. Biorheology 1993; 30:49–61.
35. Gil J, Weibel ER. Extracellular lining of bronchioles after perfusion-fixation of rat lungs for electron microscopy. Anat Rec 1971; 169:185–200.
36. Van As A. Pulmonary airway clearance mechanisms: a reappraisal [editorial]. Am Rev Respir Dis 1977; 115:721–726.
37. Boucher RC, Stutts MJ, Bromberg PA, Gatzy JT. Regional differences in airway surface liquid composition. J Appl Physiol 1981; 50:613–620.
38. Boucher RC. State of the art: human airway ion transport. Am J Respir Crit Care Med 1994; 150:271–281, 581–593.
39. Widdicombe JH. Ion and fluid transport by airway epithelium. In: Takishima T,

Shimura S, eds. Airway Secretion: Physiological Bases for the Control of Mucus Hypersecretion. New York: Marcel Dekker, 1994:399–431.

40.   Govindaraju K, Cowley EA, Eidelman DH, Lloyd DK. Analysis of proteins in micro samples of rat airway surface fluid by capillary electrophoresis. J Chromatog B Biomed Sci Appl 1998; 705:223–230.

41.   King M. Role of mucus viscoelasticity in cough clearance. Biorheology 1987; 24: 589–597.

42.   King M, Brock G, Lundell C. Clearance of mucus by simulated cough. J Appl Physiol 1985; 58:1776–1782.

43.   Zahm JM, King M, Duvivier C, Pierrot D, Girod S, Puchelle E. Role of simulated repetitive coughing in mucus clearance. Eur Respir J 1991; 4:311–315.

3

Regulation of Airway Mucus Secretion

J. H. WIDDICOMBE

University of California–Davis
Davis
and Cardiovascular Research Institute
University of California–San Francisco
San Francisco, California, U.S.A.

I. Introduction

This chapter first briefly summarizes the many components and sources of mucous secretions. The correspondingly varied array of preparations and techniques for measuring mucus output is then discussed. Finally, the regulation of mucus secretion is reviewed. The chapter deals only with the secretory apparatus of the trachea and bronchi. Nasal secretions and their regulation are similar to those of the large airways (1). Little is known about regulation of secretion in the bronchioles (2,3).

II. Components of Mucus

Mucus, as defined by Rose (4), is "any viscid, slimy, viscoelastic gel-like material covering biological surfaces." The function of airway mucus is primarily to protect the underlying epithelium. Inhaled particles are trapped in the mucus, which is continuously removed from the lungs by the beating of the underlying cilia (5).

Mucus has properties of both a solid and a liquid; in rheological terms it possesses both viscosity and elasticity (6). It is mucins that confer these peculiar viscoelastic properties. These glycoproteins are 150–7000 kDa in size and 55–90% by weight carbohydrate. They can be either secreted or attached to the cell surface. Other complex glycoconjugates of mucous secretions include proteoglycans and N-glycoproteins. They are distinguished in part from mucins by the form of the chemical linkage between carbohydrate and amino acid (4).

Eight mucin (MUC) genes have been identified in normal respiratory-tract epithelia (7). Interestingly, gland mucous cells and goblet cells of the surface epithelium express mRNA for different sets of mucins (8). Furthermore, the types of mucins expressed changes in disease (9). Thus, the mucin content of the airway mucous blanket may vary considerably with variations in pathophysiological status. It is not yet known how such variation affects the viscoelasticity and other properties of the mucous blanket.

In addition to mucins and other high-molecular-weight glycoconjugates, mucous secretions contain salts, proteins actively secreted by the airway epithelium such as secretory IgG, lactoferrin and lysozyme (10), and a long list of secreted low-molecular-weight components including ATP (11,12), and plasma exudate (13).

Under all conditions, water probably comprises between 90 and 98% of mucous secretions (14), with the exact volume of these secretions being regulated by water movement down transepithelial osmotic and hydrostatic pressure gradients. These gradients can be generated in several ways. In gland serous cells (and perhaps also in serous cells of surface epithelium), active secretion of Cl generates a lumen negative potential difference that draws Na, and generates an osmotic gradient locally across the epithelium (15). As airway epithelium has a high hydraulic conductivity (16,17), this gradient is probably small, and transepithelial liquid movements are approximately isotonic (18,19). Inflammatory extravasation raises hydrostatic pressure beneath the surface epithelium, increases the hydraulic conductivity of the epithelium (20), and drives water flow into the airway lumen down the transepithelial gradient in hydrostatic pressure (21–23). Active Na absorption across the surface epithelium mediates absorption of isotonic saline solution at $\sim 5 \ \mu L/cm^2/h$ (24,25). Hydration of newly released mucous granules may also draw water into the lumen (26). Alterations in the balance of these water flows result in excessively dilute or concentrated mucous secretions, and the associated changes in viscoelasticity can markedly affect mucociliary clearance. This is illustrated most clearly in cystic fibrosis. Here decreased Cl secretion from gland serous cells (27) coupled with increased Na absorption across the surface epithelium (28) results in highly concentrated mucous secretions (29,30) and a virtual failure of mucociliary clearance (30,31).

III. Sources of Mucous Secretions

In human cartilaginous airways (i.e., the trachea and bronchi), the mucus-secreting apparatus consists mainly of glands and of goblet cells in the surface epithelium. Glands are not present in the cartilage-free airways (i.e., bronchioles). By contrast, goblet cells are present in both bronchi and conducting bronchioles, where they account for about one-fifth of the columnar cells of surface epithelium, with most of the rest being ciliated (32). In the respiratory bronchioles, goblet cells are replaced by Clara and serous cells (33,34), neither of which are known to secrete mucins (3,35). However, goblet cells are formed in human respiratory bronchioles in response to chronic irritation (36).

There are about 100 gland openings per cm^2 of surface area in a healthy adult human trachea (37), with each gland containing $\sim$15 secretory tubules (38). In human bronchi the volume of mucous granules in submucosal glands is $\sim$40 times that in the goblet cells of the surface epithelium (39). In humans and other large mammals, individual glands are approximately 100 nL in volume (40,41). However, the numbers and size of human glands decrease progressively with increasing airway generation number, till by the eighth generation gland volume per unit luminal surface area is only 1/20 that of the trachea (41).

Gland secretory tubules empty into a dilated collecting duct, which connects to the airway surface via a narrow ciliated duct (38). Each secretory tubule is lined with mucous cells and terminates in acini lined with serous cells (42). This latter cell type is believed to secrete the fluid that serves to flush out the mucins released by the more proximal mucous cells (43). Serous cells are also the primary source of several natural antibiotics such as lactoferrin and lysozyme (35). They also contain proteoglycans (44,45) and mucins (46,47).

In general, the larger the airway, the more likely it is to have glands and goblet cells. Thus, numbers of glands and goblet cells in trachea and bronchi in the larger mammalian species (ox, dog, horse, sheep, goat, pig, monkey, cat, ferret) resemble those of humans (40). Smaller species either lack glands (rabbit, mouse) or have them confined to the upper part of the trachea (rat) (40,48). In these small species, goblet cells are often replaced by other cell types, e.g., serous cells in rat trachea (49) and Clara cells in mouse trachea (50). However, chronic irritation or inflammation increases the numbers of goblet cells or induces them in species and airways where they are normally absent (36).

IV. Methods for Measuring Mucous Secretions

Mucins may be measured directly. However, other parameters of mucous secretions are often measured, and it is generally assumed that the rate of secretion of mucins will change in parallel. The various parameters that have been used as indices of mucous secretions are listed in Table 1.

Florey et al. (51) were the first to provide quantitative estimates of the volume of airway mucous secretions. They attached cannulas to both ends of a section of cat trachea in vivo. The tracheal lumen was filled with oil, one cannula was sealed, and movement of the oil's meniscus along the other cannula monitored. Another approach avoids filling the tracheal lumen with liquid (52). A trachea is mounted laryngeal end down in a conventional muscle bath. Its uppermost (i.e., caudal) end projects above the surface of liquid in the bath. The bottom end is cannulated with a Perspex tube connected to a conical collecting well. Secretions collect in the well under the influence of gravity and mucociliary transport, and are weighed at set intervals. Secretion rates of individual glands can also be measured. In one approach, the tip of a constant bore capillary tube, previously flared out by heating, is placed over an individual gland opening visualized by the vital dye neutral red (53). A tight seal between pipette tip and surface epithelium permits the gland secretions to flow directly into the tube. Alternatively, the mucosal surface can be overlaid with mineral oil, and beads of secretion visualized with a dissecting microscope (54,55). Because beads are generally approximately spherical, it is easy to estimate the rates of volume secretion from the change in bead diameter (55). A similar technique

Table 1 Measurements of Mucous Secretions

Parameter	Technique
Volume of gland secretions	Liquid-filled trachea
	In vitro collection by gravity
	Micropipette sampling from gland openings
	"Hillocks" and "beads"
	Dual-capacitance probe technique on cell cultures
Net NaCl secretion	Radioisotopes in Ussing chambers
Radiolabeled high-molecular-weight glycoconjugates	Sampling from tracheal lumen
	Organ culture
	Ussing chambers
	Isolated cells
	Cell culture
Mucins	Colorimetry
	ELISA
	ELLA (enzyme-linked lectin assay)
Lactoferrin/lysozyme	Bacteriolysis/ELISA
Granule discharge/vacuolization	Histochemistry/electron microscopy/ videomicroscopy

involves coating the airway surface with a layer of tantalum dust; gland secretions are visualized as upswellings, or "hillocks," in the tantalum (56). Cell cultures of glands are valuable in that they convert the complex tubulo-acinar geometry of the airway gland into a planar sheet. Liquid movement has been measured across such cultures from human trachea using a double-capacitance probe technique (15,24). This approach is potentially useful in studies on the regulation of fluid secretion and its relationship to mucus release. However, it is not possible to relate with any accuracy the volume flows measured across cultures to secretory flows from intact glands.

The liquid transported by epithelia is not water but salt solution. Thus, estimates of liquid flow can be made by measuring the net fluxes of radioactive Na and Cl across sheets of tracheal wall mounted between half-chambers in vitro (25,57). Glands secrete and surface epithelium generally absorbs liquid (15,24). Net NaCl fluxes across a sheet of tracheal wall will reflect the balance between these two processes. However, under certain conditions, such as during cholinergic stimulation, it is reasonably safe to assume that changes in net fluxes of Na and Cl reflect gland secretion.

A commonly used approach to estimating mucin secretion is to incubate cells or tissues with radioactive precursors of mucins such as $^{35}SO_4$, ^3H-galactose-N-acetylgalactosamine, or ^3H-serine (58). After sufficient time has elapsed to allow incorporation of the radiolabel into mucins, the luminal or bathing medium is collected, and the high-molecular-weight radiolabeled compounds separated by a variety of techniques, including dialysis, precipitation with a mixture of trichloracetic and phosphotungstic acids, and exclusion chromatography. Ion exchange chromatography, hydroxyl apatite chromatography, and lectin-affinity chromatography have also been used (10). In general, exclusion chromatography seems the quickest and most reliable way to isolate the radiolabeled high-molecular-weight material (58,59).

The use of radiolabeled high-molecular-weight glycoconjugates as an index for mucus secretion has some disadvantages. First, not all pools of mucins may reach equilibrium levels of labeling, and in nonsterile conditions the time needed for complete labeling could exceed the tissue preparation's life span. Second, the molecular-weight cut-off is arbitrary; small mucins might be lost from the sample. Third, high-molecular-weight compounds other than mucins will be labeled, proteoglycans in particular. These can be removed from the samples by enzymatic digestion or density-gradient centrifugation (10), but these procedures are tedious. A seldom discussed disadvantage of the radiolabeling approach is its poor time resolution. Sampling periods must be long enough to obtain sufficient counts in the sample to accurately determine changes between successive periods. Counts can be increased, and the duration of sampling periods reduced, by increasing the amount of radioactivity present during labeling, although financial and safety considerations argue against this approach. In practice, sampling periods have varied from 15 minutes to 24 hours. Thus, if stimulation of mucin release is transient and of shorter duration than the collecting period, the maximal increase in the rate of mucin release will be underestimated. In fact, other techniques have suggested that gland secretion is maximal within 10 minutes of cholinergic or adrenergic stimulation, and then rapidly declines to considerably lower sustained levels (54,55,60,61).

There are assays for mucins that do not involve radiolabeling. These include enzyme-linked immunosorbent assays (ELISA) (62–64), enzyme-linked lectin assays (ELLA) (60), and a colorimetric approach using Alcian blue (65). The ELLA and colorimetric assays suffer from a certain lack of specificity, as both potentially cross-react with proteoglycans. In addition, the ELLA may fail to react with all mucins, and even mucin molecules derived from the same gene may vary in their content of the carbohydrate recognized by the lectin. Mucin antibodies are generally against carbohydrate epitopes, so ELISAs may suffer from some of the same disadvantages as ELLAs. However, the potential of ELISA for differentiating between the products of the various MUC genes is appealing.

Lactoferrin and lysozyme are present predominantly in serous gland cells (66,67). They have thus been frequently used as markers of serous cell discharge and, by implication, of the volume of gland secretions. Nowadays, ELISAs are generally used to measure these bactericidal compounds, but bacteriolytic assays are also available.

At one time, cytology was the only approach potentially specific for particular cell types. Loss of material stained with Alcian blue or PAS has been used to measure goblet cell and gland mucous cell discharge by light microscopy (68,69). Autoradiographic analysis of the loss of material labeled with radioactive mucus precursors (70,71) is an alternative. Immunocytochemical staining for lysozyme has been used to monitor serous cell discharge (72). The electron microscope has been used for morphometric analysis of mucous granule depletion and related changes in gland structure (68,73), as well as mediator-induced vacuolization of serous cells (74). A particularly exciting new development is the use of videomicroscopy of living explants to visualize the discharge of individual mucous granules from goblet cells (75,76) and of secretion from individual glands (61). Of course, all these microscopic approaches suffer from being laborious, and they are often only semiquantitative.

V. Preparations for Measuring Mucus Secretion

Some preparations contain both gland and surface epithelium, whereas others exclude one or other of these cell types (see Table 2).

Table 2 Cell and Tissue Preparations for Measurement of Mucous Secretions

Preparation	Cellular source of secretions
Perfused trachea (in vitro or in vivo)	Glands and goblet cells
Chronic tracheal pouch	Glands and goblet cells
Explant/tissue sheet in vitro	Glands, surface epithelium, and connective tissue
Isolated subepithelial tissue	Glands and connective tissue
Gland openings	Serous and mucous gland cells
Single isolated glands	Serous and mucous gland cells
Dispersed gland cells or acini	Serous and mucous gland cells
Cultured gland cells	Serous and/or mucous gland cells
Isolated surface epithelium	Goblet and ciliated cells
Dispersed isolated surface cells	Goblet, ciliated, and basal cells
Cultured surface epithelium	Goblet and/or ciliated cells

Secretions collected from the lumen of intact tracheas come from both glands and surface epithelium. The lumen may be perfused either in vivo or in vitro (51,77,78). Perfusion can be avoided if the trachea is mounted in vitro with the cephalic end down and the secretions draining from its open end collected (52). Wardell et al. (79) developed the "tracheal pouch," in which a segment of cervical trachea is separated and formed into a pouch opening to the surface of the neck, allowing repeated long-term collection of mucus from unanesthetized animals.

Organ cultures have the disadvantage over intact tracheas that high-molecular-weight glycoproteins in the culture medium may come from connective tissue as well as glands and goblet cells. Not being sterile, tissues studied in Ussing chambers have a shorter life span than those in organ culture. However, the intact surface epithelium prevents products of the connective tissue from appearing in the mucosal bath. Another advantage of Ussing chambers is that transepithelial ion transport (or even water movement) can be measured simultaneously with mucus secretion.

In studies of radiolabeled HMG release from cell sheets in vitro, it is often assumed that release is from the glands rather than goblet cells for two reasons. First, in most of the larger mammalian species, the total volume of mucus in tracheal glands is much greater than in goblet cells (39,40), although the rhesus monkey and horse are exceptions (36,80). Second, goblet cells are refractory to many neurohumoral agents (see below). However, it is comparatively easy to separate the surface epithelium from the underlying glands (81–85) and measure HMG release from the subepithelial tissues. When this was done in the ferret, the secretory responses to methacholine of intact and epithelium-free tissues were the same, but the isolated surface epithelium was unresponsive (84).

Oxygenation of glands embedded in the connective tissue of an explant may be poor, and their viability may suffer. Microdissected airway glands therefore represented both a major technical achievement and a considerable refinement as an experimental preparation. Initially these were obtained from cats (86), but more recently have come from humans (87). They have been used extensively by Shimura and colleagues, but technical difficulties and the small amount of material obtained have prevented general adoption of this approach. Interestingly, these isolated glands sometimes behave differently from other gland preparations. Thus, VIP stimulated HMG release from isolated glands by as much as 300% but failed to affect HMG release from explants (88). Similar results have been obtained with substance P (89). Such differences could reflect reduced viability of glands in explants. However, Sasaki et al. (90) have shown that addition of isolated epithelium to isolated glands depresses their secretory responses to the same level as that of explants. The identity of the epithelial-derived inhibitory factor remains to be determined, but it is evidently short-lived, as supernatant from epithelial cell cultures does not have an inhibitory action (90).

Isolated cells from airway surface epithelium are readily obtainable by mild enzymatic digestions (91,92). Cultures obtained from these cells now show excellent levels of mucociliary differentiation (93–95), with clearly distinguishable goblet and ciliated cells. For studies of mucus secretion, Kim and colleagues have developed a set of conditions that produces cultures of hamster tracheal epithelium consisting of >90% goblet cells (96,97). Cell cultures are often grown on solid plastic surfaces. However, it is comparatively easy to grow cells in porous-bottomed inserts and measure transepithelial resistance with a "chopstick" voltmeter (98). A measurable transepithelial resistance is present only if the cells form tight junctions and polarize into apical and basolateral membranes. This simple measurement of resistance is not often made, but it would seem important to document that any epithelial cell cultures used for studies of mucin secretion had indeed differentiated into a functional polarized epithelium. Further, we have recently shown that cells grown on solid substrates show much lower levels of differentiation than cells grown with an air interface on porous supports (99).

Recently, a cell line (SPOC-1) has been described that is derived spontaneously from primary cultures of rat tracheal epithelium, and consists exclusively of cells resembling goblet cells (100,101). Although there are many other cell lines from surface airway epithelium (92,102), none shows true mucociliary differentiation, and most do not even have tight junctions.

Several groups have obtained dispersed airway gland cells and acini by enzymatic digestions (103–108) that are long and strenuous compared with those needed to acquire surface epithelial cells. These preparations have generally been used to initiate cell cultures, but Dwyer et al. (60) describe an elegant superfusion technique for collecting mucus released from dispersed gland cells.

So far, most primary airway gland cell cultures are of nondescript phenotype with rudimentary features of both serous and mucous gland cells (92). The inhibition by amiloride of short-circuit current across these cultures suggests that they may also have features of duct cells (109). Alteration in culture conditions has shifted these cultures toward a mucous phenotype (110), but it is proving difficult to obtain cultures of highly differentiated serous phenotype (W. E. Finkbeiner, personal communication). Growth in collagen gels dramatically improves the differentiation of gland cultures (111), but this preparation is less convenient than cell sheets.

In 1986, Finkbeiner et al. established a cell line from bovine tracheal gland cells, which had small numbers of electron-dense secretory granules resembling those of serous cells (105). Since then, cell lines of airway gland cells have been used with increasing frequency (92,102), but in general they are even less well differentiated than the primary gland cultures. The Calu-3 cell line, derived from a lung carcinoma, is exceptional in that it forms tight junctions, and resembles serous cells in its high levels of the cystic fibrosis transmembrane conductance regulator (CFTR) (112,113). However, it also contains large electron-opaque granules closely resembling those of mucous cells (113).

VI. Neurohumoral Regulation of Mucus Secretion by Surface Epithelium

In experimental preparations of surface epithelium (explants, mucociliary cultures, mucous cultures), baseline secretion of radiolabeled glycoconjugates is generally at least 50% that achieved with even the most potent secretagogues (114,115). Even in cultures enriched with goblet cells, this resting secretion may come from somewhere other than secretory granules as microscopy shows that baseline degranulation of goblet cells is negligible (75,76,116). Neutrophil elastase releases glycocalyx without affecting goblet cell discharge (117). Furthermore, after a pulse label, the amount of material spontaneously released from hamster tracheal cultures (which are enriched in goblet cells) declines with a half-life of about 30 minutes, but the amount of label released by neutrophil elastase is constant for up to 1.5 hours after the pulse (117). Thus, in addition to secretory granules, at least two other pools of secretory material are indicated. One is spontaneously released and turns over rapidly. The other turns over more slowly and is released by neutrophil elastase. Ciliated cells may contribute to the rapidly turning-over pool. Thus, following labeling of ferret tracheal explants with $^{35}SO_4$, autoradiographic silver grains were detected over ciliated and goblet cells of surface epithelium as well as serous and mucous cells of the glands (70,118). On removal of isotope, the grains over the surface epithelium fell by about half over 4 hours. Glands and cartilage showed no apparent loss of label over the same period. Neurotransmitter agents (bethanecol, phenyleph-rine, and isoproterenol) decreased grain density over the gland cells but had no effect on cartilage or epithelium. In cultured dog tracheal cells, the half-life for equilibration of $^{35}SO_4$ with the elastase-releasable surface pool is ~7.5 hours. The half-life for loss of radiation from the pool is ~4.5 hours (118).

Cholinergic and adrenergic nerve fibers have been found in close proxim-ity to goblet cells of surface epithelium (119,120). However, goblet cell dis-charge in humans, cats, cows, and hamsters is usually not affected by either adrenergic or cholinergic agonists (51,78,121–123), although Niles et al. (124) reported a slight inhibition of HMG release from hamster tracheal organ cultures by isoproterenol and a small stimulation (34%) by pilocarpine. By contrast, in rats and guinea pigs, vagal stimulation causes loss of PAS-positive material from goblet cells (69,125). Although substance P is involved in these responses, atropine is inhibitory (116), suggesting a direct effect of acetylcholine on guinea pig goblet cells (69).

Table 3 summarizes the agents known to stimulate mucin secretion from the surface epithelium. In some cases, discharge of goblet cell granules has been demonstrated by microscopic techniques, such as differential interference microscopy in vivo (75,76) or loss of material stained with Alcian blue/PAS (69,126). In many cases, however, mucin release has been measured without any cytological assessment. The material so measured is often assumed to come from goblet cell mucous granules but could represent constitutive secretion (i.e., nongranular) or release of glycocalyx.

ATP is perhaps the most potent direct secretagogue of goblet cells, and it has been shown recently that this agent is released into the airway lumen by mechanical strain (11). Other agents that may act directly to induce goblet cell degranulation in vivo include leukotrienes, prostaglandin $F_{2\alpha}$, substance P, hista-mine, stretch, and extremes of pH. However, in cultured hamster epithelium, histamine, prostaglandins, and leukotrienes had no effect on mucus release (122,127), suggesting that their actions in vivo and on organ cultures may de-pend on the presence of cell types in addition to goblet cells. Depending on species, PAF acts either directly or by release of leukotrienes (59,128). Results from Adler's laboratory (114,129) suggest that NO plays a pivotal role in the signaling pathways by which diverse inflammatory mediators provoke mucus release from guinea pig tracheal epithelium.

Bacterial proteases degranulate goblet cells (130), but human neutrophil elastase does not (131). Instead, the latter acts by digesting away mucins and proteoglycans bound to the cell surface (117,131–134).

Macrolide antibiotics inhibit the goblet cell discharge and neutrophil migration induced by lipopolysaccharide (LPS) in vivo (135); it is unclear whether LPS directly stimulates goblet cell discharge or whether this is caused by the neutrophil migration. Dexamethasone likewise has been shown to inhibit the release of mucins in response to antigen challenge (136).

In summary, goblet cells in humans and most other mammalian species are not under neuronal control, but secrete directly or indirectly in response to a wide variety of luminal irritants. In addition, constitutive secretion and release of glycocalyx may make important contributions to the content of airway mucous secretions.

VII. Regulation of Goblet Cell Secretion by Second Messengers

Elevation of $[Ca^{2+}]_i$ with Ca ionophores does not affect mucin release from hamster goblet cells in tracheal cultures (137,138). Similarly thapsigargin (an agent that releases Ca from intracellular stores) and BAPTA-AM (an agent that prevents increases in $[Ca^{2+}]_i$) had no effects on mucus secretion, nor did they alter the stimulation by ATP (138). However, Ca ionophores do cause granule exocytosis from goblet cells in explants of human and canine tracheal epithelium (139) and mucin secretion by rabbit tracheal explants (140,141).

Surprisingly, there seems to have been only one attempt to test for the effects of elevating intracellular cAMP, in which it was found that a permeable analogue of cAMP did not alter mucin secretion from primary cultures of hamster tracheal epithelium (122). This is consistent with the comparatively few reports of a lack of effect of adrenergic agents and adrenergic nerve stimulation (69,122). Elevation of cAMP with permeable analogues of cAMP, forskolin, or phosphodiesterase inhibitors is without effect on mucus discharge from the rat goblet cell line SPOC-1 (139).

Kim and coworkers suggested that ATP-dependent mucin secretion from cultured hamster goblet cells involves, at least in part, coupling of the ATP receptor to phospholipase C via GTP-binding proteins sensitive to pertussis toxin (PTX) (115). The same group has implicated protein kinase C (PKC) in the stimulation of mucin release by ATP (138). Thus, release was stimulated by phorbol myristate acetate (PMA), an activator of PKC, and this stimulation was partially blocked by inhibitors of the kinase. Furthermore, desensitization of PKC by prolonged exposure to PMA resulted in partial inhibition of ATP-induced mucin release. Similar findings were obtained by others (142). The effects of PAF on mucin release from primary cultures of cat tracheal epithelium may also be mediated by PKC, as suggested by several findings (143). First, the effects of PAF are blocked by inhibitors of PKC. Second, PAF causes trans-

Table 3 Stimulators of Surface Epithelial Mucin Secretion

Agent	Preparation[a]	Granule discharge	Species	Mechanism[b]	Ref.
Tobacco smoke	IV, OC	Y	Rat Guinea pig	Ach and SP from nerves	126,255
SO_2	IV	Y	Dog	pH	256
NH_3	IV	?	Cat	pH	78
Leukotrienes C_4 and D_4	IV, OC	Y	Guinea pig	Direct?	128,257
Lipopolysaccharide (endotoxin)	IV	Y	Guinea pig Rat	Neutrophils	258,259
pH <4 or >9	CC	?	Hamster	Direct	260
Histamine	IV, OC	Y	Guinea pig	Direct and cholinergic reflex	114,261,262
Substance P	IV, OC	Y	Guinea pig	Direct	75,263
$PGF_2\alpha$	OC	?	Guinea pig	Direct?	264
Platelet-activating factor (PAF)	OC, CC	?	Rat Rabbit Human Dog Guinea pig Cat	Direct?, LTs, NO, HETEs	128,194,220,265,266

			Species	Mediator	References
Superoxide and reactive oxygen species	OC, CC	?	Guinea pig Rat	NO, PGF$_2$?, LTs	264,267
ATP	OC, CC	Y	Hamster Dog Human	Direct	76,115,116,122
Hypo-osmolarity	CC	?	Hamster	Stretch	127
Mechanical strain	CC	?	Hamster	ATP?	268
Bacterial proteases	IV, OC, CC	Y	Rabbit Guinea pig Hamster	Direct?	130,269
Human neutrophil elastase	IV, OC, CC	N	Hamster		117,124,131,270
TNF-α	CC, OC	?	Guinea pig Human	NO	114,271,272
Antigen	IV	Y	Guinea pig	Neutrophil elastase	136,273,274

[a]IV = in vivo; OC = Organ culture; CC = cell culture.
[b]ACh = acetylcholine; SP = substance P; LTs = leukotrienes; NO = nitrous oxide; HETE = hydroxyeicosatetranoic acids.

location of PKC from the cytosol to the cell membrane and increases the activity of membrane-bound PKC.

Kim found hamster goblet cells to be unresponsive to cholinergic agents (122). More recently, however, Steel and Hanrahan (137), using the same preparation, found that carbachol increased release of high-molecular-weight glycoconjugates radiolabeled with ^{3}H-N-acetyl-glucosamine by 70%. Their results indicate that this increase in secretion is coupled to a PTX-sensitive G protein and requires activation of a phorbol ester–insensitive isoform of PKC.

SPOC-1 cells are a continuous cell line spontaneously derived from rat tracheal epithelium (100). When grown in xenographs in vivo (a technique in which a trachea is denuded of its own epithelial cells, seeded with SPOC-1 cells, and then transplanted beneath the skin of an immunodeficient nude mouse), the cells contained typical mucous granules, which stain strongly with mucin antibodies (101). SPOC-1 cells resemble canine and human goblet cells (but differ from hamster) in that they secrete mucins in response to Ca ionophore and thapsigargin (139). As for primary hamster cells, mucin secretion from SPOC-1 cells may involve activation of PKC. Thus, they secrete acutely in response to PMA, and prolonged exposure to PMA blunts their responses to ATP and UTP (139). Further studies on SPOC-1 cells permeabilized with streptolysin O showed that mucin secretion was regulated by both Ca^{2+}-insensitive PKC-dependent and Ca^{2+}-dependent PKC-potentiated pathways (144).

VIII. Neural Mediation of Gland Secretion

In the cat, glands receive a dense autonomic innervation. In the region within 10 μm of the glands, there are nine times as many cholinergic varicosities as adrenergic ones (145). Human bronchial glands are also densely innervated, but with approximately equal numbers of adrenergic and cholinergic nerve terminals (146,147). Nerves containing VIP, peptide histidine isoleucine (PHI), substance P, GRP, galanin, and neuropeptide Y have also been discerned in the vicinity of airway glands (2,148,149). Autoradiography and ligand-binding studies have demonstrated muscarinic, α-adrenergic, β-adrenergic, and peptidergic receptors on airway gland cells (1,2,150,151).

In 1896, Kokin reported that stimulation of the vagal nerves of dogs caused gland secretions to appear as drops of secretion on the tracheal surface (152). Kountz and Koenig confirmed this result, and showed in addition that sympathetic stimulation was without effect (153). In anesthetized cats, Florey et al. (51) filled a section of trachea with oil, sealed one end, and attached an open cannula to the other. There was no movement of oil along the cannula under resting conditions. However, stimulation of the vagal nerves caused liquid to move from the trachea into the cannula. After the contribution of smooth-muscle contraction to this movement was eliminated by treatment with atropine (which had no effect on the position of the meniscus under resting conditions), the vagally induced fluid secretion was calculated as ~250 µL/h. Histological analysis showed depletion of glands by vagal stimulation but no change in the numbers or appearance of goblet cells. Forty years later, secretion from individual cat glands was monitored, and two separate groups reported cholinergically mediated increases in gland secretion of ~10 nL/min/gland (53,54). A piece of trachea of the size used by Florey et al. will have a surface area of ~2.5 cm^2. In the cat, there are ~200 gland openings per cm^2 (53). At ~10 nL/gland, the predicted total secretion becomes 288 µL/h, very close to the 250 µL/h measured by Florey et al. In fact, Florey and colleagues' estimate of gland secretion will be an underestimate as surface epithelium absorbs liquid at ~5 µL/cm^2/h (24,154). However, the volume flow across the entire surface epithelium of the tracheal segment (~12.5 µL/h) will be small compared with gland secretion.

Neural regulation of gland secretion in the cat was revisited by Gallagher et al. in 1975 (155). An in vivo tracheal segment was filled with saline, and $^{35}SO_4$ was delivered intravenously or intraluminally. The saline in the tracheal segment was removed every 15 or 30 minutes and replaced with fresh medium. Radiolabeled HMG in the tracheal luminal liquid were determined, and their rate of appearance became constant after about 2 hours. Stimulation of the peripheral cut ends of the vagal nerves at this point increased mucus output by 150%, and this increase was blocked by intravenous atropine. Stimulation of the stellate ganglion (containing the cell bodies of the sympathetic postganglionic nerves to the trachea) increased mucus secretion by 65%, an effect blocked by propranolol, a β-adrenergic blocker, but not by α-adrenergic blockers. Similar results were obtained when the peripheral cut ends of the cervical sympathetic nerves were stimulated. These results suggest that the parasympathetic cholinergic innervation is more potent than the sympathetic adrenergic innervation at stimulating airway gland secretion.

In contrast to their initial result (155), a later study by the same group (156) failed to find a block of vagal stimulation with atropine. Nor did a combination of atropine, phentolamine (an α-adrenergic blocker), and propranolol (a β-adrenergic blocker) significantly affect vagally mediated output of HMG. The authors concluded that a large part of the vagal response was mediated by noncholinergic, nonadrenergic transmitter(s). However, the extreme variability of the control response to vagal stimulation (+14 to +447% for ^{35}S-HMG) would have made it very difficult to detect any significant effects of pharmacological blockade.

Several studies have used electrical field stimulation (EFS) to evoke transmitter release from nerves within the tracheal wall or around isolated glands of ferrets and cats (84,157–160). Involvement of nerves in secretion is indicated by the block of EFS-induced secretions with tetrodotoxin. The resulting gland secretion has been measured as hillocks or as output of radiolabeled glycoconjugates or lysozyme. Experiments with blockers suggest that the increases in mucin secretion induced by EFS are mediated by cholinergic, α- and β-adrenergic nerves. However, in the presence of blockers of all three types of receptor, some EFS-induced mucin secretion remains (84,157,160). Fung et al. (157) have taken this to indicate the presence of nonadrenergic noncholinergic (NANC) nerve terminals in the tracheal wall. These authors rightly point out that the conclusions drawn when using blockers depend on their effectiveness, and justify the blocker concentrations they used by pointing out that they completely block the stimulatory effects of supramaximal doses of cholinergic or adrenergic agents. However, at the more intimate contacts between nerve and gland, transmitter concentrations may reach levels higher than the highest concentration of exogenously added agent. In other words, concentrations of antagonists that successfully block the action of exogenously added agent may not ensure complete block of transmitter released from nerve terminals. Shimura et al. (160) have suggested that the types of nerves activated may depend on the duration of EFS. Thus, the secretory response to 3 minutes or less of EFS was blocked by atropine. However, responses to 30 minutes of EFS were not completely blocked by a combination of atropine, phentolamine, and propranolol. The authors concluded that short stimulations acted via cholinergic nerves, but that NANC nerves became important with longer stimulations. Again, an alternative interpretation of this result is that prolonged EFS causes progressive increases in neurotransmitter concentrations that override the pharmacological blockade.

Baker et al. (159) studied release of HMG into the mucosal medium of sheets of human bronchi mounted between lucite half-chambers. The collection periods were 15 minutes long, and EFS induced a 50% increase in mucin release. The corresponding changes for unstimulated tissues and for stimulated tissues pretreated with atropine were 17% and 18%, respectively. Thus, these results provide evidence for cholinergic innervation of human bronchial glands but not for NANC. However, sheets of ferret trachea used in the same study showed a 365% increase in secretion in response to EFS, calling into question the viability of the human tissues used; no tests of viability are mentioned by the authors.

Using the hillocks technique, there have been several reports of cholinergically mediated reflex stimulation of gland secretion in dogs and piglets (161–168), with the reflexes being initiated by airway stretch receptors, irritant receptors, pulmonary C-fibers, hypoxemic stimulation of the carotid, and gastric irritation. Central control of gland secretion has been demonstrated by studies in which intracisternal application of substance P (169,170) or direct stimulation of the ventral surface of the medulla with nicotine (171) induced the formation of hillocks in dog trachea.

IX. Effects of Cholinergic Agents on Gland Secretion

Cholinergic agents are the most potent releasers of mucins from airway glands of humans and other mammals. On maximal cholinergic activation, stimulated gland flows are ~15 nL/gland/min in all the larger species studied (55). However, individual glands in rodents are much smaller (48), and presumably also have smaller flows. This statement may also apply to the horse, which has tracheal glands only about 1/10 the volume of those in other large mammals (80). Resting gland secretions are <1 nL/gland/min (55), except that basal secretory rates of ~10 nL/gland/min have been reported when secretions have been sampled by placing micropipettes over the gland opening (53,163,172). However, the high basal rates seen in the latter type of study may be an artifact of the "negative pressures needed to initiate flow into the pipette" (53).

In an early study on mucus secretion from human airway glands, rings of human bronchi were maintained in organ culture (71). After 4 hours of incubation with ^{3}H-glucose, the tissues were fixed, sectioned, and analyzed by autoradiography. In control tissues, ~25% of the gland mucous cells were secreting radiolabeled material into the gland lumen. This fraction was increased by methacholine in a dose-dependent fashion such that with 100 µg/mL of acetylcholine ~70% of the cells were secreting. Atropine reduced the number of basally secreting cells by ~45% and blocked the effects of acetylcholine. Shelhamer et al. (173) collected radiolabeled macromolecular secretions from explants of human bronchi over a 4-hour period. Compared to control, untreated explants, those incubated with methacholine showed a 60% increase in the rate of secretion, an increase that was completely blocked by atropine. However, as discussed earlier, the very long collection periods used in this study may have resulted in much smaller values for methacholine-induced secretion than the true maximum. Cholinergic stimulation of mucin release from explants of human bronchus has also been demonstrated using ELISA (62).

Regulation of gland mucous secretion has been studied most thoroughly in the cat, in which cholinergic agents have been shown to increase total tracheal volume secretion (51), secretion from individual glands (53,54,172), output of radiolabeled HMG (88,155), and vacuolization of serous cells (74). In isolated cat glands, Shimura et al. (88) found the $K_{0.5}$ for secretion of radiolabeled ^{3}H-HMG by methacholine to be ~2×10^{-7} M, and maximal rates of secretion to be ~250% greater than baseline. Shimura et al. (86) have also indicated that cholinergically induced contraction of myoepithelial cells may be important in stimulation of gland volume secretion. Cholinergic effects on glands are mediated predominantly by M3 receptors (174–176).

The ferret is another heavily studied species in which cholinergic agents cause increases in total tracheal secretion (177), fluid secretion from individual glands (158), release of HMG (84), lysozyme secretion (177,178), degranulation of mucous cells (68), and degranulation and vacuolization of serous cells (73).

Evidence for stimulation of gland secretion by cholinergic agents also exists for tracheas from dog (57,179,180), pig (60,61,81,165,175), cow (123), and sheep (181). In the dog, Marin et al. (57) found that acetylcholine increased net flows of Na and Cl toward the lumen by $\sim$1.5 μEq/cm^2/h. If this represents secretion of isotonic NaCl solution by the glands, then it corresponds to 10 μL/cm^2/h.

X. Effects of Adrenergic Agents on Gland Secretion

Airway glands contain α_1-, α_2-, β_1-, and β_2-adrenergic receptors (85,182,183). In human glands, β_2 receptors are 10 times as frequent as β_1 (183).

Quantitative estimates of adrenergically mediated gland secretion are summarized in Table 4. In the cat, α-adrenergic agents stimulate volume flows to

Table 4 Comparison of α- and β-Andrenergic Responses

Species	Method	% Cholinergic response			
		α	β	$\beta + \alpha$	Ref.
Human	Granule discharge	0	0		71
	^{35}S-HMG			80	185
	^{3}H-HMG	79	0	0	173
	"Beads" of gland secretion	5			55
Dog	3H-HMG	0	0		179
Pig	"Beads"	7			55
Sheep	"Beads"	5	9		55
Cat	Micropipette	128			53
	Micropipette	55	42	76	172
	Micropipette	65	5	8	54
	"Beads"	100			55
	^{3}H-HMG			29	85
	Serious cell vacuolization	$\sim$100	$\sim$50	$\sim$50	74
	^{35}S-HMG			30	185
	^{3}H and ^{35}S-HMG			60–79	156
Ferret	^{35}S-HMG	42	22	52	84
	^{35}S-HMG	120	70	58	68
	Mucous cell volume	0	61		68
	Lysozyme release	31	13	42	178
	Lysozyme release	56	0	0	177
	Total volume of secretions	22	11	50	177
	Serous granule discharge	85	23 (ns)	27	73

approximately the same degree as cholinergic agents. Thus, it is to be expected that they also cause serous cell granule discharge and vacuolization (74). However, they have little effect on mucous cell ultrastructure. The selective stimulation of liquid-secreting elements explains the finding that cat gland secretions induced by α-adrenergic stimulation have lower viscosity than cholinergically induced secretions (172). Surprisingly, given the apparent absence of mucous granule discharge, α- adrenergic agents are quite potent at increasing the output of radiolabeled HMG. Perhaps these HMG are proteoglycans derived from serous cells, and contribute less to the viscosity of mucous secretions than mucins. α-adrenergic agents have little action on gland secretions in species other than the cat (55).

In several species, β-adrenergic agents induce lower volumes of secretions than either cholinergic or α-adrenergic agents (Table 4), and similar nonquantitative findings have also been described for the rat (184). These agents cause mucous cell degranulation and release of radiolabeled HMG, but have little effect on the ultrastructure of serous cells. The mucous secretions are therefore presumably low in water and high in mucus (i.e., comparatively concentrated), consistent with the finding in the cat that β-adrenergic agents induce higher viscosity gland secretions than either cholinergic or α-adrenergic agents (172).

Isoproterenol has generally been used as the β-adrenoreceptor agonist in studies of mucus secretion. However, release of ^{35}S-HMG from human bronchial explants is stimulated with equal effectiveness by specific β_1- and β_2-agonists (185). The endogenous mixed β- and α-agonists epinephrine and norepinephrine are also effective secretagogues, being generally about as effective as pure α- or β-agonists (i.e., less effective than cholinergic agents) (85,186). In one case, however, norepinephrine was twice as effective as acetylcholine and five to eight times as effective as pure α- or β-agonists (84).

The selectivity of α-adrenergic agents for serous cells and of β-adrenergic agents for mucous cells is reflected in the distribution of adrenergic receptors in the cat trachea, with β-adrenergic receptors being more numerous on mucous cells and α-receptors on serous cells (182).

α_2-adrenergic agents inhibit stimulation of mucus secretion by β-adrenergic agents (85). This effect has been described in other systems, and may be due to inhibition of membrane-bound adenylate cyclase (187). The α-adrenergic agent phenylephrine increased the fluxes of radioactive Na and Cl toward the lumen of cat tracheal sheets by ~5.5 μEq cm^{2}h, equivalent to a secretion of isotonic NaCl solution of 37 μL/cm^2/h (188).

XI. Regulation of Gland Secretion by NANC Agents

Substance P, neurokinin A (NKA), NKB, neuropeptide Y (NPY), calcitonin gene–related peptide (CGRP), and gastrin-releasing peptide (GRP) have all been identified in airway sensory nerve terminals (1) and stimulate mucus release following their release by axon reflexes (189,190). Neurokinin and VIP receptors have been found on airway glands (191,192). A large number of lipid mediators released from both leukocytes (1) and epithelial cells (193) are also known to stimulate mucus secretion. These and the other NANC agents that have been demonstrated to increase mucus secretion are summarized in Table 5. It is important to remember that all the studies on human airways, and many of those on experimental animals, were done by measuring release of radiolabeled HMG from explant cultures. In most such cases the exact source of the

Table 5 NANC Gland Secretagogues

Agent	Species	Ref.
Platelet-activating factor (PAF)	Ferret, cat, human	77,128,195–197
Prostaglandins	Human, ferret	198,199,212,227,275
Arachadonic acid	Human	198
HETE	Dog, human	198,276
Substance P	Cat, ferret, dog	68,89,200,206,277–279
Prostaglandin-generating factor of anaphylaxis	Human	201
LTC$_4$ and LTD$_4$	Dog, cat, human	280–283
VIP	Cat, ferret	72,88,284
Histamine	Ferret, human	173,203
Pseudomonas proteases/rhamnolipids/ alginate	Human, cat, ferret	285,286,287
Neutrophil elastase	Human, dog, ferret	288,212
Bradykinin	Cat, human, ferret	87,207
Endothelin	Cat, ferret	202,289
ECP (eosinophil cationic protein)	Cat, human	222
Kallidin	Dog	206
Physaelleimin	Dog	206
CGRP (calcitonin gene–related peptide)	Cat	230
GRP (gastrin-releasing peptide)	Cat	290
PHI/NKY	Ferret	291
ATP	Cat, ferret	208,212
NO	Cat, human	87
Endorphins	Cat	292
Ozone	Sheep	293
Monocyte/macrophage mucous secretagogue	Human	209,210
Complement component C3a	Human	294
Antigen	Sheep, human	173,211
Cold and hypertonicity	Pig, cat	215,216

secretions has not been determined, although it is generally assumed to be glands based on the difference in total volume between glands and surface goblet cells.

Pharmacological studies indicate that in tracheal explants, PAF acts by releasing leukotrienes (LTs) (194–196). In isolated cat glands (197), PAF requires platelets to have an effect, indicating that the LTs mediating PAF's effects in explants come from a cell source other than mucous glands. Prostaglandin $F_{1\alpha}$, PGE_1, thromboxane B_2, and PGI_2 all had no effect on release of radiolabeled HMG from human bronchial explants (198). In one study on human tracheal explants, PGE_2 was inhibitory (198); in another it had no effect (199). Substance P apparently acts via release of LTs (200), as may also the prostaglandin-generating factor of anaphylaxis (201) and endothelin (202). In addition to its stimulatory actions, VIP modulates the effects of autonomic agents. In ferret trachea, Webber and Widdicombe found that VIP increased the release of lysozyme in response to phenylephrine but not in response to methacholine (203). By contrast, in isolated cat glands, VIP augments cholinergically induced glycoconjugate secretion (88). Coles et al. (204) reported that VIP inhibits the release of acid-precipitable HMG and lysozyme from explants of human bronchial mucosa. CGRP is another agent that modulates the effects of secretagogues (205). Bradykinin has been reported to have no effect on mucin secretion from dog trachea or feline tracheal explants (206,207) and comparatively small effects on ferret and human tracheal sheets. However, more recently, Nagaki et al. (87) reported that it induces mucus release from isolated human and cat tracheal glands by a mechanism that involves release of NO. Adenosine does not affect mucus output from isolated feline gland, but ATP does (208). This indicates that the purinergic receptors in glands are the P_2 rather than the P_1 subtype. Monocyte and macrophage mucous secretagogues are 2-kDa peptides released from monocytes and macrophages that induce release of radiolabeled HMG from human tracheal explants (209,210). The effect of antigen on mucus release seems to be mediated largely by histamine released from mast cells (173,211). Human neutrophil elastase is a potent stimulator of gland secretion (212).

Excess airway mucus is a feature of patients dying in status asthmaticus (213), and levels of mucus in airway secretions correlate with the severity of this disease (214). The role of mucin secretion in the form of asthma triggered by breathing cold, dry air during exercise has been investigated using animal models. Breathing dry air should concentrate airway surface liquid by evaporation. Accordingly, Peatfield et al. (215) tested hyperosmolar solution instilled into the tracheal lumen of the cat and found that it increased the output of radiolabeled HMG. Passage of ambient air warmed to body temperature was also stimulatory unless it had previously been saturated with water vapor at that temperature. Instillation of cold saline had no effect. Increased osmolarity stimulated mucin secretion from isolated pig gland cells (216). In addition, there was a marked increase in mucin release on restoring the cells to isotonic medium. Decreasing the temperature of the incubating solution from 37 to 32°C increased baseline secretion threefold.

Dexamethasone (217–219) and erythromycin (220) inhibit baseline gland secretion and its stimulation by other agents. Ramnarine et al. (221) found that inhibitors of NO synthase markedly increased mucus release from ferret trachea in vitro. Thus, in contrast to the stimulatory effects of NO on feline glands (87) and on goblet cells (114), they concluded that NO derived from constitutive NO synthase acts as an endogenous inhibitor of mucous secretion in the ferret. Major basic protein of eosinophils inhibits release of HMG from explants of human and feline trachea (222).

XII. Regulation of Gland Mucus Secretion by Second Messengers

There is evidence that mucin secretion by gland mucous cells can be regulated by both cAMP- and Ca-dependent pathways.

Whimster and Reid determined that both addition of cAMP and inhibition of phosphodiesterase with theophylline increased release of radiolabeled macromolecules from organ cultures of human bronchus (223). Later, Liedtke et al. (186) showed that β-adrenergic agents stimulate secretion of radiolabeled HMG from strips of cat tracheal wall while elevating intracellular cAMP. Permeable analogues of cAMP and block of phosphodiesterase both caused mucin release. Finally, 8-N_3-[^{32}P]cAMP bound to proteins of the correct electrophoretic mobility to be type I and type II cAMP-dependent protein kinase, and this binding was inhibited by adrenergic agents. Furthermore, permeable analogues of cAMP stimulate glycoprotein secretion from cat submucosal glands (90), and immunocytochemistry has shown that prostaglandins, β-adrenergic agents, and VIP all increase cAMP in gland cells (224,225). In isolated cat glands glycoprotein secretion is stimulated by dibutyryl-cAMP (90), although, surprisingly, β-adrenergic stimulation is without effect (63). In general, however, the evidence suggests that β-adrenergic modulation of mucus is effected by cAMP and involves the activation of cAMP-dependent protein kinase.

Influx of calcium and release of calcium from intracellular stores are both involved in the stimulation of mucus secretion by cholinergic and other agents. An early study (226) found that extracellular Ca was required for methacholine-induced secretion of mucus from dog tracheal organ cultures. Also in dog, verapamil (a Ca-channel blocker) failed to influence the secretory response to cholinergic agents, but TMB-8 (a blocker of Ca release from the endoplasmic reticulum) was inhibitory (227). Removal of Ca from the bathing medium inhibits the secretory response of isolated cat tracheal glands to methacholine (88). Ishihara et al. (228) showed that the secretagogues, methacholine, phenylephrine, and substance P all increased $[Ca^{2+}]_i$ in cat glands, but that isoproterenol and VIP did not. ATP, CGRP, endothelin, bradykinin, and tachykinins also increase gland $[Ca^{2+}]_i$ (202,208,229,230). The methacholine-induced increase in $[Ca^{2+}]_i$ seems to involve M3 receptors (174) and is abolished by monoclonal antibodies to the IP_3 receptor (231). Involvement of IP_3 in the mediator-induced increases in $[Ca^{2+}]_i$ is also suggested by the finding that the same secretagogues that increase $[Ca^{2+}]_i$ also increase intracellular levels of IP_3 (82). The change in $[Ca^{2+}]_i$ in response to methacholine is biphasic, with a large transient 10-fold increase followed by a smaller sustained increase. The former may reflect release from stores, the latter influx from the outside (228).

There is cross-talk between the Ca- and cAMP-dependent pathways. Thus, Shimura et al. (160) have shown that isoproterenol enhances ATP-induced mucus secretion and whole-cell Cl currents in cat tracheal explants. In human airway explants, Shelhamer et al. (173) have reported that α-adrenergic and cholinergic stimulation both increase cGMP levels and that 8-bromo-cGMP increases mucin secretion.

XIII. Gland Water Secretion

Gland water secretion is presumably coordinated in some way with mucus secretion, as secretion of both is necessary for effective mucociliary clearance. However, the two processes occur in different cell types, with distal serous cells providing the liquid that flushes out the mucous secreted by the proximal mucous cells.

Liquid secretion by glands is secondary to active secretion of Cl by serous gland cells (43). Sodium follows (between the cells) by electrical attraction, and water flows down the resulting transepithelial osmotic gradient. In cystic fibrosis, lack of functional CFTR, a cAMP-activated Cl channel, in the apical membrane of serous gland cells (232) leads to failure of gland water secretion (15), and the secretions, which are now presumably abnormally concentrated, accumulate within the glands, markedly dilating their lumens (233). Animal experiments suggest that the reduction in mucociliary transport seen in cystic fibrosis (234) almost certainly reflects changes in the rheology of gland mucus secretions. Thus, when pig tracheas were treated with Cl transport inhibitors, plugging of duct lumens occurred (235). Furthermore, with Cl transport inhibited, the mucus secreted was threefold more concentrated in solids and of greater rigidity (236), changes that would be expected to inhibit mucociliary clearance.

Active secretion of Cl is effected as follows (237,238). Net movement of Cl into the cells across the basolateral membrane is via a NaK_2Cl cotransporter.

The K that enters by cotransport with Cl (and Na) recycles to the basolateral medium via K channels. Intracellular Na concentration is kept low by the NaK-ATPase, which is found exclusively on the basolateral membrane. Net Cl exit across the apical membrane is down an electrochemical gradient via Cl channels. One of these Cl channels is CFTR, and serous gland cells have much higher levels of CFTR than any other airway cell type (232). Calcium-activated Cl channels are also present (181,231,239), and may be activated directly by Ca without the involvement of protein kinases (240).

Sustained increases in Cl secretion require increases in the turnover of Cl channels in the apical membrane and the NaK-ATPase, NaK_2Cl cotransporter and K channels in the basolateral. The NaK-ATPase is probably not directly regulated by second messengers but responds to changes in $[Na]_i$. However, CFTR, basolateral K channels, and NaK_2Cl cotransport are all stimulated by cAMP via activation of protein kinase A (238). Likewise, calcium activates Cl and K channels and the cotransporter (238). Serous cells contain IP_3 receptors in their apical poles (231), and in response to methacholine, Ca rises first in the apical region before diffusing to the basolateral. Thus, Cl currents increase before basolateral K currents (231). However, Ca-activated Cl channels are not necessary for Ca to increase Cl secretion; activation of basolateral K channels will hyperpolarize the cell and increase the driving force for Cl movement through CFTR.

Mucous cells probably do not secrete much liquid. They do not have detectable levels of CFTR (232), and in culture a shift toward a mucous phenotype is associated with a marked decline in Cl secretion (110).

XIV. Secretion by Gland Cell Cultures

A bovine cell line has been derived from primary cultures of gland acini, which have many features of serous cells. The cells are homogeneous, contain electron-dense granules, neutral and acidic polysaccharides, stain with antibodies specific for serous cells, and release HMG (predominantly chondroitin sulfate) in response to β-adrenergic and other agents (44,105,241). The dose-response relationships for stimulation of mucin secretion and elevation of cAMP by isoproterenol are essentially superimposable in these cells (242). Furthermore, permeable analogues of cAMP mimicked the response to isoproterenol, increased the activity of cAMP-activated protein kinase, and markedly increased phosphorylation of proteins in the soluble fraction (242). However, perhaps the most potent stimulators of secretion from these cells are neutrophil elastase and cathepsin G (a related protease from mast cells) (106). Surprisingly, the secretion induced by these agents does not involve any of the classical second messengers (243). By contrast, in the same cells, cAMP, cAMP-dependent protein kinase, protein kinase C, and $[Ca^{2+}]_i$ have been implicated in the response to histamine, whereas bradykinin apparently acts via IP_3, PKC, and $[Ca^{2+}]_i$ (243,244).

In direct contrast to the above results, other workers have found that neutrophil elastase promotes rapid exocytosis from primary cultures of human airway gland cells by producing oscillations in cytosolic $[Ca^{2+}]_i$ (245). These cultures did not show exocytosis in response to ATP (a secretagogue of isolated feline glands), and may most closely resemble serous cells of the native gland (208). The same group has reported similar results with the human tracheal gland cell line MM39 (246).

Merten and Figarella (247) have reported that acetylcholine stimulates and norepinephrine inhibits mucin secretion of bronchial inhibitor (BrI) from primary cultures of human airway glands. These secretagogue-mediated effects were blunted in cells from patients with cystic fibrosis, but basal levels of secretion for BrI, lysozyme, and lactoferrin were all elevated 10–50 times in cystic fibrosis.

XV. Conclusions

The airways of healthy adults breathing clean humid air may be virtually free of mucous secretions (248). However, in response to environmental insults, the airway wall defends itself by producing a mucous blanket. This can happen very rapidly. Stimulation of gland secretion in bovine trachea, for instance, increases the depth of airway surface liquid from 20 to 75 μm within 2 minutes (123). There are several mucin genes in airway cells (7) and at least four sources of mucins: glands, goblet cells, glycocalyx, and constitutive secretion by the surface epithelium. The secretory response to insult thus has the potential for fine regulation. It is known, for instance, that the rheology of gland secretions varies quite markedly between secretagogues (172). However, although attempts are being made to study the interaction of the individual components of mucociliary transport (30,249–252), the precise role that the different sources of mucus and water play in the overall system is as yet little understood. But at the most basic level, it is clear that the exact water content of mucous secretions is critical. All the diseases characterized by accumulation of airway mucous secretion—bronchitis, asthma, and cystic fibrosis—have one thing in common: the ratio of mucus-secreting to water-secreting cells increases. In cystic fibrosis, secretion of water by serous cells in bronchioles and tracheobronchial glands is greatly reduced by the absence of functional CFTR in the apical cell membranes. In all three diseases there is an increase in the numbers of goblet cells in the surface epithelium (36) and a conversion of serous cells to mucous cells may occur in the glands (253,254). Thus, development of therapies for disorders of mucus clearance will be aided by an understanding not only of mucus secretion by airway epithelium but also of ion and water transport.

References

1. Johnson CW, Larivee P, Shelhamer JH. Epithelial cells: regulation of mucus secretion. In: Busse WW, Holgate SH, eds. Asthma and Rhinitis. Oxford: Blackwell Scientific Publications, 1995:584–598.
2. Finkbeiner WE, Widdicombe JH. Control of nasal airway secretions, ion transport, and water movement. In: Parent RA, ed. Treatise on Pulmonary Toxicology. Vol. 1. Comparative Biology of the Normal Lung. Boca Raton, FL: CRC Press, 1992:633–657.
3. Plopper CG, Hyde DM, Buckpitt AR. Clara cells. In: Crystal RG, West JB, Weibel E, Barnes PJ, eds. The Lung: Scientific Foundations. Philadelphia: Lippincott-Raven, 1997:517–534.
4. Rose MC. Mucins: structure, function, and role in pulmonary diseases. Am J Physiol 1992; 263:L413–L429.
5. Sleigh MA, Blake JR, Liron N. The propulsion of mucus by cilia. Am Rev Respir Dis 1988; 137:726–741.
6. Yeates DB, Besseris GJ, Wong LB. Physicochemical properties of mucus and its propulsion. In: Crystal RG, West JB, Weibel ER, Barnes PJ, eds. The Lung: Scientific Foundations. Philadelphia: Lipinott-Raven, 1997:487–503.
7. Rose MC, Nickola TJ, Voynow JA. Airway mucus obstruction: mucin glycoproteins, MUC gene regulation and goblet cell hyperplasia. Am J Respir Cell Mol Biol 2001; 25:533–537.
8. Reid C, Gould S, Harris A. Developmental expression of mucin genes in the human respiratory tract. Am J Respir Cell Mol Biol 1997; 20:592–598.
9. Chen Y-C, Zhao YH, Di Y-P, Wu R. Characterization of human mucin 5B expression in airway epithelium and the genomic clones of the amino-terminal and 5′-flanking region. Am J Respir Cell Mol Biol 2001; 25:538–541.
10. Boat TF, Cheng P-W, Leigh MW. Biochemistry of mucus. In: Takishima T, Shimura S, eds. Airway Secretion. New York: Marcel Dekker, 1994:217–282.
11. Grygorczyk R, Hanrahan JW. CFTR-independent ATP release from epithelial cells triggered by mechanical stimuli. Am J Physiol 1997; 272:C1058–C1066.
12. Braga PC, Allegra L, eds. Methods in Bronchial Mucology. New York: Raven Press, 1988.
13. Persson CG, Erjefalt JS, Greiff L, Andersson M, Erjefahlt I, Godfrey RW, Korsgren M, Linden M, Sundler F, Svensson C. Plasma-derived proteins in airway defence, disease and repair of epithelial injury. Eur J Respir Dis 1998; 11:958–970.
14. Lusuardi M, Donner CF. Macromolecule and ion identification: glycoproteins. In: Braga PC, Allegra L, eds. Methods in Bronchial Mucology. New York: Raven Press, 1988.
15. Jiang C, Finkbeiner WE, Widdicombe JH, Miller SS. Fluid transport across cultures of human tracheal glands is altered in cystic fibrosis. J Physiol 1997; 501:637–648.
16. Folkesson HG, Matthay MA, Frigeri A, Verkman AS. Transepithelial water permeability in microperfused distal airways: evidence for channel-mediated water transport. J Clin Invest 1996; 97:664–671.

17. Matsui H, Davis CW, Tarran R, Boucher RC. Osmotic water permeabilities of cultured, well-differentiated normal and cystic fibrosis airway epithelia. J Clin Invest 2000; 105:1419–1427.
18. Persson BE, Spring KR. Gallbladder epithelial cell hydraulic water permeability and volume regulation. J Gen Physiol 1982; 79:481–505.
19. Diamond JM. Osmotic water flow in leaky epithelia. J Membr Biol 1979; 51: 195–216.
20. van Os CH, Wiedner G, Wright EM. Volume flows across gallbladder epithelium induced by small hydrostatic and osmotic gradients. J Membrane Biol 1979; 49: 1–20.
21. Azizi F, Matsumoto PS, Wu DX-Y, Widdicombe JH. Effects of hydrostatic pressure on permeability of airway epithelium. Exp Lung Res 1997; 23:257–267.
22. Kondo M, Finkbeiner WE, Widdicombe JH. Changes in permeability of dog tracheal epithelium in response to hydrostatic pressure. Am J Physiol 1992; 262: L176–L182.
23. Serikov VB, Jang YJ, Widdicombe JH. An estimate of the subepithelial pressure that drives inflammatory transudate into the airway lumen. J Appl Physiol 2002; 92:1702–1708.
24. Jiang C, Finkbeiner WE, Widdicombe JH, McCray PB, Miller SS. Altered fluid transport across airway epithelium in cystic fibrosis. Science 1993; 262:424–427.
25. Knowles MR, Murray GF, Shallal JA, Askin F, Ranga V, Gatzy JT, Boucher RC. Bioelectric properties and ion flow across excised human bronchi. J Appl Physiol 1984; 56:868–877.
26. Tam PY, Verdugo P. Control of mucus hydration as a Donnan equilibrium process. Nature 1981; 292:340–342.
27. Yamaya M, Finkbeiner WE, Widdicombe JH. Altered ion transport by tracheal glands in cystic fibrosis. Am J Physiol 1991; 261:L491–L494.
28. Boucher RC, Stutts MJ, Knowles MR, Cantley L, Gatzy JT. Na transport in cystic fibrosis respiratory epithelia: abnormal basal rate and response to adenylate cyclase activation. J Clin Invest 1986; 78:1245–1252.
29. Jayaraman S, Joo NS, Reitz B, Wine JJ, Verkman AS. Submucosal gland secretions in airways from cystic fibrosis patients have normal [Na(+)] and pH but elevated viscosity. Proc Natl Acad Sci USA 2001; 98:8119–813.
30. Matsui H, Grubb BR, Tarran R, Randell SH, Gatzy JT, Davis CW, Boucher RC. Evidence for periciliary liquid layer depletion, not abnormal ion composition, in the pathogenesis of cystic fibrosis airways disease. Cell 1998; 95:1005–1015.
31. Middleton PG, Geddes DM, Alton EW. Effect of amiloride and saline on nasal mucociliary clearance and potential difference in cystic fibrosis and normal subjects. Thorax 1993; 48:812–816.
32. Rhodin JAG. Ultrastructure and function of the human tracheal mucosa. Am Rev Respir Dis 1966; 93:1–15.
33. Rogers AV, Dewar A, Corrin B, Jeffery PK. Identification of serous-like cells in the surface epithelium of human bronchioles. Eur Resp J 1993; 6:498–504.
34. Boers JE, Ambergen AW, Thunnissen FB. Number and proliferation of Clara cells in normal human airway epithelium. Am J Respir Crit Care Med 1999; 159: 1585–1591.

35. Basbaum CB, Jany B, Finkbeiner WE. The serous cell. Annu Rev Physiol 1990; 52:97–113.
36. Rogers DF. Airway goblet cells: responsive and adaptable front-line defenders. Eur Respir J 1994; 7:1690–1706.
37. Tos M. Development of the tracheal glands in man: number, density, structure, shape, and distribution of mucous glands elucidated by quantitative studies of whole mounts of the tracheal glands in man. Acta Pathol Microbiol Scand 1966; 68(suppl 185): 1–130.
38. Meyrick B, Sturgess JM, Reid L. A reconstruction of the duct system and secretory tubules of the human bronchial submucosal gland. Thorax 1969; 24:729–736.
39. Reid L. Measurement of the bronchial mucous gland layer: a diagnostic yardstick in chronic bronchitis. Thorax 1960; 15:132–141.
40. Choi HK, Finkbeiner WE, Widdicombe JH. A comparative study of mammalian tracheal mucous glands. J Anat 2000; 197:361–372.
41. Whimster WF. Number and mean volume of individual submucous glands in the human tracheobronchial tree. Appl Pathol 1986; 4:24–32.
42. Meyrick B, Reid L. Ultrastucture of cells in human bronchial submucosal glands. J Anat 1970; 107:291–299.
43. Widdicombe JH, Shen B-Q, Finkbeiner WE. Structure and function of human airway mucous glands in health and disease. Adv Struct Biol 1994; 3:225–241.
44. Paul A, Picard J, Mergey M, Veissiere D, Finkbeiner WE, Basbaum CB. Glycoconjugates secreted by bovine tracheal serous cells in culture. Arch. Biochem Biophys 1988; 260:75–84.
45. Baraniuk JN, Shizari T, Sabol M, Ali M, Underhill CB. Hyaluronan is exocytosed from serous, but not mucous cells, of human nasal and tracheobronchial submucosal glands. J Invest Med 1996; 44:47–52.
46. Sharma P, Dudus L, Nielsen PA, Clausen H, Yankaskas JR, Hollingsworth MA, Engelhardt JF. MUC5B and MUC7 are differentially expressed in mucous and serous cells of submucosal glands in human bronchial airways. Am J Respir Cell Mol Biol 1998; 19:30–37.
47. Buisine MP, Devisme L, Copin MC, Durand-Reville M, Gosselin B, Aubert JP, Porchet N. Developmental mucin gene expression in the human respiratory tract. Am J Respir Cell Mol Biol 1999; 20:209–218.
48. Widdicombe JH, Chen LL-K, Sporer H, Choi HK, Pecson IS, Bastacky SJ. Distribution of tracheal and laryngeal mucous glands in some rodents and the rabbit. J Anat 2001; 198:207–221.
49. Jeffery PK, Reid L. New observations of rat airway epithelium: a quantitative light and electron microscopic study. J Anat 1975; 120:295–320.
50. Pack RJ, Al-Ugaily LH, Morris G. The cells of the tracheobronchial epithelium of the mouse: a quantitative light and electron microscopic study. J Anat 1981; 132:71–84.
51. Florey H, Carleton HM, Wells AQ. Mucus secretion in the trachea. Br J Exp Pathol 1932; 13:269–284.
52. Kyle H, Robinson NP, Widdicombe JG. Mucus secretion by tracheas of ferret and dog. Eur J Respir Dis 1987; 70:14–22.

53. Ueki I, German VF, Nadel J. Micropipette measurement of airway submucosal gland secretion: autonomic effects. Am Rev Respir Dis 1980; 121:351–357.

54. Quinton PM. Composition and control of secretions from tracheal bronchial submucosal glands. Nature 1979; 279:551–552.

55. Joo NS, Wu JV, Krouse ME, Saenz Y, Wine JJ. Optical method for quantifying rates of mucus secretion from single submucosal glands. Am J Physiol 2001; 281: L458–L468.

56. Davis B, Marin M, Fischer S, Graf P, Widdicombe J, Nadel JA. New method for study of canine mucous gland secretion *in vivo*: cholinergic regulation. Am Rev Respir Dis 1976; 113:257a.

57. Marin MG, Davis B, Nadel JA. Effect of acetylcholine on Cl⁻ and Na⁻ fluxes across dog tracheal epithelium in vitro. Am J Physiol 1976; 231:1546–1549.

58. Cheng P-W, Serman JM, Boat TF, Bruce M. Quantitation of radiolabeled mucous glycoproteins secreted by tracheal explants. Anal Biochem 1981; 117:301–306.

59. Kim KC. Epithelial cell goblet secretion. In: Takishima T, Shimura S, eds. Airway Secretion. New York: Marcel Dekker, 1994:433–450.

60. Dwyer TM, Szebeni A, Diveki K, Farley JM. Transient cholinergic glycoconjugate secretion from swine tracheal submucosal gland cells. Am J Physiol 1992; 262:L418–L426.

61. Inglis SK, Corboz MR, Taylor AE, Ballard ST. In situ visualization of bronchial submucosal glands and their secretory response to acetylcholine. Am J Physiol 1997; 272:L203–L210.

62. Logun C, Mullol J, Rieves D, Hoffman A, Johnson C, Miller R, Goff J, Kaliner M, Shelhamer J. Use of a monoclonal antibody enzyme-linked immunosorbent assay to measure human respiratory glycoprotein production in vitro. Am J Respir Cell Mol Biol 1991; 5:71–79.

63. Lin H, Carlson DM, St. George JA, Plopper CG, Wu R. An ELISA method for the quantitation of tracheal mucins from human and nonhuman primates. Am J Respir Cell Mol Biol 1989; 1:41–48.

64. Steiger D, Fahy J, Boushey H, Finkbeiner WE, Basbaum C. Use of mucin antibodies and cDNA probes to quantify hypersecretion in vivo in human airways. Am J Respir Cell Mol Biol 1994; 10:538–545.

65. Hall RL, Miller RJ, Peatfield AC, Richardson PS, Williams I, Lampert I. A colorimetric assay for mucous glycoproteins using Alcian Blue. Biochem Soc Trans 1980; 8:72.

66. Bowes D, Clark AE, Corrin B. Ultrastructural localization of lactoferrin and glycoprotein in human bronchial glands. Thorax 1981; 36:108–115.

67. Bowes D, Corrin B. Ultrastructural immunocytochemical localization of lysozyme in human bronchial glands. Thorax 1977; 32:163–170.

68. Gashi AA, Nadel JA, Basbaum CB. Tracheal gland mucous cells stimulated *in vitro* with adrenergic and cholinergic drugs. Tissue Cell Res 1989; 21:59–67.

69. Tokuyama K, Kuo HP, Rohde JA, Barnes PJ, Rogers DF. Neural control of goblet cell secretion in guinea pig airways. Am J Physiol 1990; 259:L108–L115.

70. Gashi AA, Nadel JA, Basbaum CB. Autoradiographic studies of the distribution of ³⁵sulfate label in ferret trachea: effects of stimulation. Ex Lung Res 1987; 12: 83–96.

71. Sturgess J, Reid L. An organ culture study of the effect of drugs on the secretory activity of the human submucosal gland. Clin Sci 1972; 43:533–543.

72. Gashi AA, Borson DB, Finkbeiner WE, Nadel JA, Basbaum CB. Neuropeptides degranulate serous cells of ferret tracheal glands. Am J Physiol 1986; 251:C223–C229.

73. Basbaum CB, Ueki I, Brezina L, Nadel JA. Tracheal submucosal gland serous cells stimulated in vitro with adrenergic and cholinergic agonists: a morphometric study. Cell Tissue Res 1981; 220:481–498.

74. Quinton P. Possible mechanisms of stimulus-induced vacuolation in serous cells of tracheal secretory glands. Am J Physiol 1981; 241:C25–C32.

75. Kamijo A, Terekawa S, Hisamatsu K. Neurotransmitter-induced exocytosis in goblet and acinar cells of rat nasal mucosa studied by video microscopy. Am J Physiol 1993; 265:L200–L209.

76. Davis C, Dowell M, Lethem M, Van Scott M. Goblet cell degranulation in isolated tracheal epithelium: response to exogenous ATP, ADP, and adenosine. Am J Physiol 1993; 262:C1313–C1323.

77. Hahn HL, Purnama I, Lang M, Sannwald U. Effects of platelet activating factor on tracheal mucous secretion, on airway mechanics and on circulating blood cells in live ferrets. Eur J Appl Pathol Dis 1986; 69:277–284.

78. Gallagher JT, Hall RL, Phipps RJ, Jeffery PK, Kent PW, Richardson PS. Mucus-glycoproteins (mucins) of the cat trachea: characterisation and control of secretion. Biochim Biophys Acta 1986; 886:243–254.

79. Wardell JR, Chakrin LW, Payne BJ. The canine tracheal pouch: a model for use in respiratory mucus research. Am Rev Respir Dis 1970; 101:741–754.

80. Widdicombe JH, Pecson IS. Distribution and numbers of mucous glands in the horse trachea. Eq Vet Res. 2002; 34:630–633.

81. Hartmann JF, Hutchison CF, Jewell ME. Pig bronchial mucous membrane: a model system for assessing respiratory mucus release in vitro. Exp Lung Res 1984; 6:59–70.

82. Hall IP. Agonist-induced inositol response in bovine airway submucosal glands. Am J Physiol 1992; 262:L257–L262.

83. Tandler B, Sherman J, Boat TF. EDTA-mediated separation of cat tracheal lining epithelium. Am Rev Respir Dis 1981; 124:469–475.

84. Borson DB, Charlin M, Gold BD, Nadel JA. Neural regulation of $^{35}SO_4$ macromolecule secretion from tracheal glands of ferrets. J Appl Physiol 1984; 57:457–466.

85. Culp DJ, McBride RK, Graham LA, Marin MG. Alpha-adrenergic regulation of secretion by tracheal glands. Am J Physiol 1990; 259:L198–L205.

86. Shimura S, Sasaki T, Sasaki H, Takishima T. Contractility of isolated single submucosal gland from trachea. J Appl Physiol 1986; 60:1237–1247.

87. Nagaki M, Shimura S, Irokawa T, Sasaki T, Oshiro T, Nara M, Kakuta Y, Shirato K. Bradykinin regulation of airway submucosal gland secretion: role of bradykinin receptor subtype. Am J Physiol 1996; 270:L907–L913.

88. Shimura S, Sasaki T, Ikeda K, Sasaki H, Takishima T. VIP augments cholinergic-induced glycoconjugate secretion in tracheal submucosal glands. J Appl Physiol 1988; 65:2537–2544.

89. Shimura S, Sasaki T, Okayama H, Sasaki H, Takishima T. Effect of substance P on the mucus secretion of isolated submucosal gland from feline trachea. J Appl Physiol 1987; 63:646–653.

90. Sasaki T, Shimura S, Sasaki H, Takishima T. Effect of epithelium on mucus secretion from feline tracheal submucosal glands. J Appl Physiol 1989; 66:764–770.

91. Widdicombe JH, Basbaum CB, Highland E. Ion contents and other properties of isolated cells from dog tracheal epithelium. Am J Physiol 1981; 241:C184–C192.

92. Finkbeiner WE. Respiratory cell culture. In: Crystal RG, West JB, Weibel ER, Barnes PJ, eds. The Lung: Scientific Foundations. Philadelphia: Lipincott-Raven, 1997:415–434.

93. Yamaya M, Finkbeiner WE, Chun SY, Widdicombe JH. Differentiated structure and function of cultures from human tracheal epithelium. Am J Physiol 1992; 262:L713–L724.

94. Whitcutt MJ, Adler KB, Wu R. A biphasic chamber system for maintaining polarity of differentiation of cultured respiratory tract epithelial cells. In Vitro 1988; 24:420–428.

95. Yankaskas JR, Cotton CU, Knowles MR, Gatzy JT, Boucher RC. Culture of human nasal epithelial cells on collagen matrix supports: a comparison of bioelectric properties of normal and cystic fibrosis epithelia. Am Rev Respir Dis 1985; 132: 1281–1287.

96. Kim KC, Brody JS. Use of primary cell culture to study regulation of airway surface epithelial mucus secretion. Symp Soc Exp Biol 1989; 43:231–239.

97. Wasano K, Kim KC, Niles RM, Brody JS. Membrane differentiation markers of airway epithelial secretory cells. J Histochem Cytochem 1988; 36:167–178.

98. Widdicombe JH, Azizi F, Kang T, Pittet J-F. Transient permeabilization of airway epithelium by mucosal water. J Appl Physiol 1996; 81:491–499.

99. Widdicombe JH, Sachs LA, Jang Y-J, Finkbeiner WE. Effects of growth surface on differentiation of cultures of human tracheal epithelium. In Vitro 2003; 39A: 51–55.

100. Doherty MM, Liu J, Randell SH, Carter CA, Davis CW, Nettesheim P, Ferriola PC. Phenotype and differentiation potential of a novel rat tracheal epithelial cell line. Am J Respir Cell Molec Biol 1995; 12:385–395.

101. Randell SH, Liu JY, Ferriola PC, Kaartinen L, Doherty MM, Davis CW, Nettesheim P. Mucin production by SPOC1 cells—an immortalized rat tracheal epithelial cell line. Am J Respir Cell Mol Biol 1996; 14:146–154.

102. Gruenert DC, Finkbeiner WE, Widdicombe JH. Culture and transformation of human airway epithelial cells. Am J Physiol 1995; 268:L347–L360.

103. Culp DJ, Penney DP, Marin MG. A technique for the isolation of submucosal gland cells from cat trachea. J Appl Physiol 1983; 55:1035–1041.

104. Yang CM, Farley JM, Dwyer TM. Acetylcholine-stimulated chloride flux in tracheal submucosal gland cells. J Appl Physiol 1988; 65:1891–1894.

105. Finkbeiner WE, Nadel JA, Basbaum CB. Establishment and characterization of a cell line derived from bovine tracheal glands. In Vitro 1986; 22:561–567.

106. Sommerhoff CP, Finkbeiner WE. Human tracheobronchial submucosal gland cells in culture. Am J Respir Cell Mol Biol 1990; 2:41–50.

107. Tournier JM, Merten M, Meckler Y, Hinnrasky J, Fuchey C, Puchelle E. Culture

and characterization of human tracheal gland cells. Am Rev Respir Dis 1990; 141: 1280–1288.

108. Chopra DP, Sullivan J, Wille JJ, Siddiqui KM. Propagation of differentiating normal human tracheobronchial epithelial cells in serum-free medium. J Cell Physiol 1987; 130:173–181.

109. Yamaya M, Finkbeiner WE, Widdicombe JH. Ion transport by cultures of human tracheobronchial submucosal glands. Am J Physiol 1991; 261:L485–L490.

110. Finkbeiner WE, Shen BQ, Widdicombe JH. Chloride secretion and function of serous and mucous cells of human airway glands. Am J Physiol 1994; 267:L206–L210.

111. Jacquot J, Spilmont C, Burlet H, Fuchey C, Buisson AC, Tournier JM, Gaillard D, Puchelle E. Glandular-like morphogenesis and secretory activity of human tracheal gland cells in a three-dimensional collagen gel matrix. J Cell Physiol 1994; 161:407–418.

112. Haws C, Finkbeiner WE, Widdicombe JH, Wine JJ. CFTR in Calu-3 human airway cells: channel properties and role in cAMP-activated Cl⁻ conductance. Am J Physiol 1994; 266:L502–L512.

113. Shen BQ, Finkbeiner WE, Wine JJ, Mrsny RJ, Widdicombe JH. Calu-3: a human airway epithelial cell line that shows cAMP-dependent Cl⁻ secretion. Am J Physiol 1994; 266:L493–L501.

114. Adler KB, Fischer BM, Li H, Choe NH, Wright DT. Hypersecretion of mucin in response to inflammatory mediators by guinea pig tracheal epithelial cells in vitro is blocked by inhibition of nitric oxide synthase. Am J Respir Cell Mol Biol 1995; 13:526–530.

115. Kim KC, Zheng QX, Van-Seuningen I. Involvement of a signal transduction mechanism in ATP-induced mucin release from cultured airway goblet cells. Am J Respir Cell Mol Biol 1993; 8:121–125.

116. Lethem MI, Dowell ML, Van Scott M, Yankaskas JR, Egan T, Boucher RC, Davis CW. Nucleotide regulation of goblet cells in human airway epithelial explants: normal exocytosis in cystic fibrosis. Am J Respir Cell Mol Biol 1993; 9: 315–322.

117. Kim KC, Wasano K, Niles RM, Schuster JE, Stone PJ, Brody JS. Human neutrophil elastase releases cell surface mucins from primary cultures of hamster tracheal epithelial cells. Proc Natl Acad Sci USA 1987; 84:9304–9308.

118. Iwamoto I, Nadel JA, Varsano S, Forsberg LS. Turnover of cell-surface macromolecules in cultured dog tracheal epithelial cells. Biochim Biophys Acta 1988; 966:336–346.

119. Sheppard MN, Kurian SS, Henzen-Longmans SC, Michetti F, Cocchia D, Cole P, Rush RA, Marangos PJ, Bloom SR, Polak JM. Neuron-specific enolase and s-100: new markers for delineating the innervation of the respiratory tract in man and other animals. Thorax 1983; 38:333–340.

120. Partanen M, Laitinen A, Hervonen A, Toivanen M, Laitinen LA. Catecholamine- and acetylcholinesterase-containing nerves in human lower respiratory tract. Histochemistry 1982; 76:175–188.

121. Sherman JM, Cheng P-W, Tandler B, Boat TF. Mucous glycoproteins from cat

tracheal globlet cells and mucous glands separated with EDTA. Am Rev Respir Dis 1981; 124:476–479.

122. Kim KC. Biochemistry and pharmacology of mucin-like glycoproteins produced by cultured airway epithelial cells. Exp Lung Res 1991; 17:533–545.

123. Wu DX-Y, Lee CYC, Uyekubo SN, Choi HK, Bastacky SJ, Widdicombe JH. Regulation of the depth of surface liquid in bovine trachea. Am J Physiol 1998; 274:L388–L395.

124. Niles RM, Christensen TG, Breuer R, Stone PJ, Snider GL. Serine proteases stimulate mucous glycoprotein release from hamster tracheal ring organ culture. J Lab Clin Med 1986; 108:489–497.

125. McDonald DM. Neurogenic inflammation in rat trachea. I. Changes in venules, leukocytes, and epithelial cells. J Neurocytol 1988; 17:583–603.

126. Kuo HP, Rhode JAL, Tokuyama K, Barnes PJ, Rogers DF. Cigarette smoke-induced airway goblet cell secretion: dose-dependent differential nerve activation. Am J Physiol 1992; 263:L161–L167.

127. Kim KC, Nassiri J, Brody JS. Mechanisms of airway goblet cell mucin release: studies with cultured tracheal surface epithelial cells. Am J Respir Cell Mol Biol 1989; 1:137–143.

128. Adler KB, Schwarz JE, Anderson WH, Welton AF. Platelet activating factor stimulates secretion of mucin by explants of rodent airways in organ culture. Exp Lung Res 1987; 13:25–43.

129. Wright DT, Fischer BM, Li C, Rochelle LG, Akley NJ, Adler KB. Oxidant stress stimulates mucin secretion and PLC in airway epithelium via a nitric oxide-dependent mechanism. Am J Physiol 1996; 271:L854–L861.

130. Klinger JD, Tandler B, Liedtke CM, Boat TF. Proteinases of *Pseudomonas aeruginosa* evoke mucin release by tracheal epithelium. J Clin Invest 1984; 74:1669–1678.

131. Breuer R, Christensen TG, Niles RM, Stone PJ, Snider GL. Human neutrophil elastase causes glycoconjugate release from the epithelial cell surface of hamster trachea in organ culture. Am Rev Respir Dis 1987; 779–782.

132. Cheng PW, Boat TF, Cranfill K, Yankaskas JR, Boucher RC. Increased sulfation of glycoconjugates by cultured nasal epithelial cells from patients with cystic fibrosis. J Clin Invest 1989; 84:68–72.

133. Varsano S, Basbaum CB, Forsberg LS, Borson DB, Caughey G, Nadel JA. Dog tracheal epithelial cells in culture synthesize sulfated macromolecular glycoconjugates and release them from the cell surface upon exposure to extracellular proteinases. Exp Lung Res 1987; 13:157–184.

134. Sommerhoff CP, Nadel JA, Basbaum CB, Caughey GH. Neutrophil elastase and cathepsin G stimulate secretion from cultured bovine airway gland serous cells. J Clin Invest 1990; 85:682–689.

135. Tamaoki J, Nakata J, Tagaya E, Konno K. Effects of roxithromycin and erythromycin on interleukin 8–induced neutrophil recruitment and goblet cell secretion in guinea pig tracheas. Antimicrob Agents Chemother 1996; 40:1726–1728.

136. Savoie C, Plant M, Zwikker M, van Staden CJ, Boulet L, Chan CC, Rodger IW, Pon DJ. Effect of dexamethasone on antigen-induced high molecular weight gly-

coconjugate secretion in allergic guinea pigs. Am J Respir Cell Mol Biol 1995; 13:133–143.

137. Steel DM, Hanrahan JW. Muscarinic-induced mucin secretion and intracellular signaling by hamster tracheal goblet cells. Am J Physiol 1997; 272:L230–L237.

138. Ko KH, McCracken K, Kim KC. ATP-induced mucin release from cultured airway goblet cells involves, in part, activation of protein kinase C. Am J Respir Cell Mol Biol 1997; 16:194–198.

139. Abdullah LH, Conway JD, Cohn JA, Davis CW. Protein kinase C and Ca^{2+} activation of mucin secretion in airway goblet cells. Am J Physiol 1997; 273:L201–L210.

140. Bogart BI, Conod EJ, Conover JH. The biologic activities of cystic fibrosis sputum. I. The effects of cystic fibrosis sera and calcium ionophore A23187 on rabbit tracheal explants. Pediatr Res 1977; 11:131–136.

141. Conover JH, Conod EJ. The influence of cystic fibrosis serum and calcium on secretion in the rabbit tracheal mucociliary apparatus. Biochem Biophys Res Commun 1978; 83:1595–1601.

142. Kai H, Kazuhisa Y, Isohama Y, Hamamura I, Takahama K, Miyata T. Involvement of protein kinase C in mucus secretion by hamster tracheal epithelial cells in culture. Am J Physiol 1994; 267:L526–L530.

143. Larivee P, Levine SJ, Martinez A, Wu T, Logun C, Shelhamer JH. Platelet-activating factor induces airway mucin release via activation of protein kinase C: evidence for translocation of protein kinase C to membranes. Am J Respir Cell Mol Biol 1994; 11:199–205.

144. Scott CE, Abdullah LH, Davis CW. Ca^{2+} and protein kinase C activation of mucin granule exocytosis in permeabilized SPOC1 cells. Am J Physiol 1998; 275:C285–292.

145. Murlas C, Nadel JA, Basbaum CB. A morphometric analysis of the autonomic innervation of cat tracheal glands. J Auton Nerv Syst 1980; 2:233–237.

146. Partanen M, Laitinen A, Hervonen A, Toivanen M, Laitinen LA. Catecholamine- and acetylcholinesterase-containing nerves in human lower respiratory tract. Histochemistry 1982; 76:175–188.

147. Pack RJ, Richardson PS. The aminergic innervation of the human bronchus: a light and electron microscopic study. J Anat 1984; 138:493–502.

148. Dey RD, Shannon WA, Said SI. Localization of VIP-immunoreactive nerves in airways and pulmonary vessels of dogs, cats, and human subjects. Cell Tissue Res 1981; 220:231–238.

149. Uddman R, Sundler F. Neuropeptides in the airways: a review. Am Rev Respir Dis 1987; 136:53–58.

150. Shimura S, Takishima T. Airway submucosal gland secretion. In: Shimura S, Takishima T, eds. Airway Secretion. New York: Marcel Dekker, 1994:325–398.

151. Mak JCW, Barnes PJ. Autoradiographic visualization of muscarinic receptor subtypes in human and guinea pig lung. Am Rev Respir Dis 1990; 141:1559–1568.

152. Kokin P. Ueber die secretorischen Nerven der Kehlkopf und Luftrohrenschleimdrusen. Pflugers Arch 1896; 63:622–640.

153. Kountz WB, Koenig K. Studies of bronchial secretion. J Allergy 1930; 1:429–440.

154. Evans DJ, Matsumoto PS, Widdicombe JH, Li-Yun C, Maminishkis AA, Miller SS. *Pseudomonas aeruginosa* induces changes in fluid transport across airway surface epithelium. Am J Physiol 1998; 275:C1284–C1290.

155. Gallagher JT, Kent PW, Passatore M, Phipps RJ, Richardson PS. The composition of tracheal mucus and the nervous control of its secretion in the cat. Proc Roy Soc Lond B 1975; 192:49–76.

156. Peatfield AC, Richardson PS. The control of mucin secretion into the lumen of the cat trachea by α- and β-adrenoceptors, and their relative involvement during sympathetic nerve stimulation. Eur J Pharmacol 1982; 81:617–626.

157. Fung DCK, Allenby MI, Richardson PS. NANC nerve pathways controlling mucous glycoconjugate secretion into feline trachea. J Appl Physiol 1992; 73:625–630.

158. Borson DB, Chin RA, Davis B, Nadel JA. Adrenergic and cholinergic nerves mediate fluid secretion from tracheal glands of ferrets. J Appl Physiol 1980; 49:1027–1031.

159. Baker B, Peatfield AC, Richardson PS. Nervous control of mucin secretion into human bronchi. J Physiol 1985; 365:297–305.

160. Shimura S, Sasaki T, Ishihara H, Sato M, Sasaki H, Takishima T. Autonomic innervation to feline tracheal submucosal glands for mucus glycoprotein secretion. Am J Physiol 1992; 262:L15–L20.

161. Davis B, Chinn R, Gold J, Popovac D, Widdicombe JG. Hypoxemia reflexly increases secretion from tracheal submucosal glands in dogs. J Appl Physiol 1982; 52:1416–1419.

162. Davis B, Roberts AM, Coleridge HM, Coleridge JC. Reflex tracheal gland secretion evoked by stimulation of bronchial C-fibers in dogs. J Appl Physiol 1982; 53:985–991.

163. German VF, Ueki IF, Nadel JA. Micropipette measurement of airway submucosal gland secretion: laryngeal reflex. Am Rev Respir Dis 1982; 122:413–416.

164. German VF, Corrales R, Ueki IF, Nadel JA. Reflex stimulation of tracheal mucus gland secretion by gastric irritation in cats. J Appl Physiol 1982; 52:1153–1155.

165. Haxhiu MA, Haxhiu-Poskurica B, Moracic V, Carlo WA, Martin RJ. Reflex and chemical responses of tracheal submucosal glands in piglets. Respir Physiol 1990; 82:267–278.

166. Schultz HD, Roberts AM, Bratcher C, Coleridge HM, Coleridge JC, Davis B. Pulmonary C-fibers reflexly increase secretion by tracheal submucosal glands in dogs. J Appl Physiol 1985; 58:907–910.

167. Yu J, Schultz HD, Goodman J, Coleridge JC, Coleridge HM, Davis B. Pulmonary rapidly adapting receptors reflexly increase airway secretion in dogs. J Appl Physiol 1989; 67:682–687.

168. Hejal R, Strohl KP, Erokwu B, Cherniack NS, Haxhiu MA. Pathways and mechanisms involved in the control of laryngeal submucosal gland secretion. J Appl Physiol 1993; 75:2347–2352.

169. Davis B, Tseng HC. Neural regulation of lysozyme secretion from tracheal submucosal glands of ferrets in vivo. J Appl Physiol 1991; 71:939–944.

170. Haxhiu MA, van Lunteren E, Cherniack NS. Central effects of tachykinin peptides on tracheal secretion. Respir Physiol 1991; 86:405–414.

171. Haxhiu MA, van Lunteren E, Cherniack NS. Influence of ventrolateral surface of medulla on tracheal gland secretion. J Appl Physiol 1991; 71:1663–1668.

172. Leikauf GD, Ueki IF, Nadel JA. Autonomic regulation of viscoelasticity of cat tracheal gland secretions. J Appl Physiol 1984; 56:426–430.

173. Shelhamer JH, Marom Z, Kaliner M. Immunologic and neuropharmacologic stimulation of mucous glycoprotein release from human airways *in vitro*. J Clin Invest 1980; 66:1400–1408.

174. Ishihara H, Shimura S, Satoh M, Masuda T, Nonaka H, Kase H, Sasaki T, Sasaki H, Takishima T, Tamura K. Muscarinic receptor subtypes in feline tracheal submucosal gland secretion. Am J Physiol 1992; 259:L345–L50.

175. Yang CM, Farley J M, Dwyer TM. Muscarinic stimulation of the submucosal glands in swine trachea. J Appl Physiol 1988; 64:200–209.

176. Ramnarine SI, Haddad EB, Khawaja AM, Rogers DF. On muscarinic control of neurogenic mucus secretion in ferret trachea. J Physiol (Lond) 1996; 494:577–586.

177. Webber SE, Widdicombe JG. The actions of methacholine, phenylephrine, salbutamol and histamine on mucus secretion from the ferret in vitro trachea. Agents Actions 1987; 22:82–85.

178. Tom-Moy M, Basbaum CB, Nadel JA. Localization and release of lysozyme from ferret trachea: effects of adrenergic and cholinergic drugs. Cell Tissue Res 1983; 228:549–562.

179. Chakrin LW, Baker AP, Christian P, Wardell JR. Effect of cholinergic stimulation on the release of macromolecules by canine trachea in vitro. Am Rev Respir Dis 1973; 108:69–76.

180. Reasor MJ, Cohen D, Proctor DF, Rubin RJ. Tracheobronchial secretions collected from intact dogs. II. Effects of cholinomimetic stimulation. J Appl Physiol 1978; 45:190–194.

181. Griffin A, Newman TM, Scott RH. Electrophysiological and ultrastructural events evoked by methacholine and intracellular photolysis of caged compounds in cultured ovine tracheal submucosal gland cells. Exp Physiol 1996; 81:27–43.

182. Barnes PJ, Basbaum CB. Mapping of adrenergic receptors in the trachea by autoradiography. Exp Lung Res 1983; 5:183–192.

183. Carstairs R, Nimmo A, Barnes P. Autoradiographic visualization of β-adrenoceptor subtypes in human lung. Am Rev Respir Dis 1985; 132:5541–5557.

184. Iravani J, van As A. Mucus transport in the tracheobronchial tree of normal and bronchitic rats. J Pathol 1972; 106:81–93.

185. Phipps RJ, Richardson PS, Pack RJ, Wright N. Sympathomimetic drugs stimulate the output of secretory glycoproteins from human bronchi *in vitro*. Clin Sci 1982; 63:23–28.

186. Liedtke CM, Rudolph SA, Boat TF. β-Adrenergic modulation of mucin secretion in cat trachea. Am J Physiol 1983; 244:C391–C398.

187. Gierschik P, Jakobs KH. Mechanisms for inhibition of adenylate cyclase by alpha-2 adrenergic receptors. In: Limbird LE, ed. The Alpha-2 Adrenergic Receptors. Clifton, NJ: Humana, 1988:75–114.

188. Phipps RJ, Nadel JA, Davis B. Effect of alpha-adrenergic stimulation on mucus

secretion and on ion transport in cat trachea in vitro. Am Rev Respir Dis 1980; 121:359–365.

189. Baraniuk JN, Kaliner M. Neuropeptides and nasal secretion. Am J Physiol 1991; 261:L223–L235.
190. Ramnarine SI, Rogers DF. Non-adrenergic, non-cholinergic neural control of mucus secretion in the airways. Pulm Pharmacol 1994; 7:19–33.
191. Carstairs JR, Barnes PJ. Autoradiographic mapping of substance P receptors in lung. Eur J Pharmacol 1986; 127:295–296.
192. Carstairs JR, Barnes PJ. Visualization of vasoactive intestinal peptide receptors in human and guinea pig lung. J Pharmacol Exp Ther 1986; 239:249–255.
193. Jacoby DB. Mediator functions of epithelial cells. In: Busse WW, Holgate ST, eds. Asthma and Rhinitis. Oxford: Blackwell Scientific Publications, 2000:573–583.
194. Rieves RD, Goff J, Wu T, Larivee P, Logun C, Shelhamer JH. Airway epithelial cell mucin release: immunologic quantitation and response to platelet-activating factor. Am J Respir Cell Mol Biol 1992; 6:158–167.
195. Lundgren JD, Kaliner M, Logun C, Shelhamer JH. Platelet activating factor and tracheobronchial respiratory glycoconjugate release in feline and human explants: involvement of the lipoxygenase pathway. Agents Actions 1990; 30:329–337.
196. Goswami SK, Ohashi M, Stathas P, Marom ZM. Platelet-activating factor stimulates secretion of respiratory glycoconjugate from human airways in culture. J Allergy Clin Immunol 1989; 84:726–734.
197. Sasaki T, Shimura S, Ikeda K, Sasaki H, Takishima T. Platelet-activating factor increases platelet-dependent glycoconjugate secretion from tracheal submucosal glands. Am J Physiol 1989; 257:L373–L378.
198. Marom Z, Shelhamer JH, Kaliner M. Effects of arachidonic acid, monohydroxyeicosatetraenoic acid and prostaglandins on the release of mucous glycoproteins from human airways in vitro. J Clin Invest 1981; 67:1695–1702.
199. Rich B, Peatfield AC, Williams IP, Richardson PS. Effects of prostaglandins E_1, E_2, and $F_{2\alpha}$ on mucin secretion from human bronchi in vitro. Thorax 1984; 39: 420–423.
200. Lundgren JD, Wiedermann CJ, Logun C, Plutchok J, Kaliner M, Shelhamer JH. Substance P receptor–mediated secretion of respiratory glycoconjugate from feline airways in vitro. Exp Lung Res 1989; 15:17–29.
201. Marom Z, Shelhamer JH, Steel L, Goetzl EJ, Kaliner M. Prostaglandin-generating factor of anaphylaxis induces mucous glycoprotein release and the formation of lipoxygenase products of arachidonate in human airways. Prostaglandins 1984; 28:79–91.
202. Shimura S, Ishihara H, Satoh M, Masuda T, Nagaki M, Sasaki H, Takishima T. Endothelin regulation of mucus glycoprotein secretion from feline tracheal submucosal glands. Am J Physiol 1992; 262:L208–L213.
203. Webber SE, Widdicombe JG. The effect of vasoactive intestinal peptide on smooth muscle tone and mucus secretion from the ferret trachea. Br J Pharmacol 1987; 91:139–148.
204. Coles NJ, Said SI, Reid LM. Vasoactive intestinal peptide and airway secretion. Am Rev Respir Dis 1981; 124:531–536.

205. Webber SE, Lim JC, Widdicombe JG. The effects of calcitonin gene-related peptide on submucosal gland secretion and epithelial albumin transport in the ferret trachea in vitro. Br J Pharmacol 1991; 102:79–84.
206. Baker AP, Hillegass M, Holden DA, Smith WJ. Effect of kallidin, substance P, and other basic polypeptides on the productin of respiratory macromolecules. Am Rev Respir Dis 1977; 115:811–817.
207. Baraniuk JN, Lundgren JD, Mizoguchi H, Peden D, Gawin A, Merida M, Shelhamer JH, Kaliner MA. Bradykinin and respiratory mucous membranes: analysis of bradykinin binding site distribution and secretory responses *in vitro* and *in vivo*. Am Rev Respir Dis 1990; 141:706–714.
208. Shimura S, Sasaki T, Nagaki M, Takishima T, Shirato K. Extracellular ATP regulation of feline tracheal submucosal gland secretion. Am J Physiol 1994; 267: L159–L164.
209. Marom Z, Shelhamer JH, Kaliner M. Human monocyte-derived mucus secretagogue. J Clin Invest 1985; 75:191–198.
210. Marom Z, Shelhamer JH, Kaliner M. Human pulmonary macrophage-derived mucus secretagogue. J Exp Med 1984; 159:844–860.
211. Phipps RJ, Denas SM, Wanner A. Antigen stimulates glycoprotein secretion and alters ion fluxes in sheep trachea. J Appl Physiol 1983; 55:1593–1602.
212. Kishioka C, Okamoto K, Kim J, Rubin BK. Regulation of secretion from mucous and serous cells in the excised ferret trachea. Respir Physiol 2001; 126:163–171.
213. Dunnill MS. The pathology of asthma, with special reference to changes in the bronchial mucosa. J Clin Pathol 1960; 13:27–33.
214. Fahy JV, Wong H, Liu J, Boushey HA. Comparison of samples collected by sputum induction and bronchoscopy from asthmatic and healthy subjects. Am J Respir Crit Care Med 1995; 152:53–58.
215. Peatfield AC, Richardson PS, Wells UM. The effect of airflow on mucus secretion into the trachea of the cat. J Physiol 1986; 380:429–439.
216. Dwyer TM, Farley JM. Mucus glycoconjugate secretion in cool and hypertonic solutions. Am J Physiol 1997; 272:L1121–L1125.
217. Marom Z, Shelhamer J, Alling D, Kaliner M. The effects of corticosteroids on mucous glycoprotein secretion from human airways in vitro. Am Rev Respir Dis 1984; 129:62–65.
218. Shimura S, Sasaki T, Ikeda K, Yamauchi K, Sasaki H, Takishima T. Direct inhibitory action of glucocorticoid on glycoconjugate secretion from airway submucosal glands. Am Rev Respir Dis 1990; 141:1044–1049.
219. Lundgren JD, Hirata F, Marom Z, Logun C, Steel L, Kaliner M, Shelhamer JH. Dexamethasone inhibits glycoconjugate secretion from feline airways in vitro by the induction of lipocortin (lipomodulin) synthesis. Am Rev Respir Dis 1988; 137:353–357.
220. Goswami SK, Kivity S, Marom Z. Erythromycin inhibits respiratory glycoconjugate secretion from human airways in vitro. Am Rev Respir Dis 1990; 141:72–78.
221. Ramnarine SI, Khawaja AM, Barnes AJ, Rogers DF. Nitric oxide inhibition of basal and neurogenic mucus secretion in ferret tracheal in vitro. Br J Pharmacol 1996; 118:998–1002.
222. Lundgren JD, Davey RJ, Lundgren B, Mullol J, Marom Z, Logun C, Baraniuk

JN, Kaliner MA, Shelhamer JH. Eosinophils and mucus airway secretion: eosinophil cationic protein stimulates and major basic protein inhibits secretion from airway organ culture. J Allergy Clin Immunol 1991; 87:689–698.

223. Whimster WF, Reid L. The influence of dibutyryl cyclic adenosine monophosphate and other substances on human bronchial mucous discharge. Exp Mol Pathol 1973; 18:234–240.

224. Lazarus SC, Basbaum CB, Barnes PJ, Gold WM. cAMP immunocytochemistry provides evidence for functional VIP receptors in trachea. Am J Physiol 1986; 251:C115–C119.

225. Lazarus SC, Basbaum CB, Gold WM. Prostaglandins and intracellular cyclic AMP in respiratory secretory cells. Am Rev Respir Dis 1984; 130:262–266.

226. Coles SJ, Judge J, Reid L. Differential effects of calcium ions on glycoconjugate secretion by canine tracheal explants. Chest 1982; 81:34S.

227. Barsigian C, Barbieri EJ. The effects of indomethacin and prostaglandins E_2 and $F_{2\alpha}$ on canine tracheal mucus generation. Agents Actions 1982; 12:320–327.

228. Ishihara H, Shimura S, Sato M, Masuda T, Ishide N, Miura M, Sasaki T, Sasaki H, Takishima T. Intracellular calcium concentration of acinar cells in feline tracheal submucosal glands. Am J Physiol 1990; 259:L345–L350.

229. Nagaki M, Ishihara H, Shimura S, Sasaki T, Takishima T, Shirato K. Tachykinins induce a $[Ca^{2+}]_i$ rise in the acinar cells of feline tracheal submucosal gland. Respir Physiol 1994; 98:111–120.

230. Nagaki M, Sasaki T, Shimura S, Satoh M, Takishima T, Shirato K. CGRP induces $[Ca^{2+}]_i$ rise and glycoconjugate secretion in feline tracheal submucosal gland. Respir Physiol 1994; 96:311–319.

231. Sasaki T, Shimura S, Wakui M, Ohkawa Y, Takishima T, Mikoshiba K. Apically localized IP_3 receptors control chloride current in airway gland acinar cells. Am J Physiol 1994; 267:L152–L158.

232. Engelhardt JF, Yankaskas JR, Ernst S, Yang Y, Marino CR, Boucher RC, Cohn JA, Wilson JM. Submucosal glands are the predominant site of CFTR expression in the human bronchus. Nature Genet 1992; 2:240–247.

233. Sturgess J, Imrie J. Quantitative evaluation of the development of tracheal submucosal glands in infants with cystic fibrosis and control infants. Am J Pathol 1982; 106:303–311.

234. Yeates DB, Sturgess J, Kahn S, Levison H, Aspin N. Mucociliary transport in the trachea of patients with cystic fibrosis. Arch Dis Child 1976; 51:28–33.

235. Inglis SK, Corboz MR, Taylor AE, Ballard ST. Effects of anion transport inhibition on mucus secretion by airway submucosal glands. Am J Physiol 1997; 272: L372–L377.

236. Trout L, King M, Feng W, Inglis SK, Ballard ST. Inhibition of airway liquid secretion and its effect on the physical properties of airway mucus. Am J Physiol 1998; 274:L258–L263.

237. Welsh MJ. Electrolyte transport by airway epithelia. Physiol Rev 1987; 67:1143–1184.

238. Widdicombe JH. Ion transport by airway epithelia. In: Crystal RG, West JB, Weibel E, Barnes PJ, eds. The Lung: Scientific Foundations. New York: Raven Press, 1996:39.1–39.12.

239. Ikeda K, Wu D, Takasaka T. Inhibition of acetylcholine-evoked Cl currents by 14-membered macrolide antibiotics in isolated acinar cells of the guinea pig nasal gland. Am J Respir Cell Mol Biol 1995; 13:449–454.

240. Clancy JP, McCann JD, Welsh MJ. Evidence that calcium-dependent activation of airway epithelial chloride channels is not dependent on phosphorylation. Am J Physiol 1990; 259:L410–L414.

241. Sommerhoff CP, Finkbeiner WE, Nadel JA, Basbaum CB. Prostaglandin D_2 and prostaglandin E_2 stimulate ^{35}S-labeled macromolecule secretion from cultured bovine tracheal gland serous cells. Am Rev Respir Dis 1987; 135:A363.

242. Finkbeiner W, Widdicombe J, Hu L, Basbaum C. Bovine tracheal serous cell secretion: role of cAMP and cAMP-dependent protein kinase. Am J Physiol (Lung Cell Mol Physiol) 1992; 262:L574–L581.

243. Sommerhoff CP, Fang KC, Nadel JA, Caughey GH. Classical second messengers are not involved in proteinase-induced degranulation of airway gland cells. Am J Physiol 1996; 271:L796–L803.

244. Paul A, Mergey M, Veissiere D, Hermelin B, Cherqui G, Picard J, Basbaum CB. Regulation of secretion in cultured tracheal serous cells by protein kinases A and C. Am J Physiol 1991; 261:L172–L177.

245. Maizieres M, Kaplan H, Millot JM, Bonnet N, Manfait M, Puchelle E, Jacquot J. Neutrophil elastase promotes rapid exocytosis in human airway gland cells by producing cytosolic Ca^{2+} oscillations. Am J Respir Cell Mol Biol 1998; 18:32–42.

246. Jacquot J, Merten M, Millot JM, Sebille S, Menager M, Figarella C, Manfait M. Asynchronous dynamic changes of intracellular free Ca^{2+} and possible exocytosis in human tracheal gland cells induced by neutrophil elastase. Biochem Biophys Res Commun 1995; 212:307–316.

247. Merten MD, Figarella C. Constitutive hypersecretion and insensitivity to neurotransmitters by cystic fibrosis tracheal gland cells. Am J Physiol 1993; 264:L98–L99.

248. Bhaskar KR, O'Sullivan DD, Seltzer J, Rossing TH, Drazen JM, Reid LM. Density gradient study of bronchial mucus aspirates from healthy volunteers (smokers and nonsmokers) and from patients with tracheostomy. Exp Lung Res 1985; 9: 289–308.

249. Seybold ZV, Mariassy AT, Mariassy D, Kim CS. Mucociliary interaction in vitro: effects of physiological and inflammatory stimuli. J Appl Physiol 1990; 68:1421–1426.

250. Winters SL, Yeates DB. Interaction between ion transporters and the mucociliary transport system in dog and baboon. J Appl Physiol 1997; 83:1348–1359.

251. Winters SL, Yeates DB. Roles of hydration, sodium, and chloride in the regulation of canine mucociliary transport system. J Appl Physiol 1997; 83:1360–1369.

252. Matsui H, Randell SH, Perretti SW, Davis CW, Boucher RC. Coordinated clearance of periciliary liquid and mucus from airway surfaces. J Clin Invest 1998; 102:1125–1131.

253. Glynn AA, Michaels L. Bronchial biopsy in chronic bronchitis and asthma. Thorax 1960; 15:142–152.

254. Bedrossian CW, Greenberg SD, Singer DB, Hansen JJ, Rosenberg HS. The lung

in cystic fibrosis: a quantitative study including prevalence of pathologic findings among different age groups. Hum Pathol 1976; 7:195–204.

255. Jones R, Bolduc P, Reid L. Goblet cell glycoprotein and tracheal gland hypertrophy in rat airways: the effect of cigarette smoke with or without the anti-inflammatory agent, phenylmethyloxadiazole. Br J Exp Pathol 1973; 54:229–239.

256. Spicer SS, Chakrin LW, Wardell JR. Effect of chronic sulfur dioxide inhalation on the carbohydrate histochemistry and histology of the canine respiratory tract. Am Rev Respir 1974; 110:13–24.

257. Hoffstein ST, Malo PE, Bugelski P, Wheeldon EB. Leukotriene D_4 (LTD_4) induces mucus secretion from goblet cells in guinea pig respiratory epithelium. Exp Lung Res 1990; 16:711–725.

258. Tamaoki J, Takeyama K, Yamawaki I, Kondo M, Konno K. Lipopolysaccharide-induced goblet cell hypersecretion in the guinea pig trachea: inhibition by macrolides. Am J Physiol 1997; 272:L15–L19.

259. Steiger D, Hotchkiss J, Bajaj L, Harkema J, Basbaum C. Concurrent increases in the storage and release of mucin-like molecules by rat airway epithelial cells in response to bacterial endotoxin. Am J Respir Cell Mol Biol 1995; 12:307–314.

260. Kim KC, Opaskar-Hincman H, Bhaskar KR. Secretions from primary hamster tracheal surface epithelial cells in culture: mucin-like glycoproteins, proteoglycans and lipids. Exp Lung Res 1989; 15:299–314.

261. Takeyama K, Tamaoki J, Nakata J, Konno K. Effect of oxitropium bromide on histamine-induced airway goblet cell secretion. Am J Respir Crit Care Med 1996; 154:231–236.

262. Tamaoki J, Nakata, J, Takeyama, K, Chiyotani, A, Konno, K. Histamine H2 receptor-mediated airway goblet cell secretion and its modulation by histamine-degrading enzymes. J Allergy Clin Immunol 1997; 99:233–238.

263. Kuo HP, Rohde JAL, Tokuyama K, Barnes PJ, Rogers DF. Capsaicin and sensory neuropeptide stimulation of goblet cell secretion in guinea-pig trachea. J Physiol 1990; 431:629–641.

264. Adler KB, Holden-Stauffer WJ, Repine JE. Oxygen metabolites stimulate release of high-molecular-weight glycoconjugates by cell and organ cultures of rodent respiratory epithelium via an arachidonic acid–dependent mechanism. J Clin Invest 1990; 85:75–85.

265. Adler KB, Akley NJ, Glascow WC. Platelet-activating-factor provokes release of mucin-like glycoproteins from guinea pig respiratory epithelial cells via a lipoxygenase-dependent mechanism. Am J Respir Cell Mol Biol 1992; 6:550–556.

266. Larivee P, Rieves RD, Levine SJ, Shelhamer JH. Airway inflammation and mucous hypersecretion. In: Takishima T, Shimura S, eds. Airway Secretion: Physiological Bases for the Control of Mucous Hypersecretion. New York: Marcel Dekker, 1994:469–511.

267. Last JA, Jennings MD, Schwartz LW, Cross CE. Glycoprotein secretion by tracheal explants cultured from rats exposed to ozone. Am Rev Respir Dis 1977; 116:695–703.

268. Kim KC, Lee BC, Brody JS. Effect of floating a gel matrix on mucin release in cultured airway epithelial cells. J Cell Physiol 1993; 156:480–486.

269. Adler KB, Hendley DD, Davis GS. Bacteria associated with obstructive pulmonary disease elaborate extracellular products that stimulate mucin secretion by explants of guinea pig airways. Am J Pathol 1986; 125:501–514.

270. Takeyama K, Agusti C, Ueki I, Lausier J, Cardell LO, Nadel JA. Neutrophil-dependent goblet cell degranulation: role of membrane-bound elastase and adhesion molecules. Am J Physiol 1998; 275:L294–L302.

271. Levine SJ, P L, Logun C, Angus CW, Ognibene FP, Shelhamer JH. Tumor necrosis factor-alpha induces mucin hypersecretion and MUC-2 gene expression by human airway epithelial cells. Am J Res Cell Mol Biol 1995; 12:196–204.

272. Fischer BM, Krunkosky TM, Wright DT, Dolan-O'Keefe M, Adler KB. Tumor necrosis factor-alpha (TNF-alpha) stimulates mucin secretion and gene expression in airway epithelium in vitro. Chest 1995; 107(suppl 3):133S–135S.

273. Hayes JP, Kuo HP, Rohde JA, Newman-Taylor AJ, Barnes PJ, Chung KF, Rogers DF. Neurogenic goblet cell secretion and bronchoconstriction in guinea pigs sensitized to trimellitic anhydride. Eur J Pharmacol 1995; 292:127–134.

274. Agusti C, Takeyama K, Cardell LO, Ueki I, Lausier J, Lou YP, Nadel JA. Goblet cell degranulation after antigen challenge in sensitized guinea pigs: role of neutrophils. Am J Respir Crit Care Med 1998; 158:1253–1258.

275. Yamatake Y, Yanura S. New method for evaluating bronchomotor and bronchosecretory activities: effects of prostaglandins and antigen. Jpn J Pharmacol 1978; 28:391–402.

276. Johnson HG, Mcnee ML, Sun FF. 15-Hydroxyeicosatetraenoic acid is a potent inflammatory mediator and agonist of canine tracheal mucus secretion. Am Rev Respir Dis 1985; 131:917–922.

277. Coles SG, Neil KH, Reid LN. Potent stimulation of glycoprotein secretion in canine trachea by substance P. J Appl Physiol 1984; 7:1323–1327.

278. Borson DB, Corrales R, Varsano S, Gold M, Viro N, Caughey G, Ramachandran J, Nadel JA. Enkephalinase inhibitors potentiate substance P–induced secretion of $^{35}SO_4$ macromolecules from ferret trachea. Exp Lung Res 1987; 12:21–36.

279. Rogers DF, Aursudkij B, Barnes PJ. Effect of tachykinins on mucus secretion in human bronchi *in vitro*. Eur J Pharmacol 1989; 174:283–286.

280. Johnson HG, Chinn RA, Chow AW, Bach MK, Nadel JA. Leukotriene-C_4 enhanced mucus production from submucosal glands in canine trachea in vivo. Int J Immunopharmacol 1983; 5:391–396.

281. Peatfield AC, Piper PJ, Richardson PS. The effect of leukotriene C_4 on mucin release into the cat trachea in vivo and in vitro. Br J Pharmacol 1982; 77:391–393.

282. Marom Z, Shelhamer JH, Alling D, Kaliner M. Slow-reacting substances, leukotrienes C_4 and D_4 increase the release of mucus from human airways in vitro. Am Rev Respir Dis 1982; 126:499–451.

283. Shelhamer JH, Marom Z, Sun F, Bach MK, Kaliner M. The effects of arachinoids and leukotrienes on the release of mucus from human airways. Chest 1982; 81:36S.

284. Peatfield AC, Barnes PJ, Bratcher C, Nadel JA, Davis B. Vasoactive intestinal peptide stimulates tracheal submucosal gland secretion in ferret. Am Rev Respir Dis 1983; 128:89–93.

285. Somerville M, Taylor GW, Watson D, Rendell NB, Rutman A, Todd H, Davies JR, Wilson R, Cole P, Richardson PS. Release of mucus glycoconjugates by *Pseudomonas aeruginosa* rhamnolipid into feline trachea *in vivo* and human bronchus *in vitro*. Am J Respir Cell Mol Biol 1992; 6:116–122.

286. Somerville M, Richardson PS, Rutman A, Wilson R, Cole PJ. Stimulation of secretion into human and feline airways by *Pseudomonas aeruginosa* proteases. J Appl Physiol 1991; 70:2259–2267.

287. Kishioka C, Okamoto K, Hassett DJ, de Mello D, Rubin BK. *Pseudomonas aeruginosa* alginate is a potent secretagogue in the isolated ferret trachea. Pediatr Pulmonol 1999; 27:174–179.

288. Schuster A, Ueki I, Nadel JA. Neutrophil elastase stimulates tracheal submucosal gland secretion that is inhibited by ICI 200,355. Am J Physiol 1992; 2 62:L86–L91.

289. Yurdakos E, Webber SE. Endothelin-1 inhibits prestimulated tracheal submucosal gland secretion and epithelial albumin transport. Br J Pharmacol 1991; 104:1050–1056.

290. Lundgren JD, Ostrowski NL, Baraniuk JN, Shelhamer JH, Kaliner M. Gastrin-releasing peptide stimulates glycoconjugate release from feline tracheal explants. Am J Physiol 1990; 258:L68–L74.

291. Webber SE. The effects of peptide histidine isoleucine and neuropeptide Y on mucus volume output from the ferret trachea. Br J Pharmacol 1988; 95:49–54.

292. Lundgren J, Kaliner MA, Logun C, Shelhamer JH. The effects of endorphins on mucous glycoprotein secretion from feline airways in vitro. Exp Lung Res 1987; 12:303–309.

293. Phipps RJ, Denas SM, Sielczak MW, Wanner A. Effect of 0.5 ppm ozone on glycoprotein secretion, ion and water fluxes in sheep trachea. J Appl Physiol 1986; 60:918–927.

294. Marom Z, Shelhamer J, Berger M, Frank M, Kaliner M. Anaphylatoxin $C_{3\alpha}$ enhances mucous glycoprotein release from human airways *in vitro*. J Exp Med 1985; 161:657–668.

4

Outcomes for Trials of Mucoactive Therapy

BRUCE K. RUBIN

Wake Forest University School
of Medicine
Winston-Salem, North Carolina, U.S.A.

CEES P. VAN DER SCHANS

University for Professional Education
"Hanzehogeschool"
Groningen, The Netherlands

I. Introduction

One of the difficulties in assessing the efficacy of mucus clearance therapy is selecting relevant outcome variables for therapeutic trials that accurately reflect direct therapeutic effects like mucus transport and secondary effects of changes in mucus transport such as the frequency and duration of illness exacerbation (including the difficult issue of defining "exacerbation"), time in hospital, change in pulmonary function, and quality of life. Patients often tell their physicians that they feel better after initiating mucoactive therapy without there being documented improvement in spirometry or chest radiographs. Distinguishing a placebo effect from the effects of intervention is critically important if we are to determine the most appropriate use of mucoactive medications or devices. As well, the most appropriate outcome measurements are different for in vitro, preclinical, and clinical studies and at different stages of the disease process.

II. In Vitro Testing

In vitro testing of mucoactive agents can help to define a primary mechanism of action and to determine the dose that needs to be achieved in vivo for a desired effect (1). If an intervention is thought to have a directly measurable effect on sputum properties (e.g., a mucolytic) or on sputum clearability (e.g., a mucokinetic medication) and if these changes cannot be demonstrated in vitro, it is unlikely that they will be observed in clinical trials. In some cases, in vitro testing can also provide an indication of onset and duration of action for a putative mucoactive agent. This is very important in determining the appropriate dosage and frequency of administration for initial animal and clinical trials. Therefore, in vitro testing is useful for screening some mucoactive medications. However, this does not imply that if an effect is seen in vitro, a similar effect will necessarily be demonstrated with clinical use.

Many patients with chronic airway disease take several different medications, including anti-inflammatory agents, antibiotics, and bronchodilators as well as mucoactive medications. In vitro testing is also useful for identifying potential medication interaction. For example some mucolytic agents (particularly the thiol-containing agents that sever disulfide bonds) may also inactivate other medications such as peptides with disulfide bridges (2). In vitro testing suggests that the azalide antibiotic azithromycin can decrease the effectiveness of dornase alfa, while other antibiotics do not seem to do this (3).

Generally, in vitro testing is performed on expectorated sputum. Expectorated sputum is the most easily obtained airway secretion, and therefore it has been best studied. Sputum is a complex and heterogeneous mixture of periciliary fluid, mucus glycoprotein gel, inflammatory cells, effete epithelial cells, inflammatory mediators, bacteria, and salivary contamination. While at this time no sputum properties have been identified that can convincingly distinguish one pulmonary disease from another, certain sputum characteristics are associated with specific disease processes and changes in properties that would be associated with the successful application of mechanical or pharmacological mucokinetic therapy (4).

For purposes of in vitro testing, it could be extremely useful to have a standard artificial mucus with composition and biophysical properties closely approximating that of "real" sputum. Such an artificial sputum should contain polymerized mucin and DNA, and its composition and properties should be readily modified to be representative of specific disease states. This simulant should be readily and consistently available in quantities that make standardized testing possible.

III. In Vitro Measurements

Changes in the biophysical properties of sputum can indicate the mechanism of a drug effect on sputum and suggest effective dose ranges. The primary bulk biophysical properties are rheology (viscoelasticity) and cohesivity (approximated by the measurement of spinnability).

For most mucolytic or mucokinetic agents, the most important in vitro tests to conduct are sputum transportability measurements. The mucociliary transportability (MCTR) of sputum is usually measured on the mucus-depleted frog palate (5) or on an excised mammalian trachea (6). To date, only a few studies have been published evaluating MCTR in a mammalian airway. Colc and colleagues have reported a significantly slower MCTR on the bovine trachea than on the frog palate, but there was no correlation between the two systems (6).

The rheology of mucus is its capacity to undergo flow and deformation (7). A Hookian (ideal) solid responds to a stress with a finite deformation that is completely recovered after the stress is removed. This stored energy is described by elasticity (G'). A Newtonian liquid responds to a stress by deforming (flowing) while a stress is applied, and after removing the stress, flow ceases and there is no strain recovery. This energy loss is viscosity (G''). A gel such as mucus initially stores energy like a solid and with continued stress will flow like a liquid.

The viscoelastic behavior of mucus is thought to be one of the major determinants of mucociliary clearance rate. Studies using mucus simulant gels (made from crosslinked vegetable gums) indicate that mucociliary transport on the frog palate (MCTR) is impeded by increasing mucus mechanical impedance (G^*) but increases with greater mucus recoil (8). However, the relationship between the properties of actual airway secretions and MCTR is unclear. Giordano et al. studied the tracheal mucus velocity of dogs and found a negative correlation between the tracheal clearance rate and the elasticity of mucus secreted in a tracheal pouch (9). Puchelle and colleagues calculated the rheological conditions for mucociliary transport in a small group of patients with chronic bronchitis (CB). Optimal transport was associated with an apparent viscosity (h0) of 25–180 poise, a strain recovery of 4–12 units, and an elastic modulus (G') of 4–8 dyne/cm-cm (10). More recently, this same group studied sputum collected from 29 patients with cystic fibrosis (CF). Significant negative correlations between MCTR and sputum elasticity ($r = -0.63$, $p < 0.01$), and between the cough transport and contact angle of the sputum ($r = -0.81$, $p < 0.0001$) were demonstrated (11). Although these studies suggest that elasticity or the viscosity/elasticity ratio of mucus is inversely correlated with MCTR, recent studies have shown no relationship between MCTR and rheology (12). These earlier studies were observational, correlative, and conducted in a small number of patients. In each, there were differences in instruments used to evaluate sputum properties and large standard deviations in measured variables.

In vitro cough transportability (CTR) can be measured in a simulated cough machine (13). There is a consensus that sputum surface properties are critically important for CTR but that there is little dependence on viscoelasticity (14–17). The absence of a strong relationship between sputum viscosity and cough clearability can be understood by the following analogy. If a pea shooter is taken to represent the airway, a longer shot (better cough) is obtained using a whole pea rather than pea soup, which acts like mucus that has been thinned by a mucolytic. Extending the analogy, the pea will go further if it is first lubricated.

Sputum cohesivity has been correlated positively with mucociliary clearance on the frog palate (18), but negatively with cough clearability (CTR) using a simulated cough machine (14). Tenacity is the force of separation (in dynes), and we calculate this as the product of cohesivity and adhesive work (W_{ad}). If we assume that mucus is a liquid that wets the solid epithelium below, then Young's equation allows us to calculate W_{ad} between the mucus and epithelial surfaces as $\gamma (1 + \cos \theta)$, where γ is the interfacial tension of secretions in air and θ is the contact angle of mucus on the epithelium. The contact angle measures the wettability of a solid surface with surface energy of the airway epithelium. Interfacial tension at an air/gel interface is most accurately measured using the de Noüy platinum ring method. We have recently modified this technique to enable us to measure the interfacial tension of microliter quantities of secretions (16). This permits us to directly calculate W_{ad} and tenacity. These studies confirm that sputum tenacity is the strongest predictor of in vitro CTR (19).

IV. Animal and Tissue Studies

Techniques for growing a well-differentiated epithelium at an air/liquid interface have permitted some studies to first be performed in cell culture systems. For example, the effect of ion or water transport modifiers can be evaluated by measuring the bioelectric properties of airway tissue culture (20). Cell culture systems are of limited use in assessing mucus secretion and clearance.

Evaluating the efficacy of mucoregulatory agents requires the assessment of mucus secretion in both the normal and the inflamed airway. This can be done using whole animals or airway tissue explants (21). The secretory cells of the human airway include surface goblet cells and submucous glands, both contributing to the mucus layer covering a profuse ciliary blanket. Smaller experimental animals such as mice, rats, hamsters, and guinea pigs have a simple airway secretory epithelium, unlike that of larger animals. Thus, whole-animal or explant studies are generally performed using ferrets, dogs, cats, sheep, or primates. Whole-animal studies are particularly valuable for the evaluation of inflammatory mediator release in the inflamed airway and suppression of inflammation-associated hypersecretion by drugs (such as anti-inflammatory drugs or cytokines) that are biological response modifiers. These whole-organ studies also allow the simultaneous measurement of mucociliary clearance and ciliary beat frequency in the same tissue preparation.

V. In Vivo and Clinical Testing

The purpose of clinical testing is to establish the safety and efficacy of an intervention such as the administration of a mucoactive agent. Unfortunately, there are few animal models of chronic airway disease, and the response of nonhuman species can be quite different from that of humans.

Testing should assess the potential toxicity of medications, bioavailability including sputum penetrance, pharmacokinetics, and pharmacodynamics, which may well be different in the airway than systemically, and patient tolerance of both the drug and the delivery system, as this can strongly can influence adherence to therapy.

In clinical trials, one of the difficulties is determining the most appropriate population to study. The clinical variability of the disease studied must be taken into account. In patients with very slowly changing disease, the duration of therapy and the duration of observation will likely need to be much greater than in those with rapidly progressive disease. In many diseases this can be confounded by age, gender, and even by cultural differences (e.g., the social acceptability of sputum expectoration). Thus, it is important to define a disease as clearly as possible. Chronic obstructive pulmonary disease (COPD) encompasses both emphysema and chronic bronchitis, but mucoactive agents will be more effective in those persons with a predominantly chronic bronchitis clinical profile.

One of the more difficult questions is if evaluation should be done while the patient is clinically stable or during an "acute exacerbation" of disease. This is confounded by conflicting definitions of exacerbation. Outcome measures during an acute exacerbation could include the duration of the exacerbation, need for hospital admission, and rapidity of resolution, but many of these are highly subjective and might be influenced by medications given concomitantly during the acute illness.

Older patients with COPD often have confounding diseases such as cardiac disease or diabetes. Either these diseases or the medications used to control these medical conditions could affect the outcome of a clinical trial, as could unanticipated medication interactions. Adherence to a medical regimen becomes more difficult if a patient is taking a large number of medications, especially if he or she has trouble understanding how and why medications are to be used. Difficulty with adherence could be as straightforward as refusal to take medication as prescribed or as complex as ineffective use of medication-delivery devices. This has been reported to be a particularly difficult problem when patents use aerosol devices to administer medications—an important issue when using topical mucoactive medications.

Because the efficacy of a novel therapy is often best assessed during a clinical trial in a homogeneous population likely to be adherent to a therapeutic protocol, CF patients are often chosen to be the first group studied when evaluating a novel mucoactive medication or device (22). However, CF can be widely variable in presentation and outcome, there are genetic differences in the CFTR gene and socioeconomic differences that could influence outcomes, and confounding concurrent diseases, such as liver disease or diabetes, both more common in the CF population. In fact, something as simple—and variable—as different degrees of airway obstruction among patients can influence airway deposition and clearance and thus the efficacy of an aerosol medication.

Identification of an appropriate control population may be more important than identifying a uniform patient population to study. Comparisons of a specific therapy to another medication or especially against another airway clearance technique can be very difficult. It is particularly difficult to monitor protocol adherence and to devise appropriate masking (blinding), if possible, for the assessment of mucus clearance devices (23).

In clinical trials, power calculations are generally made for a single primary outcome variable. This presupposes foreknowledge of the most sensitive and specific outcome of interest as well as sufficient baseline or longitudinal data in a similar population to evaluate measurement variability. There are few large longitudinal studies evaluating any outcome other than pulmonary function testing, making this the most commonly used clinical endpoint to evaluate mucoactive therapy. However, as discussed elsewhere, it is clear that lung volume and flow correlate poorly with other measures of efficacy.

Because of these difficulties, other surrogate endpoints have been used to evaluate mucoactive therapy. These have included both fairly precise measurements of radioaerosol deposition and clearance as well as theoretically attractive but poorly standardized measures such as quality of life. Both of these measurements are discussed in greater detail later in this chapter. Other clinical measures that have been used for studies of therapeutic agents in chronic lung disease include days in hospital or days of IV antibiotic therapy during the duration of the study, the frequency and length of exacerbations of pulmonary disease, and the rate of pulmonary function decline over time.

Measuring the frequency and severity of exacerbations (COPD or CF) and disease-related mortality requires studies of long duration with large numbers of patients. This is not only costly, but may miss other clinically important outcomes.

Finally, changes in the concentration of inflammatory mediators or DNA in sputum may reflect improved mucus clearance because expectoration will decrease the burden of pro-inflammatory stimuli in the airway. Pilot studies suggest that the sputum concentration of some mediators associated with neutrophilic inflammation (e.g., interleukin-8, DNA, myeloperoxidase) may correlate with temporal changes in pulmonary function, but further research is needed before these can be recommended as reliable outcomes for clinical trials of mucoactive agents.

VI. In Vivo Outcome Variables in Short-Term Studies

A. Pulmonary Function Changes

It has often been assumed that mucus has a measurable effect on pulmonary function and that improvement of mucus transport will improve pulmonary function. Retention of mucus can theoretically have several effects on lung function depending on the amount and localization of mucus. Relatively small amounts of mucus in small peripheral airways may reduce airway diameter and contribute to airflow obstruction. Therefore, in many studies, forced expiratory flow variables are used to evaluate the effect of airway clearance interventions. However, the relationship between mucus in the airways and pulmonary function is weak. Mucous gland size can be assessed by the gland:wall ratio (Reid index) (24), by absolute gland area, and by the volume proportion of glands. The volume of sputum expectorated has been reported to be significantly related to the volume proportion of mucous glands ($R = 0.53$) and to the absolute gland area ($R = 0.49$), but not to the Reid index ($R = 0.35$). Neither the Reid Index nor the volume proportion of glands was related to the forced expiratory volume in one second (FEV_1), and the measurements were not significantly related to each other. Also, the measurement of forced expiratory airflow does not seem to reflect changes in mucus transport or retention of mucus. The effects of sputum on pulmonary function were investigated by Cochrane et al. (25). These authors assessed pulmonary function before and after the application of chest physiotherapy and found that after chest physiotherapy specific conductance (SG_{AW}) was reduced without a significant change in FEV_1. The improvement in SG_{AW} was not related to the volume of mucus that was expectorated. These authors speculated that redistribution of mucus throughout the airways due to chest physiotherapy was responsible for the reduction in SG_{AW}. In many other studies no effect of airway clearance was seen on expiratory flow variables (26–33)

Mucus can also completely obstruct some airways and thus influence static lung volumes and volume of trapped gas. Regnis et al. (34) found in CF patients a significant correlation between mucus transport and the RV/TLC ratio ($R = -0.39$), indicating that slow mucus transport is associated with relatively high RV/TLC ratio. The relatively low correlation coefficients make it unlikely that changes in mucus transport due to intervention can be detected by measurement of lung volumes alone, especially in studies with a relatively small number of subjects.

The popularity of using pulmonary function tests is based more on the availability of the instruments than on a theoretical basis related to the question of evaluating changes in mucus transport or mucus retention.

B.   Radiography

Severe retention of mucus in the airways may result in complete obstruction of the airway (mucus plugging) (35). Evaluation of measures to remove the mucus plug, such as bronchoscopy, endotracheal suctioning, or chest physiotherapy, is sometimes done by chest radiography. However, studies have shown that radiography is insensitive for detecting this "mucus-plugging syndrome" and is thus insensitive for detecting improvement of mucus plugging. Pham et al. (36) studied eight patients with complete interruption of ventilation to an entire lung. These authors found that chest radiography failed to reveal the extent of the obstruction. Bray and colleagues (37) also studied a group of patients with major bronchial obstruction by mucous plugs. The chest radiographs of these patients generally did not reflect the severity of the airway obstruction and in some instances were completely normal. Dee et al. (38) described two quadriplegic patients with clinical and ventilation scan signs of severe mucus plugging. Both patients had normal chest radiography.

C.   Volume of Expectorated Sputum

Intuitively, the straightforward measurement of expectorated sputum volume might be a useful method to evaluate the effectiveness of therapeutic interventions directed toward improving mucus clearance. Measuring the volume of expectorated mucus can give a global impression of transport assuming that mucus production in the airways is stable during the time of the measurements. However, sputum volume measurements are highly variable and nonreproducible, at best, and usually inaccurate because of patient reticence to expectorate, inadvertent swallowing of secretions, and salivary contamination of secretions that are expectorated. Contamination with saliva can be partially corrected by drying the mucus and taking the dry weight for analysis, but interventions that stimulate mucus secretion can change the hydration of expectorated secretions by more than 50%, making wet-to-dry weight calculations of expectorant invalid. The actual volume of secretions expectorated is extremely variable from day to day and even at different times of the day, with greater volumes generally produced in the early morning. Finally, increased volumes of collected secretions could as easily represent increased production of mucus as increased clearance.

The correlation between the volume of expectorated mucus and mucus transport in the airways has been reported to be poor but statistically significant ($R = 0.39$, $p < 0.05$) (39). An explanation for the poor correlation is that mucus transport and sputum volume measure intrinsically different things. There is little difference in the transport velocity of a thick mucus layer and a thin mucus layer, but the volume of sputum expectorated may be very different.

D. Local Tracer Imaging

Timing the transport rate of a local tracer that is deposited onto the bronchial mucus layer can assess the transport velocity of mucus in the human airways (40). A bolus of tracer is deposited on the large airways through a bronchoscope or by inhalation. The movement of the tracer can be visualized by bronchoscopy or measured by scintigraphy if radiolabeled particles are used. Using this technique care should be taken that airway cilia are not damaged because this will disturb mucus transport. Zwas et al. (41) investigated local mucus transport rate in healthy subjects. In this study the mean (s.d.) transport rate of mucus was reported to be 4.7 (1.3) mm/min. The authors report that the variance is smaller using this technique as compared to other radioactive tracer techniques to measure mucus transport velocity.

E. Whole-Lung Tracer Imaging

The transport of mucus in the whole lung can be measured by using a tracer that is deposited in the central as well as the peripheral airways. Theoretically, two types of tracers can be used: a radiopaque tracer or a radioactive tracer.

When using a radiopaque tracer, usually tantalum, the tracer is usually introduced as an aerosol through an endotracheal tube and is deposited in the airways. The clearance of the tracer is monitored radiographically. The amount of tracer remaining in the lungs after a given time interval is expressed as a percentage of the initial amount. This technique is invasive, can potentially damage the airways, and uses a relatively high radiation dose depending on the number of chest radiographs.

To measure mucus clearance using a radioactive aerosol tracer, the tracer aerosol is inhaled and deposits on the airway surface. The effect of the radioactivity on mucus transport seems to be minimal. The amount of radioactive tracer is counted using a gamma camera or scintillation counters. Using a gamma camera for recording the tracer has the disadvantage that relatively more radioactivity is necessary, but one advantage is that the initial deposition pattern can be visualized. Thereby, corrections can be made for deposition in the esophagus or stomach, and this permits recording radioactivity in different regions of interest, allowing quantification of the initial deposition pattern and estimation of regional clearance. Assessment of regional clearance is limited because only two-dimensional images can be obtained.

In general, the transport (clearance) rate measured using a tracer technique is dependent on the site of deposition (42). The site of deposition can be quantified by calculating the ratio between peripheral and central deposition (P/C) or by measuring the retention after 24 hours representing alveolar deposition. Using the P/C ratio, the outer regions the lungs are visualized with an 81 Krm ventilation image or a transmission scan (43). The P/C ratio and 24-hour retention are equally accurate to quantify the site of deposition (42). The P/C ratio has the advantage that it is less time consuming. The site of deposition of an aerosol in the bronchial tree depends on the inspiratory maneuver and the characteristics of the aerosol. Inspiratory flow is inversely related to the depth of the deposition such that high inspiratory flow increases central deposition. Particle size influences the deposition pattern; larger particles are deposited more centrally, but there is little effect on mucus transport (42).

The reproducibility of the radioactive tracer technique has been investigated in healthy subjects, asymptomatic smokers, asthmatics, persons with chronic bronchitis, and patients with bronchiectasis (44). There was an intersubject coefficient of variation of 13% for the healthy subjects and of 28–39% for the other groups. The intrasubject coefficient of variation was about half of these values.

VII. In Vivo Outcome Variables: Long-Term Studies

A. Decline in Pulmonary Function

It can be hypothesized that improved mucus clearance may affect the rate of decline in pulmonary function over the years by reducing the number of pulmonary infections and exacerbations. This is supported by epidemiological data from the Copenhagen study (45–47). In this study it was found that chronic mucus hypersecretion is associated with excess decline in pulmonary function, with more frequent hospitalization, and with COPD-related death due to pulmonary infection. In a small number of studies, comparing different forms of chest physiotherapy, the rate of decline in pulmonary function was used as an outcome variable (48–51). Differences between different treatment protocols were found, but no specific form of chest physiotherapy could be considered as superior to others.

In order to evaluate the rate of change in pulmonary function over time, clinical trials with long observation times and large numbers of patients are needed.

B. Exercise Capacity

Exercise capacity is related to adequate ventilation, gas exchange, blood circulation, oxygen transport, and muscle mass. Airway mucus retention can affect ventilation and gas exchange and can lead to gas trapping (increased RV/TLC), in part, by decreasing the efficiency of the diaphragm. Tests to measure functional exercise capacity include both laboratory tests like treadmill or bicycle ergometry and field tests like the 6- or 12-minute walking tests (52), the shuttle run or walking test (53), and the step test (54). The 6-minute walking test is most frequently used to evaluate functional exercise capacity. The minimal clinically relevant difference in 6-minute walking distance is probably greater than 50 m (55). Smaller changes may theoretically be a more sensitive indicator of mucus clearance than usual pulmonary function measurements.

C. Dyspnea

Dyspnea is a common symptom in those patients with pulmonary disease and compromised pulmonary function. The sensation of dyspnea is complicated, but receptors in the inspiratory muscles and the lungs are thought to be involved (56). The relationship between dyspnea airway mucus retention is unclear. When mucus has a measurable effect on pulmonary function, a link to dyspnea can be hypothesized. Common measures to quantify dyspnea include the Borg score, MRC score, oxygen cost diagram, and baseline dyspnea index (57).

D. Quality of Life Scores

Hypersecretion, reduced mucus transport, and airflow obstruction are impairments, while chronic coughing and sputum expectoration or dyspnea can limit the patient in daily or recreational activities and can therefore be classified as disability. Chronic coughing, expectoration, and dyspnea can also limit the patient in his or her social functioning and thus lead to a handicap. Thus, the effects of mucoactive drugs or mucus clearance techniques can also be evaluated as these relate to disability or handicap. An intervention might decrease the impairment severity by improving bronchial mucus transport but could paradoxically have negative effects on disability or handicap due to dependence on another person or a complicated device or the need to regularly take medication. This in turn might limit adherence to therapy. There are few data concerning the psychological and social aspects of mucoactive therapy and mucus clearance techniques.

E. Quality of Life Scores: Generic Questionnaires

These questionnaires can be used either in the general population or in patients with disease. An advantage to these questionnaires is that comparisons can be made between patients and healthy subjects. However, the questions in these questionnaires do not address the specific problems of patients, and the sensitivity for change due to mucoactive therapy is thus low. Examples of generic questionnaires are the SF-36 (58) and the NHP (59,60).

F. Quality of Life Scores: Disease-Specific Questionnaires

Disease-specific questionnaires have been developed to evaluate health-related quality of life. In contrast to generic questionnaires, comparison between groups of patients and healthy subjects is usually not possible. Examples of disease-specific health-related quality of life (QOL) questionnaires are the St. George Respiratory Disease Questionnaire (SGRQ), the Chronic Respiratory Disease Questionnaire (CRDQ), the Breathing Problem Questionnaire (BPQ), and the questionnaire for patients with breathing problems.

The SGRQ was developed by Jones at al. (61) and has been validated in many countries and in different languages. The SGRQ contains questions across four dimensions: symptoms, activity, impact, and a total score. Some of the questions in the symptom dimension are related to mucus expectoration. However, only the presence or absence of the symptom is scored.

The CRDQ was developed by Gyatt et al. (62) for patients with chronic airflow limitation. The CRDQ contains 20 items, which are categorized into four dimensions: dyspnea, fatigue, emotion, and mastery. The BPQ was developed by Hyland et al. (63) and covers 13 domains.

None of these questionnaires has been validated for the specific use of measuring the efficacy of mucoactive therapy.

G. Quality of Life Scores: Symptom-Specific Questionnaires

Another category of questionnaires is developed specifically for a major symptom or symptom complex. One disease-specific questionnaire specifically for problems related to mucus is the Petty score (64). Petty and colleagues developed a questionnaire specifically designed to evaluate the clinical impact of mucoactive therapy in patients with chronic bronchitis. We have extensively evaluated this tool in patients with CF or chronic bronchitis and found that while there appears to be correlations with sputum physical properties and clearability, the Petty score is not sensitive for detecting changes in clinical status related to effective mucoactive interventions (65).

H. Days in Hospital, Days of Additional Therapy

Improvement of bronchial mucus transport is thought to reduce the retention of infected secretions and thus the frequency of respiratory tract infections. As a consequence it could be expected that the frequency of respiratory tract infections is related to days in hospital. Reisman and colleagues compared a breathing technique (which they termed the forced expiratory technique, although this differs from the FET as described in the literature) and "conventional chest physiotherapy" in a cohort of patients with CF, and no differences were found in the frequency of hospitalization (50). Although in two studies assessing the effect of PEP breathing there were fewer exacerbations (48,66), in another study of PEP (49) this could not be confirmed.

VIII. Summary

Mucus secretion and clearance is a complex physiological interaction that is greatly affected by disease, medical therapy, and a variety of nonmedical and cultural factors. Most of the time we cannot determine in advance which patients are likely to benefit from mucoactive therapy, and the effectiveness of therapy in an individual patient can be difficult to assess. When a patient feels significantly better and there is clear improvement in measured airflow and/or a reduction in trapped thoracic gas, this judgment is easy. However, changes in FEV_1, while excellent for assessing acute bronchodilator response in asthma, only poorly reflect clinical improvement with mucoactive therapy. Thus, clinical trials to assess the efficacy of mucoactive therapy must take into account this complexity, and assessment outcomes will differ depending upon the therapy being evaluated, the stage of evaluation (phases of drug or device development), the patient population being studied, and the comparison or control group being compared.

References

1. Rubin BK. An in vitro comparison of the mucoactive properties of guaifenesin, iodinated glycerol, surfactant, and albuterol. Chest 1999; 116:195–200.
2. Kim JS, Hackley GH, Okamoto K, Rubin BK. Sputum processing for evaluation of inflammatory mediators. Pediatr Pulmonol 2001; 32:152–158.
3. Ripoll L, Reinert P, Pepin LF, Lagrange PH. Interaction of macrolides with alpha dornase during DNA hydrolysis. J Antimicrob Chemother 1996; 37:987–991.
4. King M, Rubin BK. Mucus physiology and pathophysiology. In: Derenne JP, Whitelaw WA, Similowski T, eds. Acute Respiratory Failure in Chronic Obstructive Pulmonary Disease. New York: Marcel Dekker, 1996:391–411.
5. Rubin BK, Ramirez O, King M. Mucus-depleted frog palate as a model for the study of mucociliary clearance. J Appl Physiol 1990; 69:424–429.
6. Wills PJ, Garcia-Suarez MJ, Rutman A, Wilson R, Cole PJ. The ciliary transportability of sputum is slow on the mucus-depleted bovine trachea. Am J Respir Crit Care Med 1995; 151:1255–1258.
7. King M, Rubin BK. Mucus rheology, relationship with transport. In: Takishima T, Shimura S, eds. Airway Secretion: Physiological Bases for the Control of Mucous Hypersecretion. New York: Marcel Dekker, 1994:283–314.
8. King M. Relationship between mucus viscoelasticity and ciliary transport in guaran gel/frog palate model system. Biorheology 1980; 17:249–254.
9. Giordano A, Shih CK, Holsclaw DS, Khan MA, Litt M. Mucus clearance: in vivo canine tracheal vs. in vitro bullfrog palate studies. J Appl Physiol 1977; 42:761–766.
10. Puchelle E, Zahm JM, Girard F, Bertrand A, Polu JM, Aug F, et al. Mucociliary transport in vivo and in vitro. Relations to sputum properties in chronic bronchitis. Eur J Respir Dis 1980; 61:254–264.
11. Deneuville E, Perrot-Minot C, Pennaforte F, Roussey M, Zahm JM, Clavel C, et al. Revisited physicochemical and transport properties of respiratory mucus in genotyped cystic fibrosis patients. Am J Respir Crit Care Med 1997; 156:166–172.
12. Macchione M, King M, Lorenzi-Filho G, Guimaraes ET, Zin WA, Bohm GM, et al. Rheological determinants of mucociliary transport in the nose of the rat. Respir Physiol 1995; 99:165–172.
13. Agarwal M, King M, Rubin BK, Shukla JB. Mucus transport in a miniaturized

simulated cough machine: effect of constriction and serous layer simulant. Biorheology 1989; 26:977–988.

14. King M, Zahm JM, Pierrot D, Vaquez-Girod S, Puchelle E. The role of mucus gel viscosity, spinnability, and adhesive properties in clearance by simulated cough. Biorheology 1989; 26:737–745.

15. Zahm JM, Pierrot D, Vaquez-Girod S, Duvivier C, King M, Puchelle E. The role of mucus sol phase in clearance by simulated cough. Biorheology 1989; 26:747–752.

16. Albers GM, Tomkiewicz RP, May MK, Ramirez OE, Rubin BK. Ring distraction technique for measuring surface tension of sputum: relationship to sputum clearability. J Appl Physiol 1996; 81:2690–2695.

17. Girod S, Galabert C, Pierrot D, Boissonnade MM, Zahm JM, Baszkin A, et al. Role of phospholipid lining on respiratory mucus clearance by cough. J Appl Physiol 1991; 71:2262–2266.

18. Puchelle E, Zahm JM, Duvivier C. Spinability of bronchial mucus. Relationship with viscoelasticity and mucous transport properties. Biorheology 1983; 20:239–249.

19. Rubin BK. Surface properties of respiratory secretions: relationship to mucus transport. In: Baum GL, Priel Z, Roth Y, Liron N, Ostfeld EJ, eds. Cilia, Mucus, and Mucociliary Interactions. New York: Marcel Dekker, 1998:317–324.

20. Wooten R. Biophysical properties and polymeric structure of artificial mucus and sputum produced by copolymerizing mucin and DNA. 2000.

21. Kishioka C, Okamoto K, Kim J, Rubin BK. Regulation of secretion from mucous and serous cells in the excised ferret trachea. Respir Physiol 2001; 126:163–171.

22. Rubin BK, Tomkiewicz RP, King M. Mucoactive agents. In: Wilmott RW, ed. The Pediatric Lung. Basel, Switzerland: Birkhauser Publishing, 1997:155–179.

23. van der Schans CP, Postma DS, Koeter GH, Rubin BK. Physiotherapy and bronchial mucus transport. Eur Respir J 1999; 13:1477–1486.

24. Reid L. An experimental study of hypersecretion of mucus in the bronchial tree. Br J Exp Path 1963; 44:437–445.

25. Cochrane GM, Webber BA, Clarke SW. Effects of sputum on pulmonary function. Br Med J 1977; 2:1181–1183.

26. Oldenburg FA Jr, Dolovich MB, Montgomery JM, Newhouse MT. Effects of postural drainage, exercise, and cough on mucus clearance in chronic bronchitis. Am Rev Respir Dis 1979; 120:739–745.

27. May DB, Munt PW. Physiologic effects of chest percussion and postural drainage in patients with stable chronic bronchitis. Chest 1979; 75:29–32.

28. Maloney FP, Fernandez E, Hudgel DW. Postural drainage effect after bronchodilator inhalation in patients with chronic airway obstruction. Arch Phys Med Rehabil 1981; 62:452–455.

29. Mazzocco MC, Owens GR, Kirilloff LH, Rogers RM. Chest percussion and postural drainage in patients with bronchiectasis. Chest 1985; 88:360–363.

30. Gallon A. Evaluation of chest percussion in the treatment of patients with copious sputum production. Respir Med 1991; 85:45–51.

31. van Hengstum M, Festen J, Beurskens C, Hankel M, van den Broek W, Buijs W, et al. The effect of positive expiratory pressure versus forced expiration technique

on tracheobronchial clearance in chronic bronchitics. Scand J Gastroenterol Suppl 1988; 143:114–118.

32. Sutton PP, Gemmell HG, Innes N, Davidson J, Smith FW, Legge JS, et al. Use of nebulised saline and nebulised terbutaline as an adjunct to chest physiotherapy. Thorax 1988; 43:57–60.

33. van Hengstum M, Festen J, Beurskens C, Hankel M, van den Broek W, Corstens F. No effect of oral high frequency oscillation combined with forced expiration manoeuvres on tracheobronchial clearance in chronic bronchitis. Eur Respir J 1990; 3:14–18.

34. Regnis JA, Alison JA, Henke KG, Donnelly PM, Bye PT. Changes in end-expiratory lung volume during exercise in cystic fibrosis relate to severity of lung disease. Am Rev Respir Dis 1991; 144(3 pt 1):507–512.

35. Vereen LE, Payne DK, George RB. Unilateral absence of ventilation and perfusion associated with a bronchial mucous plug. South Med J 1987; 80:391–393.

36. Pham DH, Huang D, Korwan A, Greyson ND. Acute unilateral pulmonary nonventilation due to mucous plugs. Radiology 1987; 165:135–137.

37. Bray ST, Johnstone WH, Dee PM, Pope TL, Jr., Teates CD, Tegtmeyer CJ. The "mucous plug syndrome": a pulmonary embolism mimic. Clin Nucl Med 1984; 9: 513–518.

38. Dee PM, Suratt PM, Bray ST, Rose CE, Jr. Mucous plugging simulating pulmonary embolism in patients with quadriplegia. Chest 1984; 85:363–366.

39. Mortensen J, Falk M, Groth S, Jensen C. The effects of postural drainage and positive expiratory pressure physiotherapy on tracheobronchial clearance in cystic fibrosis. Chest 1991; 100:1350–1357.

40. Konrad FX, Schreiber T, Brecht Kraus D, Georgieff M. Bronchial mucus transport in chronic smokers and nonsmokers during general anesthesia. J Clin Anesth 1993; 5:375–380.

41. Zwas ST, Katz I, Belfer B, Baum GL, Aharonson E. Scintigraphic monitoring of mucociliary tracheo-bronchial clearance of technetium-99m macroaggregated albumin aerosol. J Nucl Med 1987; 28:161–167.

42. Ilowite JS, Smaldone GC, Perry RJ, Bennett WD, Foster WM. Relationship between tracheobronchial particle clearance rates and sites of initial deposition in man. Arch Environ Health 1989; 44:267–273.

43. Bjure J. Ergometry and physical training in pediatrics with special reference to pulmonary function. Acta Paediatr Scand Suppl 1971; 217:56–59.

44. Thomson ML, Pavia D. Particle penetration and clearance in the human lung. Results in healthy subjects and subjects with chronic bronchitis. Arch Environ Health 1974; 29:214–219.

45. Vestbo J, Prescott E, Lange P. Association of chronic mucus hypersecretion with FEV1 decline and chronic obstructive pulmonary disease morbidity. Copenhagen City Heart Study Group. Am J Respir Crit Care Med 1996; 153:1530–1535.

46. Lange P, Vestbo J, Nyboe J. Risk factors for death and hospitalization from pneumonia. A prospective study of a general population. Eur Respir J 1995; 8:1694–1698.

47. Prescott E, Lange P, Vestbo J. Chronic mucus hypersecretion in COPD and death from pulmonary infection. Eur Respir J 1995; 8:1333–1338.

48. Christensen EF, Nedergaard T, Dahl R. Long-term treatment of chronic bronchitis with positive expiratory pressure mask and chest physiotherapy. Chest 1990; 97: 645–650.

49. Christensen HR, Simonsen K, Lange P, Clementsen P, Kampmann JP, Viskum K, et al. PEEP-masks in patients with severe obstructive pulmonary disease: a negative report. Eur Respir J 1990; 3:267–272.

50. Reisman JJ, Rivington Law B, Corey M, Marcotte J, Wannamaker E, Harcourt D, et al. Role of conventional physiotherapy in cystic fibrosis. J Pediatr 1988; 113: 632–636.

51. McIlwaine PM, Wong LT, Peacock D, Davidson AG. Long-term comparative trial of conventional postural drainage and percussion versus positive expiratory pressure physiotherapy in the treatment of cystic fibrosis. J Pediatr 1997; 131:570–574.

52. McGavin CR, Gupta SP, McHardy GJ. Twelve-minute walking test for assessing disability in chronic bronchitis. Br Med J 1976; 1:822–823.

53. Singh SJ, Morgan MD, Scott S, Walters D, Hardman AE. Development of a shuttle walking test of disability in patients with chronic airways obstruction. Thorax 1992; 47:1019–1024.

54. Balfour-Lynn IM, Prasad SA, Laverty A, Whitehead BF, Dinwiddie R. A step in the right direction: assessing exercise tolerance in cystic fibrosis. Pediatr Pulmonol 1998; 25:278–284.

55. Redelmeier DA, Bayoumi AM, Goldstein RS, Guyatt GH. Interpreting small differences in functional status: the Six Minute Walk test in chronic lung disease patients. Am J Respir Crit Care Med 1997; 155:1278–1282.

56. Killian KJ, Gandevia SC, Summers E, Campbell EJ. Effect of increased lung volume on perception of breathlessness, effort, and tension. J Appl Physiol 1984; 57: 686–691.

57. Mahler DA, Rosiello RA, Harver A, Lentine T, McGovern JF, Daubenspeck JA. Comparison of clinical dyspnea ratings and psychophysical measurements of respiratory sensation in obstructive airway disease. Am Rev Respir Dis 1987; 135: 1229–1233.

58. Mahler DA, Mackowiak JI. Evaluation of the short-form 36-item questionnaire to measure health-related quality of life in patients with COPD. Chest 1995; 107: 1585–1589.

59. Congleton J, Hodson ME, Duncan Skingle F. Do Nottingham Health Profile scores change over time in cystic fibrosis? Respir Med 1998; 92:268–272.

60. Congleton J, Hodson ME, Duncan Skingle F. Quality of life in adults with cystic fibrosis. Thorax 1996; 51:936–940.

61. Jones PW, Quirk FH, Baveystock CM, Littlejohns P. A self-complete measure of health status for chronic airflow limitation. The St. George's Respiratory Questionnaire. Am Rev Respir Dis 1992; 145:1321–1327.

62. Guyatt GH, Berman LB, Townsend M, Pugsley SO, Chambers LW. A measure of quality of life for clinical trials in chronic lung disease. Thorax 1987; 42:773–778.

63. Hyland ME, Singh SJ, Sodergren SC, Morgan MP. Development of a shortened version of the Breathing Problems Questionnaire suitable for use in a pulmonary rehabilitation clinic: a purpose-specific, disease-specific questionnaire. Qual Life Res 1998; 7:227–233.

64. Petty TL. The National Mucolytic Study. Results of a randomized, double- blind, placebo-controlled study of iodinated glycerol in chronic obstructive bronchitis. Chest 1990; 97:75–83.
65. Piquette CA, Clarkson L, Okamoto K, Kim JS, Rubin BK. Respiratory-related quality of life: relation to pulmonary function, functional exercise capacity, and sputum biophysical properties. J Aerosol Med 2000; 13:263–272.
66. McIlwaine PM, Wong LT, Peacock D, Davidson AG. Long-term comparative trial of conventional postural drainage and percussion versus positive expiratory pressure physiotherapy in the treatment of cystic fibrosis. J Pediatr 1997; 131:570–574.

5

Adherence with the Use of Clearance Techniques

JANICE ABBOTT

University of Central Lancashire
Preston, England

**MARY E. DODD and
A. KEVIN WEBB**

Wythenshawe Hospital
Manchester, England

I. Introduction

The primary host defense mechanisms for removing respiratory secretions and inhaled debris are the mucociliary escalator and the cough. When these defense mechanisms are impaired by dysfunction (primary ciliary dyskinesia) or decreased airflow (airways obstruction) or overwhelmed by hypersecretion (chronic bronchitis, bronchial asthma, bronchiectasis, and cystic fibrosis), mucus is expectorated or retained in the airways. Airway clearance techniques (Table 1) are then introduced to improve mucociliary transport, reduce mucus retention, and improve the efficiency and effectiveness of expectoration (1). Various forced and unforced expiratory maneuvers are applied to mobilize and remove secretions, and the techniques are conventionally defined as "chest physiotherapy." Airway clearance may be prescribed in the short term for acute symptoms or prophylactically on a daily basis when hypersecretion becomes chronic. The value of chest physiotherapy on mucociliary clearance is well established for both patients who expectorate large volumes of sputum (2) and those who do not expectorate mucus (3). Exercise has become a recognized airway-clearance technique. It has been shown to improve mucociliary clearance (4) and sputum expectoration (5,6).

Table 1 Airway Clearance Techniques

Active cycle of breathing techniques
Positive expiratory pressure
High-pressure PEP
Flutter
Autogenic drainage
Exercise
Intrapulmonary percussive ventilation
High-frequency chest wall oscillation
Postural drainage and percussion

When regular chest physiotherapy is considered as a necessary treatment to prevent or delay pulmonary decline, patients are taught individualized techniques, tailored to their lung disease and lifestyle. It is then usually accepted that this program of care is continued by the patient until the patient dies or receives a transplant. For some, this period of time is their lifetime. Integrating daily chest physiotherapy into a normal lifestyle and maintaining the treatment over many years can be difficult, and the reasons for not complying are complex. This chapter discusses the many issues surrounding adherence and nonadherence: why it is important, how it is measured, the barriers to and the predictors of treatment adherence, the clinical and psychosocial consequences of nonadherence, the effectiveness of interventions, and strategies to enhance adherence.

II. Why Is Treatment Adherence Important?

When a patient is prescribed a particular course of treatment, it is based on knowledge from empirical sources and consequently the expectation that the treatment will enhance the patient's clinical status, prevent deterioration, and delay progression of the disease. It is therefore logical to presume that poor treatment adherence is likely to be clinically detrimental. Research has shown that a single session of airway clearance improves sputum expectoration (2,7) and over a 3-day period can improve lung function (8). It is considered that airway clearance by removing bacteria and inflammatory products can reduce the host's inflammatory response and thus break the "vicious circle" that leads to disease progression (9). To date it has been considered unethical to perform a randomized controlled trial of treatment versus no treatment because airway clearance has become an integral part of the respiratory management (10) and the short-term benefits are well established. Studies have attempted to link poor treatment adherence with faster disease progression in cystic fibrosis. Over a

10-year period, adherence to daily chest physiotherapy and regular 3-monthly clinic follow-up predicted a better trend in forced expiratory volume in one second (FEV_1) (11).

The possible adverse outcomes of poor adherence behavior can affect the patient and their family, the multidisciplinary team, the National Health Service (NHS) Trust purchasers, and pharmaceutical companies. Such adverse outcomes include (a) increased infective exacerbations, (b) faster disease progression, (c) cost to the NHS of wasted drugs and the preparation of medications, increased outpatient visits, hospital admissions, and domicilary care, (d) cost to the patient and family of lost time in education or work and the worry of health problems, and (e) possible erroneous conclusions about the efficacy of the treatment.

Even though these commonly assumed consequences of poor adherence have been acknowledged, there is a paucity of direct evaluation. There are two major reasons for this: first, adherence has not been routinely or systematically measured in clinical trials, and second, the relationship between adherence and health outcomes in clinical trials is complex. Clinical trials are designed to assess the efficacy of a treatment, and, therefore, adherence to the regimen is paramount. It could be assumed that adherence to an active treatment was more important than adherence in patients who received a placebo. There is substantial evidence that in double-blind, randomized placebo-controlled trials, patients who adhere to treatment, even when the treatment is a placebo, have better outcomes than patients whose adherence is poor (12). A possible explanation for such baffling results is that adherence may create an expectation that the treatment will be effective, and patients may engage in other health behaviors that will enhance clinical health outcome.

III. Levels of Adherence

Treatment adherence is a common problem even with life-threatening disorders. An early review of the literature indicated that of 537 studies, the range of adherence for long-term preventative regimens was 33–94% with a mean adherence rate of 57%. Similarly, for long-term treatments the range was 41–61% with a mean adherence rate of 54% (13). Studies of airway clearance are consistent with these findings. In cystic fibrosis (CF), studies have demonstrated that adherence is treatment specific. Fifty-three percent of patients were adherent to their physiotherapy, 75% were considered to be exercising to a beneficial level, and 83% and 46% of patients reported that they always took their enzymes and vitamins, respectively (14). The work of other researchers also supports the notion of treatment-specific adherence (15–18). Bronchiectatic patients reported failure to comply with chest clearance in 23 of 50 cases (9), and studies of CF patients have been consistent with adherence around 40–50% (14–18). In terms of airway clearance therapies, chest physiotherapy was the most frequently omitted treatment in patients with CF, but it is encouraging that patients were more adherent with their exercise regimen (14,15). However, although only 53% of patients were adherent with their chest physiotherapy, 67% believed that the amount of physiotherapy they engaged in was "about right," with only 25% reporting that they did not do enough. In contrast, 75% were found to be exercising to a beneficial level, although only 37% believed that the amount of exercise they performed was "about right," with 58% believing that they did not do enough (14). It is likely that adolescents and young adults with CF perceive exercise in a different way from their other treatments. Exercise is an activity that identifies them with rather than segregates them from their peers. Similarly, data collected from 222 physical therapists indicated that 35% of patients reported themselves to be fully adherent to their exercise regimen, but this increased to 76% when including those partially adherent (19). These data appear to suggest that determining the rate of patient adherence and nonadherence is straightforward. In reality, the area is fraught with difficulties, both conceptually and methodologically. One of the most pervasive problems is the lack of consistency in the definition and measurement of adherence.

IV. Definition of Adherence

Although there is a consensus among health professionals that adherence to chest physiotherapy and exercise is desirable, the definition of adherence is currently a contentious subject. There is little agreement regarding the terminology. Although the terms adherence and compliance have different connotations, they tend to be used interchangeably, and the recently coined terms of cooperation (20) and concordance (21) are also in use. It is beyond the scope of this review to fully debate the issue of terminology; we only note that there is increasing recognition of a need for partnership between patient and health professional when formulating treatment regimens.

Adherence to treatment has been defined in many ways: not taking enough medication or completing the course, taking too much medication, not observing the correct interval between doses, not observing the correct duration of treatment, not performing the treatment correctly, and taking additional nonprescribed medication. How do we define a nonadherent or an adherent patient? Is a patient who misses one dose of medication or one session of physiotherapy nonadherent? Again, there appears to be a lack of consensus. Adherence has been defined differently for different methods of assessment. For example, adherence was said to be achieved for a course of penicillin when 75% of urine tested positive for the drug (22), good adherence was defined as 85% by pill count (23), and adherence to chest physiotherapy was considered good when patients occasionally missed their treatment (14). In some disorders adherence is very complex, for example, in cystic fibrosis there are many treatment regimens to follow (chest physiotherapy, exercise, oral, inhaled, nebulized, and intravenous medication to aid the respiratory system, and pancreatic enzymes, vitamins, and nutritional supplements to aid gastrointestinal malabsorption and growth) (Table 2). Research has not yet identified which treatment is the most beneficial for an individual patient at any level of disease severity.

V. Measurement of Adherence

The assessment of adherence is a complex task. Obtaining accurate measures of adherence behaviors is problematic, and it is unfortunate that little empirical attention has been paid to this issue. This has led to a constant disquiet concerning the validity and reliability of the data. The inconsistent findings reported in the literature regarding predictors of adherence behavior are likely to be a product of the methodological limitations and problematic data interpretation concerning the measurement instruments, outcome measures, and study designs employed.

A. Measurement Instruments

The vast majority of studies have evaluated adherence using self-report methodology (questionnaires or interview). Various direct (blood or urine assays) and indirect (pill counts, mechanical devices, physician estimates, and self-reports) methods have previously been used to assess treatment adherence. Each method has problems and disadvantages (24–26). There is evidence of overreporting by

Table 2 Daily Timetable of Treatment for Patients with Cystic Fibrosis

A.M.	Inhaled bronchodilators	Antibiotics
	Chest clearance	Enzymes
	Inhaled steroids	Vitamins
	Nebulized antibiotics	Bronchodilators
Midday	Inhaled bronchodilators	Antibiotics
	Nebulized DNase	Enzymes
Evening	Inhaled bronchodilators	Antibiotics
	Chest clearance	Enzymes
	Nebulized antibiotics	
	Exercise	
P.M.	Inhaled bronchodilators	Antibiotics
	Inhaled steroids	Bronchodilators

Plus dietary supplements, nebulizer-compressor care, insulin, overnight feeding, nasal ventilation.
WORK, FURTHER EDUCATION, SOCIALIZE, NORMAL LIFE!

patients of self-administered medication compared with electronic devices that record nebulizer inhalation or pill counts and blood or urine assays (27,28). When patient reports have been compared with objective methods of measurement, patients have responded accurately when they report poor adherence (29). When patients claim to have adhered to their treatment regimen as prescribed, often these reports are not confirmed by objective records (30). Approximately one-quarter of peak flow diary entries were either invented or done retrospectively when, unknown to the patient, they used a peak flow meter containing an electronic timing device (31). Teenagers have been found to be less reliable in their recording than adults (32). There are several reasons why patients might underreport poor adherence: they may wish to deceive the health professional so that they are perceived favorably, they may not understand the regimen and therefore not realize that they are nonadherent, or they may forget instances of nonadherence (33). However, as long as patients inaccurately report their self-care, recommendations made on the basis of this incorrect information are likely to result in suboptimal self-care.

In mucus-clearance disorders, adherence to behavioral treatments (physiotherapy and exercise) require evaluation. Since the relationship between the rate of decline in clinical status and levels of treatment adherence in individuals is unclear, we currently have to rely on measures of reported adherence against which there are no appropriate objective measures to validate the data. Although there is a need to be mindful of inflated self-reported adherence rates, it is encouraging that those who report nonadherence rarely lie (26), and only this group has responded consistently to interventions (13). More recently, the development of an inflatable vest, ThAIRapyR, has enabled measurement of adherence by electronic monitoring in the device. Although patients were aware of the device, self-reported hours of adherence overestimated actual hours of use (0.81 hr/day vs. 0.45 hr/day) (34). In the future, this concept may be incorporated into other mechanical devices, e.g., flutter and PEP mask. Activity monitors designed to measure movement rather than heart rate are now used to determine activity levels, and these may prove to be a useful addition to the armamentarium of objective measurement devices.

Different ad hoc questionnaires/interviews are problematic. With ad hoc questioning, researchers design their own questionnaires, and it is evident that there is a lack of expertise in the development and validation of psychometric measures. It is often difficult to ascertain exactly what has been measured, making comparability with similar work difficult or impossible. Within the CF literature, there are currently two favored ways of measuring adherence. The first is based on self-report questionnaires, for example, the Manchester Adult Cystic Fibrosis Compliance Questionnaire (14). This device was developed to measure the rates of adherence to treatments and medical advice, the reasons for nonadherence, and the patients' perception of their level of adherence. It has been used with CF adolescents and young adults and family members and has been adapted for use by others (15). Second, the Medical Compliance Incomplete Stories Test (M-CIST) (35) is an assessment tool composed of five incomplete stories in which the main character is confronted with a dilemma as to whether he or she should follow specific medical advice. The patient is asked to complete the story and predict the outcome for the main character in each given situation. The instrument incorporates important concepts of self-efficacy, optimism, and coping mechanisms. Even though interrater reliability was satisfactory, it is uncertain as to what extent the perceptions of the raters influence the interpretation of adherence behavior. There is a desperate need to further develop and validate instruments for both children and adults with airway disorders. The M-CIST approach may be most appropriate for use with children, and self-report questionnaire/interview methods most suited to young adults.

B. Outcome Measures

In addition to the direct and indirect methods of determining adherence levels, outcome measures may be useful in identifying patients who fail to reach treatment goals or respond as expected to treatment. A major difficulty with this approach concerning airway clearance is that the positive relationship between adherence and health outcome, although often assumed, is not absolute. Complete compliance does not guarantee excellent health, and it is acknowledged that poor compliers remain well because individuals respond differently to treatment (36). Health professionals expect patients to adhere to burdensome lifelong treatments, yet we are unable to provide information as to the level of adherence that will result in a specified beneficial outcome. No studies to date have evaluated the benefits of once- versus twice-a-day treatment, 15- versus 20-minute treatments, airway clearance during acute exacerbations only versus continuous treatment, or treatment for large versus small sputum production. Outcome data (pulmonary function and/or sputum weight) from studies involving pre-post designs which attempt to evaluate the efficacy of a specific airway clearance technique or compare different clearance modalities may be problematic. The validity of sputum weight as a measure of airway clearance is unclear since there is the potential for it to include saliva or for unknown quantities to have been swallowed (7). A comparison of wet and dry sputum did, however, produce similar weights (2). Pulmonary function tests chosen as objective measures of improved outcome associated with sputum clearance may be appropriate short-term measures of outcome, but confounding intervening variables (infection, natural progression of the disease) may invalidate the assumed treatment-outcome association in longer-term studies (37).

Furthermore, when investigating group differences, changes in outcome may not be particularly responsive to changes in adherence. For example, if a change in adherence needs to be approximately 25% for a measurable change in outcome, this method will be unable to detect quite large changes in adherence behavior. Even so, the inclusion of outcome measures in adherence studies may help to determine the level of adherence necessary to ensure efficacy of the treatment. Additionally, at present it is not possible to ascertain the direction of causality: does adherence lead to better outcome or does improved outcome reinforce good adherence? Longitudinal work is needed to answer such questions.

C. Study Design

The measurement of adherence has also suffered from poor experimental designs. These have included (a) data collected from patients only while in the hospital and therefore not reflecting their typical adherence behaviors, (b) data obtained from medical records alone, and (c) adherence ratings based solely on the perceptions of physicians and health professionals. Insensitive scoring systems have also been problematic. Many studies have assessed several treatment regimens and have subsequently combined the data to provide an overall adherence score, thereby losing specific treatment data (38–40). Such a score, however, fails to recognize that patients may adhere to one aspect of their treatment but not to others. The demands of the different aspects of treatment vary enormously in terms of behaviors, skills required, or time needed (41). Chest physiotherapy is likely to be the most neglected of treatments in CF, but it is probably the most time consuming and onerous of all the treatments, even worse than the disease itself (10). Furthermore, children (some with parental reporting) and adults have been combined in data analyses (16,40,42), yet reports of patient and parent are not necessarily similar.

It is of great concern that the data are almost totally drawn from cross-sectional or short-term studies. It is important to understand adherence behaviors over time, and to recognize the specific times during the patient's life when a high level of adherence is more difficult to accomplish. There is an urgent need for more research linking treatment adherence with trends in clinical and psychosocial functioning, although the inherent difficulties of controlled studied have been acknowledged.

VI. Reasons for Poor Adherence

From the literature it is evident that there are numerous contraindications to adherence, some of which are considered more important than others. As yet, no consistent single reason or set of predictor variables have emerged to explain why patients engage in adherent or nonadherent behaviors. From a theoretical viewpoint, several reasons for poor adherence may be cited. These include lack of information, poor memory, poor doctor-patient communication, patient's beliefs and cognitions, characteristics of the patient, characteristics of the health professional, and characteristics of the treatment.

From the patient's perspective, however, there are perfectly understandable reasons why one might not adhere to treatment. A list of patient-perceived barriers to treatment and reasons for poor adherence is presented in Table 3. The airway-clearance techniques of chest physiotherapy and exercise have the hallmarks that make poor adherence predictable. Little reward is perceived for good self-care, and there is little motivation for the possible long-term benefits (14,43). Treatment is a daily reminder of being different from peers (44) and of the disease itself (45), together with the time-consuming and disruptive aspects of life that are never-ending, with clinical deterioration inevitable (46). Patients are also willing to tolerate symptoms (47). Parents may feel they are inflicting pain and upsetting their babies and young children with percussion techniques and therefore decide to be nonadherent.

When CF adults are asked directly, consistent reasons for missing physiotherapy have emerged from separate studies (14,15,18). These reasons can be grouped into four areas:

Table 3 Patient-Perceived Barriers to Chest Physiotherapy and Reasons for Poor Adherence

---

Well without physiotherapy
Not enough time
Can't be bothered
Less serious than others
Interrupts social life
Simply forget
Exercise instead
It's embarrassing
Feel different from friends
Daily reminder of the disease
No immediate benefit
Little motivation for long-term benefit
Willing to tolerate symptoms
Distasteful and unhygienic
Have to rely on someone to help
Don't believe it does any good
Have too many treatments and physiotherapy is the least important
Don't understand why I need to do physiotherapy
Don't know how to do physiotherapy
Have difficulty doing my own physiotherapy
Makes me feel worse
Resent having to do it

---

1. Health reasons, e.g., I feel well without treatment; I'm not as serious as others with CF; I don't feel any benefit; I do an alternative "treatment"—for example, exercise instead of physiotherapy.
2. Social reasons, e.g., interferes with social life, embarrassing doing physiotherapy. Patients with bronchiectasis report distaste, unhygienic aspects, and sputum disposal as additional reasons (9).
3. Time is a problem: not enough time; I forget; I am too busy.
4. Emotional reasons: I resent it; I can't be bothered; it makes me feel different from my friends.

Similarly, three major factors for poor adherence to exercise have been identified:

1. Patient-perceived barriers: time, forgetting, pain, lack of motivation
2. Lack of positive feedback
3. Perceived helplessness: those who believe that they are unable to do the treatment and/or that the exercise will not help them (19)

There is a problem concerning the meaning of adherence from the perspective of the patient and his or her family. What is considered nonadherence by health professionals may represent a rational, well-thought-out cost-benefit decision by the patient (48). There is usually the whole family to consider (49), so to sustain healthy family relationships, minor deviations from treatment regimens may not be problematic—at least psychologically (50). In asthma research the concept of adaptive nonadherence has been introduced since the patient and family often decide what is practicable in their home situation (51).

Koocher and colleagues (52) have explored the reasons for nonadherence in CF in a more systematic way. Three typologies of nonadherence have been described based on knowledge and beliefs. The first is inadequate knowledge (e.g., a lack of understanding of CF). The second is psychosocial resistance (e.g., struggle for control, peer pressure, difficult home circumstances, denial and depression), and the third type is educated nonadherence (e.g., a personal cost-benefit analysis based on informed choice and quality of life issues), similar to Deaton's concept of adaptive nonadherence (51). Based on behavior rather than cognition, Lask (53) has identified three groups of nonadherent patients. The categories reflect honesty in reporting adherence. The first group have been called refusers and appear similar to previously defined educated/adaptive nonadherence groups (51,52) (admit nonadherence, require control, consider treatment worse than symptoms). Procrastinators will admit to some nonadherent behavior while deniers will not. This type of categorization may be useful in aiding interventions; rather than a blanket intervention program, work can be tailored to the patients' specific difficulties. The CF team must be careful, however, not to pigeonhole patients and thereby restrict professional thinking and approaches to problems of nonadherence. Neither should these typologies be seen as totally distinct entities, since it is likely that more than one of these cognitive or behavioral processes can operate together to produce nonadherent behaviors.

VII. Demographic and Clinical Predictors of Adherence

Demographic and clinical factors have been evaluated as possible predictors of adherence in cystic fibrosis with equivocal results. Increased adherence has been associated with increasing age (39,50), although another study has demonstrated the opposite (40). There may be several confounding factors here, given that some studies focus on adolescents and young adults while others employ children and adolescents incorporating parental involvement and reporting. There are also discrepant gender data. Concerning chest physiotherapy, females have been shown to be less adherent in one study (39) but not in another (14), and, contradictorily, males have reported themselves to be less adherent than females (11). It is not surprising that young females are unwilling to expectorate sputum in the company of their partner or spouse and therefore suppress coughing. It is both unfeminine and more socially unacceptable for females. Interesting gender differences in the determinants of exercise adherence in healthy adolescents have been identified. "Perceived romantic appeal" was predictive of male exercise adherence, whereas perceived competency, self-worth, and physical appearance was predictive of female exercise adherence (54). It is interesting to note that decreased survival in females may be attributed to poor exercise performance (55).

It is a simplistic notion that knowledge of the disease will show a positive linear relationship with treatment adherence. There is a notorious lack of association between knowledge and medical advice, which is best illustrated by the relationship between knowledge of the harmful health effects of cigarette smoking and smoking behavior. Knowledge may be viewed as an important aid to adherence, but it cannot be assumed that a person with a high level of knowledge about CF will adhere to treatments. Some studies have reported a positive relationship (39,50), although Conway et al. (18) report virtually a zero correlation between knowledge and adherence in CF adults. It is, however, essential that knowledge is appraised to correct any misconceptions (56). Patients' perception of their knowledge of airway clearance techniques overestimated their actual knowledge (57). Individualized teaching specific to their lung disease improved their knowledge and reported adherence.

It was initially assumed that greater disease severity would be associated with a greater degree of adherence. Work with cancer patients (58), individuals with asthma (59), and patients with cystic fibrosis have not supported this assumption (17,18). In contrast, a negative correlation between disease severity and adherence has been reported by two independent groups of CF researchers, indicating that the most severe patients, as measured by lung function, are less likely to adhere to their treatments (60,61). It has been argued that the treatment regimens may eventually become too arduous to maintain (39). However, patients may not share the same perceptions as the CF team concerning the severity of their CF (60). This is not surprising because clinicians determine severity by the objective measures of impairment and patients measure severity by disability. It is well known in CF that some patients continue in employment until transplantation.

Additionally, adherence was not associated with employment status, age at diagnosis, the number of years practicing physiotherapy, in- or outpatient status, or the frequency of clinic visits. Patients who produced large amounts of sputum were more likely to adhere (14) and a subgroup of bronchiectatic patients who found chest physiotherapy helpful between exacerbations produced significantly more sputum than the remainder of the whole group (9). Short-term relief of symptoms influenced adherence in those patients whose chest felt better following chest physiotherapy and exercise. Those who received help with their physiotherapy were shown to be more adherent (14). Independence with chest clearance, which is considered an essential component of adherence (62), may be a mixed blessing because patients miss the companionship of the "helpers" (63). Loneliness and social isolation have been shown to be associated with low levels of adherence (15), enforcing the notion that social support is important in encouraging adherence behaviors (44).

VIII. Psychosocial Predictors of Adherence

A. Perceptions and Health Beliefs

It has been demonstrated that patients and physicians perceive disease severity and self-care differently. From the physician's viewpoint, patients underestimate the severity of the disease and overestimate their level of self-care (60). Figure 1 illustrates that over a 2-year period both patients and physicians were constant in their ratings of patient self-care and thereby maintained the doctor-patient discrepancy. From these data it is reasonable to assume, in accordance with the Health Belief Model (64), that patient-perceived disease severity is more likely to predict treatment adherence than objective clinical measures of severity. Reported adherence, however, was not influenced by patients' perceptions of their past, current, or future disease severity or their perceived susceptibility to recurrent infection (65). In other conditions, perceived severity has been shown to predict adherence (66,67). For life-threatening diseases or conditions with a shortened life expectancy, the association between perceived severity and adherence may be more complex than a simplistic positive linear relationship. Perceived disease severity may be related to adherence in an inverted-U-shaped manner; adherence being low when severity is perceived as high or low and

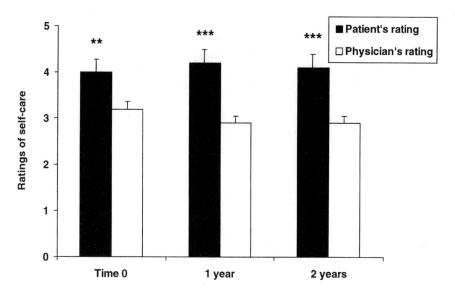

Figure 1 Mean (SE) values of ratings of patient self-care by patients and their physicians over a 2-year period. $**p < 0.01$, $***p < 0.001$ when compared to physician's rating.

greatest when severity is seen as moderate (68–70). If their perceived disease severity becomes too great to acknowledge, some individuals may avoid thoughts and behaviors that compel them to confront the seriousness of their situation. For many patients avoidance or denial may be an adaptive way of coping with CF, and the value of such strategies remain to be evaluated.

Worrying about CF (Fig. 2) and the perception of having little personal control over the disease has been shown to facilitate treatment adherence with chest clearance but not exercise (65). In contrast, exercise was associated with personal control over the disease (Fig. 3). Theoretically, patients with internal control beliefs would be expected to take control of their own self-care and thereby adhere to their treatment regimens to a greater extent that those who report having little control over the disease. It is possible, however, that those who believe they have control over their CF may make a rational decision to adhere to exercise but not chest clearance, enabling a balance between treatment regimens and life quality.

B. Coping

The early studies that attempted to evaluate the relationship between coping and adherence were blighted by inappropriate methods. Coping was initially rated by physicians, and it is strongly argued that the patient is the best judge of their

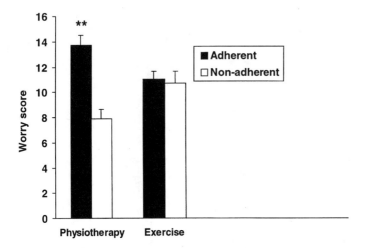

Figure 2 Mean (SE) worry score for adherent and nonadherent groups for chest physiotherapy and exercise. **$p < 0.01$ when compared to nonadherent with chest physiotherapy.

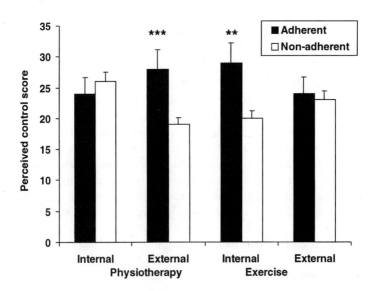

Figure 3 Mean (SE) scores for perceived internal and external control beliefs for adherent and nonadherent groups for chest physiotherapy and exercise. ***$p < 0.001$ when compared to nonadherent with chest physiotherapy, **$p < 0.01$ when compared to nonadherent with exercise.

CF coping behaviors (the ways in which they feel, think, or act). Employing the ratings of physicians, Moise et al. (71) reported no relationship between coping style and treatment adherence.

The notion of an optimistic way of coping with CF and adherence to treatment has received some attention. Higher levels of optimism were related to greater treatment adherence in CF adolescents and adults. Optimism was measured by the M-CIST, for which additional validity and reliability data are required given that the alpha coefficient for the health optimism subscale was low (39). Similarly, Gudas et al. (61) reported that greater optimism (measured simply on a five-point Likert scale) was associated with increased adherence to physiotherapy and medication-taking in children and young adults. These findings are consistent with recent work employing a well-validated—and currently the "gold standard"—self-report measure of optimism: the Life Orientation Test (LOT) (72). Using this instrument, higher levels of optimism were positively correlated with greater treatment adherence (15).

Employing the Manchester Cystic Fibrosis Compliance Questionnaire (14) and the recently developed Manchester Cystic Fibrosis Coping Scale (73), research has identified differences in coping behavior between adherent and nonadherent patients (Fig. 4). The latter scale recognizes two distinct styles of coping: hope-

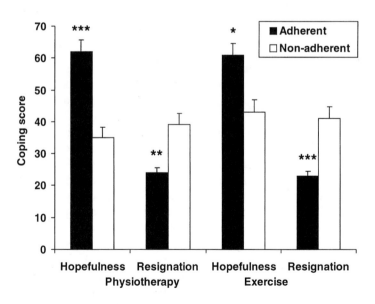

Figure 4 Mean (SE) coping scores for hopefulness and resignation for adherent and nonadherent groups for chest physiotherapy and exercise. *$p < 0.05$, **$p < 0.01$, ***$p < 0.001$ when compared to nonadherent.

Table 4 Determinants of Adherence: Summary of the Evidence

Factors not associated with adherence or evidence inconclusive
    Gender
    Employment status
    Age at diagnosis
    Objective and perceived disease severity
    Perceived susceptibility to recurrent infection
    Knowledge of the disease
    Number of years practicing airway clearance
    Frequency of clinic visits
Factors associated with increased adherence
    Large sputum production
    Receive help with physiotherapy
    Personal control over the disease
    Worrying about the disease
    Optimistic ways of coping
Factors associated with decreased adherence
    Age (decreased adherence during adolescence)
    Loneliness and social isolation
    Avoidant ways of coping

---

fulness (an optimistic, determined, and positive way of acting, thinking, and feeling) and resignation (an avoidant, passive, and helpless way of acting, thinking, and feeling). Those patients adherent with their chest physiotherapy and exercise regimens reported more optimistic and positive ways of coping with CF. These data are supported by work previously described (15,39,61). In contrast, those nonadherent with physiotherapy and exercise scored higher on the resignation scale than did adherent patients. In this respect, an avoidant and passive coping style may be viewed as maladaptive if it interferes with adequate self-care. However, this is rather a naive clinical assumption which treats avoidance behavior as rebellious, a rejection of medical advice, and self-neglect. It is also reasonable to assume that avoidance and denial may enable patients to adapt, control, and deal with CF in their own way, and in this respect enhance their quality of life. As yet, there is little empirical support for this, although based on the ratings of physicians, a decrease in psychological distress and an increase in self-esteem were associated with avoidant coping (71). An avoidant coping style may improve psychosocial health, but its effect on clinical health also requires evaluation. Table 4 lists the determinants of adherence. These data demonstrate the complexity of human behaviors, emotions, and cognitions in treatment adherence.

IX. Evidence for the Effectiveness of Intervention

The aim of measuring and seeking determinants of adherence must be to understand, intervene, and improve adherence behaviors. The questions of how this should be achieved and whether it is ethical to intervene need to be addressed. The few interventions that have been evaluated have met with little success. Despite an extensive educational program in the self-management of asthma, outcome adherence was only 40% (74), but adolescents with CF who participated in a 2-week self-care camp demonstrated improvements in FEV_1, weight, and psychosocial adjustments (75). It is unknown whether adherence behaviors continued when patients returned to their normal life. A measure of CF self-management behaviors (76) was employed with children and adolescents who received self-management training. Eight weeks following training, patients demonstrated an increase in weight and increased adherence to aerosol and chest physiotherapy treatments (77).

The literature on adherence behavior has raised ethical questions regarding the management of nonadherence. In order to change adherence behavior, there is a need to change the perceptions, beliefs, and ways of coping with CF that facilitate nonadherence. The identification of beneficial coping strategies to aid both psychological and clinical well-being may improve our ability to manage nonadherence in the most appropriate way. However, this may mean that patients have to face the stark clinical reality of their condition. The current data suggest that psychologically this approach may be more harmful than beneficial. It is well documented that poor psychological well-being can have a detrimental effect on physiological functioning (78–80), the onset and progression of disease (81,82), and morbidity and mortality (83,84).

On a positive note, in combination with physiotherapy, exercise has been shown to be beneficial as an airway clearance technique. It is encouraging from studies of patients with COPD that exercise interventions are meeting with some success. It was noted that those most active at the outset were most likely to adhere to an exercise regimen (85), and this may be related to a person's self-efficacy. A person's perception that he or she is capable of performing a given behavior successfully to produce a certain outcome is defined as self-efficacy expectation. The strength of a person's convictions about his or her ability to produce a specific outcome (exercise) determines whether or not that person attempts to deal with the situation (86). It has been demonstrated that increases in self-efficacy correlate with adherence to prescribed activities (e.g., smoking cessation, weight control, and exercise). Little research has addressed methods specifically aimed at enhancing self-efficacy in patients with chronic lung disease. Breathlessness during exercise is a barrier to patients with chronic lung disease. Individuals avoid activities that they believe are beyond their coping capabilities. Zimmerman et al. (87) have reported that it is possible to enhance self-efficacy in COPD patients [measured by the COPD self-efficacy scale (88)]. Self-efficacy beliefs increased following a 6-week self-management program (87). Kaplan et al. (89) examined health beliefs as determinants of change in exercise behavior in COPD. After 3 months, only those given specific training for adherence with exercise increased their adherence compared with a control group receiving attention only. These changes were mediated by changes in self-efficacy: a belief that they were able to perform the therapy. These data are reminiscent of the patient-reported reasons for poor exercise adherence: lack of positive feedback and perceived helplessness (a perceived inability to perform the exercise) (19), which have been successfully modified by this program. Similarly, a COPD outpatient pulmonary rehabilitation program attempted to assist patients in managing their breathing difficulties more effectively. An educational component, exercise training, and methods to increase self-efficacy and confidence in ability were employed. The program improved self-efficacy and enabled patients to manage or avoid breathing difficulties. The authors also argue that self-efficacy may be a factor in the decreased perception of dyspnea and increased exercise endurance (90). The association between self-efficacy and adherence to chest physiotherapy and exercise in mucus-clearance disorders remains to be evaluated.

X. Methods to Enhance Adherence

For effective intervention it is necessary to understand the particular issues for an individual and tailor the intervention to the specific needs and treatment preferences of each patient, e.g., their lifestyles, family commitments, and health beliefs. It is unlikely that a single intervention will be effective in all situations or that barriers to adherence will remain constant.

Common methods of enhancing adherence are given in Table 5. They

Table 5 Strategies to Enhance Adherence

Do not expect 100% adherence.
Assure patients that total adherence would be ideal but partial adherence is the norm.
Assure patients that you will not be angry, critical, or judgmental if they admit to
    having difficulty adhering.
Accept compromise and negotiate.
Engage in shared planning and decision making.
Simplify the regimen as much as possible.
Tailor regimen to daily routine of patient and family.
Regularly reassess barriers to adherence.
Promote self-efficacy.
Praise efforts when total or partial adherence occurs.

have included simplifying the regimen as much as possible and tailoring the regimen to the daily routine of patient and family. Tailored regimens have shown increased adherence (91) and avoid the poor adherence created from incompatibilities between regimen and lifestyle. There is a need to rethink practice and accept compromise. Some nonadherence is adaptive and positive: Deaton (51) found that flexibility was associated with better outcomes compared with strict adherence. Perceptions of adherence have been shown to differ between treatments (14) and also from the perspectives of the patient, the family, and the health professional (60). Each may have psychologically generated a different treatment-adherence cost-benefit equation. Frequent clinic visits involving shared planning and decision making, assessing and regularly reassessing the barriers to adherence, and evaluating the treatment plan in the context of the patient's lifestyle is likely to enhance the patient–health professional relationship and enable patients to be active in their self-management.

XI. Conclusion

On a pessimistic note, there are very serious problems within the current adherence literature. These problems involve deciding on the most appropriate terminology, inconsistencies in defining adherence and poor or nonadherence behaviors, and difficulties with assessment, measurement, and data interpretation. To date, the few interventions undertaken have not been very successful. On an optimistic note, however, much of this confusion may arise because we try to generalize what is not generalizable. Specific definitions of adherence may be required for particular treatments, although this may prove difficult because of a lack of empirical data to indicate the minimal amount of therapy required to be effective for an individual patient.

A future research agenda needs to address several questions. Which are the major predictive factors of short- and long-term adherence to chest physiotherapy and exercise in aiding airway clearance? What is the optimal frequency for performing exercise and chest physiotherapy for patients with mild disease versus those with severe disease in order to maintain health and prevent disease progression? Are the newer, less intrusive means of clearance therapy (flutter) associated with improved adherence compared to traditional chest physiotherapy? Several studies have shown a preference for one technique over another (6,92,93), but no studies have confirmed that preference is associated with short- or long-term compliance. Which techniques and interventions for enhancing adherence are most effective in mucus-clearance disorders? Until these questions are answered, it is important to recognize that incomplete compliance is normal behavior and a nonjudgmental approach is essential to maintain communication between patient and clinician. Assessment and education should be a continuous process with individualized specific treatment details as lung disease and lifestyle change. Most important, patients need support from family, friends, and the multidisciplinary team to maintain or improve compliance with the lifelong treatment of airway clearance.

References

1. van der Schans CP. Forced expiratory manoeuvres to increase transport of bron- chial mucus: a mechanistic approach. Monaldi Arch Chest Dis 1997; 52:367–370.
2. Sutton PP, Parker RA, Webber BA. Assessment of the forced expiration technique, postural drainage, and directed coughing in chest physiotherapy. Eur J Respir Dis 1983; 64:62.
3. Hasani A. Pavia D, Agnew JE, Clarke SW. The effect of unproductive coughing/ FET on regional mucus movement in the human lungs. Respir Med 1991; 85: 23–26.
4. Lannefors L, Wollmer P. Mucus clearance with three chest physiotherapy regimes in cystic fibrosis: a comparison between postural drainage, PEP and exercise. Eur Respir J 1992; 5:748–753.
5. Cerny FJ, Relative effects of bronchial drainage and exercise for in-hospital care of patients with cystic fibrosis. Phys Ther 1989; 69:633–639.
6. Bilton D, Dodd M, Abbott J, Webb AK. The benefits of exercise combined with physiotherapy in the treatment of adults with cystic fibrosis. Respir Med 1992; 86: 507–511.
7. Rossman C, Waldes R, Sampson D, Newhouse M. Effect of chest physiotherapy on the removal of mucus in patients with cystic fibrosis. Am Rev Respir Dis 1982; 120:131–135.
8. Webber BA, Hofmeyr JL, Morgan MDL, Hodson ME. Effects of postural drainage, incorporating the forced expiratory technique, on pulmonary function in cystic fi- brosis. Br J Dis Chest 1986; 80:353–359.
9. Currie DC, Munro C, Gaskell D, Cole PJ. Practice, problems and compliance with postural drainage: a survey of chronic sputum producers. Br J Dis Chest 1986; 80: 249–253.
10. Prasad SA, Main E. Finding evidence to support airway clearance techniques in cystic fibrosis. Disabil Rehabil 1998; 20:235–246.
11. Patterson JM, Budd J, Goetz D, Warwick W J. Family correlates of a 10 year pulmonary health trend in cystic fibrosis. Pediatrics 1993; 91:383–389.
12. Horwitz RI, Horwitz SM. Adherence to treatment and health outcomes. Arch Intern Med 1993; 153:1863–1868.
13. Sackett DL, Snow JC. The magnitude of compliance and non-compliance. In: Haynes RB, Taylor DW, Sacket DL, eds. Compliance in Health Care. Baltimore, MD: John Hopkins University Press, 1979:11–22.
14. Abbott J, Dodd M, Bilton D, Webb AK. Treatment compliance in adults with cystic fibrosis. Thorax 1994; 49:115–120.
15. Pownceby J. The Coming of Age Project: A Study of the Transition from Paediatric to Adult Care and Treatment Adherence Amongst Young People with Cystic Fibro- sis. Bromley, Kent, UK: Cystic Fibrosis Trust, 1996.

16. Passero MA, Remor B, Salomon J. Patient-reported compliance with cystic fibrosis therapy. Clin Pediatr 1981; 20:264–268.
17. Shepherd SL, Hovel MF, Harwood IR, Granger LE, Hofstettew CR, Molgaard C, Kaplan RM. A comparative study of the psychosocial assets of adults with cystic fibrosis and their healthy peers. Chest 1990; 97:1310–1316.
18. Conway S, Pond M N, Hamnett T, Watson A. Compliance with treatment in adult patients with cystic fibrosis. Thorax 1996; 51:29–33.
19. Sluijs EM, Kok GJ, van der Zee J. Correlates of exercise compliance in physical therapy. Phys Ther 1993; 73:771–782.
20. Kaplan RM, Sallis JF, Patterson TL. Health and Human Behavior. New York: McGraw-Hill, 1993.
21. Royal Pharmacological Society of Great Britian/Merck Sharpe and Dohme. From Compliance to Concordance. Achieving Shared Goals in Medicine Taking. London, 1997.
22. Gordis L, Markowitz PHM, Lilienfield AM. The inaccuracy in using interviews to estimate patient reliability in taking medications at home. Med Care 1969; 7: 49–54.
23. Maenpaa H, Javela K, Pikkarainan J, Malkone M, Heinonen OP, Manninen V. Minimal doses of digoxin: a new marker for compliance to medication. Eur Heart J 1987; 8:31–37.
24. Wright EC. Non-compliance—or how many aunts has Matilda? Lancet 1993; 342: 909–913.
25. Litt IF, Cuskey WR. Compliance with medical regimens during adolescence. Pediatr Clin North Am 1980; 27:3–15.
26. Epstein LH, Cluss PA. A behavioural medicine perspective on adherence to long-term medical regimens. J Consult Clin Psychol 1982; 50:950–971.
27. Ley P. Satisfaction, compliance and communication. Br J Clin Psychol 1982; 21: 241–254.
28. Dodd ME, Haworth CS, Moorcroft AJ, Miles J, Webb AK. Is medicine evidenced-based when there is discrepancy between patient reported and objective measures of compliance in clinical trials? Pediatr Pulmonol 1998; 17:398.
29. Fletcher RH. Patient compliance with therapeutic advice: a modern view. Mount Sinai J Med 1989; 56:453–457.
30. Spector SL, Kinsman R, Mawhinney H. Compliance of patients with an experimental aerosolised medication: implications for controlled clinical trials. J. Allergy Clin Immunol 1986; 66:65–70.
31. Chowienczyk PJ, Parkin DH, Lawson CP, Cochrane GM. Do asthmatic patients correctly record home spirometry measurements? Br Med J 1994; 309:1618.
32. Wonham K, Jenkins J, Pillinger J, Jones K. Compliance with completing peak flow charts. Asthma Gen Pract 1996; 4:7–8.
33. Ley P. Communicating with Patients. London: Croom Helm, 1988.
34. McColley SA, Boas SR, Jain M, Qualter NA, O'Malley CA. Patient adherence to and treatment satisfaction with an airway clearance technique. Pediatr Pulmonol 1998; (suppl 17):389.
35. Czajkowski DR, Koocher GP. Predicting medical compliance among adolescents with cystic fibrosis. Health Psychol 1986; 5:297–305.

36. Angst DB, Deatrick JA. Involvement in health care decisions: parents and children with chronic illness. J Family Nurs 1996; 2:174–194.
37. Steen HJ, Redmond AOB, O'Neill D, Beattie F. Evaluation of the PEP mask in cystic fibrosis. Acta Paediatr Scand 1991; 80:51–56.
38. Strauss GD, Wellisch DK. Psychological adaptation in older cystic fibrosis patients. J Chronic Dis 1981; 34:141–146.
39. Czajkowski D, Koocher G. Medical compliance and coping with cystic fibrosis. J Child Psychol Psychiatry 1987; 23:311–319.
40. Patterson JM. Critical factors affecting family compliance with home treatment for children with cystic fibrosis. Family Relat 1985; 34:79–89.
41. Meichenbaum D, Turk DC. Facilitating Treatment Adherence. New York: Plenum Press, 1987.
42. Meyers A, Dolan TF, Mueller D. Compliance and self-medication in cystic fibrosis. Am J Dis Child 1975; 129:1011–1013.
43. Eigen H, Clark NM, Wolle JM. Clinical-behavioral aspects of cystic fibrosis: directions for future research. Am Rev Respir Dis 1987; 136: 1509–1513.
44. Friedman IM, Litt IF. Promoting adolescents' compliance with therapeutic regimens. Pediatr Clin North Am 1986; 33:955–973.
45. McCracken M J. Cystic fibrosis in adolescence. In: Blum R, ed. Chronic Illness and Disabilities in Childhood and Adolescence. New York: Grune & Stratton, 1984.
46. Denning CR, Gluckson MM. Psychosocial aspects of cystic fibrosis. In: Taussig LM, ed. Cystic Fibrosis. New York: Thieme-Stratton, 1984.
47. Quirk FH, Jones PW. Patients' perception of distress due to symptoms and effects of asthma on daily living and an investigation of possible influential factors. Clin Sci 1990; 79:17–21.
48. Dugdale A. Non-compliance or rational decision? Lancet 1993; 342:1426–1427.
49. Patterson JM. A family systems perspective for working with youth with disability. Pediatrician 1991; 18:129–141.
50. Giess S, Hobbs S, Hannersley-Maercklein G, Kramer J, Henley M. Psychosocial factors related to perceived compliance with cystic fibrosis treatment. J Clin Psychol 1992; 48:99–103.
51. Deaton AV. Adaptive non-compliance in pediatric asthma: the parent as expert. J Pediatr Psychol 1985; 10:1–14.
52. Koocher GP, McGrath ML, Gudas LJ. Typologies of non-adherence in cystic fibrosis. Dev Behav Pediatr 1990; 11:353–358.
53. Lask B. Non-adherence to treatment in cystic fibrosis. J Roy Soc Med 1994; 87: 25–28.
54. Douthitt VL. Psychological determinants of adolescent exercise adherence. Adolescence 1994; 29:711–722.
55. Levison H, Tabachnik E. Pulmonary physiology. In: Hodson ME, Norman AP, Batten JC, eds. Cystic Fibrosis. London: Bailliere Tindall, 1983:52–81.
56. Conway SP, Pond MN, Watson A, Hamnett T. Knowledge of adult patients with cystic fibrosis about their illness. Thorax 1996; 51:34–38.
57. Dodd ME, Unsworth R, Davis A, Webb AK. Individualised teaching improves knowledge and adherence with airway clearance techniques. Pediatr Pulmonol 1998; (suppl 17):346.

58. Tebbi C, Cummings M, Zevon M, Smith L, Richards M, Mallon J. Compliance of pediatric and adolescent cancer patients. Cancer 1986; 58:1179–1184.

59. Christiaanse M, Lavigne J, Lerner C. Psychosocial aspects of compliance in children and adolescents with asthma. J Dev Behav Pediatr 1989; 10:75–80.

60. Abbott J, Dodd M, Webb AK. Different perceptions of disease severity and self care between patients with cystic fibrosis, their close companion, and physician. Thorax 1995; 50:794–796.

61. Gudas LJ, Koocher GP, Wypij D. Perceptions of medical compliance in children and adolescents with cystic fibrosis. Dev Behav Pediatr 1991; 12:236–242.

62. Muszynski-Kwan AT, Perlman R, Rivington-Law BA. Compliance with and effectiveness of chest physiotherapy in cystic fibrosis: a review. Physiother Canada 1988; 40:28–32.

63. McIlwaine MP, Davidson GF. Airway clearance techniques in the treatment of cystic fibrosis. Curr Opin Pulm Med 1996; 2:447–451.

64. Becker MH. The Health Belief Model and Personal Health Behavior. Thorofare, NJ: Slack, 1974.

65. Abbott J, Dodd M, Webb AK. Health perceptions and treatment adherence in adults with cystic fibrosis. Thorax 1996; 51:1233–1238.

66. Kirscht JP, Rosenstock IM. Patient adherence to antihypertensive medical regimens. J Commun Health 1977; 3:115–124.

67. Hartman PE, Becker MH. Non-compliance with prescribed regimen among chronic hemodialysis patients. Dial Transplant 1978; 7:978–985.

68. Becker M, Kabak M, Rosenstock I, Ruth M. Some influences of public participation in a genetic screening program. J Commun Health 1975; 1:3–14.

69. Hochbaum G. Why people seek diagnostic x-rays. Public Health Rep 1956; 71: 377–380.

70. Champion V. Use of the health belief model in determining frequency of breast self-examination. Res Nurs Health 1985; 8:373–379.

71. Moise JR, Drotar D, Doershuk CF, Stern RC. Correlates of psychosocial adjustment among young adults with cystic fibrosis. Dev Behav Pediatr 1987; 8:141–148.

72. Scheier MF, Carver CS. Optimism, coping and health: assessment and implications of generalised outcome expectancies. Health Psychol 1985; 4:219–247.

73. Abbott J, Dodd M, Gilling S, Webb AK. Coping styles and treatment adherence in adults with cystic fibrosis. 21st European Cystic Fibrosis Conference, Davos, Switzerland, 1997.

74. Chmelik F, Doughty A. Objective measurements of compliance in asthma treatment. Ann Allergy 1994; 73:527–532.

75. McCracken MJ, Budd J, Warick W. A study of self care intervention for adolescents with cystic fibrosis. Pediatr Pulmonol 1992; S8:114–115.

76. Bartholomew LK, Sockrider MM, Seilheimer DK, Czyzewski DI, Parcel GS, Spinelli SH. Performance objectives for the self-management of cystic fibrosis. Patient Ed Counsel 1993; 22:15–25.

77. Cottrell CK, Young GA, Creer TL, Holroyd KA, Kotses H. The development and evaluation of a self-management programme for cystic fibrosis. Pediatr Asthma Allergy Immunol 1996; 10:109–118.

78. Kiecolt-Glaser JK, Glaser R. Psychological influences on immunity. Psychosomatics 1986; 27:621–624.
79. Kiecolt-Glaser JK, Stephens RE, Lipetz PD, Speicher CE, Glaser R. Distress and DNA repair in human lymphocytes. J Behav Med 1985; 8:311–320.
80. McKinney ME, Hofschire PJ, Buell JC, Eliot RS. Hemodynamic and biochemical responses to stress: the necessary link between type A behavior and cardiovascular disease. Behav Med Update 1984; 6:16–21.
81. Spiegel D, Bloom JR, Kraemer HC, Gottheil E. Effect of psychosocial treatment on survival of patients with metastic breast cancer. Lancet 1989; 334:888–891.
82. Greer S, Moorey S, Baruch JDR, Watson M, Robertson BM, Mason A, Rowden L, Law M G, Bliss JM. Adjuvant psychological therapy for patients with cancer: a prospective randomised trial. Br Med J 1992; 304:675–680.
83. Berkman LF, Syme SL. Social networks, host resistance and mortality: a nine year follow-up study of Alameda County residents. Am J Epidemiol 1979; 109:186–204.
84. Kaplan GA, Wilson TW, Cohen RD, Kauhanen J, Wu M, Salonen JT. Social functioning and overall mortality: prospective evidence from the Kuopio Ischemic Heart Disease Risk Factor Study. Epidemiology 1994; 5:495–500.
85. Taylor AH. Evaluating GP exercise prescription schemes: findings from a randomised control trial. Brighton, UK: Chelsea School Research Centre, University of Brighton, 1996.
86. Bandura A. Self-efficacy: toward a unifying theory of behavioural change. Psychol Rev 1977; 84:191–215.
87. Zimmerman BW, Brown ST, Bowman JM. A self-management programme for chronic obstructive pulmonary disease: relationship to dyspnea and self-efficacy. Rehab Nurs 1996; 21:253–257.
88. Wigal J, Creer T, Kotses H. The COPD self-efficacy Scale. Chest 1991; 99: 1193–1196.
89. Kaplan R, Atkins C, Reinsch S. Specific efficacy expectations mediate exercise compliance in patients with COPD. Health Psychol 1984; 3:223–242.
90. Scherer YK, Schmieder LE. The effect of a pulmonary rehabilitation programme on self-efficacy, perception of dyspnea, and physical endurance. Heart Lung 1997; 26:15–22.
91. Rapoff MA, Christopherson ER. Compliance of paediatric patients with medical regimens: a review and evaluation. In: Stuart RB, ed. Adherence, Compliance and Generalization in Behavioral Medicine. New York: Brunner/Mazel, 1982.
92. Pryor JA, Webber BA, Hodson ME, Warner JO. The Flutter VRPI as an adjunct to chest physiotherapy in cystic fibrosis. Respir Med 1994; 88:677–681.
93. McIlwaine MP, Wong LT, Peacock D, Davidson GF. Long-term comparative trial of conventional postural drainage and percussion versus positive expiratory pressure physiotherapy in the treatment of cystic fibrosis. J. Pediatr 1997; 131:570–573.

6

Taxonomy of Mucoactive Medications

BRUCE K. RUBIN

Wake Forest University School of Medicine
Winston-Salem, North Carolina, U.S.A.

> *"When I use a word," Humpty Dumpty said in rather a scornful tone, "it means just what I choose it to mean—neither more nor less."*
>
> *Through the* Looking Glass by Lewis Carroll

I. Overview

The secretion and clearance of mucus is a critical defense mechanism of the respiratory tract. Mucus retention is usually due to a combination of hypersecretion and impaired clearance. Infected secretions induce an inflammatory response that can further damage the airway epithelium.

Mucoactive is the general term used for medications used to enhance secretion removal or reduce hypersecretion.

Expectorants increase the volume or hydration of airway secretions. Neither systemic hydration or classic expectorants have been clearly demonstrated to be clinically effective. Modifiers of airway ion and water transport including P_2Y agonists, gene activation, and gene transfer therapy are being investigated.

Mucolytics degrade polymers in secretions. Classic mucolytics depolymerize mucins and saccharide mucolytics disentangle mucin polymers. Peptide mucolytics break pathological filaments of neutrophil-derived DNA and F-actin.

Mucokinetics increase cough efficiency. Cough flow can be increased by bronchodilators in patients with airway hyperreactivity. Abhesives such as surfactants decrease epithelial-mucus attachment, augmenting both cough and mucociliary clearance.

Mucoregulatory agents reduce the volume of airway mucus and appear to be especially effective in hypersecretory states like bronchorrhea, diffuse panbronchiolitis, and some forms of asthma. These medications include anti-inflammatory agents, anticholinergic agents, and some macrolide antibiotics.

This classification should help us to better develop and evaluate new types of therapy and to direct therapy toward patients who are most likely to benefit.

II. Introduction

The airways are exposed to about 10,000 liters of air each day containing airborne pollutants and microorganisms. One of the most important defenses against inhaled particles is the production of bronchial secretions and the transport and removal of these secretions. In health there is only a small amount of mucus in the conducting airways. With airway inflammation, mucus production increases and mucus becomes mixed with inflammatory cells, cellular debris, and bacteria. This mixture is called sputum when expectorated. Mucus is usually cleared by airflow and ciliary interactions. Sputum is generally cleared by cough (1).

Chronic airway inflammation also leads to impaired mucociliary clearance and, in some cases, to decreased cough clearability of secretions. Airway obstruction can often be attributed to a combination of decreased clearance and increased mucus production. This can increase the resident time of infectious microorganisms and inflammatory mediators leading to ongoing inflammation. In order to break this cycle, mucoactive agents and physical therapy are used to promote secretion clearance. Secretion properties differ between diseases and at different times in the course of an illness. Understanding the properties of airway secretions and the mechanisms of action of mucoactive therapy can be important for determining the appropriate use of these medications.

Airway mucus clearance depends upon the physical properties of the mucus gel as well as interactions between mucus and airflow or mucus and cilia (2,3). Over the years, a diverse terminology has been used to describe medications that are thought to have an effect on mucus clearance (4). Some of these terms include expectorants, mucolytic, mucoactive, or mucokinetic medications, mucus regulators, mucus modifiers, mucus mobilizers, and mucociliary enhancers.

Many and diverse definitions have been proposed for each of these terms. Although some authors have used "mucolytic" as a general term for mucoactive agents, it is clear that many of these medications mobilize secretions by mechanisms other than by the direct lysis or "thinning" of mucus. Indeed, the simple reduction of sputum viscosity without a concomitant reduction in adhesion might actually reduce the cough clearability of sputum (3,5).

There are several mechanisms whereby medications could improve the mobilization of secretions (mucokinesis) or reduce the volume of secretions in the airway (mucoregulation). These mechanisms include reducing airway inflammation, increasing ciliary beat frequency or power, decreasing sputum adhesion to the epithelium, increasing air flow, and changing the biophysical properties of the secretions. We base the classification of mucoactive agents on the primary mechanism whereby each is thought to promote mucus clearance (4). Mucoactive therapy is the general term that we will use for all medications that affect mucus properties or mucus clearance (Table 1). Each of these therapies is discussed in greater detail in separate chapters in this volume.

III. Expectorants

Expectorants are medications that increase sputum volume (secretagogues) or mucus hydration by stimulating airway ion and water secretion or by directly adding water to the airway. Dehydration of secretions is rarely a clinically significant problem except in patients with severe systemic dehydration or those who are intubated and ventilated with inadequately humidified gases (6). Moderate supplemental hydration in patients with chronic bronchitis has no significant effect on sputum volume or ease of expectoration (7). Excessive hydration can lead to mucosal edema, and this impairs mucociliary clearance (8).

Expectorant medications include glycerol guiacolate (guaifenesin) and some iodide-containing medications. Expectorants do not alter ciliary beat frequency or mucociliary clearance. Oral expectorants are posited to increase airway mucus secretion by acting on the gastric mucosa to stimulate the vagus nerve, but this effect has not been well documented. Although guaifenesin appears to be a gastric stimulant, it has little expectorant action.

The iodide-containing agents appear to directly stimulate secretion of airway fluid, and they may also stimulate a gastric vagal reflex. Iodide rapidly appears in secretions following oral administration. In vitro, iodides have a direct mucolytic effect on mucin networks similar to the effects of acetylcysteine and other inorganic salts. In vivo, iodinated glycerol has no effect on mucus

Table 1 Classification of Mucoactive Medications

Class of agent	Subclass	Action	Examples
Expectorants		**Adds airway water**	
	Classic expectorants	Induces a "vagal gastric" reflex	Guaifenesin, iodides
	Hyperosmolar aerosols	Stimulates epithelial water secretion	Hypertonic saline mannitol
Ion-transport modifiers		**Induces ion and water transport**	
	CFTR activators	Improves ability of abnormal CFTR to transport Cl^-	CPX, genistein, phenylbutyrate
	Non-CFTR agonists	Increases non-CFTR Cl^- (and water) transport	P2Y2 puringeric agonists (e.g., UTP)
	Gene transfer	Replaces abnormal CFTR cDNA	Adenovirus, AAV, liposomal mediated
Mucolytics		**Disrupts mucus or sputum polymers**	
	Classic (mucin) mucolytics	Severs mucin polymers	N-Acetylcysteine, Nacystelyn
	Saccharides	Disrupts mucin ionic interactions and breaks $[H^+]$ bonds	Heparin, LMW dextran
	Peptide mucolytics	Degrades DNA and F-actin polymers	Dornase alfa, gelsolin, thymosin $\beta 4$
Mucokinetics		**Increases sputum cough clearability**	
	Bronchodilators	Increases air flow	Beta-agonists
	Abhesives	Decreases sputum adhesivity	Surfactants
Mucoregulatory agents		**Decreases mucin production and/or secretion**	
	Anticholinergics	Decreases stimulated (neurogenic) secretion	Atropine, ipratropium bromide
	Anti-inflammatory medications	Decreases secretion $2°$ to inflammation	Glucocorticosteroids, indomethacin, rSLPI
	Macrolide antibiotics	Unknown; possibly anti-inflammatory	Erythromycin, clarithromycin

properties, pulmonary function, or quality of life in patients with chronic bronchitis (9).

Sputum induction using hypertonic saline inhalation has been used to obtain specimens for diagnosing airway infection. The inhalation of hypertonic saline or mannitol can increase mucociliary clearance (10,11), and the addition of small amounts of salt can significantly increase the mucociliary clearability of sputum (12). Hypertonic saline is inexpensive and readily available, making this a potentially attractive form of therapy, but there is concern about the inactivation of a tracheal antimicrobial peptide at the airway surface in the presence of high salt concentration. This might increase the long-term risk of airway infection (13). The very short duration of action of all hyperosmolar aerosols might limit their clinical effectiveness as expectorants.

IV. Ion Transport Modifiers

A. Cystic Fibrosis Transmembrane Regulator Modifiers

The cystic fibrosis (CF) protein cystic fibrosis transmembrane regulator (CFTR) is a large membrane-bound epithelial ion regulator protein. In the normal human trachea, the CFTR immunolabeling is along the apical and basolateral plasma membranes of glandular mucous cells. CFTR is most strongly associated with the membrane of the secretory granules of glandular serous cells (14). Cyclic AMP–dependent opening of this apical Cl^- channel is triggered by the phosphorylation of CFTR at one of six protein kinase A domains. Although more than 800 abnormalities of the CF gene have been described, a single three-base deletion removing a phenylaline residue at position 508 of CFTR, the $\Delta F508$ mutation, is most commonly found in the Caucasian population, and this deletion is found on approximately 70% of abnormal CF chromosomes.

For the CFTR protein to function as a chloride channel, it must properly assembled and glycosylated and then must be transported intact and inserted into the cell membrane. The $\Delta F508$ CFTR protein accumulates in the cytosol of epithelial cells in the epithelium and is disassociated from the outer cell membranes, suggesting a defect in intracellular trafficking. The improperly assembled CFTR may be degraded before it reaches the cell membrane. Because the $\Delta F508$ protein retains some channel function when it is inserted into the cell membrane, there is interest in finding ways to get more mutant $\Delta F508$ protein glycosylated and to the cell surface. Even a small increase in CFTR function goes a long way as partial normalization of CFTR function is capable of restoring epithelial chloride transport (15).

CPX (8-cyclopentyl-1,3-dipropylxanthine) and DAX (1,3-diallyl-8-cyclohexylxanthine) are xanthine A_1 adenosine receptor antagonists that can directly activate ΔF508 CFTR (16). This process involves an increase in the frequency and duration of channel opening (Po) events. Genistein is a tyrosine kinase inhibitor that activates both wild-type and ΔF508 CFTR chloride secretion by binding directly to NBD-2 and also prolongs the Po. This effect is increased in the presence of forskolin and appears to be unrelated to tyrosine kinase inhibition. Genistein may also help to move CFTR to the cell surface (17).

Phenylbutyrate (sodium 4-phenylbutyric acid) is a urea scavenger that is approved for the therapy of urea cycle disorders. It is a transcription regulator that increases the amount of CFTR mRNA and thus the amount of CFTR protein that becomes glycosylated and reaches the cell surface. Phenylbutyrate decreases degradation, increases the glycosylated form of ΔF508 CFTR, and increases cAMP-activated chloride efflux through CFTR channels in cell culture. In a preliminary clinical trial at a maximum dose of 19 g orally per day there was an improvement in cAMP-activated chloride current in the nose but no change in sweat chloride values (18).

CFTR channel activity can be partially regulated by hydrolysis by phosphodiesterases. Milrinone and amrinone are class III cyclic phosphodiesterase inhibitors and activators of G proteins. They can activate mutant CFTR by increasing levels of cAMP, particularly when administered in combination with an adenylate cyclase agonist such as forskolin (19).

Improper folding of CFTR in the endoplasmic reticulum prevents proper activity. Molecular chaperones recognize improperly folded proteins and degrade them through the Golgi apparatus. Agents that stabilize proteins in their native conformation and inhibit thermal denaturation may be effective in preserving activity. Cellular osmolites like trimethylamine *N*-oxide appear to have the ability to help CFTR protein achieve the properly folded state for activity (20).

B. Non-CFTR Channel Activation

According to one hypothesis, abnormal ion and water transport in CF epithelia dehydrates the mucous gel layer and reduces the periciliary fluid depth. According to this hypothesis, blocking sodium reabsorption at the epithelium with agents like amiloride should correct the CF defect. Initial clinical trials of aerosolized amiloride appeared promising (21), but later studies demonstrated that amiloride is not effective in promoting sputum clearance in patients with CF (22).

Chloride conductance through the Ca^{+2}-dependent chloride channel is preserved in the CF airway (23). The tricyclic nucleotides UTP and ATP regulate ion transport through P_2Y_2 purinergic receptors that increase intracellular calcium. UTP aerosol, alone or in combination with amiloride, increases transepithelial potential difference and the clearance of inhaled radioaerosol (24). Because UTP is metabolized in less than 30 minutes, it may not be ideal for long-term use as a mucoactive agent, but it may be useful for sputum induction.

C. Gene Transfer Therapy

Successful and permanent gene transfer is the ultimate in correcting ion transport abnormalities in the airway. The potential for gene transfer therapy has been best studied using the CFTR gene. Early trials have identified several problems with the first generation of gene therapy vectors. The first vectors used were replication-deficient adenoviruses (25), and there was an unacceptable host immune response to this virus and an inflammatory response in vivo (26).

There are potential safety issues related to the possibility of insertional mutagenesis with both the adeno-associated virus (AAV) and the lentiviruses. AAV is a small single-stranded DNA parvovirus that is naturally replication defective. When AAV infects a cell it usually requires co-infection with a helper virus to replicate and propagate.With wild-type AAV alone, the virus tends to become latent by stably integrating into a specific area on chromosome 19, minimizing the risk of insertional mutagenesis. AAV *rep* gene products appear to be needed for site-specific integration, meaning that AAV vectors without regulatory elements integrate at multiple sites and may not integrate at all unless the cell divides. Furthermore, AAV has a small package capacity with not much room for CFTR cDNA and regulatory elements (27).

Lentiviruses (retroviruses, of which the HIV is an example) can transfect airway progenitor cells potentially leading to stable and permanent integration of the cDNA into the host cells. At this time, the potential for both insertional mutagenesis and for viral spread are unacceptably great (28). Liposomal-mediated gene transfer is attractive as it does not involve the use infectious vectors. However, the efficiency of the liposomal vectors will need to be increased for effective gene transfer (29).

At this time, and with all vectors, there are some problems related to gene targeting (surface epithelium vs. glands vs. airway progenitor basal cells), gene expression, gene persistence, and protein production that need to be optimized. Evaluating changes in the physical and transport properties of airway secretions after gene complementation is a potentially useful objective endpoint for determining the physiological effects of this therapy.

V. Mucolytics

The physical characterization of secretions includes both bulk physical (rheological) and surface properties. Rheology (viscoelasticity) measurements describe how a material responds to an applied stress. Mucus is a viscoelastic or non-Newtonian fluid because it has both liquid-like (viscous) and solid-like (elastic) properties. *Viscosity* is the resistance to flow and represents the capacity of a material to absorb and dissipate applied energy (stress). *Elasticity* is the capacity of a material to store applied energy. An ideal, or Hookian, solid responds to a stress with a finite deformation (strain), which is recovered after the stress is removed. An ideal liquid responds to a stress by flowing during the time that the stress is applied. After removing the stress, flow ceases and there is no recovery of energy. Mucus responds to stress with an initial, elastic storage of energy followed by a viscoelastic deformation and finally by a period of liquid-like steady flow in which the rate of deformation is fairly constant (3). The secretion and transport of mucus requires that mucus exhibit this non-Newtonian behavior. If mucus were an ideal solid it could not be extruded from the glands, and if mucus were an ideal liquid there could be no efficient transfer of energy from beating cilia. Nevertheless, mucus with too great a viscosity or elasticity, or too low an elasticity, is poorly transported by cilia (3,5,30).

Mucolytic medications reduce viscosity by disrupting polymer networks in the secretions. Classic mucolytic agents work through the severing of di-sulfide bonds, binding of calcium, depolymerizing mucopolysaccharides, and liquefying proteins. Saccharide mucolytics dissociate the mucin entanglements without depolymerizing the mucin filaments. Peptide mucolytics degrade patho-logical filaments of DNA and F-actin (4,31).

A. Classic Mucolytics

Classic mucolytic medications disrupt mucin glycoproteins. Agents containing free sulfhydryl groups reduce the disulfide bridges crosslinking mucin mole-cules. *N*-Acetyl L-Cysteine (NAC) is the general example of this class of drugs. Evidence for the efficacy of NAC is weak (32,33), and inhaled NAC can cause bronchospasm and airway inflammation. There are no data that clearly support the use of this or similar agents as mucolytics.

Nacystelyn (*N*-acetylcysteine lysinate) is a newer agent combining NAC with the amino acid lysine. This agent is more pH neutral than NAC (pH 6.2 vs. 2.2), potentially reducing the risk of airway inflammation after aerosol ad-ministration. In experiments comparing the effects of NAC and nacystelyn ad-ministered by aerosol to healthy anaesthetized dogs, nacystelyn also appeared to have greater mucolytic activity than NAC (34). Clinical trials of this medica-tion for the therapy of CF are underway in Europe.

The protein backbones of mucins are encoded by MUC genes. Of the nine human MUC genes identified to date, seven are expressed in the respiratory tract. MUC5/5AC and MUC4 are generally localized to goblet cells, while MUC5B, MUC8, and MUC7 localize to submucosal glandular cells. MUC5/ 5AC is the predominant mucin mRNA expressed in the airway, and there is increased airway MUC2 expression induced by inflammation. Because mature mucins are heavily glycosylated, it is has been difficult to raise antibodies specific for naked protein stretches of specific MUC mucins that would enable us to associate increased MUC mRNA with increased MUC protein. As these antibodies become available, we may find that increases in specific MUC mucins may be fairly specific markers that identify the nature of airway injury and these may be targets for specific mucolytic or mucoregulatory therapy (35).

B. Low Molecular Weight Saccharide Compounds

Mucins are glycoconjugates in which carbohydrate side chains are linked to a polypeptide backbone by *O*-glycosidic bonds between *N*-acetylgalactosamine and serine or threonine. The individual glycoprotein chains are held together by low-energy, noncovalent bonds (ionic, hydrogen, and Van der Waals forces) forming a tangled network. Saccharide compounds might osmotically pull fluid into the airway, thus increasing mucociliary clearance. This effect should be maximal for monosaccharides and decrease with increasing molecular size. Saccharides may also dissociate mucin polymers by affecting ionic charge interactions and hydrogen bonds, thus altering mucin crosslink density without reducing polymer length. This mechanism is probably optimal for saccharide units that match the length of mucin oligosaccharides (36).

C. Peptide Mucolytics

Sputum contains products of inflammation including neutrophil-derived DNA and filamentous actin (F-actin). High molecular weight DNA is present in CF sputum in concentrations up to 15 mg/mL. DNA and F-actin copolymerize to form a rigid network entangled with the mucin gel (37). Peptide mucolytics degrade these abnormal filaments.

Recombinant human DNase I (dornase alfa) was the first mucolytic agent approved in the United States for the treatment of CF lung disease. In a multicenter study, 320 patients with stable CF lung disease and a forced vital capacity (FVC) of less than 40% predicted were given an aerosol of either 2.5 mg dornase alfa once daily or excipient alone for 12 weeks. In patients receiving dornase alfa there was a 12.4% improvement in FEV_1 above baseline compared with a 2.1% increase in those receiving placebo. Therapy was safe and well tolerated, but dyspnea was more common in the dornase alfa group and the presence of dyspnea was associated with a decreased response (38). Dornase alfa aerosol has not been demonstrated to be effective for the therapy of other airway diseases such as chronic bronchitis (39) or bronchiectasis (40).

Actin is the most prevalent cellular protein in the body, playing a vital role in maintaining the structural integrity of cells. Under proper conditions, G-actin polymerizes to form F-actin. Extracellular F-actin contributes to the viscoelasticity of sputum (41). F-actin concentration in CF sputum has been reported up to 0.15 mg/mL, and there is an increased ratio of F-actin to G-actin in CF sputum when compared to normal secretions. Gelsolin is an 85 kDa (577 residue) actin-severing peptide that reduces the viscosity of CF sputum at low shear rate (41). Thymosin β4 is a small (43-residue) peptide that binds G-actin, both inhibiting the formation of F-actin and shifting the polymerization kinetics to promote the rapid depolymerization of F-actin (42).

VI. Mucokinetic Agents

Cough clearability is independent of sputum viscoelasticity but is strongly influenced by the surface properties of secretions (43,44). Mucus adheres to the cilia and epithelium. Mucokinetic agents improve sputum clearance either by increasing air flow or by reducing adherence of the sputum to the epithelium.

A. Bronchodilators

The relationship between bronchodilatation, improved airflow, and sputum mobilization is complex. Improved sputum clearance leads to improved airflow, just as efficient cough requires adequate airflow. Bronchodilators increase airflow in asthma and CF, and this alone will increase mucus clearance. If airways are unstable, as in some patients with bronchiectasis or tracheomalacia, bronchodilators can further destabilize the airway and hinder sputum clearance (45).

B. Surfactant

There are components of a surfactant layer between the mucous gel and the periciliary fluid. Physiologically, this layer separates the periciliary fluid from the mucous gel and facilitates mucus spreading after secretion from the mucous glands. Exogenous surfactant improves the cough clearance of secretions by decreasing the sputum-epithelium interaction without altering sputum viscoelasticity (43). Some of the expectorant activity of classic mucolytics may also be attributed to their ability to exert their activity on the sputum from the outside inward. Although it would be of little theoretical benefit to reduce the viscosity of an entire mucous plug, by "thinning" the surface it may be possible to "unstick" the secretions from the ciliated epithelium.

As a lubricant (abhesive), surfactant increases the efficiency of energy transfer from the cilia to the mucous layer. Aerosolized surfactant increases mucociliary transport in the canine trachea in vivo (46), and in clinical trials of aerosol surfactant there was a 12% increase in FEV_1 and a decrease in trapped thoracic gas associated with increased sputum transportability (47).

Ambroxol was thought to mobilize secretions in part by stimulating surfactant secretion. This medication has been used for many years in Europe for the management of chronic bronchitis but has not been approved in the United

States or Canada. A double-blind, randomized, placebo-controlled trial in 90 patients with chronic bronchitis who had difficulty clearing secretions showed no clinical benefit (48).

VII. Mucoregulatory Agents

Mucoregulatory agents decrease mucus production or mucus secretion. These agents have been most thoroughly studied for the therapy of bronchorrhea and for diffuse panbronchiolitis, a chronic hypersecretory airway disease seen almost exclusively in Japan and Korea.

A. Anticholinergics

Anticholinergic medications reduce the volume of stimulated secretions without increasing viscosity (49). They have no demonstrable effect on constitutive (unstimulated) mucus secretion (50). Quaternary anticholinergic medications such as ipratropium bromide reduce the volume of stimulated secretions without changing their viscoelastic or transport properties (51). In patients with chronic bronchitis, regular treatment with oxitropium improves airflow limitation and reduces sputum production, probably through the inhibition of both mucus secretion and water transport (52). It is possible that more specific M3 receptor antagonists may provide better control of mucus hypersecretion (53).

B. Anti-inflammatory Medications

Many inflammatory mediators are potent secretagogues, and chronic inflammation leads to mucous gland hyperplasia. There is experimental evidence that steroids are effective in reducing the volume of secretions (54,55). There are no published data on the use of inhaled steroids as mucoregulatory agents, but it is likely that this mode of delivery would also be effective. Steroids also reduce the severity of CF lung disease. Side effects seen at the higher dose of 2 mg/kg of prednisone per day has limited the use of this therapy (56), but at a dose of 1 mg/kg/day, side effects are minimal and clinical benefit is equivalent to that of ibuprofen therapy (see below).

Ibuprofen at a peak peak plasma concentration of 50–100 µg/mL has specific activity against neutrophils. In a 4-year trial of ibuprofen in patients with mild CF lung disease, there was a slower decline in pulmonary function and better body weight in the ibuprofen group, and the effect was most pronounced in younger patients (57). With more widespread use of ibuprofen there are reports of gastrointestinal and bleeding problems. Plasma concentrations must be tightly controlled. At higher doses there is an increased risk of side effects, and at concentrations lower than the therapeutic range there is a risk of paradoxically increased neutrophil activation.

Indomethacin is an anti-inflammatory agent that has been administered by aerosol for the treatment of mucus hypersecretion associated with diffuse panbronchiolitis (58). Pentoxifylline is a xanthine that inhibits the synthesis of TNFα and IL-1β, probably by inhibiting phosphodiesterase activity. In a preliminary study in CF patients receiving 1600 mg/day for 6 months, there was no change in bronchial neutrophil elastase, but there was an increase in those taking placebo (59).

Tyloxapol is an alkylaryl polyether alcohol polymer, nonionic detergent, and antioxidant that was used with a mixture of other mucolytic agents for the treatment of chronic bronchitis in the United States until 1981. Tyloxapol has been reported to inhibit the nuclear transcription factor, NF-κB, scavenge oxygen radicals, and reduce cystic fibrosis sputum viscosity in vitro (60).

C. Macrolide Antibiotics

Some of the 14-carbon macrolide antibiotics, particularly erythromycin and clarithromycin, appear to be able to reduce mucus secretion (61–64) and improve mucus clearability (65). This action is unrelated to antibacterial activity and may be due to an anti-inflammatory action (66,67). Tamaoki and colleagues studied the effect of clarithromycin on sputum properties in patients with chronic lower respiratory tract infections (63). Clarithromycin was given at 100 mg twice daily for 8 weeks and compared with placebo. They reported that clarithromycin decreased sputum production from 51 to 24 g/day and the percent solids of the sputum increased from 2.44 to 3.01% in patients given clarithromycin, with no effect in patients given a placebo.

VIII. Clinical Use of Mucoactive Therapy

Mucoactive therapy is used to reduce airway obstruction due to abnormal secretions. The majority of diseases that have been potential targets for mucoregulatory therapy are associated with hypersecretion and poor clearance of airway secretions. By decreasing the volume of airway secretions, gas trapping is reduced and there is improved performance of the muscles of respiration. Mucus overproduction and retention could be due to epithelial damage with disrupted clearance, increased secretion production, and abnormal secretion properties. Thus, therapy should be directed at reducing infection and inflammation, minimizing exposure to airway irritants, using mucoregulatory medications to decrease mucus production, and employing medications, physical therapy, and mechanical devices to assist the patient with sputum expectoration.

Patients most likely to benefit from mucoactive therapy usually have a history of increased sputum expectoration and preserved airflow. Theoretically, when airflow is profoundly compromised, mucolytic agents could reduce sputum clearance due to the retrograde flow of airway secretions. Also, patients with acute mucus retention may be less responsive to mucoactive medications due to decreased airflow and to muscular weakness caused by the infection, further reducing airflow-dependent clearance mechanisms.

Knowledge of the physical and transport properties of airway secretions has given us improved tools to better understand the mechanisms of pulmonary disease, to develop and assess new therapeutic agents, and to identify those patients who are most likely to benefit from mucoactive therapy.

References

1. King M, Rubin BK. Mucus physiology and pathophysiology: therapeutic aspects. In: Derenne JP, Similowski T, Whitelaw WA, eds. Chronic Obstructive Lung Disease. New York: Marcel Dekker, 1996:391–411.
2. Wanner A, Salathé M, O'Riordan TG. Mucociliary clearance in the airways. Am J Respir Crit Care Med 1996; 154:1868–1902.
3. King M, Rubin BK. Mucus rheology: relationship with transport. In: Takishima T, ed. Airway Secretion: Physiological Bases for the Control of Mucus Hypersecretion. New York: Marcel Dekker, 1994:283–314.
4. Rubin BK, Tomkiewicz RP, King M. Mucoactive agents: old and new. In: Wilmott RW, ed. The Pediatric Lung. Basel: Birkhäuser, 1997:155–179.
5. Rubin BK, MacLeod PM, Sturgess JM, King M. Recurrent respiratory infections in a child with fucosidosis: is the mucus too thin for effective transport? Ped Pulmonol 1991; 10:304–309.
6. Iotti GA, Olivei MC, Palo A, et al. Unfavorable mechanical effects of heat and moisture exchangers in ventilated patients. Intensive Care Med 1997; 23:399–405.
7. Shim C, King M, Williams MJ. Lack of effect of hydration on sputum production in chronic bronchitis. Chest 1987; 92:679–682.
8. Marchette LC, Marchette BE, Abraham WM, Wanner A. The effect of systemic hydration on normal and impaired mucociliary function. Pediatr Pulmonol 1985; 1: 107–111.
9. Rubin BK, Ramirez O, Ohar JA. Iodinated glycerol has no effect on pulmonary function, symptom score, or sputum properties in patients with stable bronchitis. Chest 1996; 109:348–352.
10. Eng PA, Morton J, Douglass JA, Riedler J, Wilson J, Robertson CF. Short term efficacy of ultrasonically nebulized hypertonic saline in cystic fibrosis. Pediatr Pulmonol 1996; 21: 77–83.
11. Daviskas E, Anderson SD, Brannan JD, Chan HK, Eberl S, Bautovich G. Inhalation of dry-powder mannitol increases mucociliary clearance. Eur Respir J 1997; 10: 2449–2454.
12. Wills PJ, Hall RL, Chan WM, Cole PJ. Sodium chloride increases the ciliary transportability of cystic fibrosis and bronchiectasis sputum on the mucus-depleted bovine trachea. J Clin Invest 1997; 99:9–13.

13. Smith JJ, Travis SM, Greenberg EP, Welsh MJ. Cystic fibrosis airway epithelia fail to kill bacteria because of abnormal airway surface fluid. Cell 1996; 85:229–236.
14. Jiang Q, Engelhardt JF. Cellular heterogeneity of CFTR expression and function in the lung: implications for gene therapy of cystic fibrosis. Eur J Hum Gene 1998; 6:12–31.
15. Dorin JR, Farley R, Webb S, et al. A demonstration using mouse models that successful gene therapy for cystic fibrosis requires only partial gene correction. Gene Ther 1996; 3:797–801.
16. Arispe N, Ma J, Jacobson KA, Pollard HB. Direct activation of cystic fibrosis transmembrane conductance regulator channels by 8-cyclopentyl-1,3-dipropylxanthine (CPX) and 1,3-diallyl-8-cyclohexylxanthine (DAX). J Biol Chem 1998; 273: 5727–5734.
17. Weinreich F, Wood PG, Riordan JR, Nagel G. Direct action of genistein on CFTR. Pflugers Arch 1997; 434:484–491.
18. Rubenstein RC, Zeitlin PL. A pilot clinical trial of oral sodium 4-phenylbutyrate (Buphenyl) in deltaF508-homozygous cystic fibrosis patients: partial restoration of nasal epithelial CFTR function. Am J Respir Crit Care Med 1998; 157:484–490.
19. Haws CM, Nepomuceno I, Krouse ME, Wakelee H, Law T, Xia Y, Nguyen H, Wine JJ. ΔF508-CFTR channels: Kinetics, activation by forskolin, and potentiation by xanthines. Am J Physiol 1996; 270:C1544–1555.
20. Brown CR, Hong-Brown LQ, Biwersi J, Verkman AS, Welch WJ. Chemical chaperones correct the mutant phenotype of the delta F508 cystic fibrosis transmembrane conductance regulator protein. Cell Stress Chaperones 1996; 1:117–125.
21. Knowles MR, Church NL, Waltner WE, Yankaskas JR, Gilligan P, King M, Edwards LJ, Helms RW, Boucher RC. A pilot study of aerosolized amiloride for the treatment of lung disease in cystic fibrosis. N Engl J Med 1990; 322:1189–1194.
22. Graham A, Hashani A, Alton EW, Martin GP, Marriott C, Hodson ME, Clarke SW, Geddes DM. No added benefit from nebulized amiloride in patients with cystic fibrosis. Eur Respir J 1993; 6:1243–1248.
23. Stutts MJ, Fitz JG, Paradiso AM, Boucher RC. Multiple modes of regulation of airway epithelial chloride secretion by extracellular ATP. Am J Physiol 1994; 267: C1442–C1451.
24. Bennett WD, Olivier KN, Zeman KL, Hohneker KH, Boucher RC, Knowles MR. Effect of aerosolized uridine 5′-triphosphate plus amiloride on mucociliary clearance in adult cystic fibrosis patients. Am J Respir Crit Care Med 1996; 153:1796–1801.
25. Bellon G, Michel-Calemard L, Thouvenot D, et al. Aerosol administration of a recombinant adenovirus expressing CFTR to cystic fibrosis patients: a phase I clinical trial. Hum Gene Ther 1997; 8:15–25.
26. Otake K, Ennist DL, Harrod K, Trapnell BC. Nonspecific inflammation inhibits adenovirus-mediated pulmonary gene transfer and expression independent of specific acquired immune responses. Hum Gene Ther 1998; 9:2207–2222.
27. Flotte T, Carter B, Conrad C, Guggino,W, Reynolds T, Rosenstein B, Taylor G, Walden S, Wetzel R. A phase I study of an adeno-associated virus-CFTR gene vector in adult CF patients with mild lung disease. Hum Gene Ther 1996; 7:1145–1159.

28. Goldman MJ, Lee PS, Yang JS, Wilson JM. Lentiviral vectors for gene therapy of cystic fibrosis. Hum Gene Ther 1997; 8:2261–2268.

29. McDonald RJ, Liggitt HD, Roche L, Nguyen HT, Pearlman, R, Raabe OG, Bussey LB, Gorman CM. Aerosol delivery of lipid:DNA complexes to lungs of rhesus monkeys. Pharm Res 1998; 15:671–679.

30. Puchelle E, Zahm JM, Girard F, Bertrand A, Polu JM, Aug F, Sadoul P. Mucociliary transport in vivo and in vitro. Relations to sputum properties in chronic bronchitis. Eur J Respir Dis 1980; 61:254–264.

31. Dasgupta B, King M. Molecular basis for mucolytic therapy. Can Respir J 1995; 2:223–230.

32. Millar AB, Pavia D, Agnew JE, Lopez-Vidriero MT, Lauque D, Clarke SW. Effect of oral N-acetylcysteine on mucus clearance. Br J Dis Chest 1985; 79:262–266.

33. Thomson ML, Pavia D, Jones CJ, McQuiston TA. No demonstrable effect of S-carboxymethylcysteine on clearance of secretions from human lung. Thorax 1975; 30:669–673.

34. Tomkiewicz RP, App EM, De Sanctis GT, Coffiner M, Maes P, Rubin BK, King M. A comparison of a new mucolytic N-acetylcysteine L-lysinate with N-acetylcysteine: airway epithelial function and mucus changes in dog. Pulm Pharmacol 1995; 8:259–265.

35. Rose MC, Gendler SJ. Airway mucin genes and gene products. In: Rogers DF, Lethem MI, eds. Airway Mucus: Basic Mechanisms and Clinical Perspectives. Basel: Birkhäuser, 1997:41–66.

36. Feng W, Garrett H, Speert DP, King M. Improved clearability of cystic fibrosis sputum with dextran treatment in vitro. Am J Respir Crit Care Med 1998; 157: 710–714.

37. Tomkiewicz RP, Kishioka C, Freeman J, Rubin BK. DNA and actin filament ultrastructure in cystic fibrosis sputum. In: Baum G, ed. Cilia, Mucus and Mucociliary Interactions. New York: Marcel Dekker, 1998:333–341.

38. McCoy K, Hamilton S, Johnson C. Effects of 12-week administration of dornase alfa in patients with advanced cystic fibrosis lung disease. Chest 1996; 110:889–895.

39. Bone RC, Fuchs H, Fox NL, Meinert L, Sanders C, Hyzy R, Thompson N, Fiel S. The chronic obstructive pulmonary disease mortality endpoint trial. Chest 1995; 108:R.

40. Wills PJ, Wodehouse T, Corkery K, Mallon K, Wilson R, Cole PJ. Short-term recombinant human DNase in bronchiectasis. Effect on clinical state and in vitro sputum transportability. Am J Respir Crit Care Med 1996; 154:413–417.

41. Vasconcellos CA, Allen PG, Wohl M, Drazen JM, Janmey PA. Reduction in sputum viscosity of cystic fibrosis sputum in vitro by gelsolin. Science 1994; 263: 969–971.

42. Rubin BK. Emerging therapies for cystic fibrosis lung disease. Chest 1999; 115: 1120–1126.

43. Rubin BK. Surface properties of respiratory secretions: relationship to mucus transport. In: Baum G, ed. Cilia, Mucus, and Mucociliary Interactions. New York: Marcel Dekker, 1998:317–324.

44. Agarwal M, King M, Rubin BK, Shukla JB. Mucus transport in a miniaturized

simulated cough machine: Effect of constriction and serous layer simulant. Bior-heology 1989; 26:977–988.

45. Rubin BK. Tracheomalacia as a cause of respiratory compromise in infants. Clin Pulm Med 1999; 6:1–4.

46. De Sanctis GT, Tomkiewicz RP, Rubin BK, Schürch S, King M. Exogenous surfactant enhances mucociliary clearance in the anaesthetized dog. Eur Respir J 1994; 7:1616–1621.

47. Anzueto A, Jubran A, Ohar JA, Piquette CA, Rennard SI, Colice G, Pattishall EN, Barret J, Engle M, Perret K, Rubin BK. Effects of aerosolized surfactant in patients with stable chronic bronchitis. A prospective randomized controlled trial. JAMA 1997; 278:1426–1431.

48. Guyatt GH, Townsend M, Kazim F, Newhouse MT. A controlled trial of ambroxol in chronic bronchitis. Chest 1987; 92:618–620.

49. Lopez-Vidriero MT, Costello J, Clark TJ, Das I, Keal EE, Reid L. Effect of atropine on sputum production. Thorax 1975; 30:543–547.

50. King M, Cohen C, Viires N. Influence of vagal tone on rheology and transportability of canine tracheal mucus. Am Rev Respir Dis 1979; 120:1215–1219.

51. Wanner A. Effect of ipratropium bromide on airway mucociliary function. Am J Med 1986; 81:23–27.

52. Tamaoki J, Chiyotani A, Tagaya E, Sakai N, Konno K. Effect of long term treatment with oxitropium bromide on airway secretion in chronic bronchitis and diffuse panbronchiolitis. Thorax 1994; 49:545–548.

53. Barnes PJ. Muscarinic receptor subtypes: implications for therapy. Agents Actions Suppl 1993; 43:243–252.

54. Moretti M, Giannico G, Marchioni CF, Bisetti A. Effects of methylprednisolone on sputum biochemical components in asthmatic bronchitis. Eur J Respir Dis 1984; 65:365–370.

55. Marom Z, Shelhamer J, Alling D, Kaliner M. The effects of corticosteroids on mucous glycoprotein secretion from human airways in vitro. Am Rev Respir Dis 1984; 129:62–65.

56. Eigen H, Rosenstein BJ, FitzSimmons S, Schidlow DV. A multicenter study of alternate-day prednisone therapy in patients with cystic fibrosis. Cystic fibrosis foundation prednisone trial group. J Pediatr 1995; 126:515–523.

57. Konstan MW, Byard PJ, Hoppel CL, Davis PB. Effect of high-dose ibuprofen in patients with cystic fibrosis. N Engl J Med 1995; 332:848–854.

58. Tamaoki J, Chiyotani A, Kobayashi K, Sakai N, Kanemura T, Takizawa T. Effect of indomethacin on bronchorrhea in patients with chronic bronchitis, diffuse panbronchiolitis, or bronchiectasis. Am Rev Respir Dis 1992; 145:548–552.

59. Aronoff SC, Quinn FJ Jr, Carpenter LS, Novick WJ Jr. Effects of pentoxifylline on sputum neutrophil elastase and pulmonary function in patients with cystic fibrosis: preliminary observations. J Pediatrics 1994; 125:992–997.

60. Ghio AJ, Marshall BC, Diaz JL, Hasegawa T, Samuelson W, Povia D, Kennedy TP, Piantadosi CA. Tyloxapol inhibits NF-κB and cytokine release, scavenges HOCL, and reduces viscosity of cystic fibrosis sputum. Am J Respir Crit Care Med 1996; 154:783–788.

61. Tamaoki J, Takeyama K, Yamawaki I, Kondo M, Konno K. Lipopolysaccharide-

induced goblet cell hypersecretion in the guinea pig trachea: inhibition by macrolides. Am J Physiol 1997; 272:L15–L19.

62. Suez D, Szefler SJ. Excessive accumulation of mucus in children with asthma: a potential role for erythromycin? A case discussion. J Allergy Clin Immunol 1986; 77:330–334.
63. Tamaoki J, Takeyama K, Tagaya E, Konno K. Effect of clarithromycin on sputum production and its rheological properties in chronic respiratory tract infections. Antimicrob Agents Chemother 1995; 39:1688–1690.
64. Suga T, Sugiyama Y, Fujii T, Kitamura S. Bronchoalveolar carcinoma with bronchorrhoea treated with erythromycin. Eur Respir J 1994; 7:2249–2251.
65. Rubin BK, Druce H, Ramirez OE, Palmer R. Effect of clarithromycin on nasal mucus properties in healthy subjects and in patients with purulent rhinitis. Am J Respir Crit Care Med 1997; 155:2018–2023.
66. Tamaoki J, Sakai N, Tagaya E, Konno K. Macrolide antibiotics protect against endotoxin-induced vascular leakage and neutrophil accumulation in rat trachea. Antimicrob Agents Chemother 1994; 38:1641–1643.
67. Khair OA, Devalia JL, Abdelaziz MM, Sapsford RJ, Davies RJ. Effect of erythromycin on Haemophilus influenzae endotoxin-induced release of IL-6, IL-8 and sICAM-1 by cultured human bronchial epithelial cells. Eur Respir J 1995; 8:1451–1457.

7

Mucoactive Drug Delivery

ISRAEL AMIRAV

R. Sieff Hospital
Kfar Hanassi, Israel

MICHAEL T. NEWHOUSE

Nektar Therapeutics
San Carlos, California, U.S.A.

I. Introduction

Respiratory-tract secretions consisting of mucus, surfactant, and periciliary fluid are vital components of respiratory defenses since they trap, absorb, dilute, and, by virtue of their contained lysozyme, antibodies, etc., assist in destroying noxious biological and nonbiological invaders. Acute and chronic airway injury results in inflammatory changes, which are usually associated with hypersecretion from goblet cells and mucous glands. The resulting secretions can also be physically abnormal, particularly when they become infected, and this can lead to mucus inspissation, postobstructive atelectasis, and pneumonitis. A vicious circle leading to airway and parenchymal injury and/or destruction with bronchiectasis and pulmonary fibrosis may result and can lead to severe pulmonary dysfunction and death unless the excessive and/or abnormal secretions are eliminated.

For many years physicians have employed a variety of agents as "mucolytics" and "expectorants" in an attempt to improve mucus clearance. Because mucolysis is only one of the ways to alter mucus clearance, they have been more appropriately called "mucoactive" drugs. By definition, a mucoactive drug is one that possesses as its primary action the capability of modifying mucus volume (mucoregulation), modifying physical characteristics to thin excessively tenacious secretions (mucolysis) and/or improve the mobilization of secretions (mucokinesis) (1). Most of the original mucoactive drugs were manufactured as oral preparations designed to either decrease mucus production or accelerate mucus clearance. Because of its many advantages, the oral route has been the "traditional" method of administering these medications. Dosing of oral preparations is relatively precise—the dose delivered to the body is consistent, although absorption is not necessarily efficient, and swallowing a pill is an easy task for most adults. Some mucoactive agents—for example, the macrolide antibiotics—appear to be effective only when given orally. Other drugs may best target effector cells if given orally. This is the case with the expectorant guaifenesin (glycerol guiacolate), which may stimulate mucus secretion via a gastric vagal reflex (2). If applied directly to the epithelium (e.g., by aerosol) it may even be ciliotoxic (3). In general, compliance with oral administration may be better than with other forms of administration.

An ideal oral mucoactive agent should be:

1. Easily ingested (in terms of both dose and taste)
2. Well absorbed from the gastro-intestinal tract
3. With minimal and minor (ideally no) side effects
4. Effective in decreasing secretions and improving mucus clearance

In practice, systemically administered agents used to treat airway diseases are often only marginally effective because of a poor therapeutic ratio. This is because only 1–2% of the systemic dose actually reaches the airways (4). Thus, in recent years, there has been an increasing trend toward airway drug targeting by means of aerosol inhalation. The advantage of inhaling mucoactive medications is that they are directed at the target organ (the airways), are likely to have a more rapid onset of action, and cause fewer side effects due to reduced systemic absorption and hemodilution. A large number of newer compounds are peptides and proteins, which are easily broken down by enzymes in the stomach; if taken orally, they would never reach their destination. Furthermore, compared with oral or intravenous administration, the dose of inhaled drug for equivalent therapeutic benefit in the airways can be substantially decreased.

The targeting of mucoactive drugs to the respiratory tract is critically dependent on the delivery system. As the oral route has, with rare exceptions (5), been largely ineffective—in particular with mucolytic agents (6)—this chapter is devoted mainly to the inhaled route of administration, likely to be most effective for the majority of mucoactive agents. We first present an overview of available aerosol delivery systems followed by examples of the application of these systems to therapy with aerosolized mucoactive drugs.

II. Aerosol Delivery Systems

Therapeutic aerosols may be generated and delivered by small-volume liquid nebulizers (SVNs), pressurized metered-dose inhalers (pMDIs), or dry-powder inhalers (DPIs). SVNs and pMDIs are considered "active" devices, which generate the aerosol independent of the patient's effort, deaggregated and suitable for inhalation. DPIs can be either "active" or "passive" devices. Passive devices require vigorous suction by the patient to deaggregate the powder and simultaneously inhale the medication (Table 1).

A. Small-Volume Nebulizers

Jet Nebulizers

The majority of currently used commercial nebulizers were developed from squeeze-bulb devices. They utilize compressed gas to generate liquid aerosol droplets by means of a Venturi that operates on the Bernoulli principle—

Table 1 Aerosol Generation and Delivery Devices

Small-volume liquid nebulizers (SVNs)
  Jet
  Ultrasonic
  Electrohydrodynamic (Batelle Pharma, Columbus, Ohio)
  Atomizers*
    Reservoir (e.g., Respimat, Boehringer Ingelheim Pharma, Ingelheim am Rhein, Germany)
    Unit dose blister (e.g., AeRx, Aradigm Corp., Hayward, California)
Metered-dose inhalers (pMDIs)
  Press and breathe
  Breath-activated (e.g., Autohaler, 3M, St. Paul, Minnesota)
pMDI with Accessory Devices
  Spacers—simple extension tubes
  Valved holding chambers (VHCs)
Dry-powder inhalers (DPIs)
  Passive (e.g., Rotahaler or Diskus, Glaxo Wellcome, Ware, England; Clickhaler, ML Labs, St Albans, England; FO2, Boehringer Ingelheim, Ingelheim, Germany; Turbuhaler, Astra, Lund, Sweden)
  Active*
    Battery-powered turbine (e.g., Spiros, Dura Parmaceuticals, Berkeley, California)
    Compressed air–driven (e.g., Powder Delivery System, Inhale Therapeutic Systems, San Carlos, California)
    Mechanical (spring-driven) scraper (Maghaler, Frankfurt, Germany)

*All still experimental.

namely, acceleration of gas through a small orifice directed across a liquid-filled capillary tube (7). This causes a fall in pressure at the capillary orifice that results in the drug solution being forced through the capillary from a reservoir by atmospheric pressure. The liquid is thus turned into a heterodisperse aerosol containing droplets of a range of sizes with a geometric standard deviation (GSD) greater than 1.22. The larger droplets are removed by baffles, while particles below 10 μm, down to approximately 0.5 μm, mass median aerodynamic diameter (MMAD) are inhaled into the lower respiratory tract (LRT) with increasing probability as their aerodynamic diameter decreases. LRT delivery efficiency peaks at about 80–90% for particles of approximately 1–2 μm delivered to the mouth in normal adults inhaling at ~0.5 L/sec from functional residual capacity to total lung capacity (8). The major problem with jet nebulization is that the primary droplets are relatively coarse. In order to filter out the larger droplets (over 5μm) and limit the output, as much as possible, to the lung-targetable dose (MMAD <~ 3 μm), inertial filtration is used. Nebulizers that deliver fine aerosols do so by baffling out and recirculating coarse droplets. This produces smaller particles better suited for targeting to the LRT and reduces oropharyngeal deposition. The disadvantage is long nebulization times that may lead to reduced compliance, especially among children and adolescents. Overall LRT deposition is usually no more than 8–10%, due mainly to the nebulizer "dead volume" (residual drug in the nebulizer reservoir and on the walls) and aerosol losses to the environment during exhalation with continuously operating devices or on exhalation with aerosols below about 1 μm.

Increasing the fill volume increases the overall drug delivery efficiency (DDE) to the mouth but prolongs the nebulization time. Using undiluted, very concentrated drug solutions may reduce the nebulization time for a given dose but is wasteful in medication. However, this may not be an important issue with inexpensive agents.

Advantages of SVNs include relative ease of use (patients can inhale from nebulizers by tidal breathing without the need to coordinate inspiration and aerosol delivery) and ability to aerosolize large volumes (up to 15–20 mL/hr with large-volume nebulizers) and deliver medications (e.g., large peptides) that are not formulated for delivery by pMDIs or DPIs.

The disadvantages of SVNs include: cost—the compressors required to drive the nebulizers are expensive ($120–150); longer administration time—an average treatment lasts 10–15 minutes; discomfort—younger children may not tolerate the tightly fitting mask and the compressor noise for more than a few seconds and may cry, thus getting little, if any medication (9); inconvenience—compressor-driven nebulization systems are bulky, not readily portable, and need a power source and frequent cleaning to prevent contamination (10). Another disadvantage of nebulizers is their lack of standardization that has led to considerable (as much as 10- to 20-fold) inter- and intramodel variability, the latter suggesting poor quality control (11,12). Having recognized that a serious problem exists in this regard, European and North American committees have been formed to develop standards for nebulizers.

Ultrasonic Nebulizers

Ultrasonic nebulizers (USNs) produce aerosol particles by means of high-frequency vibration of a piezoelectric crystal (7). The advantage of USNs is that they may deliver a large volume of aerosol over a reasonably short period of time. When choosing USNs, it is important to ensure that they are sufficiently powered to produce therapeutic aerosols of particle size appropriate for efficient airway and lung deposition. Some of the earlier, underpowered USNs generated inappropriately large particles, most of which were deposited in the oropharynx (e.g., manufactured by Siemens-Bosch, Munich). The LRT deposition efficiency of such devices rarely exceeds 3%. Durability of USNs has been an ongoing problem because saline tends to crystallize around the circuitry of the USN, causing malfunction. As the USN empties, there is considerable stress on the crystal, which may cause it to crack and fail. Current designs use a number of electronic tricks such as load sensing and automatic frequency matching to control crystal temperature and increase reliability. Other disadvantages of USN devices is their tendency to denature peptide medications due to relatively high temperatures, their inefficiency for nebulizing drug suspensions (13), their generally larger droplet size, and their high cost.

Small-Volume Nebulizers: Drug Delivery Efficiency

A major problem with nebulizers is that they have a large internal "dead volume" and up to 50% of a 3-ml fill can remain trapped inside the nebulizer body on the walls and baffles and in the tubing (14). Overall lower respiratory tract drug delivery efficiency (LDE) varies greatly between 5 and 15% (rarely ≥ 10–15%) and nebulization time varies between ~5 and 15 minutes. Most nebulizers deliver aerosol continuously whereas patients only inhale for approximately 30–50% of the respiratory cycle. Thus, the dose available to be inhaled into the LRT is half or less of that delivered to the mouth. In general, only about 10% or less of the drug dose placed in the nebulizer actually deposits within the lower respiratory tract even with optimal inhalation technique.

There is room for improvement in nebulizer design and standardization. Some newer nebulizers have interrupters or inspiratory control valves that allow synchronization of aerosol delivery and inspiration. Others have holding chambers, or "reservoirs," that fill during exhalation and are emptied on inspiration. Newer designs incorporate an extra vent into the nebulizer in such a way that the negative pressure generated by the expansion of compressed air at the Venturi sucks air into the chamber via the vent as well as fluid for atomization from the feeding capillary tubes. This "open-vent" design results in greater airflow through the chamber, thus delivering more small particles and shortening nebulization time as a result of increased evaporation. Other designs have (e.g., Optineb, Air Liquide, Paris) used electronic or manual interrupters. The latter require coordination by the patient and, due to the time required to achieve maximum flow, will initially generate larger particles, reducing LDE while at the same time somewhat prolonging the duration of administration.

The recent generation of nebulizers was designed to combine the convenience of continuous operation and the efficiency of intermittent nebulization. One design (Pari LC Plus, Pari, Germany) nebulizes continuously, but a valve on top of the device opens only during inspiration, allowing extra air to be drawn through the nebulizer. As with the open-vent nebulizers, it is claimed that this air will draw a greater number of lung-targetable particles into the inspired air stream. During exhalation the inspiratory valve closes, decreasing the flow of air through the chamber to that from the compressor only. This limits losses of aerosol during exhalation to that from a conventional jet nebulizer. Likewise, the Ventstream (Inspired Medical Products, Pagham, West Sussex, England) has a valve that opens only during inspiration, allowing air to be drawn through the nebulizer to increase drug output. On exhalation this valve closes as exhaled air passes out of the device through a separate expiratory pathway. These "breath-assisted, open-vent" nebulizers increase the LDE and reduce wastage (15). Another recent development by Trudell Medical International (London, Ontario) is an inexpensive, disposable jet nebulizer that mechanically generates aerosol on demand only (16). This device uses a spring-loaded diaphragm to separate the drug solution–containing feed tube from the air jet during exhalation. At the onset of inhalation the liquid feed tube and air jet are aligned by the negative pressure and aerosol generation is initiated.

B. Pressurized Metered-Dose Inhalers (pMDIs)

pMDIs are small spray cans that have been the standard for about half a century for targeting most aerosolized drugs to the pulmonary airways. pMDIs have traditionally used chlorofluorocarbon (CFC) 12 and 114 with high vapor pressure at room temperature as the power source and CFC 11, which is liquid at room temperature, as the suspending liquid, or solvent for the drug. pMDIs are by far the most popular aerosol generators, accounting for about 70% of the 500 million aerosol therapy devices sold annually worldwide. They accurately and reproducibly deliver a metered dose of CFC-pressurized drug suspension or solution. CFCs are gradually being replaced by newer, more ozone-friendly propellants such as hydrofluoro alkane (HFA) 134a or 227. The HFA 134a beclomethasone formulation (QVAR) developed by 3M allows relatively small uniform droplet aerosols (MMAD of ~ 1.1 μm and GSD ~ 2) to be generated, with an

LDE of 50–60%. This fine aerosol more efficiently deposits not only in large but also in small airways and alveoli even in the presence of airflow obstruction because particles ≤1.0 μm behave increasingly like a gas as their MMAD decreases. On a dose-per-dose basis this superfine aerosol is more than twice as effective as the coarser CFC formulation and has a similar safety profile (17).

pMDIs consists of three major components: a reservoir containing drug particles in suspension or drug solution in pressure-liquefied inert gas propellant; a metering valve, which when depressed reliably delivers a fairly precise quantity of the reservoir contents; and a spray actuator, which together with the stem of the metering valve comprises a twin orifice expansion chamber and spray nozzle that directs the aerosol toward the mouthpiece of the pMDI.

The main advantages of pMDIs are their small size, multidose convenience, versatility (with appropriate attachments), higher LDE, dose reproducibility from puff to puff, freedom from bacterial contamination, and self-contained power source. Additional important benefits include ergonomic similarity from manufacturer to manufacturer, multiple-dose capability, rational drug combinations within the same canister (e.g., sympathomimetic with parasympatholytic or with corticosteroids), and lower cost per dose.

The main disadvantages of pMDI, especially in young children and the elderly, is that, when used alone, patients and caregivers may find them difficult to use because they require considerable hand–breath coordination to achieve optimal benefit. Breath-activated pMDIs that provide medication only on inspiration have recently been introduced and may prove useful in older children (>6 years) as well as in adults with poor coordination who can reliably achieve the inspiratory flow of 25–30 L/min necessary to activate them. Another disadvantage is release of aerosol at high velocity (~100 kph). This ballistic effect, more marked with the larger, high-inertia aerosol droplets, causes deposition of approximately 65% of the medication from CFC-driven devices (~30% with HFA) in the upper respiratory tract (URT) (mouth, oropharynx, and larynx). This URT dose contributes considerably to increased systemic absorption and side effects, including local side effects (hoarseness, gagging or burning sensation, candidiasis, bad taste) in the oropharynx and larynx (18). The low temperature of the CFCs or HFAs discharged from a pMDI frequently causes children to abruptly stop inhaling (cold freon effect). The possible contribution of CFCs to destruction of the stratospheric ozone layer has been an increasing environmental concern. The Montreal protocol is an international agreement to ban the manufacture and use of CFCs in developed countries, with a year-to-year exemption for any remaining essential medical purposes, starting in 2005 (in Third World nations by 2012). It was this that caused the chemical and pharmaceutical industries to develop innovative substitutes using HFA 134a (also used increasingly for refrigeration, foaming plastics, etc.) and 227 instead of CFC12 and 114.

Unfortunately, there is no ready substitute for CFC 11, which has made reformulation of pMDIs very challenging.

pMDI Accessory Devices: Spacers and Valved Holding Chambers

Over the past 20 years, these "low-tech" and inexpensive pMDI add-on units have evolved into highly sophisticated patient- and task-specific devices that have had a major impact on aerosol delivery at home and in hospital practice. The addition of valved holding chambers (VHCs) to pMDIs reduces problems of hand–breath coordination, by dissociating aerosol discharge and inhalation. They also considerably decrease (by up to 90%) ballistic deposition in the oropharynx and total body dose by 75%, improve the LDE by 30–50%, increase the therapeutic ratio, and facilitate patient- and task-specific aerosol delivery (19).

MDI accessory devices began as simple tubes or containers (e.g., coffee cups, toilet rolls, modified 1–1.5-liter plastic flasks), which were appropriately named spacers. The main benefit of spacers is that they allow the larger aerosol particles that have little or no therapeutic benefit to decelerate and deposit about 50% in the spacer, thus reducing ballistic and inertial impaction of particles in the URT. This decreases systemic absorption and local side effects. The main rationale behind the development of pMDI accessory devices was to provide a reservoir of aerosol, from which the patient could breathe, removing the need to coordinate the actuation of the inhaler with inspiration. While spacers still require hand–breath coordination, the development of relatively simple and practical VHCs almost completely overcame this problem. Furthermore, VHCs with masks enabled pMDIs to be used instead of nebulizers in relatively uncooperative, tidal breathing patients such as the confused elderly and adults or children with severe shortness of breath (e.g., during acute severe asthma). The addition of a face mask to the VHC also allowed pMDIs to be used successfully in infants and children from birth to 3–4 years of age who are too young to breath through a mouthpiece. Using a VHC also allows more CFC or HFA to evaporate and traps excipients such as oleic acid. This results in a greater mass (by up to 40%) of smaller drug particles (20), which not only enhances drug penetration but increases the dose delivered to more peripheral airways, improving clinical outcomes (21).

Some larger MDI accessory devices (up to 750 ml) are relatively bulky and children will usually be reluctant to use them in school. Large VHCs provide only slightly greater output in particles under 2–3 μm than 150 mL devices (22), nor have they been shown to produce additional clinically relevant benefit (23,24). Indeed, for treating infants with low tidal volumes, chambers of approximately 150 mL are superior in LDE to those over 200 mL (25,26). Several other factors, such as mask fit (27), dead space, and electrostatic charge (28–30), are also important in holding-chamber design.

III. Dry-Powder Inhalers

Currently dry-powder inhalers (DPIs) are all "passive" devices that require vigorous rapid inspiration by the patient to release and deaggregate the drug. Active (powdered) and highly efficient DPIs now undergoing clinical trials will probably be available within 2 years. However, because of their greater cost, they are unlikely to be substituted for current devices unless the medication itself is very expensive.

In principle, the drug formulated as a dry powder is dispersed in the inspiratory airstream when the patient inhales rapidly and vigorously through the device. Since the drug is aerosolized and delivered only during inspiration, "hand–lung" coordination is ensured. DPIs have therefore found considerable popularity. However, with most of these DPIs the high initial airflow required to disperse the drug powder creates a ballistic effect and URT deposition quantitatively similar to those with pMDIs. DPIs are small and unobtrusive, and their use is thought to be relatively easy to teach although, in practice, they may be used suboptimally by patients about as commonly as pMDIs (31). The Bricanyl (terbutaline) and Pulmicort (budesonide) Turbuhalers contain only pure drug without the lactose carrier common to most other formulations. Some Turbuhalers have recently been formulated with a lactose carrier (e.g., Inspiryl), to increase the total mass metered. This should improve the reliability of dosing compared with pure powder devices, which have had considerable difficulty meeting FDA requirements for dose and fine-particle fraction reproducibility between and within batches mainly due to the minute amounts of drug being metered. Whereas the first-generation DPIs were single-dose inhalers (Rotahaler, Glaxo Wellcome, England; FO2, Boehringer Ingelheim, Germany; and Spinhaler, Fisons, Loughborough, England), in recent years multidose devices (e.g., Turbuhaler, Astra Draco, Lund, Sweden; Diskhaler and Diskus, Glaxo Wellcome, Ware, England; Clickhaler, ML Labs, St Albans, England; and Easyhaler, Orion, Helsinki, Finland) have become available. With most passive DPIs, an inspiratory airflow of 15–60 L/min must be generated rapidly to adequately disperse the powder into small particles (at least 60 L/min in the case of Turbuhaler, which is particularly flow-sensitive). Small children under 6 years of age and older patients with severe airflow obstruction may not be able to generate sufficient inspiratory flow to efficiently disperse the powder. Other disadvantages include powder clumping, particularly under conditions of high humidity, and relatively low flow, especially with devices with a drug reservoir that is exposed to the environment and with hygroscopic drugs (e.g., Bricanyl Turbuhaler) (32–34). There is also the limitation of airway irritation and coughing (particularly with devices that use large doses of lactose as a dispersant), and the limited pharmacological spectrum currently available as DPIs. This results in another problem that arises from the ergonomic variety among DPIs from various manufacturers as well as the marked differences in inhalation technique between passive DPIs and pressurized pMDIs that will doubtless confuse many patients and adversely impact compliance and therapeutic outcome. Also, the cost per dose tends to be higher than with pMDIs. The main advantage of DPIs is that they are inherently breath-actuated since they deliver drug only when the patient inhales. Paradoxically, this is also a potential disadvantage. The deaggregation and LDE are critically dependent on the patient's ability to generate a sufficiently high flow within 100–200 milliseconds, a particular problem with small children or patients in severe acute respiratory distress, especially with high-resistance devices such as the FO2 and Turbuhaler.

With active or powered DPIs, the energy required for powder deaggregation is provided by compressed air, a battery-driven turbine, or vacuum. The aerosol can then be inhaled at a low inspiratory flow by the patient. These devices are still experimental but hold considerable promise because they may be able to replace SVNs for providing the relatively high payloads of mucoactive medications, antibiotics, and drugs for systemic therapy such as insulin, as appropriate formulations become available. With DPIs, therapy could be accomplished in 1–2 minutes in contrast to the 10–20 minutes required for SVNs. Furthermore, the LDE is likely to be three- to fourfold greater, thus reducing the 75% or more medication wastage resulting from the nebulizer and tubing dead volume and continuous operation.

IV. Aerosolized Mucoactive Drugs

Currently available clinical and/or experimental (*) aerosolized mucoactive drugs are summarized in Table 2. With the exception of nalcystelin and some members of the miscellaneous group that have been formulated as pMDIs, only SVNs are currently capable of providing treatment with these agents. No other mucoactive agents are commercially available as pMDIs or DPIs, but it is anticipated that with time these more convenient, efficient, and portable delivery systems will become available for delivering at least some of these agents.

A. Selecting the Best Delivery System

Many factors must be considered when choosing a specific aerosol delivery system. This issue can best be illustrated by considering the mucolytic dornase alfa (Pulmozyme, Genentech, South San Francisco). Aerosolized dornase alfa cleaves long strands of DNA into shorter fragments, facilitating mucolysis and expectoration. Neutrophil-derived DNA contributes to mucus adhesivity and viscosity, especially in chronic inflammatory airway diseases such as cystic fibrosis (CF). Placebo-controlled clinical trials in patients with CF have shown that regular treatment with aerosolized dornase alfa significantly but modestly

Table 2 Aerosolized Mucoactive Drugs

Mucolytics
Dornase alfa, N-acetyl-L-cysteine (NAC), N-acetylcysteine
L-lysinate(NAL),* thymosin β4*
Osmolar agents
Hypertonic saline
Mannitol, lactose,* dextran*
Surfactants
Ion-transport regulators
Sodium-channel blockers (e.g., amiloride*)
Chloride secretagogues
Miscellaneous
Antibiotics
Bronchodilators
Anti-inflammatory agents

*Experimental.

improves lung function and reduces the frequency of respiratory tract infections and hospitalization (35–37). During the clinical development of Pulmozyme a number of nebulizer systems were used. Initially the Hudson T Up-Draft (Hudson Respiratory Care Inc., Temecula, California) and the Marquest Acorn II (Englewood, Colorado), both driven by Pulmo-Aide (DeVilbiss Health Care Inc., Somerset, Pennsylvania) compressors, were shown to be effective. These systems have similar delivery characteristics, with an MMAD about 5 μm and an overall LDE of about 12%. In a subsequent study these devices were compared with a third nebulizer, the Pari LC jet (Pari Werk GmbH, Starnberg, Germany). All three nebulizers were shown to be equivalent with regard to total dose and fine-particle fraction delivered (38).

The effect of droplet size on safety and efficacy has been investigated in two more recent studies. In one study, carried out at the Royal Brompton Hospital, the Hudson T UP-Draft II nebulizer driven by a Pulmo-Aide compressor was compared with the reusable Medicaid Sidestream (Inspired Medical Products, Pagham, West Sussex, England) driven by a CR50 compressor (39). These systems deliver aerosols with an MMAD of 5 and 2.1 μm, respectively, with similar total LDE. Although no statistical difference was observed, there was a trend toward a greater response, as measured by FVC and FEV_1, for the Sidestream's "finer" aerosol. In the second study, from the United States and Canada (40), the Hudson T UP-Draft II nebulizer driven by a Pulmo-Aide compressor was compared to the Medicaid Sidestream nebulizer driven by a MobileAire compressor. The two nebulizer systems were significantly different in terms of aerosolized drug delivery. The Sidestream/MobileAire system took 1.3–2.0 minutes to deliver aerosolized dornase alfa with an MMAD of 2.1 µm. The Hudson Up-Draft II/Pulmo-Aide system took 8.1–10.3 minutes to deliver aerosolized dornase alfa with an MMAD of 4.9 µm. Again no significant FEV_1 difference was observed. However, as might be expected, there was a trend toward a greater response with the "finer" aerosol.

Not all nebulizers that provide similar aerosol delivery characteristics can be used with Pulmozyme. For example, Cipolla et al. (41) have shown that some ultrasonic devices may denature dornase alfa, causing protein aggregation and loss of activity. Patient-related factors such as the degree of airway patency and compliance also need to be accounted for. In patients with airflow obstruction it may be difficult to deliver drugs such as dornase alfa to the most severely affected regions by inhalation as shown by radiolabeled deposition studies (42). Nevertheless, it may be still be possible to reach these poorly ventilated areas even in the presence of mucus plugging, by diffusion through the mucus plug.

The choice of a particular nebulizer system for the delivery of a therapeutic agent is a compromise between physicochemical considerations (such as droplet size and physicochemical properties), dose and delivery requirements, and patient compliance issues related mainly to the duration of often multiple aerosol therapies. The clinical efficacy of nebulizing mixtures of medications (e.g., dornase alfa and antibiotics), a practice that may enhance compliance, has also not been evaluated in vivo although in vitro studies (see below) suggest that this would not be efficacious. These issues must all be kept in mind during clinical development programs. When economically and pharmacologically feasible, mucoactive agents should be formulated as pMDIs and DPIs since such devices are invariably more patient-friendly, much faster to administer and clean, and usually more cost-effective than SVNs.

B. N-Acetyl-L-Cysteine

N-acetyl-L-cysteine (NAC) induces expectoration through an irritant effect on the bronchial mucosa which stimulates hypersecretion of watery mucus via vagal afferents. Its main use has been in patients with COPD and CF. NAC is thought to liquify sputum by disrupting the intermolecular disulfide bonds of mucin glycoproteins (43). It may improve mucus clearance by disrupting and loosening impacted mucus plugs, yet its effectiveness in changing the viscosity of the sputum has been challenged (44). A recent systematic review on the use of NAC in CF (45) found only three randomized controlled trials on nebulized NAC, none of them showing a statistically significant or clinically relevant beneficial effect (46–48).

Nebulization of NAC may induce bronchospasm, and the routine addition of a bronchodilator to the NAC solution in the nebulizer has been advocated (49). It has an unpleasant taste and "rotten egg" odor and is generally disliked by patients, who are therefore likely to be nonadherent. It is now used infrequently.

N-acetylcysteine was attached to the basic amino acid lysine in order to increase the pH and increase topical tolerability. N-acetylcysteine L-lysinate (NAL) improved tracheal mucus velocity and reduced viscoelasticity compared with NAC (50). It has also been administered as a pMDI (50–52).

C. Thymosin β4

An interesting and potent mucolytic in vitro, this 4.8-kD peptide depolymerizes filamentous actin from disintegrating inflammatory cells to globular actin, thus reducing the viscosity of purulent secretions. It has a synergistic effect when administered with dornase alfa (53). It has not been studied in vivo in animals or humans.

D. Osmolar Agents

Aerosols of isotonic saline have been shown to improve lung clearance of secretions in "normal" subjects (54). King et al. (55) examined the effects of 3% hyperosmolar saline compared with normal saline on mucus viscosity in vitro. Hyperosmolar saline reduced spinnability and sputum "rigidity" and improved calculated mucus clearability in vitro more than dornase alfa. In a recent study, Eng et al. (56) found significant clinical improvement, with a 15% increase in FEV_1 after 2 weeks of daily hyperosmolar saline inhalation in CF patients using a portable ultrasonic nebulizer (Omron NE-U 07, Osaka, Japan). The effect was dose-dependent up to a concentration of 12% (57).

Although administered by USNs for speedier delivery, hyperosmolar saline can also be administered by SVNs. It should be stressed that in patients with airway hyperreactivity bronchodilators should be administered 15 minutes before hyperosmolar saline inhalation to avoid bronchospasm (58).

Mannitol is a naturally occurring sugar that is not absorbed in the gastrointestinal tract and is not metabolized to any appreciable extent when injected. A dry-powder formulation of mannitol has been used as a hyperosmolar stimulus to increase mucociliary clearance in adults (59,60). Inhalation of mannitol from a DPI immediately increased mucociliary clearance (MCC), the increase for 60 minutes after the start of mannitol inhalation being 26.4% and 18.1% compared with placebo, in asthmatic and healthy subjects, respectively. The increase in MCC in response to mannitol inhalation by DPI was similar to the increase observed following hyperosmolar saline. The increase was not related to induced cough, as the number of coughs was low and similar to that on the placebo day.

E. Surfactants

Surfactants are essential for normal lung function, since they maintain bronchiolar and alveolar patency during exhalation. Originally, natural and synthetic surfactants were developed for intratracheal instillation in intubated premature infants with hyaline membrane disease due to surfactant deficiency. They were shown to also increase mucociliary clearance (61–63). However, direct tracheal instillation is clearly impractical for most patients with reduced MCC. Furthermore, this mode of administration is inefficient and very costly because of non-uniform distribution of the instillate, resulting in the need to administer a very large dose of the surfactant that greatly exceeds the total endogenous surfactant pool. An appealing alternative is surfactant delivery by aerosol with the potential for reducing the therapeutically equivalent dose 50- to 100-fold (64). Surfactant dysfunction has recently been implicated in the pathophysiology of chronic bronchitis and asthma (65,66). Additionally, it is likely to play an important part in the pathophysiology of bronchopulmonary dysplasia in neonates due to the leakage of serum proteins into the lumen of injured and inflamed airways. Indeed, this may account for the recent observation that the incidence of bronchopulmonary dysplasia was not reduced by administering inhaled beclomethasone dipropionate to high-risk neonates for 4 weeks, although the need for systemic steroid and duration on assisted ventilation were significantly decreased (67). It is tempting to speculate that continuous administration of surfactant in addition to steroids might have diminished mucosal injury and at least some of the chronic changes of bronchopulmonary dysplasia.

In a recent randomized clinical trial, Anzueto et al. (68) examined the effects of exogenous surfactant on sputum clearance and pulmonary function in patients with severe but stable, relatively fixed airflow obstruction due to chronic bronchitis. A synthetic surfactant (Exosurf, GlaxoWellcome Inc., Research Triangle Park, North Carolina), containing dipalmitoyl phosphadidylcholine (DPPC), and surface-spreading components, tyloxapol and hexadecanol, was administered as an aerosol using a jet nebulizer (Pari LC) with the formulation diluted to 5 mL with normal saline. The authors evaluated the effects on several in vitro parameters of sputum characteristics, pulmonary function, and symptoms in patients with chronic bronchitis. DPPC surfactant aerosol treatments resulted in a modest but statistically significant improvement in pulmonary function (11.4% increase in FEV_1) and in mucociliary transportability of expectorated secretions in the frog palate model. These results are comparable to the effects reported for dornase alfa in CF. Exosurf did not significantly improve patients' symptoms. As emphasized by the authors, larger studies are needed to confirm these results. Assessing symptoms, the frequency of exacerbations, hospitalizations, the rate of decline of pulmonary function, and other clinical parameters over a longer period, particularly in less severely obstructed patients, will be important in determining whether surfactant will have a role in long-term therapy of patients with chronic bronchitis. Jarjour and Enhorning (69) showed that surfactant underwent a fivefold decrease in its ability to maintain in vitro capillary patency in patients subjected to specific antigen challenge. Since it was shown that as bronchoalveolar lavage fluid protein increased, patency decreased, these authors postulated that the antigen-induced inflammation caused protein to leak into the airways, thus impairing the function of surfactant.

A major disadvantage of using jet nebulizers to aerosolize surfactants is foaming. Schermuly et al. (70), by means of an ultrasonic nebulizer (Portasonic II, Devilbiss, Langen, Germany), were able to increase the inhaled surfactant "load" approximately eightfold as compared with standard jet nebulizers maintaining functionally active surfactant after nebulization. Whereas surfactant instillation did not improve severe ventilation-perfusion mismatch in an isolated lung model of acute lung injury, nebulized surfactant markedly reversed it. This therefore appears to be a promising and economical approach for providing surfactant therapy, at least in patients with ARDS. In this study the MMADs (GSD) were 4.5 µm (2.6), predicting a lung dose of 10 mg surfactant/kg body weight per hour, a 30-fold smaller dose than is traditionally administered by instillation (50–500 mg/kg).

DPI administration of surfactant would be a potentially advantageous alternative with possibly more rapid and efficient administration and elimination of foaming. Egan and colleagues' recent study of fetal lambs with IRDS demonstrated that a single dose of engineered aerosolized surfactant powder one-eighth of the dose usually instilled rapidly and significantly improved gas exchange. However, the duration of action was less than 1 hour, and a single dose 30 times larger was not more effective (70a). Studies in which sequential small doses are administered to attempt to extend the duration of action would be of interest.

F. Ion-Transport Regulators

Sodium Channel Blockers

Knowles et al. (71) conducted an initial crossover study to determine whether blocking Na+ absorption across the respiratory epithelium with aerosolized amiloride, a sodium-channel-blocking diuretic, would affect the course of lung disease in CF. Mean loss of FVC over time was significantly reduced (1.44 mL per day) during the 25-week treatment with amiloride as compared with placebo (3.39 mL per day). A subsequent analysis of sputum from these same patients by Tomkiewicz et al. (72) demonstrated that nebulized amiloride treatment decreases sputum viscoelasticity threefold. While Na+ and Cl− content were altered significantly, solid and liquid content and K+ levels were unchanged. The authors speculated that the clinical effectiveness of the treatment might have been due to the improvement it produced in the rheological properties of airway secretions, which might have resulted in improved peripheral airway patency and decreased gas trapping. A third study (73) failed to replicate the clinical benefits of amiloride. Methodological differences make it difficult to reconcile the contradictory findings.

Of interest is that amiloride is one of the only mucoactive drugs that has been experimentally micronized and delivered by DPI (Turbuhaler) (74). The in vitro doses of amiloride generated were similar to those delivered by SVN.

Chloride Secretagogues

Patients with CF have impaired chloride secretion in the airway through the CFTR chloride channel. P2Y purinergic agonists (e.g., adenosine triphosphate [ATP], uridine triphosphate [UTP]) activate calcium-dependent Cl– channels and are promising candidates for normalizing the composition of the periciliary fluid in CF. Because ATP and its metabolites provoke bronchospasm, UTP was initially chosen for clinical studies. Phase I clinical data (75) suggested that aerosolized UTP is safe for use in CF patients and enhances mucociliary clearance following acute inhalation in normal subjects. Despite their earlier promise and a decade of research, these agents are not available clinically. The same investigators demonstrated by scintigraphy that UTP produced a 50% improvement in cough clearance of secretions in patients with absent mucociliary transport due to primary ciliary dyskinesia. The benefit was attributed to increased chloride secretion and mucin release from goblet cells (76).

In the past few years there has been considerable controversy about the link between defects in the CF transmembrane conductance regulator gene and retained, infected secretions. One hypothesis attributes recurring and persistent infection to hypotonic–low salt/defensin levels while another postulates that the final common path is loss of periciliary fluid and the resulting ciliary dysfunction. Determining the correct pathophysiological "model" could have important therapeutic implications. If the major problem is loss of airway surface liquid and a reduction in the depth of the periciliary fluid, then addition of isotonic saline should improve mucus clearance. This was demonstrated in CF epithelial tissue cultures and suggests that isotonic saline aerosol therapy should be effective, particularly if initiated early in the course of the disease (76a,76b).

G. Antibiotics

Antibiotics are routinely used to treat bacterial pulmonary infections. To the degree that they are successful in reducing the inflammatory stimulus for the secretion of mucus into the airways, antibiotics may play an important role in the management of excessive and purulent airway secretions and the associated inflammation. The inhaled route provides greater access to infected secretions, reduces systemic toxicity, and permits long-term dosing to the airways at sputum concentrations that should be capable of overwhelming even "drug-resistant" pathogens by concentrations up to 50 times the minimum inhibitory concentration (MIC) (4). Concerns about drug resistance have somewhat curbed enthusiasm for the long-term use of inhaled antibiotics, but the apparent safety and effectiveness of high-dose intermittent therapy, and the potential for long-term antibiotic prophylaxis starting with the first evidence of infection, are leading to renewed interest in this strategy. This is particularly the case since an antibiotic "holiday" or the use of antibiotics of different classes in rotation has been shown to delay the development of bacterial antibiotic resistance and often restores sensitivity after a few weeks. A common approach to the therapy of chronic *Pseudomonas aeruginosa* (Psa) infection in CF is to alternate 4 weeks on and off inhaled tobramycin. A recent multicenter study demonstrated that this intermittent approach was well tolerated. There was improved pulmonary function (FEV$_1$ increased 12% during the first month but had decreased to only 4% above baseline by the sixth month), a marked decrease in the density of Psa in sputum initially, and a decrease in the risk of hospitalization in patients with CF (77). However, over the 6 months of the study (3 months on active therapy and 3 months on placebo), there appeared to be a progressive loss of Psa sensitivity to tobramycin. This was reflected in reduced bacterial killing (colony counts at 6 months were only slightly less than placebo and baseline preantibiotic levels) but an apparently slower decline in FEV$_1$ nevertheless. Clinicians have also alternated tobramycin inhalations with the oral fluoroquinolone ciprofloxacin, administered for 2–4 weeks of each in rotation. However, long-term studies to demonstrate the benefits, safety, and emergence of resistance with this therapy are not available.

An earlier 3-month crossover CF study demonstrated the safety and efficacy of aerosolized tobramycin administered in a large nebulized dose of 600 mg three times a day with what was probably a relatively inefficient nebulizer (78).

It had previously been shown, in a pilot study, that micronized gentamicin could be administered as a dry-powder aerosol using the Rotahaler DPI (79). In a recent study from our laboratory, Labiris et al. (4) compared bacterial killing capacity of inhaled and intravenous (IV) gentamicin in adult patients with bronchiectasis who were chronically infected with Psa. Patients received a single dose of either gentamicin 160 mg via DPI (Clickhaler, ML Laboratories, St Albans, England) or SVN (Pari LC, Pari-Werk GmbH, Starnberg, Germany), or gentamicin 5 mg/kg ($\sim$350 mg) by IV infusion. After 2 hours, inhaled gentamicin significantly decreased the sputum Psa density almost 10-fold, even though the DPI was only 15% as efficient in achieving LRT delivery as the SVN (sputum gentamicin concentrations of 13 μg/g sputum vs. 97 μg/g sputum, respectively). No significant decline in bacterial counts was observed after IV gentamicin. When gentamicin was inhaled, blood concentrations were minimal, well below concentrations known to cause systemic toxicity. Thus, given efficient formulations and delivery devices, inhaled, but not IV, gentamicin has the potential for overcoming Psa resistance and possibly sterilizing the LRT. More aggressive antibiotic therapy early in the course of airway infection and before the development of marked parenchymal lung injury due to chronic Psa infection might actually sterilize the LRT and maintain freedom from infection as long as antibiotic prophylaxis is continued (80). This would predictably preserve lung function much more effectively over the long term unless infection with more aggressive and resistant organisms supervened. By eliminating airway infection and maintaining the integrity of the lung tissue, reinfection and the development of resistant organisms is less likely.

H. Bronchodilators

Bronchodilators, such as beta-agonists and anticholinergic agents, increase mucus production and ciliary beat frequency and force and may augment mucociliary clearance (81–84). They can also significantly improve cough clearance inpatients with asthma and COPD, probably by virtue of their ability to increase expiratory flow in intermediate and large airways and possibly gas-liquid "pumping" in peripheral airways (85).

I. Anti-Inflammatory Agents

By reducing airway mucosal inflammation, anti-inflammatory agents may restore epithelial integrity, improve airway caliber, and decrease retained secretions. In asthma and other inflammatory airway diseases, the airway mucosa is inflamed and the epithelium may desquamate. Secretions may increase in volume, protease content, DNA concentration, and filamentous actin from inflammatory cells, mainly granulocytes, resulting in plugging of airways.

Treatment with low doses (1 mg/kg) oral corticosteroids improved the clinical course of CF patients, but was associated with adverse effects when higher (2 mg/kg) doses were used (86).

Trials using inhaled corticosteroids show conflicting results. Fluticasone propionate (400 µg/day) given as a DPI for 6 weeks, failed to decrease sputum inflammatory markers, lung function, and symptoms in CF (87). On the other hand, 1500 µg of beclomethasone dipropionate given by MDI and spacer improved lung function in children with CF (88). Daily inhalation of 1600 µg/day of budesonide for 6 weeks induced a small but significant improvement in bronchial hyperresponsiveness to histamine and in symptoms of cough and dyspnea in both adult (89) and pediatric (90) CF patients.

For management of COPD, current guidelines (91,92) recommend a trial of inhaled steroids only in the small (~5%) number of patients who show objective benefit during a 2–3-week systemic steroid trial. Few methodologically sound studies (93,94) are available to support these guidelines.

Indomethacin is another anti-inflammatory agent that has been effectively administered by nebulizer for the treatment of mucus hypersecretion associated with diffuse panbronchiolitis (95). It has decreased sputum volume and increased sputum solids content.

Leukotriene modifiers are a new class of agents whose place in treatment of asthma is currently being defined. As leukotrienes are important mediators causing mucus secretion, it is possible that leukotriene receptor antagonists and biosynthesis inhibitors will be adjuvant anti-inflammatory agents with mucoactive properties (96).

There is currently considerable interest in airway-targeted antioxidant and antiprotease therapy as a means of reducing tissue injury in a variety of pulmonary diseases. If effective, such therapies might be capable of reducing secretion volume and purulence.

J. Aerosolized Drug Translocation Through Airway Mucus

Delivery of aerosolized medication to patients with impaired mucus clearance involves more than just delivering the drug to the airways. Optimal drug delivery must take into account the decreased drug transport rate across infected secretions in addition to drug losses due to binding to the glycoproteins, inactivation by various components of the mucus, and inefficient delivery to more peripheral airways due to mucus plugs. Only a few in vitro studies have looked into these complex interactive mechanisms.

The rate of diffusion through purified extracellular alginate from Psa was measured for 12 beta-lactam antibiotics (97). The diffusion rate decreased as the antibiotic molecular weight increased, but the range of diffusion rates exhibited by the common anti-Pseudomonal penicillins was relatively small. The diffusion of ticarcillin through mixtures of alginate and purified mucus glycoprotein (mucin) from sputum of CF patients showed that, at equivalent concentrations, alginate represented the greater barrier to penetration. However, if the mucin concentration was increased to 4.0% w/v, a more realistic physiological concentration, the diffusion of ticarcillin was retarded to a greater extent than in 1% w/v alginate, and the effect was compounded by other sputum components such as DNA. The results suggest that the antibiotic diffusion barrier represented by mucin may be significant in vivo, particularly for inhaled antibiotics.

Since antibiotic bioactivity may be reduced by sputum, and glycoproteins (mucins) and high-molecular-weight DNA make up 2–3% and 3–10% of the dry weight of sputum, respectively, it was assumed that treating sputum with dornase alfa would increase antibiotic bioactivity. However, this was not the case when tobramycin activity was studied in vitro (98), although it was found that the binding of tobramycin to the sputum had increased. In contrast to that study, the degree of antibiotic binding to whole CF sputum was shown to be dependent on the DNA concentration and the presence of acidic mucins in the sputum (99).

K. Combination Therapy

Combination therapy may consist of either two different medications aerosolized together or in tandem or two different and simultaneously administered therapeutic modalities. Commonly used is the combination of antibiotic and bronchodilator solutions by patients with CF. The rationale behind this combination is that some airways may be narrowed or closed by bronchospasm so that bronchodilation may improve pulmonary distribution of the antibiotic. Furthermore, bronchodilator therapy is part of routine care, and concurrent administration is time-saving to the patient and thus may improve compliance. Unfortunately, clinical studies to assess the merit of this practice are lacking. In vitro studies have shown that addition of albuterol solution to tobramycin lowered the surface tension of the solution in the nebulizer and resulted in a greater output of tobramycin (100). The magnitude of this effect varied among different nebulizers and different nebulization techniques.

In comparison to individual treatments, combined treatment with flutter-valve oscillations and dornase alfa significantly reduced mucus rigidity in vitro, suggesting the possibility of increased mucus clearability (101,102). These in vitro results suggest that a combination of biochemical treatment (e.g., dornase alfa, hyperosmolar saline, mannitol) and mechanical oscillation may have a better therapeutic potential for mucus clearance in CF lung disease than either modality alone.

Another possible combination is two chemical formulations such as Na-cystelyn with dornase alfa (103). Combination therapy at half the concentration of each drug significantly decreased in vitro sputum spinnability more than either treatment alone. This suggests additive effects with these two mucolytics. Similar effects were observed with the combination of hyperosmolar saline and dornase alfa (55).

V. The Future

As our understanding of the role of mucoactive agents in a variety of inflammatory conditions affecting the airways increases, it should be possible to devise more effective therapies. These are likely to include gene transfection to "cure" the disease. Both CFTR gene–laden liposomes and modified adenoviral vectors have been unsuccessfully attempted in CF (104,105). Furthermore, better delivery devices and methods should improve aerosol delivery efficiency and compliance. Active DPIs or atomizer devices capable of aerosolizing small volumes (50–100 µL) of highly concentrated drug solutions within a few seconds are most likely to accomplish this goal with particles of about 1–3 μm MMAD (GSD ~2). The key to success will be development of appropriate engineered drug formulations that can be readily dispersed and targeted to the large and small airways using improved and increasingly simple, relatively inexpensive aerosolization systems.

References

1. Rubin BK, Tomkiewicz RP, King M. Mucoactive agents: old and new. In: Wilmott RW, ed. The Pediatric Lung. Basel, Switzerland: Birkhauser Verlag, 1997: 155–179.
2. Thomson ML, Pavia D, McNicol MW. A preliminary study of the effect of guaifenesin on mucociliary clearance from human lung. Thorax 1973; 8:742–747.
3. Rubin BK. An in vitro comparison of the mucoactive properties of guaifenesin, iodinated glycerol, surfactant, and albuterol. Chest 1999; 4116:195–200.
4. Labiris NRC, Holbrook AM, Chrystyn H, Macleod SM, Newhouse MT. Dry powder versus intravenous and nebulized gentamicin in cystic fibrosis and bronchiectasis: pilot study. Am J Respir Crit Care Med 1999; 160.1711–1716.
5. Rubin BK, Druce H, Ramirez OE, Palmer. Effect of clarithromycin on nasal mucus properties in healthy subjects and in patients with purulent rhinitis. Am J Respir Crit Care Med 1997; 55:2018–2023.
6. Guyatt GH, Townsend M, Kazim F, Newhouse MT. A controlled trial of ambroxol in chronic bronchitis. Chest 1987; 92:618–620.
7. Johnson CE. Principles of nebulizer-derived drug therapy for asthma. Am J Hosp Pharm 1989; 46:1845–1855.
8. Finlay WH, Stapelton KW, Zuberbuhler P. Comparison between inhaled fine particle fraction and lung dose for nebulized aerosols. J Aerosol Med 1998; 11(suppl 1):S65-S72.
9. Murakami G, Igarashi T, Adachi Y, Matsuno M, Adachi Y, Sawai M, Yoshizumi A, Okada T. Measurement of bronchial hyperreactivity in infants and preschool children using method. Ann Allergy 1990; 64:383–387.
10. Barnes KL, Clifford R, Holgate ST, Murphy D, Comber P, Bell E. Bacterial contamination of home nebulizers. Br Med J 1987; 295:812.
11. Hollie MC, Malone RA, Skufca RM, Nelson HS. Extreme variability in aerosol output of the DeVilbiss jet nebulizer. Chest 1991; 100:1339–1344.
12. Alvine GF, Rodgers P, Fitzsimmons KM, Ahrens RC. Disposable jet nebulizers: how reliable are they? Chest 1992; 100:316–319.
13. Nikander K, Turpeinen M, Wollmer P. The conventional ultrasonic nebulizer proved inefficient in nebulizing a suspension. J Aerosol Med 1992:47–53.
14. O'Callaghan C, Barry PW. The science of nebulized drug delivery. Thorax 1997; 52:(suppl 2):S31-S44.
15. Newnham DM, Lipworth BJ. Nebulizer performance, pharmacokinetics, airways and systemic effects of salbutamol given via a novel nebulizer system (Ventstream). Thorax 1994; 49:762–770.

16. Verdun AM, Mitchell JP, Nagel MW. Performance of a new breath-actuated small volume nebulizer (BA-SVN) when used with oxygen as driving gas under conditions of hospital use. Am J Respir Crit Care Med 1998; 157:A638.

17. Busse W, Colice G, Donnel D, Hannon S. A dose-response dose-comparison of HFA-BDP and CFC-BDP based on FEV1 and FEF 25–75%. Eur Respir J 1998; 12(suppl 28):61S.

18. Salzman GA, Pyszczynski DR. Oropharyngeal candidiasis in patients treated with beclomethasone diproprionate delivered by metered-dose inhaler alone and with AeroChamber. J Allergy Clin Immunol 1988; 81:424–428.

19. Newhouse MT. Asthma therapy with aerosols: are nebulizers obsolete? A continuing controversy. J Pediatr 1999; 135:5–8.

20. Corr D, Dolovich M, McCormack D, Ruffin R, Obminski G, Newhouse M. Design and characteristics of a portable breath actuated, particle size selective medical aerosol inhaler. J Aerosol Sci 1982; 13:1–7.

21. Chua HL, Chambers CB, Newhouse MT. Comparison of the effect of four MDI add-on devices on lung deposition and function in asthmatics. Am Rev Respir Dis 1994; 149:A217.

22. Wildhaber JH, Devadason SG, Hayden MJ, Eber E, Summers QA, LeSouef PN. Aerosol delivery to wheezy infants: a comparison between a nebulizer and two small volume spacers. Pediatr Pulmonol 1997; 23:212–216.

23. Konig P, Gayer D, Kantak A, Kreutz C, Douglass B, Hordvik NL. A trial of metaproterenol by metered-dose inhaler and two spacers in preschool asthmatics. Pediatr Pulmonol 1988; 5:247–251.

24. Crimi N, Palermo F, Cacopardo B, Vancheri C, Oliveri R, Palermo B, Mistretta A. Bronchodilator effect of Aerochamber and Inspirease in comparison with metered dose inhaler. Eur J Respir Dis 1987; 71:153–157.

25. Everard ML, Clark AR, Milner AD. Drug delivery from holding chambers with attached facemask. Arch Dis Child 1992; 67:580–585.

26. Campbell R, Dolovich M, Chambers C, Newhouse M. Holding chamber volume/salbutamol dose delivered through an endotracheal tube at low tidal volumes. J Aerosol Med 1992; 5:304.

27. Amirav I, Newhouse MT. Aerosol therapy with valved holding chambers in young children: importance of the facemask seal. Pediatrics 2001; 108:389–394.

28. Bisgaard H. A metal aerosol holding chamber devised for young children with asthma. Eur Respir J 1995; 8:856–860.

29. Bisgaard H, Anhoj J, Klug B, Berg E. A non-electrostatic spacer for aerosol delivery. Arch Dis Child 1995; 73:226–230.

30. Pierart F, Wildhaber JH, Vrancken I, Devadason SG, Le Souef PN. Washing plastic spacers in household detergent reduces electrostatic charge and greatly improves delivery. Eur Respir J 1999; 13:673–678.

31. Kesten S, Elias M, Cartier A, Chapman KR. Patient handling of a multidose dry powder inhalation device for albuterol. Chest 1994; 105:1077–1081.

32. Meakin BJ, Cainey JM, Woodcock PM. Simulated in-use and mis-use aspects of the delivery of terbutaline sulphate from Bricanyl Turbohaler dry powder inhalers. Int J Pharm 1995; 19:103–108.

33. Tseng M, Kennedy A, Chambers C, Newhouse MT. Bricanyl turbuhaler: high relative humidity and low inspiratory flow cause severe impairment of terbutaline deaggregation. Am J Respir Crit Care Med 1999; 159:A117.

34. Newhouse M, Kennedy A, Tseng M, Stepner N. Ventolin Discus vs Inspiryl Turbuhaler under conditions of varying flow and relative humidity. Am J Respir Crit Care Med 1999; 159:A117.

35. Fuchs HJ, Borowitz DS, Christiansen DH, Morris EM, Nash ML, Ramsey BW, Rosenstein BJ, Smith AL, Wohl ME. Effect of aerosolized recombinant human DNase on exacerbations of respiratory symptoms and on pulmonary function in patients with cystic fibrosin. N Engl J Med 1994; 331:637–642.

36. Shah PL, Scotts F, Geddes DM, Hodson ME. Two years experience with recombinant human DNase 1 in the treatment of pulmonary disease in cystic fibrosis. Respir Med 1995; 89:499–502.

37. Wagener JS, Rock MJ, McCubbin MM, Hamilton SD, Johnson CA, Ahrens RC. Aerosol delivery and safety of recombinant human deoxyribonuclease in young children with cystic fibrosis: a bronchoscopic study. J Pediatr 1998; 133:486–491.

38. Fiel SB, Fuchs HJ, Johnson C, Gonda I, Clark AR. Comparison of three jet nebulizer aerosol delivery systems used to administer recombinant human DNase I to patients with cystic fibrosis. Chest 1995; 108:153–156.

39. Shah PL, Scott SF, Geddes DM, Conway S, Watson A, Nazir T, Can SB, Wallis C, Marriott C, Hodson ME. An evaluation of two aerosol delivery systems for rhDNase. Eur Respir J 1997; 10:1261–1266.

40. Geller DE, Eigen H, Fiel SB, Clark A, Lamarre AP, Johnson CA, Konstan MW. Effect of smaller droplet size of dornase alfa on lung function in mild cystic fibrosis. Dornase Alfa Nebulizer 9 Group. Pediatr Pulmonol 1998; 25:83–87.

41. Cipolla DC, Clark AR, Chan H-K, Gonja I, Shire SJ. Assessment of aerosol delivery systems for recombinant human deoxyribonuclease. STP Pharma Sci 1994; 4:50–62.

42. Sanchis J, Dolovich M, Rossman C, Wilson W, Newhouse MT. Pulmonary mucociliary clearance in cystic fibrosis. N Engl J Med 1973; 288:651–654.

43. Peters JA, Peters BA. Pharmacology for respiratory care. In: Scanlan CL, Spearman CB, Sheldon RL, eds. Fundamentals of Respiratory Care. 5th ed. Philadelphia: CV Mosby, 1990:455–482.

44. Wallace CS, Hall M, Kuhn RJ. Pharmacologic management of cystic fibrosis. Clin Pharm 1993; 12:657–674.

45. Duijvestijn YCM, Brand PLP. Systematic review of N-acetylcysteine in cystic fibrosis. Acta Paediatr 1999; 88:38–41.

46. Howatt WF, DeMuth GR. A double-blind study of the use of acetylcysteine in patients with cystic fibrosis. Univ Mich Med Cent J 1966; 32:82–85.

47. Teclin JS, Holsclaw DS. Bronchial drainage with aerosol medications in cystic fibrosis. Phys Ther 1976; 56:999–1003.

48. Romano C, Gargani GF, Minicucci L, Nantron M. Studio Clinico controllato sulli-attivitadi un nuovo farmaco mucoregolatore nella patologia astruttiva bronchiale a marcata impronta ipersecretiva. Minerva Pediatr 1984; 36:127–138.

49. Dano G. Bronchospasm caused by acetylcysteine in children with bronchial asthma. Acta Allergol 1971; 26:181–190.

50. Tomkiewicz RP, App EM, De Sanctis GT, Coffiner M, Maes P, Rubin BK, King M. A comparison of a new mucolytic N-acetylcysteine L-lysinate with N-acetylcysteine: airway epithelial function and mucus changes in dog. Pulm Pharmacol 1995; 8:259–265.

51. Baran D, App EM, King M, Hochstrasser K, Coffiner M, Fossion J, et al. Acute, single dose study for efficacy and safety of a new mucolytic agent Nacystelyn (NAL) in metered dose inhaler for the treatment of lung disease cystic fibrosis [poster]. Proceedings 19th Conference European Working Group for Cystic Fibrosis, Paris, May 29-June 3, 1994.

52. Malfroot A, Baran D, Dab I, App EM, Maes P. Coffiner M. Efficacy and safety of acystelyn (NAL) metered dose inhalation in CF: an acute, single dose study over 24 hours [poster]. In: Proceedings 20th Conference European Working Group for Cystic Fibrosis, Brussels, June 1995:18–21.

53. Rubin BK, Kater AP, Dian T, Ramirez OE, Tomkiewicz RP, Goldstein AL. Effects of thymosin beta on cystic fibrosis sputum. Pediatr Pulmonol 1995; 12(suppl):134.

54. Daviskas E, Anderson SD, Gonda I, Eberl S, Meikle S, Seale JP, Bautovich G. Inhalation of hypertonic saline aerosol enhances mucociliary clearance in asthmatic and healthy subjects. Eur Respir J 1996; 9:725–732.

55. King M, Dasgupta B, Tomkiewicz RP, Brown NE. Rheology of cystic fibrosis sputum after in vitro treatment with hypertonic saline alone and in combination with recombinant human 17 deoxyribonuclease I. Am J Respir Crit Care Med 1997; 56:173–177.

56. Eng PA, Morton J, Douglass JA, Riedler J, Wilson J, Robertson CF. Short-term efficacy of ultrasonically nebulized hypertonic saline in cystic fibrosis. Pediatr Pulmonol 1996; 21:77–83.

57. Robinson M, Hemming AL, Regins JA, Wong AG, Bailey DL, Bautovitch GJ, King M, Bye PT. Effect of increasing doses of hypertonic saline on mucociliary clearance in patients with cystic fibrosis. Thorax 1997; 52:900–903.

58. Smith CM, Anderson SD. Inhalational challenge using hypertonic saline in asthmatic subjects: a comparison with responses to hyperpnoea, methacholine and water. Eur Respir J 1990; 3:144–151.

59. Daviskas E, Anderson SD, Brannan JD, Chan HK, Eberl S, Bautovich G. Inhalation of dry-powder mannitol increases mucociliary clearance. Eur Respir J 199; 10:2449–2454.

60. Daviskas E, Anderson SD, Eberl S, Chan HK, Bautovich G. Inhalation of dry powder mannitol improves clearance of mucus in patients with bronchiectasis. Am J Respir Crit Care Med 1999; 159:1843–1848.

61. Rubin BK, Ramirez O, King M. Mucus rheology and transport in neonatal respiratory distress syndrome and the effects of surfactant therapy. Chest 1992; 101:1080–1085.

62. Allegra L, Bossi R, Braga P. Influence of surfactant on mucociliary transport. Eur J Respir Dis 1985; 142:71–76.

63. Girod de Bentzmann S, Pierrot D, Fuchey C, Zahm JM, Morancais JL, Puchelle E. Distearoyl phosphatidylglycerol liposomes improve surface and transport properties of CF mucus. Eur Respir J 1993; 6:1156–1161.

64. Lewis JF, Goffin J, Yue P, McCaig LA, Bjarneson D, Veldhuizen RA. Evaluation of exogenous surfactant treatment strategies in an adult model of acute lung injury. J Appl Physiol 1996; 80:1156–1164.
65. Hohlfeld JM, Ahlf K, Enhorning G, Balke K, Erpenbeck VJ, Petschallies J, Hoymann HG, Fabel H, Krug N. Dysfunction of pulmonary surfactant in asthmatics after segmental allergen challenge. Am J Respir Crit Care Med 1999; 159:1803–1809.
66. Griese M. Pulmonary surfactant in health and human lung diseases: state of the art. Eur Respir J 1999; 13:1455–1476.
67. Cole CH, Colton T, Shah BL, Abbasi S, MacKinnon BL, Demissie S, Frantz ID 3rd. Early inhaled glucocorticoid therapy to prevent bronchopulmonary dysplasia. N Engl J Med 1999; 340:1005–1010.
68. Anzueto A, Jubran A, Ohar JA, Piquette CA, Rennard SI, Colice G, Pattishall EN, Barrett J, Engle M, Perret KA, Rubin BK. Effects of aerosolized surfactant in patients with stable chronic bronchitis: a prospective randomized controlled trial. JAMA 1997; 278:1426–1431.
69. Jarjour NN, Enhorning G. Antigen-induced airway inflammation in atopic subjects generates dysfunction of pulmonary surfactant. Am J Respir Crit Care Med 1999; 160:336–341.
70. Schermuly R, Schmell T, Gunter A, Grimminger F, Seeger W, Walmarth D. Ultrasonic nebulization for efficient delivery of surfactant in a model of acute lung injury; impact on gas exchange. Am J Respir Crit Care med 1997; 56:445–453.
70a. Tareen L, Candela Z, Swartz D, Forrestel R, Gordon MS, Kadrichu N, Holm BA, Eagan EA. Delivery of effective surfactant therapy by inhalation. Am J Respir Crit Care Med 2002; 165:A80.
71. Knowles MR, Church NL, Waltner WE, Yankaskas JR, Gilligan P, King M, Edwards LJ, Helms RW, Boucher RC. A pilot study of aerosolized amiloride for the treatment of lung disease in cystic fibrosis. N Engl J Med 1990; 322:1189–1194.
72. Tomkiewicz RP, App EM, Zayas JG, Ramirez O, Church N, Boucher RC, Knowles MR, King M. Amiloride inhalation therapy in cystic fibrosis. Am Rev Respir Dis 1993; 148:1002–1007.
73. Graham A, Hasani A, Alton EW, Martin GP, Marriott C, Hodson ME, Clarke SW, Geddes DM. No added benefit from nebulized amiloride in patients with cystic fibrosis. Eur Respir J 1993; 6:1243–1248.
74. Everard ML, Devadson SG, Sunderland VB, Le Souef PN. An alternative aerosol delivery system for amiloride. Thorax 1995; 50:517–519.
75. Noone PG, Olivier KN, Knowles MR. Modulation of the ionic milieu of the airway in health and disease. Annu Rev Med 1994; 45:421–434.
76. Noone PG, Bennett WD, Regnis JA, Zeman KL, Carson JL, King M, Boucher RC, Knowles MR. Effect of aerosolized uridine-5'-triphosphate on airway clearance with cough in patients with primary ciliary dyskinesia. Am J Respir Crit Care Med 1999; 160:144–149.
76a. Matsui H, Grubb BR, Tarran R, Randell SH, Gatzy JT, Davis WC, Boucher RC. Evidence for periciliary layer depletion not abnormal ion composition in the pathogenesis of cystic fibrosis airways disease. Cell 1998; 95:1005–1015.
76b. Tarran R, Grubb BR, Gatzy JT, Davis WC. The relative roles of passive surface

forces and active ion transport in the modulation of airway surface liquid volume and composition. J Gen Physiol 2001; 118:223–236.

77. Ramsey BW, Pepe MS, Quan JM, Otto KL, Montgomery AB, Williams-Warren J, Vasilejev-K M, Borowitz D, Bowman CM, Marshall BC, Marshall S, Smith AL. Intermittent administration of inhaled tobramycin in patients with cystic fibrosis. N Engl J Med 1999; 340:23–30.
78. Ramsey BW, Dorkin HL, Eisenberg JD, Gibson RL, Harwood IR, Kravitz RM, Schidlow DV, Wilmott RW, Astley SJ, McBurnie MA, et al. Efficacy of aerosolized tobramycin in patients with cystic fibrosis. N Engl J Med 1993; 328:1740–1746.
79. Goldman JM, Bayston SM, O'Connor S, Meigh RE. Inhaled micronised gentamicin powder: a new delivery system. Thorax 1990; 45:939–940.
80. Johansen HK, Kovesi TA, Koch C, Corey M, Hoiby N, Levison H. *Pseudomonas aeruginosa* and *Burkholderia cepacia* infection in cystic fibrosis patients treated in Toronto and Copenhagen. Pediatr Pulmonol 1998; 26:89–96.
81. Tamaoki J, Chiyotani A, Tagaya E, Sakai N, Konno K. Effect of long term treatment with oxitropium bromide on airway secretion in chronic bronchitis and diffuse panbronchiolitis. Thorax 1994; 49:545–548.
82. Ziment I. Pharmacologic therapy of obstructive airway disease. Clin Chest Med 1990; 11:461–486.
83. Matthys H, Daikeler G, Krauss B, Vastag E. Action of tolubuterol and fenoterol on the mucociliary clearance. Respiration 1987; 51:105–112.
84. Chambers CB, Corrigan BW, Newhouse MT. Salmeterol speeds mucocilary transport in healthy subjects [abstract]. Am J Respir Crit Care Med 1999; 159:636.
85. Newhouse MT. Primary ciliary dyskinesia: what has it taught us about pulmonary disease? Eur J Respir Dis 1983; 64(suppl 127):151–156.
86. Eigen H, Rosenstein BJ, FitzSimmons S, Schidlow DV. A multicenter study of alternate-day prednisone therapy in patients with cystic fibrosis. Cystic Fibrosis Foundation Prednisone Trial Group. J Pediatr 1995; 126:515–523.
87. Balfour-Lynn IM, Klein NJ, Dinwiddie R. Randomised controlled trial of inhaled corticosteroids (fluticasone propionate) in cystic fibrosis. Arch Dis Child 1997; 77:124–130.
88. Nikolaizik WH, Schoni ME. Pilot study to assess the effect of inhaled corticosteroids on lung function in patients with cystic fibrosis. J Pediatr 1996; 128:271–274.
89. van Haren EH, Lammers JW, Festen J, Heijerman HG, Groot CA, van Herwaarden CL. The effects of the inhaled corticosteroid budesonide on lung function and bronchial hyperresponsiveness in adult patients with cystic fibrosis. Respir Med 1995; 89:209–214.
90. Bisgaard H, Pedersen SS, Nielsen KG, Skov M, Laursen EM, Kronborg G, Reimert CM, Hoiby N, Koch C. Controlled trial of inhaled budesonide in patients with cystic fibrosis and chronic bronchopulmonary *Pseudomonas aeruginosa* infection. Am J Respir Crit Care Med 1997; 156(4 pt 1):1190–1196.
91. American Thoracic Society. Standards for the diagnosis and care of patients with chronic obstructive pulmonary disease. Am J Respir Crit Care Med 1995; 152: S77–S120.

92. British Thoracic Society. Guidelines for the management of chronic obstructive pulmonary disease. Thorax 1997; 52(suppl 5).
93. Nishimura K, Koyama H, Ikeda A, Tsukino M, Hajiro T, Mishima M, Izumi T. The effect of high-dose inhaled beclamethasone dipropionate in patients with stable COPD. Chest 1999; 115:31–37.
94. Paggiaro PL, Dahle R, Bakran I, Frith L, Hollingworth K, Efthimiou J. Multicentre randomized placebo controlled trial of inhaled fluticasone propionate in patients with chronic obstructive pulmonary disease. Lancet 1998; 351:773–780.
95. Tamaoki J, Chiyotani A, Kobayashi K, Sakai N, Kanemura T, Takizawa T. Effect of indomethacin on bronchorrhea in patients with chronic bronchitis, diffuse panbronchiolitis, or bronchiectasis. Am Rev Respir Dis 1992; 145:548–552.
96. Liu YC, Khawaja AM, Rogers DF. Effects of the cysteinyl leukotriene receptor antagonists pranlukast and zafirlukast on tracheal mucus secretion in ovalbumin-sensitized guinea-pigs in vitro. Br J Pharmacol 1998; 124:563–571.
97. Bolister N, Basker M, Hodges NA, Marriott C. The diffusion of beta-lactam antibiotics through mixed gels of cystic fibrosis-derived mucin and *Pseudomonas aeruginosa* alginate. J Antimicrob Chemother 1991; 27:285–293.
98. Hunt BE, Weber A, Berger A, Ramsey B, Smith AL. Macromolecular mechanisms of sputum inhibition of tobramycin activity. Antimicrob Agents Chemother 1995; 39:34–39.
99. Bataillon V, Lhermitte M, Lafitte JJ, Pommery J, Roussel P. The binding of amikacin to macromolecules from the sputum of patients suffering from respiratory diseases. J Antimicrob Chemother 1992; 29:499–508.
100. Coates AL, MacNeish CF, Meisner D, Kelemen S, Thibert R, MacDonald J, Vadas E. The choice of jet nebulizer, nebulizing flow, and addition of albuterol affects the output of tobramycin aerosols. Chest 1997; 11:1206–1212.
101. Dasgupta B, Tomkiewicz RP, Boyd WA, Brown NE, King M. Effects of combined treatment with rhDNase and airflow oscillations on spinnability of cystic fibrosis sputum in vitro. Pediatr Pulmonol 1995; 20:78–82.
102. Dasgupta B, King M. Reduction in viscoelasticity in cystic fibrosis sputum in vitro using combined treatment with nacystelyn and rhDNase. Pediatr Pulmonol 1996; 2:161–166.
103. Dasgupta B, Brown NE, King M. Effects of sputum oscillations and rhDNase in vitro: a combined approach to treat cystic fibrosis lung disease. Pediatr Pulmonol 1998; 26:250–255.
104. Schreier H, Gagne L, Conary JT, Laurian G. Simulated lung transfection by nebulization of liposome cDNA complexes using a cascade impactor seeded with 2-CFSMEO-cells. J Aerosol Med 1998; 11:1–13.
105. Bellon G, Michel-Calemard L, Thouvenot D, Jagneaux V, Poitevin F, Malcus C, et al. Aerosol administration of a recombinant adenovirus expressing CFTR to cystic fibrosis patients: a phase I clinical trial. Hum Gene Ther 1997; 5–25.

8

Expectorants

IRWIN ZIMENT

Olive View–UCLA Medical Center
Sylmar, California

As an introduction to this topic, it is worth pointing out that I have maintained a close interest in the use of expectorant agents in respiratory disease for over 25 years (1). Although ion-channel modifiers may prove to be useful, no other significant advances in mucoactive pharmacology have occurred during this period, and no innovative expectorant drugs have been introduced into general patient-care practices. Indeed, there is an ever-increasing interest in the use of traditional agents, some of which are being rediscovered after thousands of years of usage through incorporation in worldwide traditional folk medicine practices. However, several old drugs and some newer products that had been gaining popularity during the past quarter of a century have faded from common usage in the past few years.

Although there is little new to say about expectorants, it is worthwhile summarizing current concepts and reviewing the numerous classes of agents regarded as having some value as expectorants. It must be emphasized that old problems facing researchers who investigate old or new agents have not been solved, and that research on all mucoactive dugs remains a backwater of therapeutics (2,3). To begin this enquiry, we should consider why expectorant therapy is regarded as a phantom science, in which the need for expectorants is questioned as much as is the apparent effectiveness of specific pharmacological products recommended for enhancing expectoration.

I. What Are Expectorants?

Different definitions of expectorants are currently used. The term literally implies coughing mucoid material out of the chest, but this could apply to the end result of any form of mucokinetic therapy. A typical dictionary definition of an expectorant is an agent promoting "the ejection by spitting of mucus or other fluids from the lungs or trachea" or an agent "that promotes the ejection of mucus or exudates form the lungs, bronchi, and trachea" (4). In practice, most drugs that are recognized to be expectorants are preparations that are taken by mouth to bring about enhanced sputum production in patients who have difficulty clearing abnormal tracheobronchial secretions. These drugs do not necessarily have any direct action on mucoid secretions when added to them in vitro, and they do not generally have significant effects on ciliary function. Based on traditional concepts and their application over many years, it is reasonable to utilize the term expectorant for an oral agent that evokes a reflex activation of bronchial glands to increase their output of mucoid material; this increase in volume of respiratory tract secretions leads to increased effectiveness of clearance by the mucociliary escalator or by coughing.

In therapeutic practice, physicians are encouraged to think of expectorants as being adjunctive agents for use in treating colds and coughs of various etiologies. Thus, the *Physician's Desk Reference* lists expectorants under the headings "decongestants, expectorants and combinations" (5). *Drug Facts and Comparisons* has a section on expectorants and includes only three basic drugs: guaifenesin, terpin hydrate, and iodine derivatives (6). The American Medical Association's *Drug Evaluations* discusses expectorants, mucolytics, and hydrating agents under the category of peripherally acting antitussives and lists guaifenesin, salts, ipecac, and iodides as expectorants (7). *Martindale's Extra Pharmacopoeia* distinguishes between expectorants, which increase the volume of respiratory secretions and thereby facilitate their removal by ciliary action and coughing, and mucolytics, which act on mucus to decrease its viscosity and thereby facilitate its removal by ciliary action or expectoration (8).

The editor of this volume has written extensively on mucoactive drugs. His definition of an expectorant, however, is deliberately vague, and the focus is on the direct effect on the respiratory airway, where expectorants "increase the hydration of sputum either by direct addition of water or by stimulation of water secretion into the airway" (9). Rubin et al. (9) do not explain the mechanism by which this effect is produced, and they limit their discussion of true expectorants to water, guaifenesin, iodides, and ion-channel modifiers. This very limited acknowledgment of the pharmacology of expectorants gives piquancy to the comments of Gunn, who wrote the twentieth-century classic account of expectorants in 1927 (10). Gunn somberly declared that the therapeutics of expectorants is a department "in which little forward movement has been registered, not only in a decade, but hardly any even in the last half-century." Gunn explained why expectorants are given so little respect: it is difficult to measure the quantity of bronchial secretion (compared to urine, for instance), it is difficult to get a control and to separate saliva from the bronchial discharge, normal people are not good subjects for studies on expectorants, and animal models are not satisfactory. The perspicacious comments of Gunn over 70 years ago are equally appropriate today (1,11).

II. Mechanisms of Action of Expectorants

In former years, expectorants were classified in various categories. The most popular scheme, still followed in some current books, divides drugs into two main groups: sedative or stimulant expectorants (12–14). "Sedative expectorants" were supposed to act by stimulating gastric reflexes: examples given by one author (12) include ambroxol, ammonium salts, antimony potassium tartrate, apomorphine, bromhexine, cistenexine, farrerol, guaiacol and related drugs, ipecac syrup, potassium iodide, sodium citrate, and vasicin. "Stimulant expectorants" were credited with stimulating secretory cells of the respiratory tract; examples include angelica, creosote and its derivatives, garlic, glycosides, grindelia, licorice, mercaptoethane sulfonate, saponaria, senega, squill, and tolu balsam. Most of these substances have not been adequately studied to discern how they work—if they do work. Thus, both the classification as sedatives and stimulants and the contents of each class are of dubious relevance, although there is no doubt that gastric irritants can enhance expectoration.

Gunn, in his thoughtful review of the action of expectorants (10), credited Christison in 1842 as being the first writer "to give something of an explanation" of the major physiological effect of expectorants. Essentially, Christison believed that a "gentle stimulus" of the gastric mucous membrane by an emetic drug caused the pulmonary mucous membrane to put out increased secretion. Gunn modernized this concept by explaining that stimulant drugs irritated the gastric mucous membrane by prolonged gentle irritation, thereby stimulating sensory fibers of the vagus. This results in a reflex through the vomiting center (or possibly a center for bronchial secretion), which had efferent output through the secretory fibers of the vagus going to the bronchial mucosa, causing prolonged secretion of the serous and mucous glands. Gunn's concept was adopted by me 50 years later (15), and the mechanism was christened the "gastropulmonary vagal mucokinetic reflex," which was envisaged as being controlled by the hypothesized mucokinetic center adjacent to the respiratory and vomiting centers in the medulla (1). At the present time no better hypothesis has emerged, and, disappointingly, little has been done to evaluate Gunn's reflex explanation.

Although the existence in humans of the gastropulmonary reflex has not been stringently established, its probable existence can readily be accepted. Thus, the stomach and the tracheobronchial tree arise from the embryonic foregut, and both have similar vagal afferents and efferents connecting them with the medulla. In reality, the tenth cranial nerve, which is vague in its anatomical distribution, can be regarded as comprising several distinct nerves supplying the lungs, bowels, and heart, with each interacting and each having a reflex control over visceral movement and secretion. The tracheobronchial tree must be supplied by separate components of the vagus nerve: one mediating mucus secretion, the other causing peristaltic tracheo-bronchial muscle contraction. In the asthmatic, the gastropulmonary vagal reflex can apparently be stimulated to cause mucous secretion without inducing bronchospasm.

A number of questions could be asked about the gastropulmonary reflex:

Is the expectorant effect of drugs lost following gastrectomy and vagotomy?

Would a stronger dose of an emetic, enough to cause vomiting as well as expectoration, result in vagal induction of tracheobronchial muscle contraction in an asthmatic patient?

Does mechanical stimulation of the throat insufficient in degree to induce emesis produce expectoration, as is claimed by some pediatricians?

Demulcent, mucilaginous agents—which soothe the throat and reduce coughing—should not have any pharmacological action on mucous secretion or on mucociliary clearance. Are such agents antimucokinetic?

Are all gastric irritants, such as pungent spices, endowed with expectorant properties? And do smokers who habitually eat pungent foods suffer less from retained sputum?

Is theophylline, which is notorious for causing nausea in large doses, primarily an expectorant in bronchitis?

Are all the reputed folk medicines believed to have expectorant effects serving as gastric irritants, and would they induce vomiting if taken in larger amounts?

Are expectorant drugs capable of acting as cough suppressants by stimulating the production of secretions that soothe the irritated respiratory tract?

Does stimulation (neurological or pharmacological) of the medullary "mucokinetic" center cause an increase in respiratory tract secretion output? Apomorphine may work in this fashion.

There are many clues to suggest that the answers to these questions are in the affirmative. In contrast, the use of antiemetics, such as milk, which can counteract the action of ipecacuanha, may inhibit expectoration; this explanation could account for the finding that milk "thickens" mucus or worsens acute bronchitis.

III. Expectorant Drugs

Although expectorants are believed to work mainly by stimulating a reflex from the stomach, other mechanisms are possibly involved. Table 1 provides the suggested mechanism of action for a number of agents that could be considered to have major mucoactive properties when administered orally.

Most discussions of expectorants are limited to a few drugs (9,12), and the majority of American physicians utilize only guaifenesin as an expectorant. The prototype expectorant is ipecacuanha.

A. Ipecacuanha

Seventeenth-century Portuguese settlers became aware of the ipecacuanha plant (*Cephaelis ipecacuanha*) in Peru and Brazil, where extracts of the root were

Table 1   Possible Mechanisms of Action of Oral Mucokinetic Agents

	Expectorant site of action		Bronchial gland activator		
	Gastric emetic	CNS stimulant	Stimulant (Broncho-mucotropic)	"Normalizer" (Mucoregulator)	Improve mucociliary effectiveness
Theophylline	++		±		++
Phenols, terpenes	+++			± → ++	±
Ipecac	+++	+			+
Guaifenesin	++				++
Apomorphine		+++			
Iodides	++		+++		++
Hypertonic salts	+++				±
Mustard	+++		+	±	±
Horseradish	++		+	±	+
Garlic	− → ++		+	++	+
Radish seedlings	+		+	+	
Acetylcysteine	++			+++	+++
Other cysteines	+ → ++		+	+++	+ → ++
Bromhexine	±		±	+++	++
Ambroxol	±		±	+++	++
Herbs					
Volatile oils	++		++		+
Nonvolatile	++		±		+

used as an expectorant and as a treatment for dysentery. The plant extract, ipecac, was subsequently studied in France, where one of the relevant emetic components, emetine, was isolated; this was recognized to be a plant alkali or alkaloid (16). The popular syrup of ipecac is currently used as a potent but relatively safe emetic, and smaller doses are used for inducing expectoration. The more potent fluid extract of ipecac contains 14 times as much of the drug as the syrup (1,8).

Ipecac has been used in combinations with many other drugs (13,14). A popular old preparation for fevers was Dover's powder, consisting of ipecac and opium (8). Many old cough medicines contained ipecac with expectorant agents such as ammonia, ammonium acetate, ammonium bicarbonate, and sodium bicarbonate or with morphine, chloroform, squill, tolu, aniseed, or guaifenesin. It has been combined with antihistamines and antitussives in cough suppressants.

The expectorant dose of ipecac syrup for adults is 0.5–2 mL containing 0.7–3 mg of alkaloids (Table 2). The adult emetic dose is 15–20 mL. Half-dosages are used for children. The emetine in ipecac is known to act both centrally and on the gastric mucosa to induce vomiting. Subemetic doses have been shown to increase respiratory tract fluid production in experimental animals, but ipecac's value as an expectorant in humans has not been adequately studied.

In India, *Tylophora asthmatica* is a medical plant known as Indian ipecac. It is utilized as an emetic and is favored for treating asthma (16,17). Similarly, ipecacuanha in various forms has been advocated for asthma therapy (1). Both of these drugs may improve the asthmatic patient's ability to clear inspissated secretions. Apomorphine, an emetic, has also been used to enhance expectoration. Pilocarpine is a more definite vagal stimulant, but it has drastic side effects and is unsuitable for therapy as an expectorant.

B. Iodides

The use of iodide products as expectorants has had historical acceptance similar to that of ipecacuanha (11,16). Following the discovery of iodine early in the nineteenth century, both iodine and its salts were used in many ways to treat a multitude of diseases. In the middle of the century, potassium iodide became popular in the therapy of asthma; it was thought that by loosening up secretions, the drug could result in relaxation of bronchospasm.

Currently, potassium iodide (KI) is mostly utilized as a saturated solution (SSKI). This colorless liquid contains about 1 g/mL of KI, and it has a recognizable, persisting metallic salt taste when given in the typical dose of 10 drops (about 1 mL, containing 1 g KI) given 3–4 times a day (Table 2). There are 6 mEq of potassium per mL of SSKI, and typical dosing with 30–80 drops of this drug per day could result in a daily intake of 18–48 mEq of potassium and an equal amount of iodide (1).

In spite of its long history as an expectorant, there are no reliable studies

Table 2 Expectorant Dosages

Drug	Expectorant dosage (adult)	Toxicity
Ipecac syrup	0.5–2 mL 3–4 x/day	Nausea, vomiting, diarrhea CNS depression—with large overdose Arrhythmias—with overdose
Guaifenesin	400 mg 4–6 x/day	Nausea, sedation Potentiation of sedatives, antidepressants, and relaxants
SSKI	10–30 drops in a beverage or water, 3–6 x/day	Metallic taste, salivation, lacrimation Parotid swelling (indicates need for smaller doses) Acne (especially in children) Hypothyroidism (in up to 10% of patients; usually only appears after 6 weeks of therapy)
Acetylcysteine	100–300 mg 2–3 x/day	Gagging, nausea, vomiting—less likely with oral formulations unavailable in U.S.
Pepper sauce	10–20 drops in a beverage or water, 3–4 x/day	Gagging, choking, dyspepsia, vomiting—caution is required; some patients obtain sufficient expectorant benefit by gargling with solution
Salts, e.g., of ammonium, calcium, potassium, or sodium	300–400 mg 3–4 x/day	Nausea, vomiting, gastritis Electrolyte disturbance
Herbs (various)	No dosages established	Few side effects in most cases, other than nausea and vomiting

to show that SSKI is effective, although years of experience support its use (1,9). Large doses can cause nausea, and it is therefore reasonable to assume that the drug stimulates the gastropulmonary mucokinetic reflex. Its side effects include nasolacrimal hypersecretion, salivation, and occasionally parotid swelling; these actions suggest a stimulatory effect on exocrine glands, and this direct action on bronchial glands is termed a bronchomucotropic effect. The presence of iodide in the resulting secretions is of relevance, since in vitro studies have shown that this ion has a direct mucolytic effect and it can also stimulate the action of natural proteases to break down mucoprotein. Other actions that have been attributed to iodide include ciliary stimulation and an anti-inflammatory effect. SSKI appears to offer multiple benefits in patients with inspissated, adhesive secretions and thus results in improved mucociliary clearance (1,18).

In spite of the positive aspects of iodide therapy, many pediatricians oppose its use, partly because its effectiveness has not been proved, and partly because of side effects. Adolescents may develop acne if treated with SSKI, and there is an incidence in less than 10% of patients of thyroid depression after 6 weeks of daily therapy. Thus, in general, iodides should not be given for more than 1 month, followed by a break of a few weeks, after which another 4–6 weeks of therapy can safely be given. The majority of patients can tolerate continuous use of SSKI without developing side effects, but any suspicion of hypothyroidism should lead to investigation of thyroid function.

Sodium iodide was formerly available for intravenous administration, but it is no longer marketed. Similarly, it is not used orally, although it was formerly considered to be an alternative to potassium iodide.

Organic iodides were developed to provide more acceptable oral products. Iodopropylidine glycerol (iodinated glycerol, Organidin®) was the most widely used tablet preparation. A large multicenter trial suggested its clinical value in bronchitis, although a smaller study showed no benefit (9,19). The U.S. Food and Drug Administration (FDA) became concerned about the potential of Organidin to cause an unusual tumor in rats and chose to ban its use (it is now remarketed as Organidin NF, which is guaifenesin). In Italy, a similar drug, domiodol (4-hydroxymethyl-2-iodomethyl-1,3-dioolane) is marketed.

Other iodides, such as hydroxic acid, calcium iodide, niacinamide hydroiodide, iodostarin, lipoiodine, iodotropin, and sajodin, are no longer used (8,13). Similarly, in the past, various bromide salts were used when other agents failed.

C. Water and Salts

Undoubtedly, water and natural mineral waters have been used since ancient times in the treatment of respiratory diseases. Flavored water in the form of soups, teas, tissanes, juices, cordials, tinctures, syrups, elixirs, emulsions, and suspensions is becoming more popular since herbs and minerals that are not used in orthodox medical practice can be incorporated in attractive potions for oral imbibition.

Water taken orally in a daily amount of 2–3 L is generally believed to loosen up sticky respiratory tract secretions (17). However, this concept has been challenged (9,20,21). Shim et al. showed that in patients with chronic obstructive pulmonary disease, neither decreased nor increased daily water intake changed expectorated sputum volume (22). Thus, there is as yet no scientific evidence that oral water has an expectorant effect, which challenges the claims that expectorant drugs only work if enough water is taken simultaneously. The conclusion that water drinking does not improve expectoration correlates with Boyd's belief that the normal production of respiratory tract fluid continues even in severe dehydration (23).

Salts in general appear to increase respiratory tract fluid production in airway disease. As was discussed in the section on potassium iodide, salts given in subemetic dosages can stimulate expectoration by activating the gastropulmonary reflex. In contrast, very concentrated salt solutions given in sufficient amount will induce emesis. Numerous salt solutions have been advocated over the years as expectorants; in particular, sodium, potassium, and ammonium preparations have been favored (1,8,13,16).

Expectorant properties have been claimed for sodium chloride, sodium iodide, sodium bromide, sodium acetate, sodium bicarbonate, sodium citrate, sodium lactate, and sodium phosphate. Similarly, in addition to potassium iodide, potassium chloride, potassium citrate, and potassium acetate have been used as expectorants. Several similar salts of ammonia, such as ammonium acetate, ammonium bicarbonate, ammonium citrate, ammonium carbonate, and ammonium chloride, have been used, but since they are irritating to the stomach they were usually given in subtherapeutic amounts or in enteric-coated capsules that would prevent the drug from activating the gastropulmonary reflex. Most of these salts are no longer used, since their benefits were dubious at best. Other comparable agents such as calcium and antimony salts have also been retired from expectorant service.

Sodium chloride is favored mainly for intravenous and inhalant use in respiratory disease (1). As an inhalant it can be used to induce expectoration even from "dry" lungs, and it also serves as a useful diagnostic aerosol for evaluating the presence of hyper-reactivity. When given intravenously in dehydrated bronchitic patients, it can be expected to improve mucociliary clearance, although this has not been demonstrated in a rigorous study. Its use as a pure expectorant entails taking a saline solution orally, and there is no evidence of its effectiveness. Theoretically the appropriate product would be hypertonic saline (e.g., 20%) given in small subemetic amounts (Table 2), whereas isotonic or hypotonic saline in reasonable doses would have no effect on the gastropulmonary reflex.

Sodium bicarbonate is another salt worth considering (1). It is often used to neutralize stomach hyperacidity, and the reaction liberates carbon dioxide. The resulting distension of the stomach may irritate vagal stimulation of the gastropulmonary reflex. However, there is no evidence that oral sodium bicarbonate is a useful oral emetic, whereas it has a mucolytic effect when given by direct instillation into the tracheobronchial tree.

Antimony potassium tartrate, which has antischistomiasis properties, was known as tartar emetic. Its nauseant effect provides an explanation for favoring lower dosages of the drug as an expectorant. Zinc sulfate and copper sulfate are other salts that were recommended by nineteenth-century writers. More dangerous expectorant choices were arsenic and mercury products, which were possibly chosen for their supposed accompanying tonic and anti-infective properties.

D. Phenol Derivatives

Many phenolic agents derived from plants have been used to treat coughs, bronchitis, and asthma (16). These drugs are nauseating and thus stimulate mucokinesis by activating the gastropulmonary reflex. Most are no longer in use.

Creosote is a composite phenolic derived from beechwood; it is unpleasant to use and is toxic, as are its major constituents, phenol, creosol, and cresol. The remaining important agent that can be obtained from creosote is guaiacol (methylcatechol). It can also be obtained from guaiac wood and from coal tar, and it can be synthesized. In the mid-nineteenth century, guaiacol and several derivatives were used to treat bowel and lung infections, including tuberculosis. It was believed to act as a general stimulant of mucosal secretions and eventually was favored for use as an expectorant. The incorporation of glycerol in the guaiacol molecule resulted in the propanediol derivative glyceryl guaiacolate, which since the 1970s has been called guaifenesin. This product has come to be the most popular expectorant in the United States. Derivatives marketed as expectorants in other countries include guaiacol, guacetisal, guaiapate, guaietolin, guaimesal, and guethol (8).

Guaifenesin (methylphenoxydiol, glyceryl guaiacolate) is only given as an oral medication. In excessive doses it causes nausea and vomiting; thus, when given in lower dosages as an expectorant, it activates the gastropulmonary mucokinetic reflex (1). The drug is absorbed from the stomach into the blood stream and thereby acts on the bronchial glands and may also enter the sputum. Unsubstantiated claims have been made that guaifenesin "hydrates" the sputum and decreases its surface tension, thereby reducing its adhesiveness, but it does not have a mucolytic action on mucoprotein.

The value of guaifenesin remains a contentious issue, ever since Boyd in his classical studies found the drug to be effective only in the autumn months of the year (2–4). Several good studies have failed to show any benefit, although these authors do not stipulate which months were devoted to their observations. Other, poorly designed studies have found useful effects in up to 75% of patients, but with a placebo response in over 30% there is reason to question observed benefits in such trials (9). The conclusion to be drawn from the reported studies, and from personal experience, is that adults taking at least 2400 mg of guaifenesin a day may experience subjective improvement in expectorating viscous secretions, but objective evidence of value is inadequate (Table 2).

Guaifenesin may have a nonspecific antitussive effect in simple acute respiratory infections, but this claim has not been substantiated. Similarly, it does
not benefit bronchospasm or airways inflammation. It has a minor mucosal anesthetic effect, and it may share some of the spasmolytic and sedative properties
of the related muscle relaxant methocarbamol; some practitioners believe guaifenesin is of symptomatic benefit for fibromyalgia. The drug may inhibit platelet
aggregation, but its effects on hemostasis appear to be insignificant.

Guaifenesin is a very popular nonprescription drug that is available in
liquids, tablets, and capsules (1). It is incorporated as an expectorant in many
combination products, including cough and cold medications. The typical recommended adult dose of 200–400 mg (5–10 mL of Robitussin®) given every
4–8 hours may be sufficient for small children, but a total of 2000–3000 mg a
day is advised in adults, with the caution that larger dosages may induce nausea.
In contrast, much smaller doses, which are well tolerated, should be recognized
as merely serving a placebo purpose.

E. Terpene Derivatives

Pine and larch tree products are the source of pitch and other resinous materials,
including terpenes. However, the turpentine tree, *Pistacia terebinthus*, is the best
source of turpentine oil, from which are obtained pinenes. Hydration of these
pinenes results in terpin hydrate (16).

Terpin hydrate (dipenteneglycol) was introduced as a cough medication in
the 1880s and eventually became the only terpene used for respiratory disorders.
Although Boyd showed it to have some expectorant action in guinea pigs, terpin
hydrate gradually lost credibility as an effective drug in humans. Larger doses
of terpin hydrate, which may be effective for inducing expectoration, cause
nausea and stomach discomfort, and therefore the drug is not recommended. In
spite of terpin hydrate's popularity in preparations such as terpin hydrate and
codeine elixir for coughs, this old expectorant is no longer approved, as it was
abused for its codeine and alcohol content. A European product, Ozothin®,
containing monoterpene alcohols, aldehydes, and ketones, has been shown to
stimulate serous glands, reduce surface tension, and increase mucociliary clearance (17).

F. Pungent Spices

Over the years, mustard, peppers, horseradish, onions, garlic, cinnamon, ginger,
and other pungent spices have been used in medical therapy (1,14). Throughout
the world, ancient theories regarding the balancing of body secretions or humors
have been used as a basis for selecting medications (16). In Chinese traditional
practice, the yin-yang balance of secretions invoked concepts of hot and cold,
astringent and salty, or sweet and sour; secretions believed to be abnormal be-

cause of an excess of one of these pairs would be treated with drugs offering the opposite qualities. In the ancient ayurvedic medical practice of India, the three basic qualities were kapha (cold, phlegm-like), pitta (hot, inflamed), and vata (wind, flatulent); kapha abnormalities, such as heavy phlegm, were treated with pitta remedies, such as peppers. In Greek-Roman medical theory, the four humors included phlegm; derangements were brought into balance by "hot" drugs for disorders involving expectoration. There is thus a long tradition of treating lung disease with hot remedies that included pungent spices (Table 1). A major example of such therapy was the spicy chicken soup that Maimonides introduced in his book, *Treatise on Asthma*. In the current era, this worthy expectorant therapy has been reformulated to emphasize the beneficial effects of garlic and chile peppers (5,21,25,26).

Garlic is of particular interest, since it fulfills several requirements as a mucokinetic agent (21). When taken orally in excess, it irritates the stomach and causes nausea; subemetic amounts would stimulate the gastropulmonary reflex. Garlic is absorbed into the blood and is excreted through the epithelium of the lungs; as a potent chemical that readily causes lacrimation, rhinorrhea, or sneezing, it would be expected to have a bronchomucotropic effect and cause the bronchial glands to secrete a watery fluid that would dilute viscous secretions. Most remarkably, an active agent in garlic, S-allyl-L-cysteine, is very similar in structure to the mucolytic drug N-acetyl-L-cysteine; thus, garlic compounds or their derivatives may have a slow mucoregulator effect, as may acetylcysteine, bringing about a gradual restoration of abnormal mucoprotein secretion to a more normal, easily cleared mucus (27). Moreover, as is the case with acetylcysteine, garlic is an antioxidant. Finally, the breathing in of aromatic, garlicky flavor molecules from hot spicy chicken soup could have a bronchorrheic effect on the respiratory mucosa, resulting in transepithelial exudation of water into the tracheobronchial secretions. Although more attention has been focused by the public on the cardiovascular benefits of garlic, it is expected that its mucokinetic properties will earn garlic a greater role in protecting airways, by virtue of its mucokinetic and antioxidant properties, from damage from smoke, irritant chemicals, dusts, and infections. Onion may have a similar benefit, and both onions and garlic are used as expectorants in many parts of the world. However, an old European folk remedy, which requires that these agents be cooked in milk, may negate their mucokinetic effect. It is of interest that both onion and garlic may have anti-inflammatory properties that can be of benefit in asthma.

Peppers are capable of causing lacrimation, rhinitis, sneezing, and coughing. Capsicum peppers (e.g., chilies) contain capsaicin, which liberates substance P; this mediator is synthesized in the nodose ganglion of the vagus nerve and is released by unmyelinated branches that activate submucosal glands (28). Capsaicin can thus result in mucus release, since substance P is a potent stimulant of mucus secretion and it may also cause the myoepithelial cells that surround submucosal glands to contract and expel secretions from the glands and ducts. Pepper sauce offers a useful alternative to standard expectorants (Table 2). Black pepper (*Piper nigrum*) may have a gastropulmonary reflex effect, but it lacks the capsaicin that causes tracheobronchial gland stimulation.

Other pungent vegetables have cysteine chemicals that could offer mucokinetic benefits (24). Radish seedlings contain S-carboxymethylcysteine, which is the same chemical that is used as a mucoregulator drug, carbocysteine. Radish, mustard, horseradish, wasabi, and similar pungent herbs could act as reflex expectorants by stimulating afferent receptors in the stomach. Mustard is also used as a household emetic since it is an effective stimulant of the vomiting reflex originating from the gastric mucosa.

The less pungent spices may also have expectorant properties. However, they are less likely to have a major effect on the gastropulmonary reflex, being more likely to act directly on bronchial glands and on the respiratory mucosa. The odor of many aromatic spices is exhaled on the breath following oral ingestion, thus implying that their chemical constituents could have a chemical effect in the respiratory tract (14). *Spices* that have been used as expectorants include cinnamon and the related cassia, aniseed, fenugreek, mints, thyme, oregano, and tumeric (14,16). Cloves might also have some effect, since the main constituent, eugenol, is related to guaifenesin (16). Thus, eugenol is allyl-guaiacol: this chemical is of interest, since the allyl radical is also found in garlic. Eugenol is a local anesthetic, as is guaifenesin, and it is liberated by using clove cigarettes—the favored tobacco product in Indonesia; one wonders whether this potential mucokinetic has any protective effect on smokers of the Indonesian kretek cigarettes, which contain cloves.

G. Herbs

Numerous derivatives of herbal origin have been used to treat chest diseases (1,16). In traditional therapy, it is difficult to distinguish between medications for treating asthma, bronchitis, catarrh, and cough. Often, drugs used for these diseases seem to have only mucokinetic effects, without specific bronchodilator, decongestant, anti-inflammatory, or antitussive effects. Furthermore, there is no good evidence that most of the herbs that have persisted in use are of value. Presumably, if larger doses induce nausea and vomiting, then subemetic doses of such agents would have a reflex expectorant effect. Appropriate dosages for herbal preparations are not known.

Large numbers of remedies for respiratory diseases were described by Mesopotamian, Egyptian, Greek, and Roman writers (16). Biblical herbs of importance such as myrrh, frankincense, cinnamon, cassia, galbanum, calamus, and nard were probably used as expectorants (29). Arabic physicians recognized the value of hyssop and maidenhair fern, in addition to culinary herbs; however, some also recommended fox and hedgehog lungs as remedies for human lung disorders (16). This type of logic—i.e., using similar appearing drugs for specific organ diseases—influenced much of old pharmaceutical practice and had a directive impact on the development of homeopathy.

The Chinese have long utilized numerous herbs for mucus therapy, and new ones keep appearing. In recent years, rhododendron products (such as farrerol) have been recommended, although older drugs such as licorice are preferred (12,27,30). The Indian drugs used in traditional ayurvedic practice are most interesting. They include the familiar peppers, garlic, ginger, and licorice as well as less well-known herbs such as the malabar nut tree. This is the source of vasaka (vasicin), which has long been used for lung diseases; from this comes the modern products bromhexine and ambroxol, which are now marketed as mucokinetic agents. Other ayurvedic expectorants include *Inula racemosa* (pushkarmola), *Hypericum perforatum* (St. John's wort), omum seeds, *Abbies webbiana* (talispatra), *Barringtonia acutangula* (samudraphala), and many other agents as yet unknown in the West (1,31,32).

Mexico and the Americas were fertile areas for drug discovery, and the New World was the source not only of ipecacuanha, guaiac, and peppers, but also of cocillana (Guapi bark), yerba santa, snakeroot (senega), grindelia, and balsams (1,16,30). The huge numbers of mucokinetic herbs that have been used in many countries have been reviewed (1,16,24), and it is evident that most of them have never been subjected to any evaluation. In spite of this, many traditional drugs remain popular. An example is Friar's Balsam®, which is used orally and by inhalation in Great Britain (16). It consists of tincture of benzoin, tolu balsam, storax, aloes, and alcohol. Boyd was unable to show any benefit from this medication in laboratory studies (33). Most other popular oral balsams and products, such as Vicks' VapoRub, have not been shown to have mucokinetic effects.

The best organized assessment of herbal medications has been made in Germany by an expert committee, Commission E, established in 1978 by the Bundesgesundheitsamt (The German Federal Institute for Drugs and Medical Devices). Commission E has published drug monographs and a book, which was recently translated into English and published by the American Botanical Council (34). The Commission carefully evaluated all herbal medications and recommended over 360 as having a "reasonable certainty" of being effective, although rigorous proof in appropriately controlled trials was not required. About 115 herbs were negatively evaluated as having "no plausible evidence of efficacy" and posing "documented or suspected risk." Another 57 drugs were not approved: although they had no toxicity, they lacked evidence of benefit.

The monographs of Commission E vary in quality and do not use standardized criteria. Thus, 34 herbs are described as "expectorant" or "secretolytic" or as being of use in "catarrhs." No rationale is provided for rating an herb as effective for any of these individual functions. A popular German herbal medication for sinusitis and bronchitis, Sinupret, contains gentian, primrose (primula), sorrel (sour dock), elder, and verbena (vervain): this product appears to be an effective mucokinetic (35). The Commission E text lists gentian, primrose, and vervain as expectorant or secretolytic, while sorrel is not discussed. Books from other countries are also erratic in their inclusions and exclusions, and agreement between standard texts is poor (8,12,17).

If one scans textbooks in English from America, Europe, and Asia, one finds large lists of expectorant herbs which are distinguished mainly by the lack of agreement between authors except for a core group including eucalyptus, pine, thyme, and licorice (34,36–41). An excellent American encyclopedia of herbs (41) lists 47 expectorants; others are described for treating bronchitis, but are not classified as expectorants. Personal experience of a visit to several traditional medical schools in China reveals the same lack of uniform agreement in that country: authorities at each school presented a list of favored mucokinetic drugs, which differed greatly from those of the other schools. Table 3 lists the recommendations of several standard books on herbal medicine; there is hardly any agreement between them, and thyme is the only agent that is recommended by each. There is no reason to believe that generally favored agents are any more effective than a host of less favored ones.

Constituents of herbs—numerous active chemicals occur in medicinal plants. The ones of major interest as mucokinetic agents occur in 10 categories (36–38).

1. *Alkaloids*, predominantly basic amines, are usually insoluble in water, but their salts are soluble (37). Emetine, which is found in ipecac, is a mucokinetic alkaloid, whereas atropine is antimucokinetic.

2. *Balsams* are usually found in the resinous secretions of trees. They contain cinnamic and benzoic acids and esters (37). The common balsams such as benzoin, storax (from *Styrax officianalis*), Peru balsam, and Tolu balsam (both from *Myroxylon balsamum*) are soluble in organic solvents or alcohols. They were incorporated in older cough medications, and were formerly very popular in respiratory therapeutics, but they are of limited nonspecific value— or, as Boyd found, of no value at all (23,33).

3. *Essential oils* are also known as volatile oils or essences. They are represented by the generally pleasant odiferous contents of flowering plants or the more pungent agents in spices (37). Many of therm are derived from the basic molecule isoprene, which is synthesized from acctate. Combinations of isoprene units results in terpenoids; resins are formed by oxidation of terpenoid complexes. Other essential oils are derived from phenylpropanoids, which are generally phenols or phenol esters.

Terpenoids include terpin hydrate, camphor, cineole (also called eucalyptol, the active principle of eucalyptus and of cajuput and myrtol), menthol (which is prepared from peppermint oil), and thymol (from thyme) (16,37).

Table 3 Comparison of Herbal Expectorant Recommendations

	Ref. 34	Ref. 38	Ref. 40	Ref. 39	Ref. 36
Ammoniacum				✔	
Angelica		✔	✔		✔
Anise	✔	✔	✔	✔	
Asafetida		✔	✔		
Balm of Gilead		✔		✔	✔
Benzoin		✔			
Beth root					✔
Bittersweet					✔
Blessed thistle					✔
Bloodroot			✔		✔
Boneset				✔	
Borage	✔	✔	✔		✔
Cajeput	✔	✔			
Camphor	✔				
Caraway		✔			✔
Cedar		✔			
Chaparral		✔			
Chervil		✔			
Cocillana		✔		✔	
Cocoa		✔			
Coltsfoot	✔		✔		✔
Comfrey		✔			✔
Cornflower	✔				
Cubeb		✔			
Daisy					✔
Dog-grass		✔			
Elder	✔				✔
Elecampane			✔	✔	✔
Elemi		✔			
Epimedium		✔			
Eucalyptus	✔	✔	✔		
Euphorbia			✔		✔
Fennel	✔	✔			✔
Fenugreek			✔		✔
Fir	✔				
Galbanum		✔			
Garlic		✔	✔		✔
Gentian	✔				
Goldenseal					✔
Grindelia	✔			✔	✔
Heartsease				✔	

Table 3 Continued

	Ref. 34	Ref. 38	Ref. 40	Ref. 39	Ref. 36
Hempnettle	✔				
Holy thistle			✔		
Horehound		✔	✔	✔	✔
Horseradish	✔				
Hound's tongue	✔				
Hyssop				✔	✔
Iceland moss					✔
Irish moss					✔
Immortelle		✔			
Ipecac		✔		✔	✔
Ivy	✔		✔	✔	✔
Kava kava		✔			
Knotweed	✔				
Labdanum		✔			
Licorice	✔	✔	✔		✔
Life root			✔		✔
Linden	✔				
Lobelia		✔	✔		✔
Lovage		✔			
Lungwort					✔
Mallow			✔		✔
Marjoram					✔
Mints	✔				
Mouse-ear					✔
Mullein	✔			✔	✔
Mustard	✔				
Myrrh		✔	✔		✔
Niauli	✔				
Onion		✔			
Oregano	✔	✔			
Pansy					✔
Parsley			✔		✔
Peach leaf					✔
Pimpinella	✔				
Pine	✔	✔			
Plantain	✔				✔
Pleurisy root			✔		✔
Primula	✔		✔		✔
Queen's delight			✔	✔	✔
Quillaja		✔			
Radish	✔				
Red clover		✔	✔		✔

Table 3 Continued

	Ref. 34	Ref. 38	Ref. 40	Ref. 39	Ref. 36
Red poppy					✔
Saffron		✔			
Sanicle	✔				
Savory		✔			
Saw palmetto		✔			
Schisandra		✔			
Senega	✔		✔	✔	✔
Skunk cabbage			✔		✔
Soapwort	✔				✔
Squill		✔	✔	✔	✔
Storax		✔			
Sundew			✔		✔
Tea		✔			
Thuja					✔
Thyme	✔	✔	✔	✔	✔
Tolu	✔	✔			✔
Turpentine	✔				
Watercress	✔				
Wild cherry					✔
Verbena	✔				
Vervain					✔
Violet				✔	✔
Yerba santa		✔			

These and similar agents are often incorporated in oral and inhalational respiratory medications, and Boyd has shown that many of them have a bronchorrheic or broncomucotropic effect by stimulating the production of respiratory tract secretions (23). Larger amounts given by inhalation are less effective than smaller concentrations (the "reversal effect"), and only very small amounts are usually given orally. Their oral administration may result in a gastropulmonary mucokinetic reflex or may cause bloodborne secretory responses in the airways.

Phenylpropanoids include the essential oils cinnamaldehyde (found in cinnamon), eugenol (in cloves), myristicin (in nutmeg), anethole (in anise or aniseed and fennel), and methylsalicylate (wintergreen) (37). These agents are likely to have a significant mucokinetic effect, although they are rarely considered to be medications.

It is not clear which of the many essential oils are of value and whether combination products are of greater benefit. However, there is some evidence in humans of an expectorant effect produced by oral use of menthol, camphor, eucalyptus oil, and conifer oil and constituents such as anethole, cineole, citral, citronella, geraniol, isoeugenol, limonene, nerol, phellandrane, and pinene (17, 23,37). It is of interest that menthol may also have antitussive and broncho-spasmolytic effects. Many other agents in western cough mixtures may have expectorant effects, e.g., sweet flag, skunk cabbage, euphorbia species, hore-hound, marshmallow, wild lettuce, squills, cascara, sanguinaria, pleurisy root, chloroform, and even alcohol (1,7,36–41).

4. *Resins*, which are oxidation products of terpenes, often occur in mix-tures with volatile oils: the material is insoluble in water. Mucokinetic resins are found in sources such as capsicum, ginger, pine, and turpentine (37,38). Resins can also occur mixed with gums, which are water-soluble carbohydrate derivatives from oleogum resins. Eriodictyon (yerba santa) is a traditional ex-pectorant: it contains several resins such as eriodictyol. Oleogum resins used as mucokinetic agents include myrrh and asafetida; these ancient respiratory drugs are still used in some countries (29).

5. *Saponins* are soap-like agents that may foam when shaken with water. They are derivatives of glycosides, which are sugar complexes, usually with a terpenoid aglycone component (37). Topically, they may have a surfactant effect in the respiratory tract. However, they are usually irritating when given either by inhalation or orally. Their nauseant effect implies that low doses would be expectorants. Traditional saponin-containing herbs that are used orally include *Grindelia* (gumweed), *Hedera* (ivy), *Polygala* (senega snake root), *Primula* (primrose, cowslip), *Quillaja* (soapbark), and *Gypsophila* (soapwort) (36–38). Licorice (*Gycyrrhiza*) may also be in this group; it contains the saponin-like glycoside glycyrrhizin, which is very sweet, but this is unlikely to have an expectorant effect, although it is claimed to be an effective antitussive.

6. *Glycosides* are similar to saponins (37). They yield one or more sug-ars (such as glucose and rhamnose) on hydrolysis, but their classification is difficult. They include cyanogenic glycosides, which yield hydrocyanic acid on hydrolysis, and isothiocyanate glycosides (or glucosinolates), which yield their aglycone isothiocyanate component on enzymatic hydrolysis.

Cyanogenic compounds are found in wild cherry bark, which yields pru-nasin; this compound may soothe cough as well as having expectorant effects. The isothiocyanate glycosides are found in herbs such as mustard (37). Black mustard contains sinigrin (allyl glucosinolate), which is hydrolyzed by the ac-companying enzyme myrosinase (myrosin) to give the pungent allyl isothiocya-nate (mustard oil). White mustard contains sinalbin (sinapine glucosinalbate), which is hydrolyzed by myrosinase to the nonvolatile but pungent product, *p*-hydroxybenzyl isothiocyanate. These isothiocyanate products have long been used for respiratory diseases—orally, as chest poultices, and in footbaths.

7. *Phenolic derivatives* include guaifenesin, salicylic acid and salicy-lates, thymol, and eugenol (16). Of this group, only guaifenesin is well recog-

nized as an expectorant. Capsaicin, from *Capsicum* peppers, could also be regarded as a phenol derivative, and its value as a secretagogue appears to be greater than its recognized effect as a topical pain therapy.

8.   *Bitters*, such as occur in gentian and white horehound, reflexly stimulate salivary flow; a similar reflex may induce mucokinesis (7,35). Other agents with a disturbing taste or a nauseating quality would be capable of having an expectorant effect. Presumably, all traditional unpleasant-tasting cough medications work in this fashion.

9.   *Demulcents*, in contrast to bitters, are soothing to the throat and may suppress a cough originating from irritated pharyngeal receptors: as such, demulcents should inhibit mucokinesis. However, demulcents are syrupy or mucilaginous, and thus they resemble mucus; this association led earlier physicians and healers to equate herbal preparations having demulcent qualities with relief of sputum. Although the belief continues to persist, there is no basis for accepting that mucilages, syrups, and so on are expectorants. Nevertheless, authors often attribute the expectorant qualities believed to exist in herbs such as coltsfoot, Irish moss, lungwort, licorice, marshmallow, mallow, mullein, and slippery elm to the demulcent effect of their polysaccharide mucilage content (41).

10.   *Astringents*, such as tannin, which are complex mixtures of polyphenols, precipitate protein and cause mucous membranes to contract or pucker. Such properties may result in the evocation of the gastropulmonary reflex, although older authors thought this action was antiexpectorant. The astringent qualities of several herbs, e.g., beth root, ground ivy, lungwort, mouse ear, plantain and wild cherry, have been correlated with their alleged expectorant properties (41).

H. European Expectorants

The European pharmaceutical industry finds an enthusiastic clinical audience for expectorant drugs (9,16,43,44). In contrast to the scene in the United States, where new drugs have not been introduced in many years, numerous agents have been made available in Europe and on other continents for oral use as mucokinetic agents. Although these may have the ability to initiate the gastropulmonary expectorant reflex, most appear to have their effect following intestinal absorption and bloodborne delivery to the bronchial glands. As such, they may be classified principally as mucolytics or mucoregulators, and they are considered in detail in other chapters. The focus in this discussion is on the expectorant effects of these drugs.

N-Acetyl-L-cysteine (NAC) is a thiol compound with an active free sulfhydryl group that ruptures disulfide bridges in mucoprotein. It is therefore a mucolytic. In the United States it is given only by inhalation for respiratory diseases. For the emergency therapy of poisoning by acetaminophen, acetylcysteine is given orally or intravenously, since it functions as a scavenger of free radicals.

In Europe, the mucolytic and antioxidant effects of NAC are appreciated for their value in lung disease, and appropriately formulated oral products (e.g., Fluimucil®) are available that lack the unpleasant sulfurous quality of the American product that is designed for aerosolization (18). A large study involving 259 patients carried out by the Swedish Society for Pulmonary Disease showed that twice-daily oral NAC given for 6 months reduced exacerbations of COPD but resulted in no improvement in pulmonary function (9,45). The trend in most other studies on oral NAC has been for clinical improvement with no objective spirometric benefit (46). In contrast, the value of aerosolized NAC has not been clearly demonstrated, partly because there is a tendency for the aerosol to induce bronchospasm (43,47). Studies of cystic fibrosis and sinusitis show some benefits, but the drug is not of clear value in asthma or in post-operative management of retained secretions. Acetylcysteine in a dose of at least 200 mg t.i.d. may serve as an expectorant as well as a mucolytic and a mucoregulator. However, recent explanations for the benefit of NAC emphasize its antioxidant (43) and immunomodulator actions (48).

Other cysteines are numerous (24,44). One useful agent is 2-mercapto-ethane sulfonate (Mesna®), which is used as a free-radical scavenger rather than as a mucokinetic (1). Methylcysteine and ethylcysteine are less effective alternatives to acetylcysteine, whereas dithiothreitol is too toxic for clinical use (44). Thiopronine is a sulfhydryl, as is acetylcysteine, but it is used as a minor mucolytic (15,44). *S*-Carboxy-methylcysteine (carbocysteine), which has a blocked thiol group, is a relatively popular choice, but is considered to be a mucoregulator rather than a mucolytic or an expectorant (18). Letosteine is a cyclic derivative of cysteine and is similar to carbocysteine; however, it is likely to cause gastric irritation and should therefore be classified as an expectorant (8).

Lysine salt derivatives of older cysteine products are being introduced, but since they are less irritating to the stomach (49), they are less likely to have an expectorant effect. Thus, nacystelyn, the lysine salt of *N*-acetylcysteine, is being evaluated as a better tolerated oral drug, but the emphasis is on its function as an antioxidant (50). Carbocysteine lysine salt monohydrate (SCMC-Lys) is a newer variant of carbocysteine, with no major differences, although it may cause less stomach irritation (49,51). Other related products, including nesosteine, methyl-diacetylcysteinate, and *N*-guanylcysteine, are of uncertain value (8). Another relatively new derivative of cysteine, cistinexine (52), has been shown to have an expectorant effect, which is only manifested in patients with severe impairment of mucus transport. Homocysteine thiolactone and its derivative, dithiosteine, are not used. A related drug, erdosteine, is a thiol derivative derived from homocysteine; it has two blocked sulfydryl groups, and it acts as a mucoregulator rather than an expectorant (53). New cysteine derivatives, such as *S*-(3-hydroxypropyl)-L-cysteine, which may have expectorant and mucoregulator properties, are under evaluation (49).

In Europe manufacturers currently market two mucokinetic drugs that are derived from a traditional Indian respiratory remedy, vasaka (vasicin), which comes from the plant *Adhatoda vasica*. The first, bromhexine, acts on bronchial glands to increase secretion, thus acting as a bronchomucotropic. It may also stimulate lysosomal enzymes to break up the mucopolysaccharide fibrils of viscous mucus (1). Although it acts like iodide, it does not appear to be a true expectorant activator of the gastropulmonary reflex. The second agent, ambroxol, was derived from bromhexine, and it has the interesting property of significantly stimulating type II alveolar cells to produce surfactant (1). Ambroxol may be a more effective mucokinetic drug, but it also seems to lack expectorant properties. Clinical studies have yielded conflicting results of effectiveness. As is the case with acetylcysteine, recent studies have focused on its anti-inflammatory and antioxidant properties in the lung (54).

Sobrerol is a derivative of pinene, and it resembles terpin hydrate; however, sobrerol is a more potent expectorant, and it also has a mucoregulator effect (16). This product deserves wider recognition as a modern expectorant. Stepronine is a drug that liberates a lytic sulfhydryl group when metabolized; it may be a mucolytic with mucoregulator properties. Similar products include stepronine lysine salt and lysine-proprionil glycine (8). Other glycine derivatives are available, such as thiopronine (α-mercaptoproprionylglycine), tasuldine (a pyrimidine product), brovanexine (a derivative of bromhexine), among others. All these drugs are of minor interest to everyone except their manufacturers.

IV. Asiatic Expectorants

A host of herbal remedies, as well as some of animal or mineral origin, are used in the traditional medical practices of China, India, Indonesia, and Japan, perhaps to a greater degree than in other countries around the world. It is difficult to sort out which of these folk medicines or traditional prescriptions are of value in respiratory disease, and it is particularly difficult to determine which function as expectorants (27,44). With the possible exception of the ayurvedic drugs derived from the plants *Tylophora asthmatica* and *Adhatoda vasica*, which have been credited with specific expectorant effects, no Asiatic drug appears to be as valuable as the traditional western drugs ipecac and guaifenesin—and since these drugs are being discounted, there is little reason to believe any other folk medicine will prove to be of clinical significance. Typical Asiatic mucokinetic drugs have been listed in detail previously, and reference can be made to these prior publications (16,24,44,55–57). New suggestions for therapy are occasionally written about in the English literature; such remedies include Qing-Fei-Tang and Mai-men-Dong Tang (4,9). The latter contains six traditional herbs— Ophiopogonis (lilyturf), Pinellia, Zizyphus (Chinese date), licorice, ginseng, and rice—which are of dubious value (27,57).

Homeopathy, which is widely used in India and is making a comeback in many other countries, does not offer a physiological basis for treating abnormal mucus (56). Homeopathic therapies are targeted at the basic causation of the disease, with relief coming from stimulation of the body's own healing powers. In addition, the theory of homeopathy is to use drugs is hugely diluted solutions to treat symptoms that the undiluted drug produces. As an example, infinitesimally diluted solutions of ipecac are used to treat vomiting, and similarly diluted atropine might be used to treat thick mucus. Thus, homeopathic theory does not allow for expectorant drugs that would initiate the gastropulmonary reflex. It is thought provoking to recognize that patients who believe in the value of homeopathic treatment appear to obtain equal mucokinetic benefit from their drugs as do allopathically treated patients who invest their confidence in the conventional expectorants discussed in this chapter.

V. Conclusions

No progress has been made in expectorant therapy over the past 70 years since the Gunn reflex theory of action was propounded. Very few agents are employed as expectorants in America, and there is little objective evidence to support the clinical impression that these drugs are useful. The limited number of quality studies on expectorant and related mucokinetic agents suggest that they offer a clinical benefit in the absence of any evidence of physiological improvement (47). As a group, however, expectorant drugs remain on the border of being noneffective, and it may require new study techniques to give objective justification to clinicians and patients who claim that they are helpful in enhancing the coughing out of abnormal airway secretions.

Most ancient cultures have a huge pharmacopeia of herbs, plant extracts, and salts that are favored as expectorants. Increasingly, patients are returning to these phytomedicines (which are advertised on the Internet) as a reaction to their dissatisfaction with orthodox mucokinetic pharmaceutical preparations. However, there is virtually no evidence to support the claims of herbalists and alternative practitioners that these traditional or "natural" medications are effective, and most could be considered to be placebos. That is why sceptical clinicians rely on treatment with bronchodilators, anti-inflammatory drugs, and antibiotics to provide expectorant therapy since these drugs produce measurable spirometric benefits with observable increases in expectoration as a secondary outcome. What more could one expect from an expectorant?

Fortunately, there is at least some reason to believe that one class of expectorant agents does offer true benefits. Thus, ingestion of pungent spices, such as chili peppers, mustard, horseradish, and wasabi, which clearly evoke a mucokinetic response in the nose and sinuses, may also stimulate the gastropulmonary expectorant reflex through the vagus. Therefore, it would seem advisable to ensure that future comparative studies on expectorant drugs utilize spicy, pungently hot chicken soup as a basic standard, using a modern updating of the 800-year-old remedy described by Maimonides (25,26). It is realistic to reflect that it may take almost as long to prove that this recipe, or any other specific drug therapy, is truly effective as an expectorant agent for mucus-impacted lungs.

References

1. Ziment I. Respiratory Pharmacology and Therapeutics. Philadelphia: W. B. Saunders, 1978.
2. Baum GL. Enhancing mucociliary clearance. Chest 1996; 110:876.
3. Lurie A, Mestiri M, Huchon G, Marcas J, Lockhart A, Strauch G, Bergogne-Berezin E, Brignon J, Carbon C, Chwalow J. Methods for clinical assessment of expectorants: a critical review. Int J Clin Pharmacol Res 1992; 12:47–52.
4. Dorland's Medical Dictionary, 24th ed. Philadelphia: W. B. Saunders, 1965:525.
5. Physicians Desk Reference. 52nd ed. Montvale, NJ: Medical Economics, 1998.
6. Drug Facts and Comparisons. St. Louis, MO: Facts and Comparisons, 1998.
7. AMA Drug Evaluations. Chicago: American Medical Association, 1995.
8. Reynold JEF, ed. Martindale's Extra Pharmacoepia. 31st ed. London: Pharmaceutical Press, 1996.
9. Rubin BK, Tomkiewicz RP, King M. Mucoactive agents: old and new. In: Wilmott RW, ed. The Pediatric Lung. Basel: Birkhauser Verlag, 1997:155–191.
10. Gunn JA. The action of expectorants. BMJ 1927; 2:972–975.
11. Ziment I. Bronchospasm, inflammation, and mucus in COPD. J Respir Dis 1993; 14(10, suppl):S9-S14.
12. Korolkovas A. Essentials of Medicinal Chemistry. 2nd ed. New York: Wiley-Interscience, 1988:334–335.
13. Brown OH. Asthma. Presenting an Exposition of the Nonpassive Expiration Theory. St. Louis, MO: C. V. Mosby, 1917.
14. Headland FW. The Action of Medicines in the System. 3rd ed. Philadelphia: Lindsay and Blakiston, 1859.
15. Ziment I. What to expect from expectorants. JAMA 1976; 236:193–194.
16. Braga PC, Allegra L, eds. Drugs in Bronchial Mucology. New York: Raven Press, 1989.
17. Schultz V, Hansel R, Tyler VE. Rational Phytotherapy. A Physicians' Guide to Herbal Medicine. 3rd ed. Berlin: Springer-Verlag, 1998.
18. Ziment I. Pharmacologic control of mucus secretion. In: Junod A, Olivieri D, Pozzi E, eds. Endothelial and Mucus Secreting Cells. Milan: Masson, 1991:269–283.
19. Rubin BK, Ramirez O, Ohar JA. Iodinated glycerol has no effect on pulmonary function, symptom score, or sputum properties in patients with stable chronic bronchitis. Chest 1996; 109:348–352.
20. Marchette LC, Marchette BE, Abraham WM, Wanner A. The effect of systemic hydration on normal and impaired mucociliary function. Pediatr Pulmonol 1985; 1: 107–111.

21. Ziment I. Hydration, humidification and mucokinetic therapy. In: Weiss EB, Stein M, eds. Bronchial Asthma. Mechanisms and Therapeutics. 3rd ed. Boston: Little, Brown, 1993:917–933.
22. Shim C, King M, Williams MH. Lack of effect of hydration on sputum production in chronic bronchitis. Chest 1987; 92:679–682.
23. Boyd EM. Respiratory Tract Fluid. Springfield, IL: Charles C Thomas, 1972.
24. Ziment I. Mucokinetic agents. In: Hollinger MA, ed. Current Topics in Pulmonary Pharmacology and Toxicology. New York: Elsevier, 1987:122–155.
25. Carper J. Food—Your Miracle Medicine. New York: Harper Collins, 1993:337–345.
26. Barnett RA. Tonics. More Than 100 Recipes That Improve the Body and the Mind. New York: Harper Perennial, 1997:67–68.
27. Ziment I. Possible mechanisms of action of traditional Oriental drugs for bronchitis. In: Chang HM, Yeung HW, Tso W-W, Koo A, eds. Advances in Chinese Medicinal Materials Research. Singapore: World Scientific, 1985:193–202.
28. Barnes PJ. Nonadrenergic, noncholinergic nerves and neuropeptides. In: Weiss EB, Stein M, eds. Bronchial Asthma. Mechanisms and Therapeutics. 3rd ed. Boston: Little, Brown, 1993:232–252.
29. Ziment I. The messianic relationship between inspiration and expectoration. In: Baum GL, Priel Z, Roth Y, Liron N, Ostfeld EJ, eds. Cilia, Mucus, and Mucociliary Interactions. New York: Marcel Dekker, 1998:383–389.
30. Ziment I. Five thousand years of attacking asthma: an overview. Respir Care 1986; 31:117–136.
31. Kapur LD. Ayurvedic medicine of India. J Herbs Spices Med Plants 1993; 1:37–219.
32. Dastur JF. Everybody's Guide to Ayurvedic Medicine. Bombay: DB Taraporevala Sons and Company, 1960.
33. Boyd EM, Sheppard EP. Friar's balsam and respiratory tract fluid. Am J Dis Child 1966; 111:630–634.
34. Blumenthal M, ed. The Complete German Commission E Monographs. Therapeutic Guide to Herbal Medicines. Austin, TX: American Botanical Council, 1998.
35. Marz RW. Evaluation of Phytomedicine. Clinical Pharmacological and Toxicological Data. Thesis. Utrecht: University of Utrecht, Faculty of Pharmacy, 1998.
36. Chevallier A. The Encyclopedia of Medicinal Plants. A Practical Reference Guide to More Than 550 Key Medicinal Plants and Their Uses. London: Dorling Kindersley, 1996.
37. Robbers J, Speedie MK, Tyler VE. Pharmacognosy and Pharmacobiotechnology. Baltimore, MD: Williams and Wilkins, 1996.
38. Leung AY, Foster S. Encyclopedia of Common Natural Ingredients Used in Food, Drugs and Cosmetics. 2nd ed. New York: John Wiley and Sons, 1996.
39. British Herbal Pharmacopoeia. 4th ed. London: British Herbal Medicine Association, 1996.
40. Newall CA, Anderson LA, Phillipson JD. Herbal Medicines. A Guide for Healthcare Professionals. London: Pharmaceutical Press, 1996.
41. Hoffman D. The Complete Illustrated Holistic Herbal. New York: Barnes and Noble, 1996.

42. Muller-Limmroth W, Frohlich HH. Effect of various phytotherapeutic expectorants on mucociliary transport. Fortschr Med 1980; 98:95–101.
43. Wills PJ, Cole PJ. Mucolytic and mucokinetic therapy. Pulm Pharmacol 1996; 9: 197–204.
44. Ziment I. Agents that affect respiratory mucus. Prob Respir Care 1988; 1:15–41.
45. Boman G, Backer U, Larsson S, Melandes B, Wahlander L. Oral acetylcysteine reduces exacerbation rate in chronic bronchitis: report of a trial organized by the Swedish Society for Pulmonary Diseases. Eur J Respir Dis 1983; 64:404–414.
46. Hansen NC, Skriver A, Brorsen-Riis L, Balslov S, et al. Orally administered N-acetylcysteine may improve general well-being in patients with mild chronic bronchitis. Respir Med 1994; 88:531–535.
47. Rubin BK. Pharmacologic management of mucus retention based on a taxonomy of mucoactive medications. In: Baum GL, Priel Z, Roth Y, Liron N, Ostfeld EJ, eds. Cilia, Mucus, and Mucociliary Interactions. New York: Marcel Dekker, 1998: 383—389.
48. De Flora S, Grassi C, Carati L. Attenuation of influenza-like symptomatology and improvement of cell-mediated immunity with long-term N-acetylcysteine treatment. Eur Respir J 1997; 10:1535–1541.
49. Miyata T, Kai H, Isohama Y, Takahama K. Current opinion of mucoactive drug research: strategies and problems. Eur Respir J 1998; 11:480–491.
50. Gillissen A, Jaworska M, Orth M, Coffiner M, et al. Nacystelyn, a novel lysine salt of N-acetylcysteine, to augment cellular antioxidant defence in vitro. Respir Med 1997; 91:159–168.
51. Allegra L, Cordaro Cl, Grassi C. Prevention of acute exacerbations of chronic obstructive bronchitis with carbocysteine lysine monohydrate: a multicenter, double-blind, placebo-controlled trial. Respiration 1996; 63:174–180.
52. Santoliciandro A, Baldi S, Giuntini C. The effect of a new expectorant drug on mucus transport in chronic bronchitis. J Aerosol Med 1995; 8:33–42.
53. Dechant KL, Noble S. Erdosteine. Drugs 1996; 52:875–881.
54. Pfeifer S, Zissel G, Kienast K, Muller-Quernheim J. Reduction of cytokine release of blood and bronchoalveolar mononuclear cells by ambroxol. Eur J Med Res 1997; 24:129–132.
55. Gershwin ME, ed. Alternative and complementary therapy for asthma. Clin Rev Allergy Immunol 1996; 14:241–355.
56. Ziment I. Alternative therapies. In: Barnes PJ, Grunstein MM, Leff AR, Woolcock AJ, eds. Asthma. Philadelphia: Lippincott-Raven, 1997:1689–1705.
57. Ziment I. The management of common respiratory diseases by traditional Chinese drugs. Orient Heal Arts Int Bull 1988; 13:133–140.

9

Mucolytics and Mucus Clearance

MALCOLM KING

University of Alberta
Edmonton, Alberta, Canada

I. Introduction

Mucus is a nonhomogeneous, viscoelastic fluid containing carbohydrates, proteins, and lipids in a watery matrix. Airway mucus is the secretory product of the mucous cells—the goblet cells of the pseudo-stratified columnar surface layer and the mucous cells of the submucosal glands. The mucus is transported from the lower respiratory tract into the pharynx by airflow and mucociliary clearance. The mucous secretion along with serous fluid forms the airway surface fluid (ASF) that provides a protective milieu for the airways. The composition and physical characteristics of ASF allow for normal ciliary activity and airway hygiene (1). When disruption of normal secretory or mucociliary clearance processes occurs, respiratory secretions can accumulate, and impair pulmonary function, reduce lung defenses, and increase the risk for infection and possibly neoplasia (2–4).

ASF consists of two phases: a superficial gel or mucous layer and a liquid or periciliary fluid layer that bathes the epithelial cilia. These two layers are probably separated by a thin layer of surfactant (5). In health, the mucous layer is about 2 to 5 μm thick in the trachea, and extends from the bronchioles to the upper airway. The serous layer lies between the cellular surface and the mucus layer at a depth that is just less than the height of a fully extended cilium. The depth and composition of normal ASF depend on secretion from airway glands, goblet cell discharge, and active ion transport across surface epithelium, as a mechanism for altering hydration (6).

The study of normal ASF involves obtaining samples from laryngectomized subjects, bronchial lavage from healthy nonsmokers, bronchial aspirates from healthy animals, or secreted material in vitro from animal trachea and human bronchial explants. Frequently, the study of airway secretions consists of examining expectorated sputum, but contaminating material or small sample size can give misleading information. Expectorated sputum is a sign of respiratory disease and indicates excessive production (hypersecretion) and/or retention (impaired clearance); these conditions occur in patients with respiratory infection, bronchitis, asthma, bronchiectasis, and cystic fibrosis (CF).

Mucoactive medications are treatments designed to enhance the clearance of mucus from the respiratory tract in disorders in which mucus-clearance impairment is an important feature (7,8). Mucoactive medications include mucolytics, designed to disrupt the structural macromolecules that give respiratory-tract mucus its physical characteristics, and other agents designed to increase mucus flow by stimulating ciliary activity or improving periciliary fluid hydration. Mucokinetic therapy combating mucus retention is a major consideration in the treatment of CF and other chronic lung diseases in which mucus hypersecretion and impaired airway clearance produce symptoms.

II. Role of Mucus in Mucociliary Clearance

Airway mucus is cleared by two major mechanisms: mucociliary clearance and airflow interaction; the latter assumes increasing importance as lung disease develops (9). According to model studies mucociliary clearance is critically dependent on maintaining the depth of periciliary fluid (10,11). The depth of mucus does not appear to vary a great deal within the bronchi, but the mucous layer may become discontinuous in the smaller airways (12,13). The normal volume of respiratory secretion arriving at the larynx is estimated to be approximately 10 mL/day. The total production of ASF throughout the airway system is not known, but is probably much higher than the volume actually reaching the larynx; this apparent reduction in airway fluid volume is believed to be due to absorption of water through the lower bronchi via active ion transport mechanisms (14,15).

The mucociliary clearance rate (MCR) is affected by ciliary, serous fluid, and mucus factors. Ciliary factors that affect MCR are mainly ciliary beat amplitude and frequency, which together determine the maximal velocity at the tips of the cilia, and hence the maximal forward velocity of the mucus layer. In principle, the faster the cilia beat, the higher the MCR, although there is little direct evidence for this in the literature. Also, longer cilia should be able to clear mucus faster because they can generate greater forward velocities. The density or spacing between cilia will also affect MCR, because the greater the distance between the cilia, the more energy will be dissipated in the mucus, reducing the net forward velocity. In smaller airways, cilia are generally shorter than in the large bronchi, and even though the cilia beat frequency may be comparable, the rate of momentum transfer to the mucus will be proportionately reduced.

Serous factors that affect MCR include viscosity and depth of serous fluid. If the serous fluid is too viscous, the cilia will not be able to move very well within it and the decreased ciliary tip velocity will lead to a reduction of MCR. This principle is well established for water-propelling cilia, but for the periciliary fluid in the two-layer mucociliary system, the serous fluid viscosity is unknown. Active ion transport and its associated transepithelial water flux (15) are likely of critical importance in modulating serous fluid viscosity. Transepithelial protein fluxes may also reasonably be expected to contribute to serous fluid viscosity (16). The efficient transfer of momentum between the cilia and the mucus layer requires that the cilia firmly contact the mucus during their forward stroke while minimally interacting with it during the return. If the serous fluid is too deep or too shallow, MCR will also decrease (11).

Mucus factors affecting MCR are the depth and viscoelastic properties of the mucus (1,17). When the mucus layer is too thick and clearance by the cilia is hindered, clearance by coughing takes over (18). Mucus needs to be both viscous and elastic. The elasticity is important for clearance by cilia because it efficiently transmits energy without energy loss. The viscosity of mucus results in energy loss, but it is necessary so that mucus can be displaced and either expectorated or swallowed. A balance between these factors must be maintained for optimal MCR.

III. Cough Clearance

In various lung diseases characterized by mucus hypersecretion and impaired airway clearance, elimination of the excess mucus by coughing becomes of paramount importance. Cough clearance derives from the high-velocity interaction between airflow and the mucus, leading to wave formation in the mucus layer, temporary reduction in crosslinking within the mucous gel, and ultimately to shearing and forward propulsion of portions of the mucus layer. The depth of mucus and the airflow linear velocity are critical determinants of cough clearance (19). Physical properties of mucus that are important to cough clearance are the viscosity or resistance to flow of the mucus, the elastic component, which impedes forward motion and results in recoil after the cough event, and the surface properties, both on the air–mucus interface and, at the interface with the periciliary layer (20). Mucus that is elastic may be efficient in mucociliary clearance, but it is inefficient in cough clearance (18), and thus a dynamic balance between mucus viscosity and elasticity may be determined by nature. The effects of mucolytic treatments on both forms of clearance should be considered in evaluating their efficacy.

IV. Mucus Viscoelasticity

Many factors contribute to the viscoelasticity of mucus. Among these are the type of mucus glycoprotein, the hydration of the secretions, and the degree of mucus crosslinking and entanglement. The latter, in turn, is influenced by the pH and ion content of the secretions, as well as the presence of inflammatory mediators and enzymes. Mucolytics reduce viscosity by disrupting polymer networks in the secretion (Figure 1). Classical mucolytic agents work through the severing of disulfide bonds, binding of calcium, depolymerizing mucopolysaccharides, and liquefying proteins. Newer, peptide mucolytics degrade pathological filaments of DNA and actin.

Breakage or reduction of the bonds within the mucous gel can be achieved through disruption of the gel network—the process known as mucolysis. Mucolysis can be achieved either through physical intervention, such as high-frequency oscillation (21), or by biochemical or pharmacological agents, such as *N*-acetylcysteine or dornase alfa. Thus, by breaking the macromolecular bonds, mucolysis will result in reducing the viscoelasticity of the mucous gel. If this process is carried out to the right extent, it will facilitate mucus clearance for the patient.

Alternative strategies for reducing the concentration of crosslinks in the mucous gel (see Figure 1) include hydration or swelling, an attractive goal in theory but difficult to achieve, and rearrangement of the macromolecules to reduce their size and degree of interpenetration, as with hypertonic saline or oligosaccharide treatments (see below).

V. A Molecular Basis for Mucolytic Therapy

In the normal state, i.e., in the absence of infection or inflammation, the respiratory mucous gel is constituted primarily by a three-dimensional crosslinked network of mucous glycoproteins, or mucins. Mucins are the product of several different genes; at least 14 human MUC gene products have been described (22), and several of them are significantly expressed in airway tissue (notably MUC2, MUC5AC, and MUC5B) (23). Of the two major airway mucins, MUC5AC appears to be

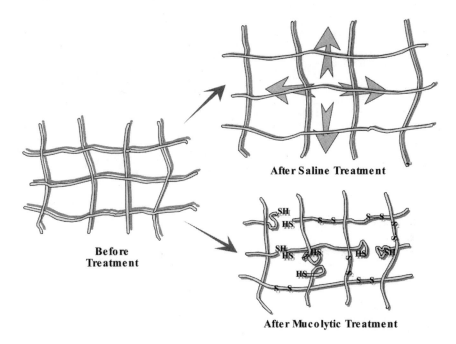

Figure 1 Two approaches to mucolysis. Direct-acting mucolytics work by disrupting network bonds; indirect mucolytic action involves rearrangement of the crosslink network.

preferentially associated with goblet cells (24), while MUC5B may be predominantly glandular. MUC1 is also expressed in airway tissue, but as a surface mucin rather than in a soluble form (as are other mucin gene products such as MUC3 and MUC4). The MUC genes all produce a similar product, namely, a protein with tandem repeat units rich in serine, threonine, and proline and heavily glycosylated; these glycosylated regions are interspersed with largely nonglycosylated units containing cysteine residues. The structure of soluble mucins can be represented in Figure 2 (8,25).

As indicated in the diagram, the three-dimensional structure that forms the mucous gel is dependent on a number of forms of bonding. The main elements include:

1. Disulfide bonds—the intramolecular, covalent links that join glycoprotein subunits into extended macromolecular chains known as mucins.
2. Because of their extended size, these mucin polymers readily form

1. COVALENT BONDS
• glycoprotein subunits are linked primarily by intramolecular S-S bonds

2. IONIC BONDS
• mucin macromolecules have both positive and negative fixed charges, which are capable of interacting

3. HYDROGEN BONDS
• H-bonds link the oligosaccharide side-chains

4. VAN DER WAALS' FORCES
• interdigitation between oligosaccharide moieties may be important

5. INTERMINGLING
• physical entanglements between mucin macromolecules

6. EXTRACELLULAR DNA & F-ACTIN
• parallel network formation in infection

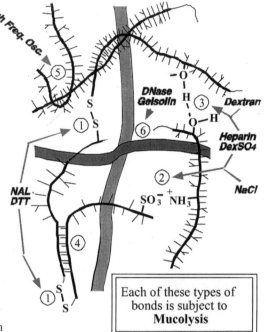

Figure 2 Types of bonds occurring in a mucous gel, and the site of interaction with various mucolytic treatments. DTT = dithiothreitol; NAC = N-acetylcysteine; rhDNase = recombinant human DNase. The mucous glycoproteins (mucins) consist of highly glycosylated subunits of about 500 kDa linked by nonglycosylated regions containing cysteines that stabilize the structure via intramolecular bonds. The oligosaccharide side chains are composed mainly of N-acetylglucosamine, N-acetylgalactosamine, galactose, fucose, and sialic acid. These glycosidic units contain numerous sites for hydrogen bonds, as well as ionic interactions. In infection, additional large macromolecules, such as undegraded DNA and actin filaments released from leukocytes and bacteria, participate extensively in the three-dimensional structure of the gel. (Adapted from Ref. 25.)

entanglements with neighboring macromolecules; these act as time-dependent crosslinks, which are susceptible to mechanical degradation.

3. The sugar units that make up the oligosaccharide side chains (about 80% of the mucin weight) form hydrogen bonds with complementary units on neighboring mucins. Although each bond is weak and readily

dissociates, the numbers of bond sites make this type of bonding potentially very important.

4. Much stronger bonds due to van der Waals attractive forces can potentially occur between complementary saccharide moieties on neighboring chains. However, the diversity of mucin oligosaccharides (26) may make such strong interactions uncommon.

5. Mucins are also ionized, containing both positively charged amino acid residues and negatively charged sugar units, principally sialic acid and sulfated residues. These increase in airway disease in general; in CF the proportion of sulfated residues is particularly elevated (27). The ionic interactions between fixed negative charges result in a stiffer, more extended macromolecular conformation, effectively increasing the polymer size and adding to the numbers of entanglements.

6. Added to this in airway diseases characterized by infection and inflammation, especially CF, are the extra networks of high-molecular-weight DNA and actin filaments released by dying leukocytes, exopolysaccharides secreted by bacteria, and glycosaminoglycans such as chrondroitin sulfate (28).

VI. General Approaches to Mucolysis

To change the physical properties of the viscous and rigid mucous gel, the direct strategy is mucolysis. Mucolysis refers to the disruption of the mucous gel, generally by altering the degree of crosslinking or the interactions between the macromolecules that form the gel. Normally it is desirable to reduce the crosslinking and viscoelasticity in the mucous gel in order to improve clearance, but occasionally the mucus will be too thin for effective transport (29,30); hence, increasing the crosslinking of the mucus by a mucospissic agent could be appropriate. Mucolytics and mucospissics are known collectively as mucotropic agents.

A. Direct-Acting Mucolytics

The most important form of crosslinking in the mucous gel is due to the physical entanglements between neighboring mucin macromolecules as their broadly coiled spheres interpenetrate at the usual mucin concentrations (about 1% by weight). A typical mucin molecule (molecular weight 2–3 million Daltons) in aqueous isotonic medium is a random coil, extended, fuzzy sphere about 400–600 nanometers in diameter (radius of gyration about 250 nm) (31), and at 1% concentration by weight (4.3×10^{-6} M), the center of each molecule lies about 70–75 nm from its nearest neighbors. Hence, mucins at physiological concentration exist as highly interpenetrating polymer coils, and the main form of cross-

linking is through intermolecular entanglements that act as time-dependent
crosslinks (see Figure 3).

The basic mucin gene products consist of long, heavily glycosylated peptide units with shorter segments of largely nonglycosylated units containing cysteine residues (23,31). Mucins are generally secreted as dimers or oligomers,
held together by –S–S– bridges derived from unpaired cysteine units near the
nonglycosylated C-terminus end of the mucin peptide, and stabilized by intramolecular –S–S– bonds that form the so-called cystine knot (32,33). Classical

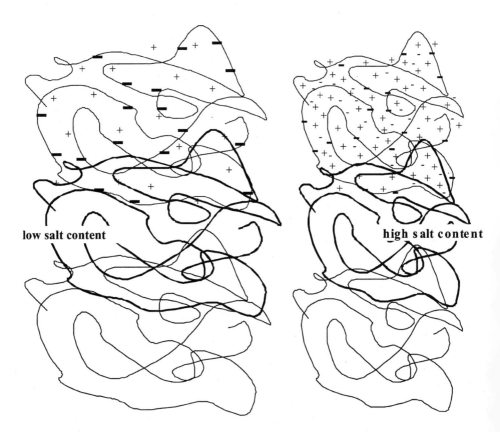

Figure 3 A model for intermolecular penetration in mucin gels. In the example shown,
the mean size of each macromolecule is decreased by the addition of salt, which shields
the fixed charges along the polymer backbone. This decreases the degree of penetration
into neighboring molecules, thereby reducing the number of gel-forming crosslinks. The
excess of fixed negative charges along the macromolecular chain is indicated by the
solid bars. Mobile ions are indicated by + and − symbols.

mucolytics, such as *N*-acetylcysteine (34) and other thiol-reducing agents, degrade the three-dimensional network that forms the mucous gel by breaking macromolecular backbone units that hold the polypeptide core together. For example, by reducing the S–S bridging unit that polymerizes a mucin dimer, the average length of the coiled mucin polymer is reduced by half, reducing its sphere of influence by perhaps a similar amount, and greatly decreasing the degree of entanglement with its neighboring macromolecules.

As indicated above, mucin macromolecules are typically 2–3 MD (mega-Daltons) and in dilute solution 400–600 nm in size. In physiological concentration (~1% mucoprotein by weight), the molar concentration of such a mucin would be 4.3×10^{-6}, i.e., 2.6×10^{12} molecules per mm^3. The space available for each molecule is therefore about 73 nm before entanglement begins to occur. Given the typical size of the mucin (~500 nm), each mucin polymer will therefore interpenetrate (entangle) with several neighboring molecules. Reducing the molecular length by 50% will greatly reduce the degree of interpenetration (from 6.8 to about 4.9 in the above example), and therefore reduce the crosslink density, which characterizes the viscoelasticity (resistance to deformation) of the gel. It is clear that it is not necessary to completely degrade the mucin molecule to greatly reduce the degree of crosslinking—only one break per mucin unit can produce a major effect (decreasing viscoelasticity to 36% of the initial value—$(4.9/6.8)^3$—in the above example, based on the number of crosslink points in a three-dimensional model (35).

The dependence of mucus gel viscoelasticity may be even greater than indicated above. Viscosity (and probably viscoelasticity) classically exhibits a 3.4-power dependence on molecular weight (35). Thus, a mere 20% reduction in molecular weight would reduce viscoelasticity to $(0.8)^{3.4}$, or 47% of the initial value. On the logarithmic scale used for viscoelasticity (log G*), this reduction would amount to 0.33 log units, which is typical for observations on mucolytics, and consistent with prediction of significant improvements in mucus clearability based on model studies (17). With hypertonic saline treatment (see below), it is assumed that there is no cleavage of intramolecular bonds and no reduction in molecular weight. However, the treatment (shielding of ionic charge) should produce substantial reductions in mean radius of gyration, hence reduced interpenetration, which will reduce the degree of entanglement coupling.

B. Oral Mucolytics: *N*-Acetylcysteine and Related Compounds

N-acetylcysteine (NAC), a derivative of cysteine, is a thiol-reducing agent. NAC has been widely used as a mucolytic agent in many countries, although not in the United States or Canada. It has been reported to reduce the viscosity of purulent sputum in both CF and chronic bronchitis patients (36), thus enhancing the removal of pulmonary secretions by ciliary action or cough.

The chemical structure of disulfide-containing proteins and peptides connected by disulfide linkages is altered by thiol compounds. Physical changes in the bronchial glycoprotein are the result of thiol reduction; they are associated with reduction in molecular size, sedimentation coefficient, and viscosity (37). NAC reduces the disulfide bond (S–S) to a sulfhydryl bond (–SH), which no longer participates in crosslinking, thus reducing the elasticity and viscosity of mucus (38,39). NAC demonstrates similar effects on both purulent and nonpurulent sputum. Other in vitro studies reported increasing mucolytic activity of NAC in solutions over the pH range of 5.5 to 8.0 (34). These mucolytic properties of NAC were tested and confirmed in in vitro experiments, in which treatment with NAC resulted a reduction in the elastic shear modulus of canine tracheal mucus (40).

A systematic review of the use of oral mucolytics for exacerbations of COPD was carried out by Poole and Black (41). Based on the results of randomized, double-blind clinical trials, treatment with NAC or related mucolytics, such as ambroxol, bromhexine, carbocysteine, and sobrerol, for at least 2 months was associated with a significant (29%) reduction in the rate of exacerbations of this condition. Another meta-analysis of oral NAC alone (42) also concluded that long-term treatment in COPD reduces exacerbations. However, maintenance treatment with mucolytic or mucoactive drugs is not associated with improvements in lung function in patients with asthma or COPD (22).

C. Aerosolized Nacystelyn

NAC, with a pKa of 2.2, has disadvantages, particularly in the area of topical or aerosol administration. It is difficult for the drug to reach more peripheral airways or poorly ventilated areas in therapeutic concentrations; also, there is the risk of bronchospasm in patients with airway hyperreactivity. NAC can be too mucolytic in its action: it can overliquefy the mucus in central airways yet underliquefy the mucus in the periphery, both instances leading to suboptimal clearability (17).

Recently, the pH-neutral lysine derivative of NAC, nacystelyn (NAL), has been shown to reduce mucus viscoelasticity, both in dogs (43) and in patients with CF (44). In dogs, nacystelyn administration by metered-dose inhaler led to a decrease in mucus viscoelasticity and an increase in tracheal mucus velocity, and was accompanied by an increase in mucus chloride content, consistent with improved hydration of the airway surface fluid (43), presumably due to its lysine component (45). As well as acting as a mucolytic agent, *N*-acetylcysteine derivatives also exhibit antioxidant and anti-inflammatory effects, for example, reducing the concentration of elastase (44) and inhibiting the nuclear transcription factors NFκB and AP1 (46). European and American clinical trials of aerosolized dry-powder NAL in CF are currently in progress (SMB & Galephar, Brussels).

D. Dornase Alfa, Gelsolin

Sputum contains products of inflammation, including cellular debris, neutrophil-derived DNA, and filamentous actin (F-actin). DNA and F-actin are colocalized in sputum to form a rigid network entangled with the mucin gel (47). Peptide mucolytics degrade these abnormal filaments, leaving the parallel glycoprotein network relatively intact. This is illustrated schematically in Figure 4.

Dornase Alfa

High concentrations of undegraded DNA (up to 15 mg/ml) have been shown to be the leading cause of the tenacious and viscous nature of the sputum (48). Although there is no direct relationship between the concentration of DNA in sputum and sputum viscosity, the addition of exogenous DNA to sputum increases both viscosity and elasticity (49). Pancreatic DNase, an enzyme-hydrolyzing DNA, was first used for the treatment of pulmonary infections more than three decades ago (50). Rcombinant human deoxyribonuclease I (rhDNase or dornase alfa, developed by Genentech, South San Francisco, Calif.) has a significant mucolytic effect on CF sputum, reducing its viscosity (51) and spinnability (21). The reduction in sputum viscosity is associated with a decrease in the size of the DNA molecules located within the sputum. In theory, dornase reduces only the excess viscoelasticity, leaving the glycoprotein gel intact (quasinormal), as illustrated in Figure 4. Hence, it is believed not to overliquefy mucus, although this could happen in some circumstances (52).

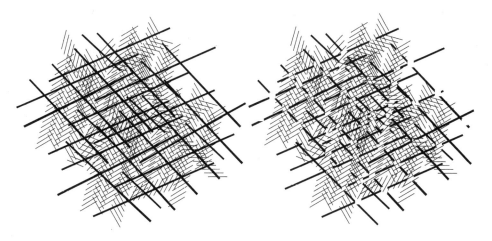

Figure 4   A model to describe the action of DNase in reducing the excess viscoelasticity in cystic fibrosis mucus. (Left) the rigidifying effect of undegraded DNA on the mucous glycoprotein network. (Right) the effect of partial degradation of the strands of DNA.

Aerosol administration of dornase alfa to patients with stable CF lung disease and preserved airflow (FEV_1 >30% predicted) improved FEV_1 by 5–7%, reduced the frequency of pulmonary exacerbations, and improved measured quality of life (53). At present, dornase alfa (Pulmozyme™, Genentech) is approved for the treatment of CF and is the only FDA-approved mucolytic medication available for prescription in the United States. Dornase alfa has not been found to be of benefit in non-CF bronchiectasis (54) or in chronic bronchitis (22).

F-Actin Depolymerizing Agents

Actin is the most prevalent cellular protein in the body, playing a vital role in maintaining the structural integrity of cells. Under proper conditions, actin polymerizes to form F-actin. Extracellular F-actin has been shown to contribute to the viscoelasticity of expectorated CF sputum (55). Concentrations of F-actin in CF sputum as high as 0.15 mg/ml have been reported, and there is an increased ratio of filamentous (F-) to globular (G-) actin in CF sputum when compared with normal secretions.

Gelsolin is an 85 kD (577-nucleotide) actin-severing peptide that has been demonstrated to significantly reduce the viscosity of CF sputum at low shear rate (55). Thymosin β4 is a small (4.8 kD, 43-nucleotide) peptide that binds G-actin, both inhibiting the formation F-actin and shifting the polymerization kinetics to promote the rapid depolymerization of F-actin (56). Dornase alfa also binds G-actin, and in the process its DNA enzymatic activity is blocked. In vitro studies with both gelsolin and thymosin β4 demonstrate that these agents are synergistic with DNase such that a greater reduction in sputum viscoelasticity and cohesiveness is seen with smaller amounts of these agents (55,57). Thus, F-actin depolymerizing agents destabilize the actin-DNA filament network as well as increase the depolymerizing activity of dornase on the DNA filaments.

DNase and gelsolin in CF sputum act in principle in a fashion similar to NAC. The mucus gel is strengthened by the addition of undegraded DNA and F-actin, acting as a reinforcing filler. The contribution of such units to viscoelasticity is highly molecular-weight-dependent, varying by a factor as high as $M^{3.4}$ (35,58). Hence, a reduction in molecular weight of just 20% (one break per four molecules on average) could result in a decrease in G* of 50% (factor of 2), which would be meaningful in terms of clearability (1).

VII. Nondestructive Mucolysis:
Ionic and Hydrogen Bonds

The other target areas illustrated in Figure 2—the ionic interaction and the hydrogen bonds—have received less attention, but are perhaps no less promising. DNase, gelsolin, and acetylcysteine derivatives are all similar in action in that they degrade the three-dimensional network by mucolysis, or macromolecular size disruption, as shown schematically in Figure 1. This tends to preferentially affect the elasticity components of the network (as opposed to viscosity), which in model studies improve cough or airflow clearance more than clearance by ciliary action (18). Agents that affect ionic charge interactions and hydrogen bonds, on the other hand, are not true mucolytic agents because they alter the crosslink density without reducing polymer chain length, the result of which is a common reduction in both elasticity and viscosity, and a preferential improvement in ciliary clearance according to model studies (59). Indeed, recent laboratory studies support the "nonmucolytic" approach to improving mucus rheology for ciliary clearance, both with ionic agents such as sodium chloride (58,60) and with nonionic agents such as dextran (61).

A. Hypertonic Saline

Hypertonic saline (HS) is not a true mucolytic treatment, but may act in part by effectively reducing the entanglements in the mucus gel. As suggested by Figure 3, HS breaks up the ionic bonds within the mucin gel, thereby reducing the effective degree of crosslinking and lowering the viscosity and elasticity (58,60). It is also believed to promote mucus clearance by extracting fluid from the respiratory-tract epithelium, thereby increasing the volume and water content of mucus (62,63). Upon administration of HS by means of a nebulizer, water from the tissues may be shifted across the epithelial membrane to dilute the saline. The diluted fluid, with altered viscoelastic properties, is then eliminated from the respiratory tree by the mucociliary escalator or by coughing.

In infected mucus, HS separates the DNA molecules from the mucoprotein, making the mucoprotein susceptible to proteolytic enzyme digestion. Lieberman reported in 1967 (50) that DNA cleavage by HS increased as the ionic strength of the solution increased beyond 0.15 M. In 1978, Pavia et al. investigated the effect of HS on chronic bronchitis patients (64). They found that, in comparison with normal saline, HS (1.21 M) doubled the rate of mucociliary clearance, with an increase in the weight of sputum expectorated. HS has been found to enhance the removal of lung secretions in patients with CF (65,66). This stimulation of mucociliary transport by saline solutions occurs in both normal individuals and chronic bronchitis patients.

HS may also function to stimulate mucociliary and cough clearance by an osmotic effect, drawing water into the mucous gel and the periciliary layer. This is clearly a short-term effect, since the epithelium has the capacity to quickly restore the salt balance. Even the coadministration of amiloride to inhibit Na-linked water resorption resulted in no additional short-term clearance benefit for CF patients (66). Perhaps longer-acting Na-channel blockers (67) might prolong the effects of inhaled osmolytes and prove beneficial. In any case, clinical trials of NaCl in CF are currently being undertaken (68.69).

VIII. Oligosaccharide Mucolytic Agents

Agents that are capable of altering the hydrogen bonding of the mucous gel can produce potentially beneficial effects on mucus clearability. Although each bond is weak, the total potential for hydrogen bonds is immense, since the oligosaccharide side chains make up about 80% of the mucin structure. This was found to be the case with dextran (61), a compound that can also block bacterial adhesion (70). Other laboratories have reported stimulation of clearance with simple mono- or disaccharides such as mannitol and lactose (71,72). In the case of mannitol, administration by dry-powder aerosol resulted in an improvement in mucociliary clearance rate in patients with bronchiectasis (71) and CF (73). In the study by Feng et al. (61), low-molecular-weight dextran treatment in vitro significantly reduced the viscoelasticity and spinnability of both CF sputum and healthy dog mucus, and increased the predicted mucociliary and cough clearability. The effects on viscoelasticity and spinnability, as illustrated in Figure 5, were greater at 4% wt/vol than at 0.4%. In dogs, dextran administered by aerosol at 65 mg/mL increased tracheal mucus velocity, but this increase was not sustained for higher concentrations (74).

These changes in mucus rheology and transportability have been attributed to disruption of network crosslinks due to hydrogen bonds between neighboring mucin macromolecules. It has been observed that the fluidifying or mucoactive effect of dextran on mucus is primarily confined to the lower-molecular-weight fractions of dextran (61), consistent with the concept that dextran does not involve true mucolysis (mucin degradation) but rather the creation of mucin–dextran hydrogen bonds that are structurally and rheologically ineffective. There are potentially two mechanisms to account for the mucokinetic effects of saccharide compounds. An osmotic mechanism, attracting fluid into the airway milieu similar to that proposed for ionic treatments (60), could account for the effects on mucus clearance. This would presumably be maximal for monosaccharides, and decrease in importance with increasing molecular size. On the other hand, the H-bond breaking mechanism is probably optimal for saccharide units matching the length of mucin oligosaccharides, i.e., 3 to 15 units (75). The reduced crosslinking of the mucous glycoprotein network should make the mucus more easily clearable by both ciliary and cough mechanisms. A clinical trial of aerosolized low-molecular-weight dextran in CF is currently in progress in Canada (BCY LifeSciences, Toronto).

Recently, we have looked at agents that might alter both the hydrogen bonds and the ionic interactions. Our initial studies found that one such agent— the charged oligosaccharide, low-molecular-weight heparin—had a greater mucolytic and mucokinetic capacity than the neutral saccharide polymer, dextran. This was seen in in vitro rheological testing and in excised frog palate clearance measurements (76). Subsequently, similar mucolytic effects were seen with

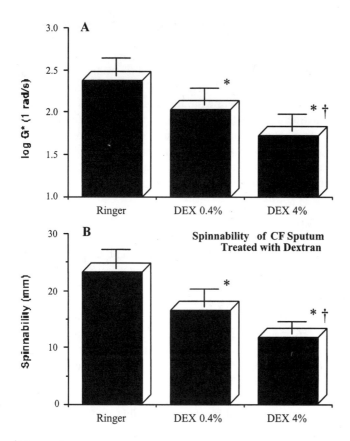

Figure 5 Effects of dextran treatment in CF sputum rheology. Sputum samples were obtained from CF patients not receiving dornase alfa. Aliquots of sputum were incubated at 37°C for 30 minutes with Ringer (10% added volume) or Dextran 4000 to achieve final concentrations of 0.4% (4 mg/ml) or 4% (40 mg/ml). Rigidity modulus (viscoelasticity) was determined by magnetic rheometry ($n = 10$), and spinnability (cohesiveness) was determined by filancemeter ($n = 8$). *significantly different from Ringer; †significantly different from DEX 0.4%. (Adapted from Ref. 61.)

aerosolized low-molecular-weight dextran sulfate, which significantly reduced tracheal mucus viscoelasticity in anesthetized dogs (77). Heparin and dextran sulfate, as charged oligosaccharides, may combine the features of hydrogen-bond disruption, as seen with low-molecular-weight, neutral dextrans, and improvement of ionic interactions, as with HS (76). Aerosolized low-molecular-weight heparin also shows promise as an antiasthmatic medication, presumably by interfering with antigen–receptor binding (78), and as an anti-inflammatory therapy in CF, reducing the content of neutrophil elastase in sputum (79) and decreasing serum IL-8 (80).

Charged oligosaccharides are believed to decrease mucus viscoelasticity by 1) interaction of their negative charges with the amino groups of the mucin molecule, thereby reducing their association with neighboring mucin sulfate or sialic acid moieties, and/or 2) interfering with intermolecular hydrogen bonding due to their oligosaccharide moieties (similar to dextran), and/or 3) ionic shielding effects of mobile counterions (principally sodium) on the polyionic moieties of the mucin molecule. Charged oligosaccharides may also stimulate the movement of ions across the epithelium, thereby increasing hydration of the airway surface fluid (63), similar to the action of chloride secretagogues (43).

IX. Physical Mucolysis: High-Frequency Oscillation

High-frequency oscillations are commonly included as part of physiotherapy methods, using devices such as the Vest (Advanced Respiratory, St. Paul, Minn.) (81), the Flutter (82), and the Cornet (83). High-frequency oscillations applied to the mucus are believed to break up the physical entanglements by reducing the degree of crosslinking within the mucous gel (84,85). Disruption and disentanglement of the mucous macromolecules reduces the crosslinks that bind the mucous glycoproteins, and thereby loosens the mucus to facilitate mucociliary clearance. However, oscillations may also break up the DNA molecules, as these molecules have an inflexible helical structure that makes them more vulnerable to high-frequency oscillation (86). Oscillation is probably unable to break hydrogen and ionic bonds as both types of bonds are reversible, and even if broken they will reform.

Our own studies indicate that oscillating CF sputum (21) results in a decrease in spinnability. The decrease in spinnability correlated in previous studies with increased transportability of mucus, particularly by cough and airflow mechanisms (84). This decrease in spinnability may be explained by the reduction of polymer size, induced through lysis of macromolecular backbone linkages. This has recently been demonstrated in studies using DNA laddering to demonstrate the breakdown of DNA after in vitro application of mechanical oscillations, with increased DNA fragmentation in sputum from CF patients receiving dornase alfa (86). These changes in the physical properties of the sputum may be considered potentially beneficial in the treatment of CF patients.

X. Airway Surface Hydration by Epithelial Ion Transport

In vivo approaches to mucoactive therapy must consider not only the direct action of mucoactive agents but also the stimulation or suppression of secretion and the postsecretory adjustment of mucus character by transepithelial salt and water transport. Therapy by amiloride or uridine triphosphate (UTP) to either block the excess absorption of sodium or stimulate secretion of chloride ion falls into this category. Amiloride is a potassium-sparing diuretic that blocks sodium resorption when applied to the apical membrane of airway epithelia (87). Although early clinical trials with inhaled amiloride showed a slower decline in lung function than with placebo (87,88), subsequent studies suggested that amiloride is ineffective in promoting sputum clearance in patients with CF (89).

Calcium-dependent chloride channels can be activated by the nucleotides ATP and UTP, which act through apical P2Y receptors in airway epithelial cells (90). UTP aerosol (with or without amiloride) was seen to increase airway mucociliary clearance in persons with CF (91). However, as the tricyclic nucleotides are also mucus secretagogues, it is possible that some of the increase in clearance was due to increased mucus secretion. Newer, more specific P2Y2 receptor agonists with extended duration have been developed (92) and are undergoing clinical testing (Inspire Pharmaceuticals, Durham, North Carolina). The combination of direct and indirect mucolysis is also possible, such as with nacystelyn, which can potentially reduce disulfide bonds as well as stimulate chloride secretion (43).

XI. Interaction Between Mucoactive Agents

Each of the elements illustrated in Figure 2 is a potential target for mucoactive therapy. The most successful therapy in CF, and the only mucoactive agent with proven efficacy, is dornase alfa, which has been found to improve lung function in a broad spectrum of patients (53). Its target, of course, is the excess DNA characteristic of CF sputum, and its attractiveness as a therapy is that it does not affect the normal glycoprotein network, meaning that it cannot overliquefy the mucus, at least in theory. However, even with such advances in mucolytic therapy, there is plenty of room for improvement. One area of great potential is the development of combination therapies, since no single mucoactive therapy may be appropriate for all patients or even for individual patients during different stages of their disease. Also, with combination approaches, there is the potential for synergism of action.

Laboratory studies have shown that DNase and mechanical oscillation have additive effects on sputum rheology (21), and clinical studies have been designed to examine the interaction in vivo. Since oscillations may serve to both rearrange crosslinks and reduce polymer size, the interaction between the methods may be synergistic. In other laboratory studies, DNase has also been combined with gelsolin to break up the actin network colocalized with the DNA (55), and with nacystelyn to degrade disulfide bonds (93,94), in both cases with

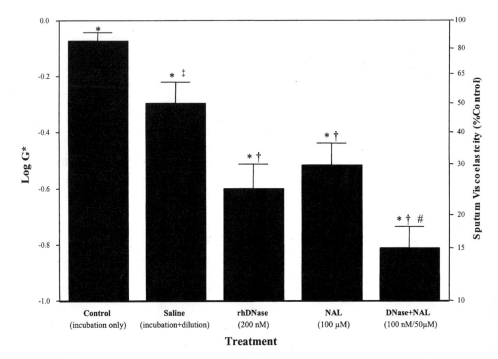

Figure 6   The additive effect of dornase alfa (Pulmozyme) and nacystelyn (NAL) on viscoelasticity (log G^*) of CF sputum in vitro. Values are expressed as the change in log G^* from the pretreatment control values (rt. ordinate: % control linear scale). Each vertical bar represents the mean value ±S.E. for 15 samples. * = Statistically significant difference from the pretreatment value. ‡ = Statistically significant difference from the control value. † = Statistically significant difference from the saline value. # = Statistically significant difference from the NAL value. (Adapted from Ref. 94.)

additivity or synergy of effect (see Figure 6). Actin also inhibits the DNA-hydrolyzing activity of DNase (95); therefore, by binding actin, the action of DNase in CF sputum may be enhanced. As further mucolytic treatments are developed, their interaction and their potential for synergy need to be examined. Ultimately, the goal is to tailor mucolytic prescriptions to suit the needs of individual patients, and to complement their other therapy.

References

1.   King M, Rubin BK. Rheology of airway mucus: relationship with clearance function. In: Takashima T, Shimura S, eds. Airway Secretion: Physiological Bases

for the Control of Mucous Hypersecretion. New York: Marcel Dekker, 1994: 283–314.

2. Wanner A. Clinical aspects of mucociliary transport. Am Rev Respir Dis 1977; 116:73–109.

3. Zayas JG, Man GCW, King M. Tracheal mucus rheology in patients undergoing diagnostic bronchoscopy: interrelations with smoking and cancer. Am Rev Respir Dis 1990; 141:1107–1113.

4. Wanner A, Salathé M, O'Riordan TG. Mucociliary clearance in the airways. Am J Respir Crit Care Med 1996; 154:1868–1902.

5. Morgenroth K, Bolz J. Morphological features of the interaction between mucus and surfactant on the bronchial mucosa. Respiration 1985; 47:225–231.

6. Widdicombe JH, Bastacky SJ, Wu DXY, Lee CY. Regulation of depth and composition of airway surface liquid. Eur Respir J 1997; 10:2892–2897.

7. Rubin BK, Tomkiewicz RP, King M. Mucoactive agents: old and new. In: Wilmott RW, ed. The Pediatric Lung. Basel, Switzerland: Birkhäuser, 1997:155–179.

8. King M, Rubin BK. Mucus controlling agents: past and present. In: Rau JL, ed. Aerosolized drugs for the respiratory tract. Respir Care Clin N Am 1999; 5:575–594.

9. King M, Rubin BK. Mucus physiology and pathophysiology: therapeutic aspects. In: Derenne JP, Whitelaw WA, Similowski T, eds. Acute Respiratory Failure in COPD. New York: Marcel Dekker, 1996:391–411.

10. Blake JR. On the movement of mucus in the lung. J Biomechanics 1975; 8:179–190.

11. King M, Agarwal M, Shukla JB. A planar model for mucociliary transport: effect of mucus viscoelasticity. Biorheology 1993; 30:49–61.

12. Gil J, Weibel ER. Extracellular lining of bronchioles after perfusion-fixation of rat lungs for electron microscopy. Anat Rec 1971; 169:185–200.

13. Van As A. Pulmonary airway clearance mechanisms: a reappraisal [editorial]. Am Rev Respir Dis 1977; 115:721–726.

14. Boucher RC, Stutts MJ, Bromberg PA, Gatzy JT. Regional differences in airway surface liquid composition. J Appl Physiol 1981; 50:613–620.

15. Boucher RC. State of the art: human airway ion transport. Am J Respir Crit Care Med 1994; 150:271–281, 581–593.

16. Govindaraju K, Cowley EA, Eidelman DH, Lloyd DK. Analysis of proteins in micro samples of rat airway surface fluid by capillary electrophoresis. J Chromatog B Biomed Sci Appl 1998; 705:223–230.

17. King M. Mucus, mucociliary clearance and coughing. In: Bates DV. Respiratory Function in Disease. 3rd ed. Philadelphia: Saunders, 1989:69–78.

18. King M. Role of mucus viscoelasticity in cough clearance. Biorheology 1987; 24: 589–597.

19. King M, Brock G, Lundell C. Clearance of mucus by simulated cough. J Appl Physiol 1985; 58:1776–1782.

20. King M, Zahm JM, Pierrot D, Vaquez-Girod S, Puchelle E. The role of mucus gel viscosity, spinnability, and adhesive properties in clearance by simulated cough. Biorheology 1989; 26:737–745.

21. Dasgupta B, Tomkiewicz RP, Boyd WA, Brown NE, King M. Effects of combined

treatment with rhDNase and airflow oscillations on spinnability of cystic fibrosis sputum in vitro. Pediatr Pulmonol 1995; 20:78–82.

22. Rogers DF. Mucoactive drugs for asthma and COPD: any place in therapy? Expert Opin Investig Drugs 2002; 1:15–35.

23. Rose MC, Gendler SJ. Airway mucin genes and gene products. In: Rogers DF, Lethem MI, eds. Airway Mucus: Basic Mechanisms and Clinical Perspectives. Basel, Switzerland: Birkhäuser, 1997:41–66.

24. Hovenberg HW, Davies JR, Carlstedt I. Different mucins are produced by the surface epithelium and the submucosa in human trachea: identification of MUC5AC as a major mucin from the goblet cells. Biochem J 1996; 318:319–324.

25. Dasgupta B, King M. Molecular basis for mucolytic therapy. Can Respir J 1995; 2:223–230.

26. Klein A, Strecker G, Lamblin G, Roussel P. Structural analysis of mucin-type O-linked oligosaccharides. Methods Mol Biol 2000; 125:191–209.

27. Chace KV, Leahy DS, Martin R, Carbelli R, Flux M, Sachdev GP. Respiratory mucous secretions in patients with cystic fibrosis: relationship between levels of highly sulfated mucin component and severity of the disease. Clin Chim Acta 1983; 132:143–155.

28. Rahmoune H, Lamblin G, Lafitte JJ, Galabert C, Filliat M, Roussel P. Chondroitin sulfate in sputum from patients with cystic fibrosis and chronic bronchitis. Am J Respir Cell Mol Biol 1991; 5:315–320.

29. Puchelle E, Zahm JM, Polu JM, Sadoul P. Drug effects on viscoelasticity of mucus. Eur J Respir Dis 1980; 61:195–208.

30. Rubin BK, MacLeod PM, Sturgess J, King M. Recurrent respiratory infections in a child with fucosidosis: is the mucus too thin for effective transport? Pediatr Pulmonol 1991; 10:304–309.

31. Thornton DJ, Davies JR, Carlstedt I, Sheehan JK. Structure and biochemistry of human respiratory mucins. In: Rogers DF, Lethem MI, eds. Airway Mucus: Basic Mechanisms and Clinical Perspectives. Basel, Switzerland: Birkhäuser, 1997:19–39.

32. Bell SL, Khatri IA, Xu G, Forstner JF. Evidence that a peptide corresponding to the rat Muc2 C-terminus undergoes disulphide-mediated dimerization. Eur J Biochem 1998; 253:123–131.

33. Perez-Vilar J, Hill RL. The strusture and assembly of secreted mucins. J Biol Chem 1999; 274:31,751–31,754.

34. Sheffner AL, Medler EM, Jacobs LW, Sarrett HP. The in vitro reduction in viscosity of human tracheobronchial secretions by acetylcysteine. Am Rev Respir Dis 1964; 90:721–729.

35. Ferry JD. Molecular theory for undiluted polymers and concentrated solutions: networks and entanglements. In: Viscoelastic Properties of Polymers. 2nd ed. New York: Wiley, 1970:268–270.

36. Ventresca GP, Cicchetti, Ferrari V. Acetylcysteine. In: Braga PC, Allegra L, eds. Drugs in Bronchial Mucology. New York: Raven Press, 1989:77–102.

37. Roberts GP. The role of disulfide bonds in maintaining the gel structure of bronchial mucus. Arch Biochem Biophys 1976; 173:528–537.

38. Sheffner AL. The reduction in vitro in viscosity of mucoprotein solutions by a new mucolytic agent, N-acetylcysteine. Ann NY Acad Sci 1963; 106:298–310.

39. Davis SS, Deverell LC. The effect of sulphydryl compounds and cross-linking agents on the viscous and viscoelastic properties of mucus. Biorheology 1975; 12: 225–232.

40. Martin R, Litt M, Marriott C. The effect of mucolytic agents on the rheologic and transport properties of canine tracheal mucus. Am Rev Respir Dis 1980; 121:495–500.

41. Poole PJ, Black PN. Mucolytic agents for chronic bronchitis or chronic obstructive pulmonary disease. Cochrane Database Syst Rev 2000; 2:CD001287.

42. Grandjean EM, Berthet P, Ruffman R, Leuenberger P. Efficacy of oral long-term N-acteylcysteine in chronic bronchopulmonary disease: a meta-analysis of published double-blind, placebo-controlled clinical trials. Clin Ther 2000; 22:209–221.

43. Tomkiewicz RP, App EM, De Sanctis GT, Coffiner M, Maes P, Rubin BK, King M. A comparison of a new mucolytic N-acetylcysteine L-lysinate with N-acetylcysteine: airway epithelial function and mucus changes in dog. Pulm Pharmacol 1995; 8:259–265.

44. App EM, Baran D, Dab I, Malfroot A, Coffiner M, Vanderbist F, King M. Dose-finding and 24-hour monitoring for efficacy and safety of aerosolized Nacystelyn in cystic fibrosis. Eur Respir J 2002; 19:294–302.

45. Sudo E, King M. Effect of lysine on tracheal mucus rheology and secretion in mice. Am J Respir Crit Care Med 1999; 159:A686.

46. Gillissen A, Jaworska M, Orth M, Coffiner M, Maes P, App EM, Cantin AM, Schultze-Werninghaus G. Nacystelyn and N-acetylcysteine augment cellular antioxidant defense in two distinctive ways. Resp Med 1997; 81:159–168.

47. Tomkiewicz RP, Kishioka C, Freeman J, Rubin BK. DNA and actin filament ultrastructure in cystic fibrosis sputum. In: Baum G, ed. Cilia, Mucus, and Mucociliary Interactions. New York: Marcel Dekker, 1998:333–341.

48. Lethem MI, James SL, Marriott C, Burke JF. The origin of DNA associated with mucous glycoproteins in cystic fibrosis sputum. Eur Respir J 1990; 3:19–23.

49. Picot I, Das I, Reid L. Pus, deoxyribonucleic acid and sputum viscosity. Thorax 1978; 33:235–242.

50. Lieberman J. Inhibition of protease activity in purulent sputum by DNA. J Lab Clin Med 1967; 70:595–605.

51. Shak S, Capon DJ, Hellmiss R, Marsters SA, Baker CL. Recombinant human DNase I reduces the viscosity of cystic fibrosis sputum. Proc Natl Acad Sci USA 1990; 87:9188–9192.

52. Zahm JM, Girod de Bentzmann S, Deneuville E, Perrot-Minnot C, Depret E, Pennaforte F, Roussey M, Puchelle E. Dose-dependent in vitro effect of recombinant human DNase on rheological and transport properties of cystic fibrosis respiratory mucus. Eur Respir J 1995; 8:381–386.

53. Fuchs HJ, Borowitz DS, Christiansen DH, et al. Effect of aerosolized recombinant human DNase on exacerbations of respiratory symptoms and on pulmonary function in cystic fibrosis. N Engl J Med 1994; 331:637–648.

54. Crockett AJ, Cranston JM, Latimer KM, Alpers JH. Mucolytics for bronchiectasis. Cochrane Database Syst Rev 2001; 1:CD001289.

55. Vasconcellos CA, Allen PG, Wohl M, Drazen JM, Janmey PA. Reduction in sputum viscosity of cystic fibrosis sputum in vitro by gelsolin. Science 1994; 263: 969–971.

56. Rubin BK, Kater AP, Dian T, Ramirez OE, Tomkiewicz RP, Goldstein AL. Effects of thymosin b4 on cystic fibrosis sputum. Pediatr Pulmon 1995; 12S:134–135.
57. Dasgupta B, Tomkiewicz RP, De Sanctis GT, Boyd WA, King M. Rheological properties in cystic fibrosis airway secretions with combined rhDNase and gelsolin treatment. In: Singh M, Saxena VP, eds. Advances in Physiological Fluid Dynamics. New Delhi, India: Narosa, 1996:74–78.
58. King M, Dasgupta B, Tomkiewicz RP, Brown NE. Rheology of cystic fibrosis sputum after in vitro treatment with hypertonic saline alone and in combination with rhDNase. Am J Respir Crit Care Med 1997; 156:173–177.
59. King M. Relationship between mucus viscoelasticity and ciliary transport in guaran gel/frog palate model system. Biorheology 1980; 17:249–254.
60. Wills PJ, Hall RL, Chan WM, Cole PJ. Sodium chloride increases the ciliary transportability of cystic fibrosis and bronchiectasis sputum on the mucus-depleted bovine trachea. J Clin Invest 1997; 99:9–13.
61. Feng W, Garrett H, Speert DP, King M. Improved clearability of cystic fibrosis sputum with dextran treatment in vitro. Am J Respir Crit Care Med 1998; 157: 710–714.
62. Ziment I. Mucokinetic agents. In: Respiratory Pharmacology and Therapeutics. Philadelphia: Saunders, 1978:60–104.
63. Winters SL, Yeates DB. Role of hydration, sodium, and chloride in regulation of canine mucociliary transport system. J Appl Physiol 1997; 83:1360–1369.
64. Pavia D, Thompson DL, Clarke SW. Enhanced clearance of secretions from the human lung after the administration of hypertonic saline aerosol. Am Rev Respir Dis 1978; 117:199–203.
65. Robinson M, Regnis JA, Bailey DL, King M, Bautovich GJ, Bye PTP. Effect of hypertonic saline, amiloride, and cough on mucociliary clearance in patients with cystic fibrosis. Am J Respir Crit Care Med 1996; 153:1503–1509.
66. Robinson M, Hemming AL, Regnis JA, Wong AG, Bailey DL, Bautovich GJ, King M, Bye PTP. Effect of increasing doses of hypertonic saline on mucociliary clearance in patients with cystic fibrosis. Thorax 1997; 52:900–903.
67. Hirsh A, Boucher RC. Absorption of Na+ channel inhibitors by cystic fibrosis airway epithelium. Pediatr Pulmonol 2000; S20:267.
68. Suri R, Wallis C, Bush A. Tolerability of nebulised hypertonic saline in children with cystic fbrosis. Pediatr Pulmonol 2000; S20:463.
69. Robinson M, Bye PTP. State of the art: mucociliary clearance in cystic fibrosis. Pediatr Pulmonol 2002; 33:293–306.
70. Barghouthi S, Guerdoud LM, Speert DP. Inhibition by dextran of *Pseudomonas aeruginosa* adherence to epithelial cells. Am J Respir Crit Care Med 1996; 154: 1788–1793.
71. Daviskas E, Anderson SD, Eberl S, Chan HK, Bautovich G. Inhalation of dry powder mannitol improves clearance of mucus in patients with bronchiectasis. Am J Respir Crit Care Med 1999; 159:1843–1848.
72. Shibuya Y, Wills PJ, Kitamura S, Cole PJ. The effects of lactose on mucociliary transportability and rheology of cystic fibrosis and bronchiectasis sputum. Eur Respir J 1997; 10:321s.

73. Robinson M, Daviskas E, Eberl S, Baker J, Chan HK, Anderson SD, Bye PTP. Effect of inhaled mannitol on bronchial mucus clearance in cystic fibrosis patients: a pilot study. Eur Respir J 1999; 14:678–685.

74. Feng W, Nakamura S, Sudo E, Lee MM, Shao A, King M. Effects of dextran on tracheal mucociliary velocity in dogs in vivo. Pulm Pharmacol Ther 1999; 12: 35–41.

75. Hirji M, Franklin R, Feng W, Boyd WA, King M. Effect of oligomeric chain length on mucolytic and mucokinetic effects of oligosaccharides. Am J Respir Crit Care Med 1998; 159:A685.

76. King M, Sudo E, Lee MM. In: Salathé M, ed. Cilia and Mucus: From Development to Respiratory Defense. New York: Marcel Dekker, 2001:277–287.

77. Sudo E, Boyd WA, King M. Effect of dextran sulfate on tracheal mucociliary velocity in dogs. J Aerosol Med 2000; 13:87–96.

78. Ahmed T, Garrigo J, Danta I. Preventing bronchoconstriction in exercise-induced asthma with inhaled heparin. N Engl J Med 1993; 329:90–95.

79. Shute J, Forsyth C, Hockey P, Carroll M. Anti-inflammatory effects of inhaled nebulised heparin in adult CF patients: results of a pilot study. Am J Respir Crit Care Med 2000; 161:A75.

80. Stockton P, Ledson MJ, Cowperthwaite C, Govin B, Gallagher MJ, Hart CA, Walshaw MJ. A double blind placebo controlled crossover study of nebulised heparin therapy in adult cystic fibrosis patients. Pediatr Pulmonol 2000; S20:278.

81. Warwick WJ, Hansen LG. The long-term effect of high frequency chest compression therapy on pulmonary complications of cystic fibrosis. Pediatr Pulmonol 1991; 11:265–271.

82. Konstan MW, Stern RC, Doershuk CF. Efficacy of the Flutter device for airway mucus clearance in patients with cystic fibrosis. J Pediatr 1994; 124:689–693.

83. Cegla UH, Bautz M, Froede G. Physiotherapy in patients with COAD and tracheobronchial instability: a comparison of two oscillating PEP systems (RC-Cornet, VRP1 Desitin). Pneumologie 1997; 51:129–136.

84. Tomkiewicz RP, Biviji AA, King M. Effects of oscillating air flow on rheological properties and clearability of mucous gel simulants. Biorheology 1994; 31:511–520.

85. App EM, Kieselmann R, Reinhardt D, Lindemann H, Dasgupta B, King M, Brand P. Sputum rheology changes in cystic fibrosis lung disease following two different types of physiotherapy: Flutter vs. autogenic drainage. Chest 1998; 114:171–177.

86. App EM, Wunderlich MO, Lohse P, King M, Matthys H. Oszillierende Physiotherapie bei Bronchialerkrankungen-rheologischer und antientzündlicher Effekt [Oscillatory physiotherapy for bronchial diseases: rheological and anti-inflammatory effects]. Pneumologie 1999; 53:348–359.

87. Knowles MR, Church NL, Waltner WE, Yankaskas JR, Gilligan P, King M, Edwards LJ, Helms RW, Boucher RC. A pilot study of aerosolized amiloride for the treatment of lung disease in cystic fibrosis. N Engl J Med 1990; 322:1189–1194.

88. App EM, King M, Helfesrieder R, Köhler D, Matthys H. Acute and long-term amiloride inhalation in cystic fibrosis lung disease. Am Rev Respir Dis 1990; 141: 605–612.

89. Graham A, Hasani A, Alton EW, Martin GP, Marriott C, Hodson ME, Clarke SW, Geddes DM. No added benefit from nebulized amiloride in patients with cystic fibrosis. Eur Respir J 1993; 6:1243–48.

90. Homolya L, Watt WC, Lazarowski ER, Koller BH, Boucher RC. Nucleotide-regulated calcium signaling in lung fibroblasts and epithelial cells from normal and P2Y(2) receptor (-/-) mice. J Biol Chem 1999; 274:26,454–26,460.

91. Bennett WD, Olivier KN, Zeman KL, Hohneker KH, Boucher RC, Knowles MR. Effect of aerosolized uridine 5′-triphosphate plus amiloride on mucociliary clearance in adult cystic fibrosis patients. Am J Respir Crit Care Med 1996; 153:1796–1801.

92. Dougherty RW, Pendergast W, Abraham WM, Sabater JR, Davis CW. Effects of P2Y$_2$ receptor agonists on cilia beat frequency in cultured human airway epithelia and on tracheal mucus velocity in sheep. Pediatr Pulmonol 2000; S20:258.

93. Dasgupta B, King M. Reduction in viscoelasticity of cystic fibrosis sputum in vitro with combined treatment by Nacystelyn and rhDNase. Pediatr Pulmonol 1996; 22:161–166.

94. Sun F, Tai S, Lim T, Baumann U, King M. Additive effect of dornase alfa and nacystelyn on transportability and viscoelasticity of cystic fibrosis sputum. Can Respir J 2002; 9:401–406.

95. Hitchcock SE, Carlsson L, Lindberg U. Depolymerization of F-actin by deoxyribonuclease I. Cell 1976; 7:531–542.

10

Modulation of Mucociliary Function by Drugs and Other Agents

JONATHAN RUTLAND, LUCY MORGAN, and ROBB DE IONGH*

Concord Repatriation General Hospital
Concord, New South Wales, Australia

I. Introduction

Mucociliary clearance (MCC) is a major function of the airway epithelium, which depends on the activity of the cilia and on the physicochemical properties of airway mucus. The latter is discussed extensively in other chapters in this book. This chapter deals with the effects of drugs and other agents on cilia. Since the interaction between cilia and mucus is complex, it is not always possible to differentiate between effects on cilia and mucus. Where studies are carried out on ciliated epithelium in vitro, effects of mucus can be largely excluded. While this allows study of the effects of drugs or agents on cilia in isolation, it also introduces the problem that cilia may behave differently when removed from an intact mucociliary system. Therefore, to take account of other modulatory influences operating in situ, various attempts have also been made to study ciliary activity in vivo. Reports of drug effects on cilia in the literature are far fewer than reports on MCC. Because of this, many reports from studies of MCC have been included in this chapter—to exclude them would be to limit the usefulness of this review. However, in many instances an effect on ciliary function has been inferred because of an effect on MCC without definite evidence of the former. As a summary of the information presented and as a quick refer-

---

Current affiliation: University of Melbourne, Parkville, Victoria, Australia.

ence point a table is presented in which are indicated drug effects on ciliary beating in humans and animals (mainly mammals) and effects on MCC (humans and animals).

II. Structure and Function

Cilia are widely distributed throughout the animal kingdom from the water-propelling cilia of unicellular protozoa to the specialized mucus transport mechanisms present in vertebrates (1) There is little phylogenetic variation in the ultrastructural features of cilia. Flagella, including sperm tails, have an internal structure almost identical to that of cilia.

Cilia and flagella first evolved in primitive unicellular organisms to propel water. Water-propelling cilia are characterized by low density or number per cell, long length, pronounced difference between effective and recovery strokes, prominent metachronal waves, and very regular rhythm. As epithelia evolved to propel mucus, cilia acquired adaptations that altered the way they operate. Where ciliated epithelium is adapted for mucus transport, as in the human respiratory tract, cilia are shorter, more numerous, and beat mainly within a low viscosity periciliary fluid layer, moving a more viscous, overlying mucus layer (2). The tips of the cilia enter the mucus layer only during the effective stroke and retract beneath the mucus layer during the recovery stroke so that the mucus is moved in one direction only. Ultrastructural studies have revealed that mucus-propelling cilia, such as those lining the human respiratory tract, have a unique structural adaptation at their apical cap. Small projections protruding from the apical cap are thought to aid in mucus propulsion by engaging the overlying mucus during the effective stroke (3).

A. Distribution of Cilia in Humans

The human tracheobronchial tree (from the larynx to the terminal bronchioles) and the nasal cavity and paranasal sinuses are lined by pseudostratified, ciliated epithelium. For both upper and lower respiratory tracts, the direction of mucus clearance is towards the oropharynx. Respiratory epithelium has a high rate of cell turnover (~4–8 weeks). Ciliated cells are also present in the middle ear, the eustachian tube, ependyma, and parts of the male (ductuli efferentes) and female (fallopian tubes) genital tracts. Modified, nonmotile cilia are also present in the olfactory epithelium and the retina, where they serve as sensory organelles. Many other cells transiently carry a single cilium during embryonic development.

B. Ciliary Structure

Human respiratory tract ciliated cells bear approximately 300 cilia on their apical surface. Cilia are elongated motile cylindrical projections of the cell membrane (~0.25 µm in diameter and 5–8 µm long). In transverse section (Fig. 1) the ciliary axoneme consists of a characteristic "9 + 2" structure of microtubules (consisting of the proteins α- and β-tubulin). The two central microtubules are each composed of 13 tubulin subunits and are surrounded and held together by the central sheath. The outer nine doublets consist of a complete microtubule ('A') with 13 tubulin subunits to which is attached a partial microtubule ('B') with 10 tubulin subunits. The peripheral subunits are linked to neighboring doublets by fine filaments of the protein nexin. Radial spokes are thicker filaments that project centrally from the 'A' microtubule towards the central sheath. Projecting at regular intervals from the 'A' microtubule towards the 'B' microtubule of the adjacent outer doublet are the inner and outer dynein arms. These are curved or hook-like filamentous structures containing proteins with ATPase activity. According to the sliding microtubule hypothesis of ciliary bending (1), the dynein arms are thought to attach intermittently to the adjacent 'B' microtubule and to change shape with a resulting sliding of doublets in relationship to each other. Such a sliding movement of different microtubule pairs in relation to each other causes ciliary bending.

The peripheral doublets extend along the length of the cilium and, at the base, continue into the cell in a modified form, becoming the triplets that form the basal body. Striated or ciliary rootlets extend from the basal extremity of

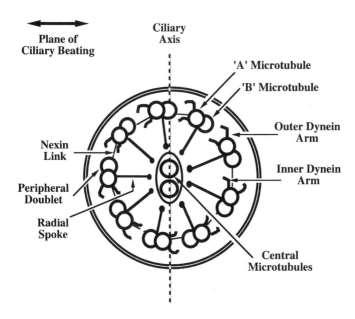

Figure 1 A cilium in transverse showing the structure of the axoneme. (Adapted from Ref. 237.)

the basal body and are in close association with the 'B' and 'C' microtubules of the triplet. These striated fibrils, which resemble collagen, consist of a protein called ankyrin and project into the apical cytoplasm. These structures, together with the basal body, anchor the cilium and maintain the orientation of its direction of beating. Projecting laterally from the basal body, in the direction of the active stroke of the cilium, is the basal foot. All basal feet in a cell and in the whole epithelium are orientated in approximately the same direction (4–6) so that the effective stroke of all cilia is in the same direction. The mechanisms that determine the parallel orientation of cilia are poorly understood but may be associated with elements of the apical cytoskeleton. Alignment appears to occur relatively late in embryonic development (7) and may be related to the commencement of ciliary beating (8).

C. Normal Ciliary Activity

Human nasal and tracheal cilia normally beat with a frequency of between 10 and 15 Hz (600–900 beats/min). Several detailed studies of the ciliary beat cycle have extended to proposing mathematical models for ciliary motion (9,10). Essentially the beat cycle comprises two phases: an effective stroke and a recovery stroke. In the effective stroke the cilium is extended and moves in a plane vertical to the surface of the cell, engaging the overlying mucus layer at its tip and moving the mucus forward. As the effective stroke is being completed, the cilium disengages from the mucus and the recovery stroke begins. During the recovery stroke the cilium retracts beneath the mucus layer and moves in the opposite direction to the effective stroke to resume its original position for the next effective stroke.

Many features of the axoneme are thought to contribute to ciliary motility. The study of mutants of *Chlamydomonas* (11) and mammals, including humans (i.e., primary ciliary dyskinesia, PCD), has led to some understanding of the function of individual components of the axoneme. Studies of invertebrate cilia led to the "sliding microtubule" hypothesis of ciliary motility (12), which proposes that the dynein arms interact with and translocate neighboring microtubules, causing them to slide. The energy for this interaction is derived from the ATPase activity of the dynein arms. The mechanochemistry of dynein in this interaction with the microtubules is very similar to that of myosin (for review, see Refs. 13 and 14). The sliding microtubule hypothesis has been further refined by the switch point hypothesis (reviewed in Ref. 14), which proposes that within the axoneme, dynein arm activity is asynchronous. During the effective stroke dynein arms on approximately half the doublets are active in producing tubule sliding and hence ciliary bending. During the recovery stroke the dynein arms on the opposite half of the axoneme are active producing ciliary bending in the opposite direction. In a single beat dynein arm activity switches from one half of the axoneme to the other. The mechanisms that regulate dynein arm activity are still under investigation.

Metachronal Activity

Ciliary beating is coordinated so that each cilium beats slightly later in the beat cycle than the one in front (constant phase difference). This results in waves of coordinated beating (metachronal pattern), which can be seen over a field of ciliated cells. The mechanisms that create such metachronal coordination in arrays of adjacent cilia are not clearly understood. It has been speculated that metachronal waves may arise from hydrodynamic coupling of adjacent cilia, presumably via the sol layer in which they beat and/or the overlying mucus (1, 15,16). Theoretical mathematical modeling has provided some support for this hypothesis (17,18).

Structure and Properties of Mucus

The physicochemical properties of airway mucus are dependent on the quality and quantity of mucus glycoproteins or mucins, which are produced by two different cell types: goblet cells of the epithelium and mucous cells of the sub-mucosal gland. The epithelial mucins are extremely hydrophobic and are associated with various macromolecules, the quality and quantity of which affect the physicochemical properties of the mucus. Secretion of epithelial mucins is stimulated by various factors, including a number of inflammatory agents (19).

The secretions of the respiratory tract are biphasic, consisting of an aqueous "sol" or periciliary layer in which the cilia beat and a more superficial "gel" layer. Due to difficulties with sampling, little is known about the physical and biochemical properties of the sol layer. The gel layer is composed of high molecular weight glycoproteins, proteins, and lipids that form a gel network with high water content (95%). The rheologic and physical properties are optimally adapted to allow effective transport by the cilia. In particular, the adhesive and elastic properties, which are influenced by lipid content and hydration, are important for effective clearance by cilia and cough. Alteration of mucus hydration or its macromolecular composition (e.g., by bacterial or cellular DNA), as occurs in obstructive airway diseases, such as cystic fibrosis, acute or chronic bronchitis, and during inflammatory and infective episodes, greatly affects its transportability by cilia and cough (for review, see Ref. 20).

Regulation of Ciliary Beating

For MCC to be effective it needs to be dynamic and to be able to respond to the many environmental changes imposed upon it. Numerous physiological and environmental stimuli can affect mucociliary clearance, in particular changes in the levels or properties of secretions in response to infection, inflammation, or allergy. Ciliated cells need to be able to respond to these changes by modulating ciliary beat accordingly. As a result, the physiology of the ciliated cell and the mechanisms that regulate ciliary beating are complex, and much remains to be elucidated. While a great deal of information about regulation of ciliary beating has been obtained from the study of invertebrate species, these data cannot always be directly extrapolated to vertebrate or mammalian respiratory tract cilia. Indeed, even studies of the effects of molecular mediators on cilia from different systems in vertebrates (e.g., frog palate vs. rabbit tracheal cilia) have led to contradictory results. For these reasons we have attempted, as much as possible, to restrict this review to studies of mammalian respiratory tract cilia.

The mucosae of the trachea and bronchial airways are innervated by nerves from the vagosympathetic trunk, dorsal root ganglia (sympathetic), and cervicothoracic ganglia. Yeates and colleagues have provided evidence that mucociliary activity in the tracheobronchial airways is regulated by a balance of inhibitory over excitatory autonomic neural activity (21). According to the model described by Yeates, the dominant neural transmission during homeostasis is inhibitory, mediated via nitric oxide–containing preganglionic fibers of the cervicothoracic ganglia acting on neuropeptide Y fibers that innervate the tracheobronchial tree. There is evidence that neuropeptide Y does have inhibitory effects on ciliary beat frequency (CBF) and can also inhibit cholinergic stimulation of CBF (see below). Excitatory pathways may be mediated through neural transmission by both the vagosympathetic trunk and the cervicothoracic ganglia, involving both adrenergic and cholinergic stimulation of ciliated cells. As discussed below, the major intracellular messenger molecules include nitric oxide and calcium.

It has been observed that in healthy volunteers but not in patients with chronic bronchitis or bronchiectasis, there is a distinct circadian rhythm of ciliary beat frequency. Cilia beat with a higher frequency in the morning than in the middle of the day (22). The function of this circadian rhythm is not known, but it is plausible that it may compensate for the depression of other clearance mechanisms, such as cough, during sleep. The mechanisms that regulate this circadian rhythm of ciliary beating are not clearly understood but may include contributions from hormones, growth factors, and the autonomic nervous system via release of neuropeptides.

Cellular Physiology of Ciliary Beating

The molecular pathways and mechanisms that regulate ciliary beating have become the subject of intense investigation over the last decade. Increasingly studies of the effects of drugs and agents on ciliary beat frequency include investigations of intracellular signaling molecules that mediate ciliary motility. As a result, rapid progress has been made in a very short time, and it is likely that further significant findings will be made in the near future.

There is considerable evidence that respiratory cilia can respond directly to physical stimuli from the environment. Rabbit tracheal cilia, which are mucus-propelling, have a compensatory mechanism when exposed to high-viscosity solutions in that they are able to maintain constant beat amplitude and CBF is only slightly decreased (23). In contrast, the CBF of water-propelling cilia decreases exponentially when exposed to high-viscosity loads (23). Extensive studies by Sanderson and Dirksen (24–26) showed, using rabbit tracheal cells grown in culture, that cilia have a mechanosensitive response. A ciliated cell, when stimulated mechanically, responds rapidly by increasing ciliary beat frequency. Furthermore, after a short delay the increase in CBF is communicated to neighboring cells. They proposed that such mechanosensitivity could provide local control of ciliary activity by increasing CBF in those regions where there is a heavy mucus load. Simultaneous analysis of cells with calcium-sensitive dyes showed that the levels of intracellular calcium increased in a spatiotemporal pattern that matched the pattern of CBF changes and suggested that the mechanosensitive response is communicated via calcium transients to neighboring cells via gap junctions. More detailed studies (see Ref. 27 for review) have elucidated aspects of the intracellular molecular events that underlie the regulation of this phenomenon. Mechanical stimulation appears to induce activation of mechanosensitive Ca^{2+} channels in the cell membrane and also activation of a membrane-bound enzyme, phospholipase C (PLC). The activated channels allow extracellular calcium to enter the cells and increase CBF rapidly in the stimulated cell(s). Activated PLC generates inositol 1,4,5-triphosphate (IP3), which can stimulate the release of intracellular stores of calcium from the endoplasmic reticulum and thus contribute to the increased CBF of the cell. Diffusion of IP3 to neighboring cells, via gap junctions, stimulates release of calcium from their endoplasmic reticulum, resulting in increased CBF. The continued diffusion of IP3 to neighboring cells generates a wave of calcium release and increased CBF that spreads radially from the stimulated cell (Fig. 2).

Two other major stimulators of CBF that have led to some understanding of the cellular physiology of ciliary beating are the purines and the cholinergics. For both of these, calcium has also been shown to be a central mediator of CBF regulation (28–31). There is evidence that the intracellular pathways utilized by both these stimulators also involve protein kinase C (PKC)– and IP3-induced release of intracellular calcium as well as involvement of the arachadonic acid pathway leading to synthesis of prostaglandins that impact on calcium release and nitric oxide.

Examination of the cholinergic signal transduction pathways (29,32) indicate that acetylcholine (ACh) or methacholine activate muscarinic (M3) receptors resulting in increased CBF and elevated intracellular calcium concentration,

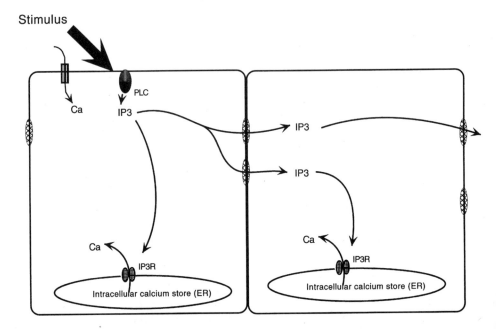

Figure 2 The intracellular molecular signaling pathways involved in mechanical stimulation of ciliary beat frequency. (Adapted from Ref. 27.)

mainly via calcium release from internal stores. It has been proposed that activation of the G-protein–linked M3 receptor leads to activation of PLC, which in turn hydrolyzes phosphatidylinositol biphosphate to diacylglycerol (DAG) and IP3 (Fig. 3) (32). The calcium released by IP3 from the endoplasmic reticulum activates nitric oxide synthase (NOS), leading to synthesis of nitric oxide from arginine. Nitric oxide in turn leads to production of cGMP via activation of guanylate cyclase. Concomitantly, DAG is degraded by DAG lipase to yield arachadonic acid, which is metabolized by the cyclo-oxygenase pathway in the synthesis of prostaglandins that, in turn, activate NOS. Yang et al. (32) also indicate that prostaglandin E_2 (PGE_2) stimulation of cyclic AMP (cAMP) production may have a role in the regulation of CBF. Prostaglandins may also directly influence the release of calcium from intracellular stores (33).

     Purines, particularly ATP, are potent stimulators of ciliary beat frequency. Korngreen and Priel have shown that, in frog cilia, purinergic stimulation results in an influx of calcium from extracellular sources as well as intracellular release of calcium from two different pools—one pool being in the apical cytoplasm near to the cilia and the other further from the cilia in the cell cytoplasm (34). In rabbit tracheal cilia they subsequently showed that ATP directly activates an

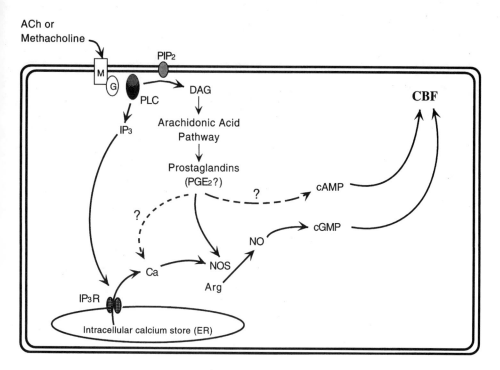

Figure 3 Diagram illustrating the intracellular molecular signaling pathways involved in muscarinic stimulation of ciliary beat frequency. (Adapted from Ref. 32.)

ion channel/P2X receptor, which may serve as a pathway for the Ca^{2+} influx (35). As for the mechanosensitive and cholinergic responses, purinergic stimulation results in activation of PLC and production of IP3 and DAG (Fig. 4). In addition, it has been shown in frog cilia that DAG activates PKC, which, in turn, induces a localized influx of extracellular calcium and also activates calcium-dependent potassium channels that mediate a potassium efflux and membrane hyperpolarization (31). Both the localized calcium influx and potassium efflux seem to be important for maintaining elevated CBF. However, the role of PKC in regulating ciliary activity is still not clear; in rabbit tracheal cilia PKC activators cause a decrease in CBF (36) rather than an increase as is seen in frogs.

Thus, it can be seen that calcium is a central regulator of ciliary beat frequency. However, it is still unclear by what mechanism changes in intracellular calcium concentration are transduced into changes in CBF. There are suggestions that elevated intracellular calcium acts via a calmodulin/calcium-dependent kinase since inhibitors of calmodulin abolish the calcium-mediated effects (37–39). There is significant evidence from studies on *Paramecium* and *Tetra-*

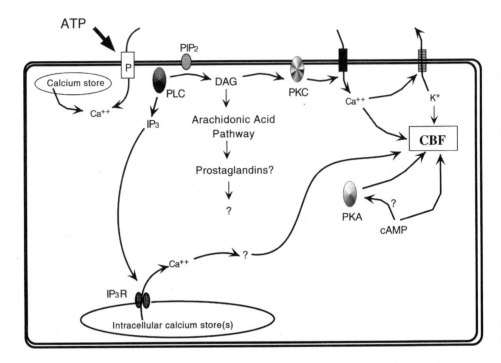

Figure 4 Diagram illustrating the intracellular molecular signaling pathways involved in purinergic stimulation of ciliary beat frequency. (Adapted from Ref. 31.)

hymena that calmodulin-dependent protein kinases and/or phosphatases interact with targets in the axoneme (see Ref. 40 for review), but as yet there is little evidence for such mechanisms in mammalian cilia. There is circumstantial evidence from immuno-electron microscopic studies that calmodulin is associated with the ciliary apparatus (microtubules, dynein arms, and basal bodies) in hamster respiratory cilia (41).

Cyclic AMP and Adrenergic Stimulation

Cyclic AMP is an important regulator of CBF. Elevated levels of cAMP have been shown to stimulate CBF of rabbit (42) and human (37) ciliated cells. In addition, adrenergic drugs that are known to increase CBF do so by raising intracellular levels of cAMP (25,43,44). The binding of adrenergic agents to β-receptors activates adenylate cyclase via G-proteins. In contrast, adenosine, which binds a specific A_1-receptor, inhibits adenylate cyclase and lowers intracellular levels of cAMP (45). The cAMP-mediated effects in rabbit and human cilia were blocked by a protein kinase inhibitor, leading to the speculation that cAMP acted via phosphorylation of specific axonemal proteins (37,42). Evidence for cAMP-mediated phosphorylation of axonemal proteins comes from studies in *Paramecium* (46) and sheep (47) cilia. In sheep cilia a 26 kD axonemal protein is phosphorylated in a cAMP-dependent fashion, but the identity of this protein is unknown (47).

Although Ca^{2+} and cAMP seem to act largely through independent pathways, it has been suggested that the pathways may converge or interact at the level of the axoneme (25,44). More recently it has been shown that in frog esophageal ciliated cells, "cross-talk" may occur at the level of protein kinase A (PKA) (48). These authors showed that elevation of cAMP by activation of adenylyl cyclase by forskolin or by treatment of cells with a membrane-permeable form of cAMP (dibutyryl cAMP) caused a rapid increase in CBF and intracellular calcium (from intracellular stores) that was due to PKA activity. PKA could also initiate a weaker but longer-term stimulation of CBF that was Ca^{2+} independent. It is not known whether a similar mechanism operates in mammalian cilia.

III. Measurement of Ciliary Function

There are a number of components of ciliary beating that could be used to describe or to measure ciliary function. These include the beat frequency, mucociliary wave frequency (similar but not identical to metachronal waves), beat direction, and shape changes of cilia during the beat cycle. Most studies of ciliary function in humans have been carried out in vitro. In practice, measurements of ciliary beat frequency are the easiest to perform.

A. In Vitro Studies

Human ciliary function in isolation from the mucus aspects of clearance may be studied in vitro. This involves obtaining intact epithelium from the subject (animal or human) and examining the cells in a nutrient medium to preserve ciliary activity. Samples of ciliated epithelium can be obtained by various techniques. These include biopsy forceps, curette, cytology brushing, and obtaining surgical specimens from the respiratory tract. We use nasal mucosal brushing (49) to provide a non-invasive means of obtaining respiratory tract epithelium. Such epithelial brushings can also be used for electron microscopy (4,49). This technique does not require local anesthesia and avoids the morbidity often associated with the use of nasal biopsy forceps. This technique rarely causes bleeding (blood may be ciliotoxic). If a patient is undergoing fiberoptic bronchoscopy, epithelial brushings may be obtained from the tracheobronchial tree. A study of 37 patients undergoing bronchoscopy revealed that nasal CBF was similar to that found in the trachea and lobar bronchi and that, in individual patients, upper and lower respiratory tract CBF was positively correlated (50).

Studies of ciliated epithelium in vitro allow a measurement of beat frequency in cilia isolated from humoral and neural influences and from mucus, providing a measurement of intrinsic ciliary activity (or drug effects on this) isolated from these factors. In some ways this may be advantageous, but it does have the disadvantage that such in vitro studies may not accurately reflect the activity of cilia in vivo. Care must be exercised in extrapolating in vitro data to the in vivo situation, in which other modulating influences may operate. In vivo and in vitro studies provide complementary information.

Various techniques have been used to study and measure ciliary beating. One of the most informative in terms of describing wave pattern as well as beat frequency is recording by high-speed cinematography (51,52). However, this technique is not easily adapted to on-line computer analysis and is relatively expensive. An alternative is high-resolution video recording (53). The laser light-scattering technique (54,55) is based on spectral analysis of a scattered laser light beam. This method, which allows complex computer analyses, is likely to come into wider use. The most commonly used technique in clinical practice is transmitted light microscope photometry, first described by Dalhamn and Rylander (56) in 1962 and subsequently employed by many other groups (49,57–59). In this technique, light passes through a wet preparation of ciliated epithelium on a slide that is viewed using a microscope and positioned so that beating cilia cross a small area from which transmitted light can be allowed to enter a photometer. As cilia interrupt light during the beat cycle, variations in light intensity are registered and transduced into an electric signal, which, after amplification, is recorded against time, allowing measurement of ciliary beat frequency. The data can be handled in various ways, such as fast-Fourier transform analysis (60). An elegant extension of this technique is the use of two optical fibers, each connected to its own photometer, and fast-Fourier transform analysis to measure velocity, wavelength, and frequency of metachronal wave propagation between two points (61).

Studies of ciliary beat pattern require either cinematography or video. Simultaneous recording and computer-aided correlation of data obtained photoelectrically and by high-speed cinematography has allowed detailed study of the phases of the ciliary beat cycle of rabbit and mussel gill cilia (59).

B. In Vivo Studies

Most in vivo studies of ciliary activity have been carried out in animal models such as the rabbit maxillary sinus (62) and canine trachea (63). However, animal studies require general anesthesia and/or surgical procedures that themselves may affect ciliary activity. In addition, some drug effects are species specific, making it difficult to extrapolate data from one species to another. The photoelectric method for assessing mucociliary activity in vitro has been further developed for use in vivo in the human (64) and rabbit (65,66) maxillary sinus. This technique measures variations in reflected light from the mucosal surface and therefore provides a measure of mucociliary wave activity rather than CBF. Laser light scattering has been used to make automated on-line objective measurements of canine tracheal ciliary activity (63). This method allowed demonstration of both magnitude and periodicity of ciliary beating and identified these two parameters as independent but coupled processes.

An in vivo photoelectric method has been developed for measuring human nasal ciliary activity and used to study the effects of pharmacological substances administered by aerosol to the nasal cavity (67). This method, similar to that used to study ciliary activity in rabbit maxillary sinus, utilizes reflected light. A rigid stainless steel probe containing optical fibers is introduced into the nasal cavity. Light from a cold light source is transmitted to the mucosal surface by an optical fiber (100 μm). The reflected light is collected and transmitted through other optical fibers to a photodiode. Variations in light intensity produced by beating cilia (recorded from a surface area of 100 μm in diameter) are registered by the photodiode and transformed into electrical signals to measure mucociliary wave activity. The method has been shown to have good reproducibility in normal subjects, but the mucociliary wave frequency did not correlate with CBF measured in vitro in ciliated epithelium from the same individuals.

C. Measurement of Clearance Rates

Many techniques have been used to measure mucociliary clearance, but most are based on two basic principles: direct measurement of the transport rate of deposited particles in an anatomically defined airway or measurement of the rate of elimination of inhaled aerosols from the tracheobronchial tree.

Direct Measurement of Transport Rate

One of the earliest methods of measuring mucociliary transport rates in a defined airway (68) used a camera attached to a bronchoscope to film and measure the transport of insufflated teflon discs along the trachea of normal human subjects as a mean tracheal mucus velocity (TMV). Values obtained ranged from 6 to 21.5 mm/min. This technique was subsequently modified by Friedman and colleagues (69), who used a fluoroscopic camera to videotape and measure the transport of bismuth-coated teflon discs that were deposited onto the tracheal mucosa bronchoscopically. They reported a mean TMV of 11.4 ± 3.8 mm/min. A similar technique has been used to measure TMV in healthy smokers (6.8 ± 5.0 mm/min) and nonsmokers (18.5 ± 6.0 mm/min) (70). The movement of radio-opaque teflon discs deposited bronchoscopically in the trachea has also been followed radiographically (71) in a study of the influence of age on TMV in healthy nonsmoking adults.

Radioisotopic variations of this technique have also been used to measure TMV. Chopra and colleagues (72) used a gamma camera to record the movement of droplets of [99]Tc -labeled albumin that had been instilled into the trachea of normal subjects at bronchoscopy. They reported a mean TMV of 15.5 ± 0.7 mm/min. Similarly, scintigraphic monitoring of ^{99}Tc-labeled macro-aggregated albumin (MAA) delivered as a relatively large particle aerosol bolus into the trachea has also been described (73). Automated computer analysis of the time-activity curves in this study produced a mean TMV of 4.7 ± 1.3 mm/min.

The advantages of measuring TMV by these various methods is that they show relatively good reproducibility, they require a short observation period (minutes), and the results are available immediately. Imaging can be done with radioactive isotopes or using radiology. However, there are disadvantages to these methods. They are limited to measurements of clearance in the large airways (such as the trachea) and hence will not reflect clearance rates in the peripheral airways. Furthermore, fiberoptic bronchoscopy is relatively invasive: it can elicit vagal stimulation and is often used with anesthetics and anticholinergics, which can influence ciliary activity and introduce artifacts. To circumvent the need for invasive bronchoscopy, we have recently adapted the method by using cricothyroid injection to deliver a small bolus of ^{99}Tc-labeled MAA (Morgan et al., unpublished data) onto the tracheal wall. Combined with the use of a gamma camera and specifically written software, this technique has permitted measurement of tracheal TMV in young (<50 years) and old (>50 years) normal subjects and patients with COPD and PCD. TMV (mean ± SD) in young normal subjects was 10.7 ± 3.5 mm/min. TMV was reduced in older subjects (6.4 ± 2.2 mm/min) and further reduced in COPD (2.4 ± 3.2 mm/min). In two patients with PCD, no clearance could be demonstrated.

Measurement of MCC by Elimination of Aerosol

Measurement of whole lung clearance, including the peripheral airways, can be achieved by aerosol clearance studies. Aerosol clearance studies rely on the inhalation and deposition of gamma-emitting radiolabeled material and have been used widely to measure clearance and transport in the lower respiratory tract (74). The clearance rate is determined by the amount of activity (corrected for isotope decay) remaining over time as detected by scintillation cameras. As ciliated airways clear more quickly than distal zones of the lung (75), clearance measured in this way in the lung is biphasic. There is an initial quick phase that is complete within 24 hours and represents clearance from the tracheo-bronchial tree, followed by a slower, later phase, which represents nonciliary alveolar clearance. Measurements of MCC by aerosol techniques are influenced by various factors, including the pattern of deposition in the airways, the inhaled particle size, and the detection system used. Tidal volume, respiratory rate, and obstructive lung pathology all influence deposition patterns. Deposition pattern is also affected by the size of the inhaled particles as particles larger than 1 μm in diameter deposit by impaction and those smaller than 0.1 μm by diffusion (76). Very large particles (>10 μm) usually deposit in the first few generations of airways, whereas small particles (1–3 μm diameter) distribute predominantly more peripherally (77). In patients with lung disease, the time required to measure lung clearance can be considerable, and over such long periods cough can have a significant impact on clearance. Intermediate-sized particles (approximately 6 μm in diameter) clear with an average half-life of 60 minutes, which is suitable for use in patient studies (78).

Technetium is the most commonly used gamma-emitting radionuclide and has been attached to a variety of carriers. Polystyrene microspheres (5 μm diameter) were used by Pavia and colleagues in a number of studies (79–81). These spheres were produced by a spinning disc aerosol generator, and after inhalation clearance from the tracheobronchial tree was monitored by suitably collimated scintillation counters, axially opposed antero-posteriorly over the midsternum of the subject. Such measurements were made over several hours.

Other particles used have included teflon (82), iron oxide (83–85), monodisperse fluorocarbon resin particles (86), human erythrocytes (87,88), and human serum albumin (88). Currently the most commonly used material is ultrasonically nebulized 3 μm particles of ^{99}Tc-albumin colloid (90).

Most studies using inhaled radiolabeled aerosols report results as a percent clearance of radiolabel with time (corrected for decay). Yeates and colleagues (91) used radiolabeled aerosols together with specific inspiratory maneuvers (inspiration from near TLC at a high flow rate) to produce deposition of aerosol boli in large central airways. They recorded movement of these boli with a gamma camera located over the trachea to produce a measure of TMV. These measurements were lower than those found using direct deposition of particles (see above). This may be related to the less invasive nature of this technique or to the particles themselves. In healthy normal subjects they reported a mean TMV of 4.4 ± 1.3 mm/min and intrapatient variability of 31.7%.

Nasal Clearance

There are fewer reports in the literature of nasal clearance than of clearance from intrathoracic airways. Although nasal clearance can be measured by inhalation of radio-aerosols (92), most studies have followed the movement of directly placed markers. These have included movement of radiolabeled particles placed in the anterior part of the nasal cavity as they move posteriorly through the nasal cavity past two collimated scintillation counters, a known distance apart (93–95). However, these techniques are not widely available. A measurement of nasal clearance can also be made by the saccharin technique, first introduced by Anderson in 1974 (96,99). This involves the placement of a saccharin particle (~1 mm^3) on the inferior turbinate. The time taken for the saccharin particles to be carried posteriorly to the oropharynx where they stimulate taste receptors can be measured as a clearance time (normal range < 30 min) (97). This technique is relatively simple and could be classed as an "office technique" but is less reproducible than other techniques. It can be used to screen for patients who may have mucociliary defects, but it has not proved sufficiently accurate for pharmacological studies (98).

IV. Drug Effects on Mammalian Cilia

Table 1 lists drug effects on cilia reported in human and nonhuman mammalian species. Because much of the information derived from the literature has consisted of drug effects on cilia presumed (not always with justification) because of effects shown on MCC, these have been listed separately. For many pharmacological agents published data are very limited.

A. Adrenergic Agents

In rats epinephrine (adrenaline) caused a dose-dependent increase in CBF between 10^{-9} and 10^{-5} M. Ephedrine had a lesser effect, causing ciliostimulation at 10^{-8}–10^{-7} M (100).

Aerosolized isoproterenol (isoprenaline) and epinephrine have been shown to accelerate mucus clearance in the human tracheobronchial tree, and this effect is independent of vasodilator or vasoconstrictor activity, parasympathetic activation, or bronchodilator activity (101). Parenteral isoproterenol caused increases in clearance similar to aerosolized isoproterenol and epinephrine. In cultured rabbit tracheal ciliated cells, isoproterenol increased CBF in a dose-dependent manner at 10^{-8}–10^{-5} M (25).

α-Adrenergic Agonists

Phenylephrine decreased human nasal CBF (102), and both phenylephrine and oxymetazoline reduced the frequency of mucociliary waves in rabbit maxillary sinus epithelium (103). The effects of xylometazoline (0.025–0.1%) have been tested on samples of human nasal epithelium in vitro and were found to significantly reduce CBF in a concentration-dependent and partially reversible manner (104). This supports the finding that xylometazoline prolongs human nasal MCC transport time in vivo using ^{51}Cr as a tracer (105).

β-Adrenergic Agonists

A number of β-adrenergic agents have been shown to stimulate ciliary activity and MCC. Van As (106) reported an increase in CBF in intact rat airway preparations and demonstrated a dose-related mean increase up to 165% of baseline

Table 1 Drugs and Agents Studied for Effects on Cilia and MCC[a]

Drug/agent	Effects on cilia — Human	Effects on cilia — Animal	Effects on MCC — Human	Effects on MCC — Animal	Comments
ADRENERGIC AGENTS					
Epinephrine (adrenaline)		↑100	↑101		Dose-dependent increase in rat CBF at 10^{-9}–10^{-5} M
Ephedrine		↑100			Increase in rat CBF with 10^{-8}–10^{-7} M
Isoproterenol (isoprenaline)		↑103	↑101		Given by aerosol and i.v. injection
					Dose-dependent stimulation of MCA in rabbit maxillary sinus epithelium (0.05–10 µg/kg i.a.)
		↑114			Blocked pyocyanin-induced cilioinhibition; propranolol blocked this effect
		↑25			Dose-dependent increase in rabbit CBF at 10^{-7}–10^{-5} M
α-Agonists					
Phenylephrine	↓102	↓103			CBF reduced in vivo in rabbits
Oxymetazoline	↓↔353	↓103			CBF reduced in vivo in rabbits
					No effect on human nasal CBF unless preservatives were present in the preparation; decreased CBF in presence of preservatives
Xylometazoline	↓104		↑105		Reduced human nasal CBF in concentration-dependent (0.025–0.1%), partially reversible manner
					Prolonged human nasal MCC
β-Agonists					
Formoterol		↑108	↑115		In vitro guinea pig trachea moderate increase (17%) in CBF using 10^{-7} M, prolonged effect
					In vivo rabbit maxillary sinus; dose-dependent 20% increase in CBF at 1 nmol/kg; at doses higher than this, weaker response was seen
					MCC (IRAT) increased in chronic bronchitis

Table 1 Continued

Drug/agent	Effects on cilia		Effects on MCC		Comments
	Human	Animal	Human	Animal	
Orciprenaline			↑112		Increased TMV in normal subjects
Salbutamol		↑103			Dose-dependent stimulation of MCA in rabbit maxillary sinus epithelium (0.05–10 µg/kg i.a.)
		↑106			Dose-dependent increase in rat CBF between 10^{-8}–10^{-4} M; max 65% at 10^{-4} M
	↑107				Cultured human bronchial cells, increase in CBF max at 10^{-4} M; blocked by propranolol 10^{-6} M
Salmeterol	↑107				Cultured human bronchial cells, increase in CBF max at 10^{-6} M; not blocked by propranolol
	↑114				Blocked pyocyanin-induced cilio-inhibition; propranolol blocked this effect
Terbutaline		↑108			Increased CBF in GP trachea (10^{-7}–10^{-3} M)
	↑↔22				CBF increased (~1 Hz) in normal subjects; not in chronic bronchitis patients
	↓109				Terbutaline 10^{-6}–10^{-12} M inhibited Ca^{2+}–induced ciliostimulation
			↑110		TMV increased in CF not in normal subjects
			↔111		No effect on MCC (IRAT) in CF
β-Blockers					
Atenolol			↔117		No effect on MCC
Metoprolol			↔89		No effect with 100 mg/day
Pindolol			↔89		No effect with 5 mg/day

Agent	Ref.	Comment
Propranolol	↓116; ↔43; ↔118	No effect on MCC in dogs
		CBF reduced in rabbit tracheal cilia by propranolol 10^{-4} M; no effect at 10^{-7} M; isoproterenol stimulation blocked by 10^{-7} M
		0.1% propranolol stopped ciliary beating in human adenoid tissue
	↔103; ↔117	No effect on MCC
		No effect on CBF but blocked ciliostimulation by isoproterenol
	↓89	MCC reduced with 80 mg/day
	↓107	Propranolol inhibited salbutamol-induced but not salmeterol-induced cilio-stimulation
ANESTHETICS: GENERAL		
Enflurane	↓122	Dose-dependent, reversible depression of TMV in dogs
Ether	↔122	No effect on MCC
Halothane	↓120; ↓121; ↓122	Dose-dependent, reversible depression of TMV in dogs
		Dose-dependent impairment of rabbit tracheal cilia
		Ferret CBF in vitro; 2% halothane—no change; >4%—reversible ciliostasis
		Human CBF reduced in vitro
Nitrous oxide	↓119; ↔123	
ANESTHETICS: LOCAL		
Cocaine	↓128	Dose-dependent impairment of human nasal CBF
Lidocaine	↓125	Lidocaine >0.25% caused dose-dependent cilio-inhibition; >4% caused ciliostasis

Table 1 Continued

Drug/agent	Effects on cilia		Effects on MCC		Comments
	Human	Animal	Human	Animal	
	↓126				Dose-related impairment of human nasal CBF; lidocaine nasal spray in clinical use did not affect CBF
		↓127			Impairment of CBF in guinea pig and bovine tracheal rings
Vadocaine	↓128	↓129			Dose-dependent impairment of human nasal CBF Reduced CBF in rat tracheal explants
ANTIBIOTICS					
Clarithromycin		↔131			Rabbit trachea explants
Erythromycin		↑130			Dose-dependent increase in rabbit tracheal CBF
		↑131			Dose-dependent increase in CBF in rabbit trachea explants—less than roxithromycin
Roxithromycin		↑131			Dose-dependent increase in CBF in rabbit trachea explants—more than erythromycin
		↑132		↑132	Oral roxithromycin given to guinea pigs for 14 days
ANTITUSSIVES					
Codeine (see Narcotics)		↔286			
Dextromethorphan (see Narcotics)		↓129			
Vadocaine (see Anesthetics, local)		↓129			
BACTERIAL PRODUCTS	↓134–175				Antibiotics inhibit bacterial product impairment of CBF (166)

Drug	Finding (ref.)
CHOLINERGICS	
Acetylcholine	↓↑177
	↓↑172 Rabbit TMV: increased at 10^{-5} M, reduced at 10^{-4} M
	Human tracheal explants; CBF reduced at concentrations >2.5%, no change at 0.01% and minor increases at 0.1–1%
Methacholine	↑178 Increased rat CBF in vivo
	↑179 Dose-dependent (0.01–2 μg/kg) acceleration of rabbit sinus MCA
	↑180,181 Increased bovine trachea CBF in vitro (10^{-7} M) and canine trachea in vivo (10^{-8}–10^{-6} M)
Pilocarpine	↑182 Increased rat MCC in vivo
ANTICHOLINERGICS	
Atropine	↓179
	↓176 Reduced rabbit TMV at 10^{-6} M
	↓183 Reduced ciliary activity at 0.1% and progressively impaired at concentrations up to 2.5%
	TMV slowed by atropine premedication 0.4 mg
	↑184 Increased TMV in anesthetized dogs in vivo; paradoxical result
	↔179 No change in rabbit MCA at 0.05–0.5 mg/kg; blocked methacholine-induced ciliostimulation
	↓185 Reduced sheep TMV; marked persistence of bacteria in trachea after inhaled aerosol of bacteria in atropinized (0.2 mg/mL) sheep
Bethanechol	↑186 Reduced MCC (IRAT)
Hyoscine	↓187 No change in dog TMV
Ipratropium	↔190 / ↔192 No change MCC (by IRAT) in normal subjects
	↔191 No change in MCC in humans (normal subjects and chronic bronchitis)
	↓188 Reduced TMV in pigeons

Table 1 Continued

Drug/agent	Effects on cilia		Effects on MCC		Comments
	Human	Animal	Human	Animal	
Methylscopolomine			↔186		
Oxitropium				↔↓188	
COMPLEMENTARY MEDICINES					
Sairei-to		↔193		↔193	At usual human doses no effect on CBF or MCC in guinea pig middle ear
		↑194		↔194	High doses (600 mg/kg) increased CBF but not MCC
Essential oils (menthol, eucalyptus, and pine needle oils)		↓195			Human nasal CBF in vitro reduced in a dose-dependent manner by menthol, eucalyptus oil, and pine needle oil at high concentrations
CORTICOSTEROIDS					
Beclomethasone dipropionate	↓196				20% decrease in human CBF at 0.005 mg/mL
Budesonide			↔199		100 µg/nasal cavity b.d. for 1 week
Corticosterone				↑198	Increased pigeon TMV by 20% after 5 mg/kg i.m. injection; no change after 1 mg/kg
Flunisolide	↓196				20% decrease in human CBF at 0.025 mg/mL
Prednisolone		↑176			Dose-dependent increase in CBF in rat trachea
DIURETICS					
Frusemide			↔200		Aerosolized frusemide 40 mg did not affect MCC
			↔201		Aerosolized frusemide 40 mg delayed the increase in MCC expected with isocapneic hyperventilation in asthmatics but not in normal subjects

Amiloride	↑202	Small, short-lived increase in human bronchial CBF (10^{-4}–10^{-3} M)
	↔203	No effect on human MCC
	↔205	
	↔204	
ETHANOL	↑↓ 207	Sheep tracheal CBF increased at 0.01%, unchanged at 0.5–1%; ciliostasis at >2%
	↔209	Bovine ciliary activity in vitro not affected; acetaldehyde, an ethanol metabolite, inhibited CBF
	↑208	Dose-dependent increase in bovine bronchial CBF (>10 mM); decrease in CBF at concentrations >1000 mM
	↔210	Ethanol caused no change in mean human MCC but did increase intrasubject variability
GROWTH FACTORS, HORMONES, AND CYTOKINES		
Adrenocorticotropin (ACTH)	↑215	Dose-dependent increase in rabbit trachea CBF (max 34% at 10^{-6} M)
Angiotensin II	↑211	Dose-dependent increase in rabbit tracheal cilia (max 36% at 5×10^{-12} M)
Atrial natriuretic factor (ANF)	↓212	Dose-dependent decrease in rabbit CBF (max 24% at 10^{-6} M)
Corticotropin-releasing factor (CRF)	↑215	Dose-dependent increase in rabbit trachea CBF (max 25% at 10^{-7} M)
Endothelin-1, -2, -3	↓216	Aerosolized ET-1 (10^{-9}–10^{-6} M) induced 54% reduction in TMV in sheep within 30 min
	↑212	Increased CBF in dog cilia
	↑218	Increase in nasal and tracheal CBF in rabbits by ET-1, but not ET-2, ET-3

Table 1 Continued

Drug/agent	Effects on cilia Human	Effects on cilia Animal	Effects on MCC Human	Effects on MCC Animal	Comments
Macrophage-stimulating protein (MSP)	↑213				Dose-dependent (1–50 ng/mL) increase in CBF (max 20%) within 30 min
Vasoactive intestinal peptide (VIP)		↑219			Dose-dependent increase in rabbit tracheal cilia (max 17% at 10^{-7} M)
HISTAMINES					
Histamine (see Inflammatory mediators)					
ANTIHISTAMINES					
Azelastine	↑220	↓221			Dose-dependent increase in human bronchial CBF 0.1% impaired CBF in rat tracheal explants
Cimetidine (H$_2$-blocker)		↓223		↑222	Small (23%) increase in canine TMV Guinea pig middle ear; cimetidine reduces the ciliostimulatory effects of histamine
Diphenhydramine (H$_1$-blocker)		↔223			Guinea pig middle ear; did not alter the ciliostimulatory effects of histamine
Hydroxyzine		↓129 ↓129			Dose-dependent reduction in rat tracheal CBF Dose-dependent reduction in rat tracheal CBF
Tramazoline hydrochloride	↔↓224				No effect on human nasal CBF at clinical doses; impaired CBF at 4 times clinical dose
INHALED SUBSTANCES					
Acetaldehyde		↓209			Slows bovine bronchial CBF
Hairspray			↓222		Transient reduction in MCC not caused by hairspray propellant alone

Agent					Effect
Nicotine		↑232		↑233	Dose-dependent, acute increase in ferret CBF 0.5–10 µg/kg accelerates MCA in rabbit maxillary sinus in vivo in a dose-dependent manner
Smoking	↔229		↓71, ↓231		Reduced TMV in smokers correlated with tobacco exposure Decreased MCC correlated with extent of smoking (pack-years) No significant difference in mean CBF between smokers, ex-smokers, or nonsmokers
Sulfuric acid		↓228			Reduced MCC in rabbits
SO_2				↓225	Reduced CBF in rabbit and rat tracheal cilia
INFLAMMATORY MEDIATORS					
Elastase	↓145, ↓150				
Histamine		↑247, ↑↓223		↓223, ↑236	7% increase in sheep cilia CBF at $>10^{-5}$ M In vitro 10^{-8}–10^{-4} M caused stimulation of CBF (6–16%), but 10^{-2} M caused inhibition In vivo—guinea pig eustachian tube 250% increase in MCA of monkeys in vivo
Neuropeptides					
Neuropeptide Y		↓238			Rabbit
Serotonin	↑244	↔178			No change in rat tracheal CBF Small increase Rabbit in vivo
Substance P	↑243, ↑246	↑241, ↑242			Dog in vivo Small change Small change in vitro

Table 1 Continued

Drug/agent	Effects on cilia		Effects on MCC		Comments
	Human	Animal	Human	Animal	
Leukotrienes					
Leukotriene C4		↑252			Sheep tracheal cilia
		↓255			Chicken
Leukotriene D4	↔256	↑252			Human adenoid
					10^{-9}–10^{-7} M stimulated CBF (13–16%) of sheep cilia at 39°C
	↓250				10^{-7} M decreased human CBF (10%) at 25°C
		↔251			No change in rabbit maxillary sinus MCA in vivo (i.v. 0.01–10 nmol/kg)
		↑248			10^{-7} M stimulated dog cilia (29%) at 37°C
	↓249				10^{-8}–10^{-6} M inhibited human eustachian tube cilia
	↑253	↑253			Dose-dependent increase in CBF but differential species sensitivity; maximum response in guinea pig 75% at 10^{-9} M; rat 119% at 10^{-7} M; human 86% at 10^{-6} M
		↑254			Stimulation of guinea pig CBF—age dependence of response
Prostaglandins					
Prostaglandin D$_2$	↔262	↑197			Increase in CBF and MCC (10^{-18}–10^{-6} M) but no dose dependence; various species rat, hamster, monkey, cat
Prostaglandin E$_1$		↑247			Dose-dependent increase (10^{-8}–10^{-6} M) in CBF, max. 25.8% at 10^{-6} M

Prostaglandin E$_2$	↑257	Increase in rabbit oviduct cilia (~7% at 10^{-8}–10^{-6} M) calcium dependent
	↑247	Dose-dependent increase in sheep tracheal cilia, max. 20% at 10^{-7} M
	↑258	In vivo increase in MCA of rabbit sinus (13.4%) at 1.0 µg/kg
	↑260	Dose-dependent increase in human nasal cilia, max. 11.9% at 10^{-6} M
	↑262	Dose-dependent increase in human adenoid cilia, max. 37% at 10^{-6} M
	↔↑262	Increase in hamster CBF at 10^{-8}–10^{-5} M. No dose-dependence; max. increase of 8% in ependymal cilia; no change in tracheal cilia
Prostaglandin F$_2$	↑257	Increase in rabbit oviduct cilia (~75%)
	↔247	No change over range 10^{-10}–10^{-6} M
	↑258	24% increase in rabbit MCC in vivo
	↑259	Dose-independent increase in CBF (10^{-8}–10^{-5} M) average increase 7% in ependymal and 13% in tracheal cilia of hamster
Hydrogen peroxide (H$_2$O$_2$)	↓266	10^{-2} M H$_2$O$_2$ reduced human CBF to 36% baseline, ciliostasis after 10 minutes; no effect at 10^{-3} M
Prostacyclin/beraprost	↑264	Dose-dependent increase in CBF from (0.5 × 10^{-7} – 10^{-5} M)
Superoxide	↑359	Rapid increase (26.8%) in human CBF after 15 s
MUCOLYTICS AND EXPECTORANTS		
Ambroxol	↑277	Rat CBF in vitro increased
	↔281	No significant effect on MCC in chronic bronchitis patients by IRAT

Table 1 Continued

Drug/agent	Effects on cilia		Effects on MCC		Comments
	Human	Animal	Human	Animal	
		↑278			Increase in CBF of guinea pig tracheal explants
			↔279		No improvement of human MCC by IRAT
		↔276			No effect on rabbit MCA in vivo
			↑275		Increased human MCC in patients with chronic bronchitis
Bromhexine			↔280		No increase in human MCC by IRAT
		↔276	↑275		Increase in MCC in patients with chronic bronchitis
		↔↑270			No effect on rabbit MCA in vivo
					Increased CBF in dog tracheal cilia at 10^{-7}–10^{-5} M
			↑282		Increased MCC in humans
Glycerol guaiacolate			↔80		No effect on MCC in normal subjects, increased MCC in bronchitic patients
			↔282		MCC human no change after single oral dose
N-Acetylcysteine		↑↓269		↑↓269	Mucus transport rate and CBF increased in rat and rabbit trachea at 10^{-12}–10^{-10} g/mL; decreased at 10^{-6} g/mL
		↑↓270			CBF increased at concentrations of 10^{-7} and 10^{-6} M in canine tracheal cilia, reductions at 10^{-4} and 10^{-3} M
				↑271	Canine TMV increased
			↑272		Human "slow clearers"—increased MCC (IRAT)
			↑275		Improved TMV in chronic bronchitis
S-carboxymethylcysteine			↔283		No change in chronic bronchitis patients
	↑285	↔285			Small increase in CBF of sinusitis patients
				↔284	Rabbit tracheal explants no change in mucus velocity

Agent	Effect	Ref.
NARCOTICS		
Morphine	↔ Human CBF in vitro; no effect of morphine 10 μmol/L	287
	↓ Reduced MCC in cats at a lower dose (0.5 mg/kg) than the cough-suppressive dose	288
Codeine	↓ Reduced canine TMV with 6 mg/kg iv	122
	↓ 5 mg/kg inhibited cat MCC; lower doses had no effect	288
	↓ Inhibition (8%–28%) of rat tracheal CBF at 10^{-7}–10^{-3} g/mL	178
Dextromethorphan	↓ Decreased CBF (rat) in vitro but not in vivo (rat and guinea pig)	286
	↓ Cilioinhibition in rat tracheal explants	129
NONSTEROIDAL ANTI-INFLAMMATORY DRUGS		
Aspirin	↓ 21% inhibition of MCC (IRAT) in healthy humans at 16 mg/kg (serum level of 80 μg/mL)	290
	↔ No effect on CBF after perfusion with aspirin (up to 200 μg/mL)	289
Indomethacin	↑ Dose-dependent increase in CBF (max. 26.5% at 0.5×10^{-7} M)	291
OSMOTIC AGENTS		
Mannitol	↑ Mannitol dry powder inhalation 50 mg/mL stimulates human MCC in normal subjects and patients with chronic bronchitis, bronchiectasis, and asthma	296, 293, 294
Hypertonic saline	↓ Hypertonic saline 7% causes reversible ciliostasis; 14% causes irreversible ciliostasis	297

Rutland et al.

Table 1 Continued

Drug/agent	Effects on cilia		Effects on MCC		Comments
	Human	Animal	Human	Animal	
PRESERVATIVES					
Benzalkonium chloride	↓298	↓298			Reduced human nasal CBF in vitro 20–200 mg/mL
Propylene glycol	↓197				
Methylparaben		↓125			Reduced ferret tracheal CBF
PURINES					
UTP			↑201		Aerosol clearance in normal subjects
Adenosine		↓45			Reduced CBF in rabbits and depletion of cAMP
		↑47			Increased sheep CBF
ATP			↑302		Increased nasal MCC
		↑45			Increased CBF in rabbit oviduct
	↑299	↑33			Dose-dependent increase in human CBF in vitro
		↑301			Increased CBF in rats/guinea pigs in vitro
	↑300	↑303			Increased MCA in dog trachea
					Increased nasal CBF and amplitude when baseline CBF is low (<8 Hz)
GTP		↑34			Extracellular ATP causes a rise in intracellular Ca and CBF in rabbit trachea
		↑303			Increased MCA of dog trachea

XANTHINES

Agent	Reference	Effect description
Aminophylline	↑309	Increase in rat tracheal CBF
	↑269	Increase in human tracheal CBF
	↑311	Improvement in MTV in canine central airways; trachea >bronchi
Theophylline	↑313	Improved MCC by IRAT in COPD
	↔↑312	By IRAT did not change but aerosol penetration increased suggesting improved MCC
	↑89	Increased MCC in asthma
	↑87	

aShown as increase (↑), decrease (↓), or no change (↔). Effects on human and animal cilia listed separately. Numbers refer to References.

in preparations incubated in 10^{-8}–10^{-4} M salbutamol (albuterol). In another animal study salbutamol induced a dose-dependent stimulation of mucociliary activity in rabbit maxillary sinus epithelium at concentrations of 0.05–10 µg/kg (103). In a similar study, Devalia and colleagues found that salbutamol increased CBF of cultured human bronchial cells (107). This was maximal at 10^{-4} M but was transient and was blocked by propranolol (10^{-6} M). These workers demonstrated that both salbutamol and salmeterol led to a release of cAMP into the culture medium that was also blocked by propranolol and suggested that activation of β-adrenocepters induces ciliostimulation via elevation of intracellular cAMP (107).

The β-adrenergic drug terbutaline has been shown to induce a dose-related (10^{-7}–10^{-3} M) increase in CBF in vitro in a guinea pig trachea preparation (108). The maximum increase in CBF was 24% at 10^{-3} M. In healthy subjects, but not in a group of 15 patients with chronic bronchitis, terbutaline induced ciliostimulation ranging from 0.1 to 1.4 Hz (22). However, in a recent study by Honeyman and colleagues, it was found that terbutaline at 10^{-6}–10^{-12} M inhibited Ca^{2+}-induced stimulation of CBF (109). This inhibition was reversed by inhibiting protein kinase A but was not reversed by simply removing terbutaline. They also found that terbutaline inhibited the increase in CBF induced by mechanical stimulation—the latter is calcium dependent. These authors suggested that terbutaline, by inhibiting calcium-mediated ciliostimulation, impairs the ability of the mucociliary system to respond to increased mucus loads. This may be particularly important in bronchitis. The possibility that this mechanism might be involved in β-agonist–related asthma deaths was raised (109).

Using direct observation of the motion of teflon discs along the tracheal mucosa, it has been shown that administration of terbutaline increased the average mucus velocity in patients with cystic fibrosis but not in control subjects (110). However, a more recent study showed, using a radio-aerosol method, that in patients with cystic fibrosis there was no significant effect of terbutaline on mucociliary clearance (111).

Using radioaerosol techniques Yeates and colleagues demonstrated that low doses of oral orciprenaline increased tracheal mucociliary transport in 12 healthy nonsmoking males but not bronchial clearance in healthy adults (112).

Not all studies of β-agonists have demonstrated ciliostimulation. For example, procaterol had no effect on MCC, as assessed by inhaled radiolabeled aerosol technique, in normal subjects or in patients with respiratory tract diseases including asthma (113). Long acting β-agonists have been shown to stimulate ciliary function. Salmeterol has been reported to stimulate CBF of cultured human bronchial epithelial cells with maximal effects at 10^{-6} M (107). The ciliostimulation occurred rapidly and was prolonged, persisting up to 24 hours. Propranolol (10^{-6} M) prevented salbutamol- but not salmeterol-induced increases in CBF.

An interesting recent finding about salmeterol is its effect on the slowing of CBF caused in vitro by pyocyanin. Pyocyanin is a phenazine pigment produced by *Pseudomonas aeruginosa* and known to impair CBF and mucus transport. Preincubation of ciliated epithelium with salmeterol prevented the pyocyanin-induced decrease in CBF, while propranolol blocked the protective effect of salmeterol (114).

Formoterol, another long-acting β-agonist, caused a dose-dependent increase in CBF in vitro in guinea pig trachea (maximum increase 17% at 10^{-7} M) (108). In vivo, formoterol stimulated ciliary activity in rabbit maxillary sinus to a maximum of 23% using 1 nmol/kg. Formoterol was 100 times more potent than terbutaline. MCC, measured by an inhaled clearance technique, was studied in stable bronchitic patients. After 6 days of treatment with formoterol aerosol, MCC was increased significantly (115).

β-Blockers

β-blockers, in general, block cilio-stimulation caused by β-adrenergic agonists but do not impair ciliary activity except at high concentrations. Propranolol at 10^{-4} M impaired CBF (43). Lower concentrations had no effect but at 10^{-7} M blocked isoproterenol-induced cilio-stimulation in rabbit tracheal cilia. Similarly, in rabbit sinus cilia, propranolol inhibited isoproterenol-induced ciliostimulation but had no effect alone.(103). However, Van de Donk and Merkus (116) found that 0.1% propranolol impaired ciliary beating within minutes, causing ciliostasis in ciliated human adenoid tissue. Propranolol (10^{-6} M) impaired ciliostimulation caused by salbutamol but not salmeterol studied in cultured human bronchial cells (107).

In a study of MCC in patients with coronary heart disease but not pulmonary disease, propranolol 80 mg daily for 3 days significantly impaired mucociliary clearance, while metoprolol (100 mg daily), a selective $β_1$-adrenoceptor blocker, had no effect (89). Pindolol, a nonselective β-blocker, like propranolol, had no effect on MCC at 100 mg daily. It was suggested that this may be because pindolol has a partial agonist effect on β2-adrenoceptors. Pavia and colleagues also studied the effects of propranolol as an example of nonselective β-antagonists after a single oral dose of 160 mg and atenolol (100 mg) as an example of a selective β-blocker. Neither affected MCC (117). Similarly, propranolol did not alter TMV in dogs (118).

B. Anesthetics

General

General anesthesia impairs mucus clearance. Some of this is due to mechanical factors such as endotracheal intubation, and some are due to drug effects. The effects of several anesthetics on ciliary activity have been investigated—halothane has been the best studied.

Exposure of human nasal ciliated epithelium to halothane in air (0.9–5.7%) resulted in a significant decrease in CBF and impaired ciliary coordination (119). In animal studies, halothane caused a dose-dependent impairment of CBF in rabbit tracheal cilia (120,121). In anesthetized dogs halothane and enflurane impaired TMV, but ether did not (122). In this study a combination of halothane and nitrous oxide impaired TMV. This impairment may have been due to the halothane since it has been shown that nitrous oxide alone does not affect TMV (123).

The mechanism by which halothane inhibits ciliary activity has been studied but not fully elucidated. Electrophysiological studies have shown that halothane alters water and ion transport, particularly chloride and sodium, in ciliated cells (124). It was suggested that these changes might reduce the volume and increase the viscosity of airway fluids, changes that could impair MCC during and after general anesthesia. It has been further speculated that halothane and other inhaled anesthetics might also deplete intracellular calcium stores and/ or reduce ATPase activity, both of which could impair ciliary beating and/or coordination, contributing to postoperative atelectasis and chest infections (119).

Local

Lidocaine (lignocaine) has been the best-studied local anesthetic. Concentrations of lidocaine as low as 0.5% were found to cause complete but reversible ciliostasis of ferret cilia. At concentrations of 1–2% this effect was not completely reversible (125). Similarly, studies with human cilia showed that concentrations of lidocaine above 0.25% caused cilioinhibition in a dose-dependent manner and that concentrations above 2% caused ciliostasis. However, application of lidocaine as a nasal spray in doses sufficient to produce local anesthesia did not inhibit CBF subsequently measured in vitro (126). Similar dose-related cilioinhibition has been demonstrated in both bovine and guinea pig tracheal rings (127).

Ingels and colleagues (128) studied the effect of varying concentrations of lidocaine on human nasal biopsy specimens and demonstrated a dose-dependent impairment of CBF similar to that shown by Rutland and colleagues (126). The same workers extended their observations to cocaine, again finding dose-related cilioinhibition, with ciliostasis occurring at a concentration of 7%. Vadocaine has also been shown to reduce CBF in rat tracheal explants (129).

Local anesthetics are in wide use as topical preparations and as such require the presence of preservatives. The effect of the preservative methylparaben on ciliary activity has been studied. Concentrations as low as 0.06 mg/mL caused reversible ciliary paralysis, but at higher concentrations (≥ 0.5 mg/mL) these adverse effects were not completely reversible. When methylparaben was combined with lidocaine, the ciliotoxic effects of the two drugs were additive (125).

C. Antibiotics

Several macrolide antibiotics have been shown to stimulate ciliary activity in animal studies. The effect of erythromycin on rabbit tracheal CBF has been studied in vitro (130). There was a dose-dependent increase, the maximum being 23% at a concentration of 6.8 mg/L. The same group found that roxithromycin caused a greater increase in CBF than erythromycin, with clarithromycin causing a nonsignificant change (131). The effects of roxithromycin and erythromycin were both dose dependent (10^{-8}–10^{-4} M) and maximal at 10^{-4} M (131). It has been reported that in guinea pigs treated with oral roxithromycin there was an increase in eustachian tube MCC and ciliary activity (132).

In the presence of infection/inflammation, macrolides may allow an increase in CBF by means of inhibition of bacteria or inhibition of recruitment of neutrophils or their production of cytokines (133). However, even in the absence of inflammation, macrolides have been shown to increase CBF. In studies using specific inhibitors, the ciliostimulatory effects of macrolides were not associated with β-adrenoreceptors, lipoxygenase products, or calcium entry into cells (130, 131). Tamaoki and colleagues studied the effects of propranolol, atropine, indomethacin, and inhibitors of protein kinases A and C as well as the effect of regulating extracellular calcium and found no effect on erythromycin-induced ciliostimulation (130). Similarly there was no effect of propranolol, verapamil, and AA-861 (lipoxygenase inhibitor) on roxithromycin-induced ciliostimulation, but indomethacin (another cyclo-oxygenase inhibitor) partly inhibited this effect. Because intracellular cAMP levels were increased by roxithromycin (10^{-5} M) at concentrations similar to those that stimulate CBF, it has been suggested that cAMP may be the major mediator of the action of roxithromycin on CBF (131).

Little has been published about the effects of other antibiotics on ciliary function. Wanner (134), in his review of the clinical aspects of mucociliary transport, referred to studies of topical penicillin and streptomycin, which had no effect or slightly stimulated mucociliary transport.

D. Antitussives

See sections on narcotics (codeine and dextromethorphan) and anesthetics (vadocaine).

E. Bacterial Products

Delayed mucociliary clearance often occurs secondary to respiratory tract disease, particularly when purulent secretions are present, such as in bronchiectasis

(135,136), cystic fibrosis (110,137), and mucopurulent sinusitis (136,138). The delayed MCC may be due to changes in the rheological properties of mucus: less elastic during viral infection (139) or more viscous in bacterial infections (134). Alternatively, impairment of MCC may be due to changes in the ciliated epithelium both structural and functional: loss of ciliated epithelium (65), absence of cilia and/or cilia with abnormal ultrastructure (140–143). Cilia sampled from areas of purulent infection have been shown to have reduced CBF and abnormal beat patterns (136).

There is increasing evidence that such secondary ciliary dyskinesia may result from bacterially produced factors (for review, see Ref. 144) and also by cell products such as elastase and proteinases liberated by leukocytes in inflammatory lung disease (145). Organisms that are known to affect ciliary activity or the integrity of the ciliated epithelium and thus affect mucociliary clearance are *Pseudomonas aeruginosa, Haemophilus influenzae, Staphylococcus aureus, Mycoplasma pneumoniae, Bordetella pertussis,* and *Streptococcus pneumoniae.*

Pseudomonas Aeruginosa

P. aeruginosa is an organism that frequently colonizes the lower airways of patients with cystic fibrosis or bronchiectasis and has been shown to produce a number of low molecular weight factors that inhibit ciliary activity. *P. aeruginosa*–derived proteases cause necrosis of the ciliated epithelium (146), disruption and digestion of axonemal components (147), and inhibition of ciliary motility (148,149). Comparison of the effects of human neutrophil elastase and *P. aeruginosa*–derived elastase and alkaline phosphatase on CBF and ultrastructure of human nasal cilia showed that *P. aeruginosa*–derived elastase and human neutrophil elastase caused epithelial disruption (20–500 µg/mL) and slowing of CBF (100 µg/mL) (150). However the *P. aeruginosa*–derived elastase required the presence of divalent metal ions to exert its cilioinhibitory effects. Alkaline phosphatase had no effect on epithelial integrity or on CBF (150).

P. aeruginosa also produces a hemolysin/rhamnolipid (148) and several phenazine derivatives (148,149,151), in particular pyocyanin and 1-hydroxyphenazine (149,151). In vitro studies showed that pyocyanin caused dose-dependent slowing of human ciliary beating and, eventually, ciliostasis and epithelial disruption at high concentrations, whereas 1-hydroxyphenazine caused a more rapid onset ciliostasis without epithelial disruption (149). In guinea pig trachea 1-hydroxyphenazine (200 ng) induced a rapid but reversible decrease in TMV with a maximum fall of 47% after 20 minutes (152). Pyocyanin (600 ng) had a slower onset, with a maximum decrease in TMV of 60% after 3 hours, and was irreversible (152). The action of these two agents in combination was additive on CBF in vitro but appeared to be synergistic on TMV in vivo. The TMV response was biphasic, with an initial rapid decrease in TMV attributed to 1-

hydroxyphenazine followed by a late-onset slowing of TMV that was significantly greater than expected for the dose of pyocyanin alone. This enhanced effect has been attributed to the 1-hydroxyphenazine inhibition of MCC, allowing greater exposure of pyocyanin to the mucosa (152). Catalase blocked the inhibitory effects of *P. aeruginosa*–derived supernatant, as well as the individual constituents pyocyanin and 1-hydroxyphenazine. This indicates that the inhibitory effects are mediated, at least in part, by the presence of neutrophils and the generation of oxygen free radicals both in vitro (153) and in vivo (154).

Very high concentrations (2.8–5.6 mg/mL) of the *P. aeruginosa*–derived hemolysin caused, in addition to ciliostasis, demembranation of the cilia, cellular disruption, and a loss of dynein arms from the axoneme of rabbit tracheal cilia (147). Similarly, high concentrations (250–10000 μg/mL) caused ciliostasis of guinea pig tracheal and human nasal cilia within 3 hours (155). However, more "pathophysiologically relevant" doses of rhamnolipid (65–125 μg/mL) did not reduce the CBF of guinea pig tracheal cilia but did reduce the CBF (26% at 100 μg/mL) of human nasal cilia. Ultrastructural examination of these cilia showed much less severe changes than observed in rabbit tracheal epithelium, with evidence of mitochondrial abnormalities and cytoplasmic blebbing at doses of 32 and 100 μg/mL. In vivo studies of MCC in guinea pig showed that a bolus dose of 5 μg/mL caused a 27% decrease in TMV over the 2-hour test period, but 10 μg/mL of rhamnolipid caused total loss of TMV after 10 minutes (155). Since rhamnolipid did not significantly affect ciliary beating at this concentration, it is likely that its influence on MCC may be via its other actions on mucus; it has been shown to act as a secretagogue in vivo in cats (156) and as an inhibitor of ion transport in sheep (156).

More recently, it has been shown that the reductions of human CBF in vitro induced by pyocyanin, 1-hydroxyphenazine, and rhamnolipid are associated with decreases in intracellular cyclic AMP and ATP (114,158,159). Agents that increase intracellular cAMP such as forskolin, isobutyl methylxanthine, and dibutyryl cAMP diminished the cilioinhibition induced by these bacterial toxins. Consistent with this, exogenous administration of ATP ameliorated depression of CBF in human cells, induced by a *P. aeruginosa*–derived lipopolysaccharide (160). β_2-Adrenoceptor agonists have also been shown to increase cAMP (107). Isoprenaline and salmeterol (a potent long-acting β_2 agonist) have been shown to inhibit the cilioinhibition and mucosal damage induced by *P. aeruginosa* infection in vitro (161) and by the *P. aeruginosa*–derived toxins by raising intracellular cAMP and ATP (114,159).

Staphylococcus Aureus

Cultures of *S. aureus* have also been shown to contain a hemolysin (rhamnolipid), which causes ciliostasis and cellular disruption in human ciliated epithelium (162).

Haemophilus Influenzae

H. influenzae has so far been shown to produce at least two products that cause inhibition of ciliary activity in vitro. The first is a heat-stable lipopolysaccharide, which caused a gradual loss of ciliary activity and disruption of the ciliated epithelium (163,164). The second product was a heat-labile compound that caused very rapid inhibition of ciliary beating (165). Interestingly, preincubation of ciliated epithelium with subminimal inhibitory concentrations (MIC) of antibiotics, such as amoxycillin, loracarbef, and ciprofloxacin (166), or macrolide antibiotics, such as dirithromycin (167), can ameliorate the loss of CBF and the structural damage caused by *H. influenzae* infection of ciliated cells in vitro. In contrast, preincubation of *H. influenzae* with sub-MIC antibiotic prior to incubation with the ciliated epithelium did not inhibit toxin-induced mucosal damage (167), suggesting that the effects of the antibiotic were directly on the epithelial cells and not on the bacteria. The mechanism of this cytoprotective effect of sub-MIC antibiotics on ciliated epithelium is not clearly understood.

Kanthakumar and colleagues (159) showed that, similar to the *P. aeruginosa*–derived pyocyanin, rhamnolipid, and 1-hydroxyphenazine, two isolates of *H. influenzae* caused falls in intracellular cAMP and ATP in human ciliated epithelial cells. Furthermore, agents that increase intracellular cAMP such as salmeterol can prevent or ameliorate this toxin-induced inhibition of CBF (159,168).

Bordetella Pertussis

Studies of nasal ciliated epithelial biopsies from patients with *B. pertussis* infection showed that *B. pertussis* associated closely with cilia and that there was a loss of cilia and ciliated cells and damage to the ciliated epithelium (169). Further studies with filtrates from *B. pertussis* cultures (170) have isolated a peptidoglycan cytotoxin that caused very similar structural effects on human ciliated epithelium in vitro (i.e., extrusion of ciliated cells, loss of cilia and ciliated cells, and toxic changes) (17,169). There were no apparent direct effects on ciliary beat frequency—the loss of CBF being attributed to the loss of cells (169).

Streptococcus Pneumoniae

Culture filtrates from *S. pneumoniae* cause slowing of CBF in human nasal and tracheal cilia (171). Further study and purification of the filtrate resulted in the identification of pneumolysin as the active agent. Purified pneumolysin caused a dose-dependent decrease in CBF with 10 μg/mL producing a 50% decrease after 4 hours in the absence of ultrastructural changes. Higher concentrations (25–50 μg/mL) of pneumolysin caused disruption of the ciliated epithelium in vitro with appearance of cytoplasmic blebs, mitochondrial swelling, cellular extrusion, and cell death. Further studies with two isogenic strains of *S. pneumoniae* that varied in their capacity to produce pneumolysin showed that the mucosal damage and decrease in CBF occurred more rapidly in the pneumolysin-sufficient than the pneumolysin-deficient strain (172).

Mycoplasma Pneumoniae

Infection with *M. pneumoniae* has been shown to slow tracheobronchial mucociliary clearance (173) and to cause disorganized and slowed ciliary beating and disruption of the ciliated epithelium (174,175). The causative molecule has not been identified.

F. Cholinergics

The effect of acetylcholine on ciliary activity was studied by observing the movement of charcoal particles in an excised rabbit trachea (176). Acetylcholine (10^{-5} M) caused an increase in TMV (mean 27%), but the opposite was seen at 10^{-4} M (a mean reduction of 33%). Similarly, studies on explants of tracheal ciliated epithelium showed that at concentrations of 0.1–1% acetylcholine increased ciliary motion, while at 2.5% CBF was decreased and at 5% there was ciliostasis (177). In vivo studies on rats showed that acetylcholine increased CBF (178).

Methacholine (0.01–2 mg/kg) caused acceleration of mucociliary waves in rabbit maxillary sinus (179). These observations were extended by Wong and colleagues (180), who found that methacholine caused an increase in CBF in bovine tracheal cilia in vitro at 10^{-7} M. Aerosolized methacholine given to anesthetized dogs also resulted in ciliostimulation at 10^{-8}–10^{-6} M (181). A recent report indicates that pilocarpine (160 mg/kg) increases rat TMV (182).

G. Anticholinergics

Atropine has been the most intensively studied of the anticholinergics, with most studies demonstrating an impairment of ciliary activity or MCC. Atropine at a concentration of 10^{-6} M impaired the movement of charcoal particles in rabbit trachea in vitro (176). Similarly, in vitro concentrations of 0.1–2.5% caused cilioinhibition (177).

The effect of atropine premedication (0.4 mg IMI) on TMV has been studied in anesthetized patients compared to controls (183). Thirty minutes after intubation, TMV was significantly slower in the atropinized patients than controls. Similar results were demonstrated in sheep with a significant decrease in TMV reported in atropinized (0.2 mg/kg hourly) animals compared to controls (185). These authors also measured tracheal bacterial counts and demonstrated that atropine resulted in marked and significant persistence of viable bacteria after inhalation of a controlled bacterial aerosol. In rabbit maxillary sinus, atropine (0.05–0.5 mg/kg) did not influence mucociliary activity but did block methacholine-induced mucociliary wave acceleration (179). In contrast, an increase in TMV has been observed in dogs following administration of 0.4 mg of atropine (184). This result, which differs from other reports in the literature on the effect of atropine, is unexplained.

Bethanechol has been shown to increase tracheobronchial clearance measured after an inhalation of teflon particles, but methylscopolomine had no effect (186).

Hyoscine (mean dose 8 µg/kg), when given to a group of normal elderly subjects and patients with airway obstruction, caused a significant impairment of lung MCC (187).

The effects of the cholinergic antagonists atropine, ipratropium, and oxitropium have been studied on mucociliary clearance in pigeons and rabbits (188). All three drugs (10^{-4}–10^{-3} g/mL) inhibited normal mucociliary transport in pigeons. They also markedly inhibited eserine-induced mucociliary transport acceleration. Neither oxitropium nor ipratropium depressed normal mucociliary clearance in rabbits, but atropine may depress it under some conditions. Wanner has reviewed anticholinergics with particular reference to ipratropium bromide (189). He suggested that while atropine depresses ciliary beat frequency and slows airway mucociliary clearance, short- and long-term administration of ipratropium bromide at doses higher than clinically recommended does not. No satisfactory explanation has thus far been offered for this difference between these two cholinergic antagonists.

Ipratropium bromide has been studied extensively and appears to have no effect on either MCC or CBF in animal and human studies even at four times the therapeutic dose (190–192).

H. Complementary Medicines

Despite their increasingly widespread use, there is little published literature on the effect of complementary medicines on ciliary function.

Sugiura and colleagues (193) cited the work of Esaki et al., which demonstrated that the herbal medicine sairei-to enhances in vitro activity of cilia from the eustachian tubes of healthy guinea pigs in a dose-dependent manner. They extended this work to in vivo studies in healthy guinea pigs and demonstrated no significant changes in either CBF or MCC following administration of 120 mg/kg of sairei-to (equivalent to the usual human dose) (193). However, at 600 mg/kg of sairei-to, CBF was enhanced, but there was no acceleration of mucociliary clearance time in the tubotympanum. They also studied guinea pigs that had otitis media with effusion secondary to intratympanic injection of lipopolysaccharide solution derived from *Klebsiella pneumoniae*. CBF and MCC were impaired significantly in these guinea pigs, and pretreatment with sairei-to did not reduce such impairment (194).

The effects of menthol, eucalyptus oil, and pine needle oil, separately and in combination, on human nasal cilia have been investigated in vitro (195). Dose-dependent decreases in CBF were reported when cilia were exposed to a vapor mixture of all three essential oils (maximum decrease of 22% at a concentration of 10 g/m^3), eucalyptus oil alone (32.5% at a concentration of 7.5 g/m^3), and pine needle oil alone (56.1% at a concentration of 9.4 g/m^3). This study was carried out in vitro; the relevance to clinical practice awaits in vivo investigation.

I. Corticosteroids

Corticosteroids, both oral and inhaled, are widely used in the treatment of both upper and lower respiratory tract diseases. Studies of the effects of different steroid preparations have produced conflicting results.

Beclomethasone diproprionate (BDP) (0.005–0.1 mg/mL) and flunisolide (0.025–0.05 mg/mL) have been shown to cause significant and dose-dependent reductions in CBF of human nasal CBF in vitro (196). Both agents were used as aqueous preparations, the formulations used in metered dose aerosol inhalers. However, BDP has been found to have no effect on the nasal saccharin clearance time in normal subjects after one week of treatment (199). Propylene glycol, the main preservative used in the flunisolide preparation, also caused cilioinhibition that was partially reversible (196). Some of the effect of the topical steroids used was due to preservative, but this did not explain all the cilioinhibition seen.

Topical BDP did not affect tracheal mucus velocity in sheep (134), but prednisolone, when applied to rat bronchial mucosa, produced a dose-related increase in CBF at concentrations of 10^{-6}–10^{-3} mg/mL, resulting in a CBF increase of 4–43% (197). Corticosterone had no effect on pigeon TMV at 1 mg/kg, but 5 mg/kg caused a small increase in TMV (198).

Since corticosteroids are used so widely, any effect on CBF or MCC may be of clinical importance. Since these drugs, given systemically, are often used for treating diseases that may themselves be associated with impaired MCC, the clinical significance of any further decrease in clearance may be compounded. On the other hand, where an improvement in MCC or CBF is caused by steroid therapy this may contribute to the drug's efficacy (e.g., in asthma, ciliostimulation may add to the anti-inflammatory effects of systemic steroids). Topical steroids and preservatives used in pharmaceutical preparations are often present at high concentrations in areas of nasal mucosa affected by the impact of aerosol sprays, and this applies also to sites of deposition of nasal drops (196). It has been suggested that impairment of CBF and MCC in patients with nasal pathology may be potentiated by the cilioinhibitory effects of topical steroids and preservatives (196). It is not known how long such cilioinhibition, which can extend to cessation of ciliary activity, persists. The clinical significance of this requires further study.

J. Diuretics

Frusemide (furosemide) is a loop diuretic that inhibits the $Na^+/K^+/Cl^-$ and NaCl co-transport systems at the basolateral membrane of epithelial cells. When inhaled, frusemide may modify the water content of the periciliary fluid layer and interfere with mucociliary clearance. Nebulized frusemide (40 mg) has no effect on lung MCC in normal and stable asthmatic subjects (200,201).

Amiloride has been shown to have a small (<10%) but statistically significant effect on human bronchial cilia studied in vitro (202). However, this increase was short-lived, and its clinical significance is doubtful. This is consistent with several studies of the effect of amiloride on MCC in patients with CF (203–205). In normal adults aerosolized UTP improved MCC, but the addition of nebulized amiloride to the UTP did not produce any further increase (206).

K. Ethanol

Studies of the effect of ethanol on the in vitro activity of sheep tracheal cilia indicate there are different effects on CBF at different concentrations. Ethanol at 0.01–0.1% caused ciliostimulation, 0.5–1% caused no change in CBF, while 2% caused ciliostasis (207).

Similarly, studies of bovine cilia showed that ethanol rapidly stimulated bovine CBF in a concentration-dependent manner (>10 mM). The effect was sustained for several hours. CBF did not decrease until concentrations of >1000 mM (208). At these concentrations ethanol stimulates the release of NO, suggesting that NO is the mediator that upregulates CBF. Propanol and isopropanol had no such effects, and methanol caused a transient rise in CBF.

Acetaldehyde is produced in physiologically significant quantities in the metabolism of ethanol and causes ciliary dysfunction. In cultured bovine bronchial ciliated epithelial cells, acetaldehyde caused a dose-dependent slowing of CBF at concentrations >15 µM and ciliostasis at concentrations above 250 µM (209). Acetaldehyde also inhibited ciliary ATPase activity above 30 µM. Similar findings were reported with other aldehydes, but ethanol itself had no effect on ciliary beating or ATPase activity in this model.

The effect of ingested ethanol (0.5 g/kg) on mucociliary clearance has also been measured by inhaled radiolabeled aerosol technique (IRAT) (210). There was no significant difference for the mean clearance rates between normal subjects who drank ethanol and a control group. However, there was increased variability in clearance rates after ethanol ingestion. The authors suggested that acute ethanol ingestion, at levels achieved during social drinking, alters MCC, with the direction and magnitude of changes varying among individuals.

L. Growth Factors, Hormones, and Cytokines

Angiotensin II is a circulating bioactive peptide that is present in the lung and airways. In vitro studies with rabbit tracheal cilia showed that angiotensin II dose-dependently stimulates CBF to a maximum of ~36% within 10 minutes (211). The effects are mediated by specific receptors and experiments with indomethacin, calcium chelators, and channel blockers indicate that the effect is dependent upon Ca^{2+} influx and subsequent activation of the arachadonic/ cyclooxygenase pathway leading to production of prostaglandin E_2. The angiotensin II effect did not involve altered levels of intracellular cAMP.

Atrial natriuretic factor (ANF) is a peptide growth factor released from heart atrium that has diuretic, natriuretic, and vasoactive properties. ANF receptors have been localized to the lung, and ANF is released in asthma and in pulmonary hypertension secondary to hypoxia. The activity of ANF is regulated, in part, by neutral endopeptidases. ANF decreases CBF of rabbit tracheal cilia up to a maximum of 24% at 10^{-6} M (212). Inhibitors of neutral endopeptidases potentiated its action, suggesting that, in vivo, these enzymes may play an important role in modulating the effects of ANF. The intracellular mechanism of ANF action involved increased levels of cGMP, implicating the involvement of a guanylate cyclase–dependent pathway. ANF did not appear to influence CBF via the arachadonic acid pathway.

Macrophage-stimulating protein (MSP) is mainly produced by hepatocytes and has structural homology to hepatocyte growth factor. Since it has been detected in bronchoalveolar lavage fluid, MSP is thought to be transported to the lung via the circulation. Expression studies show that its receptor (RON tyrosine kinase) is located on the apical surface of ciliated epithelia in the airways and oviduct (213). MSP binds with high affinity to these receptors and activates a significant and dose-dependent increase in CBF of human nasal cilia (maximum increase of 20% at 10 ng/mL). MSP exerts multiple biological effects on macrophages, but its biological significance in other cell systems is still unclear.

Calcitonin gene–related peptide (CGRP) is a neuropeptide that is released in the human nasal mucosa after trigeminal nerve stimulation. In vitro studies of the effect of CGRP on CBF of human adenoid epithelium, using computerized microscope photometry, showed that CGRP induced a significant dose-dependent (10^{-9}–10^{-6} M) stimulation of CBF with a maximum of 23% (214).

Corticotropin-releasing factor (CRF) and adrenocorticotropin (ACTH) are CNS neuropeptides that are released into the circulation and occur in various peripheral tissues, including the lung. Both CRF and ACTH dose-dependently stimulated CBF with maximal stimulation of 25% (10^{-7} M) and 34% (10^{-6} M), respectively (215). The ciliostimulatory effects were mediated by the activation of specific receptors leading to the activation of adenylate cyclase with resultant increase in cAMP. CRF- but not ACTH-induced ciliostimulation involved an influx of calcium.

Endothelins (ET) are peptides that are potent vaso- and bronchoconstrictors. Computerized photometric microscopy has been used to study the effects of ET-1, -2, and -3 on the mucociliary activity of rabbit maxillary sinus and trachea, both in vitro and in vivo. All three endothelins increased mucociliary activity of both sinus and tracheal mucosa in vivo with the effects being greater in sinus than in trachea (218). Similar ciliostimulation was found in vitro. By use of specific blockers of calcium and the cyclooxygenase pathway, it was shown that the mechanism of ciliostimulation involved prostaglandin synthesis but not release of intracellular calcium (218). However, studies of tracheal mucus velocity (TMV) in sheep showed that aerosolized ET-1 (10^{-9}–10^{-6} M) induced a significant decrease in TMV to a maximum of 54% at 10^{-6} M (216). The effects are mediated via the specific ET-A (but not ET-B) receptor and are not inhibited by indomethacin or leukotriene receptor antagonists, indicating lack of involvement of the cyclooxygenase/prostaglandin pathway or leukotrienes. In contrast, in vitro studies have shown that ET-1 stimulates CBF in dog tracheal cilia and in rabbit nasal and tracheal cilia (217). These ciliostimulatory effects are partially inhibited by indomethacin and reduction of extracellular calcium, suggesting that ET-1 stimulates CBF via calcium and prostaglandin synthesis. However, because ET-1 also stimulates chloride and mucus secretion (217), it is possible that some of the effects on TMV may be mediated by changes in the properties of the secreted mucus.

Immunohistochemical staining showed endothelins to be present in both maxillary and tracheal epithelium of the rabbit, suggesting that these molecules probably do have a biological role in these epithelia (218).

Vasoactive intestinal peptide (VIP) is known to act as a neurotransmitter in the central and peripheral nervous systems and is present in the lungs and airways. VIP causes a dose-dependent increase in CBF of rabbit tracheal cilia in vitro, with a maximum increase of ~17% at 10^{-7} M (219). The effect of VIP appears to be mediated by specific cell surface receptors and involves increases in intracellular cAMP but not the arachadonic/cyclooxygenase pathway.

M. Histamines

Histamine (see Sec. IV. P).

N. Antihistamines

Azelastine is an oral, long acting antiallergy medication that inhibits histamine release and leukotriene synthesis and has some anti-inflammatory action by suppression of inflammatory mediators. Perfusion of azelastine into preparations of human bronchial cilia in vitro has been shown to cause a dose-dependent increase in CBF (220). Azelastine inhibited the reduction in CBF produced when ciliated cells were exposed to 3 ppm SO_2 (220). In contrast, topical application of a commercially available preparation of azelastine (0.1%) nasal spray to rat tracheal preparations impaired CBF in a dose-dependent manner (221). In studies such as these there is always concern that cilioinhibition is caused by components in the topical preparation other than the drug being studied.

Diphenhydramine and hydroxyzine have both been reported to cause dose-dependent ciliostasis of CBF in rat tracheal explants (2.5 mg/mL diphenhydramine; 1.0 mg/kg hydroxyzine).

Intravenous administration of cimetidine (150 mg), an H_2 blocker, has been reported to cause small (23% after 1 h) but significant increases in TMV in anesthetized dogs (222). This study suggested that cimetidine, unlike H_1 blockers, does not depress and may possibly improve MCC. Some support for this comes from studies by Esaki and colleagues (223), who investigated the effect of diphenhydramine (10^{-6} M; H_1 blocker) and cimetidine (10^{-6} M) on the ciliary activity in the middle ear of guinea pigs in vitro and in vivo after perfusion with histamine. They reported that histamine (10^{-8} M–10^{-4} M) increased CBF. Such ciliostimulation was not affected by diphenhydramine (10^{-6} M) but was reduced by cimetidine (10^{-6} M), suggesting that histamine stimulates ciliary activity by binding to H_2 receptors.

Another antihistamine, tramazoline hydrochloride, commonly used as a topical nasal medication, did not affect human CBF measured in vitro when applied in recommended doses (224). However, at four times the clinical dose ciliostasis occurred.

O. Inflammatory Mediators

Histamine

Histamine is a potent mediator involved in the early stages of allergic reactions and inflammation. Histamine inhalation challenge (100 mL, 8 mg/mL) in anesthetized monkeys has been shown to cause a very large increase in tracheal mucociliary activity (250%) (236). In contrast, in vitro studies in sheep (223) and guinea pig middle ear cilia (247) showed only relatively small increases in CBF. These ciliostimulatory effects were apparently mediated by the H_2 receptor as they were inhibited by cimetidine. Injection of histamine into the tympanic cavity of guinea pigs resulted in reduced ciliary activity, increased mucociliary clearance time, pathological changes in the ciliary mucosa and middle ear effusions. The pathological changes included inflammatory cell infiltration, cytoplasmic vacuolation and protrusion, compound cilia, and nuclear pyknosis (247).

Proteases

Proteolytic enzymes are released in inflammatory lung disease by activated polymorphonuclear cells. Neutrophils release an elastase that has been shown to inhibit ciliary activity and to damage the respiratory epithelium (145,150). Sputum from patients with bronchiectasis inhibits human ciliary activity, and this inhibitory activity is associated with a serine protease, probably elastase (145). Similarly, human neutrophil elastase, purified from empyema, caused epithelial disruption and, at high concentrations (500 µg/mL), slowing of CBF (150).

Neuropeptide Y

Neuropeptide Y is a potent vasoconstrictor that is released from sympathetic nerves in the peripheral nervous system. The upper respiratory tract is rich in nerve fibers that are immunoreactive for neuropeptide Y. Cervin and colleagues showed in rabbit maxillary sinus in vivo that neuropeptide Y (0.1–5.0 µg/kg) caused a dose-dependent decrease in mucociliary wave activity of up to 14.6% at 5.0 µg/kg (238). The effects of neuropeptide Y were not influenced by pretreatment with α-adrenoceptor antagonists but were modulated by calcium antagonists, suggesting that the inhibitory effects are mediated via calcium and not via cAMP. These same authors, using the same system, subsequently showed that neuropeptide Y can also inhibit the cholinergic stimulation of CBF (238,239). A more recent study also indicates that neuropeptide Y has a direct inhibitory effect on CBF in vitro (240). This inhibitory effect is mediated via a novel form of PKC, but not PKA, and is Ca^{2+}-dependent.

Substance P

A number of studies have investigated the effect of substance P on mucociliary activity (see Table 1). In vivo studies in rabbit (241) and dog (242) showed large and significant increases in mucociliary activity (up to 300% in dogs). It has been further demonstrated, using various inhibitors, that this effect may be mediated via a cyclooxygenase-dependent parasympathetic reflex (242).

In vitro studies have reported conflicting results. Two studies have shown little or no effect of substance P on rabbit, guinea pig, or human cilia (243,244). They concluded that the increase in mucociliary activity seen in previous in vivo studies reflected effects of substance P on mucus and chloride secretion.

However, more recently, a very carefully controlled study by Smith and colleagues showed that substance P causes a transient, small (9%), but dose-dependent increase in CBF of human cilia (245). The increase in CBF was linked to changes in intracellular calcium concentration, and the authors suggest that methodological differences may account for the varying results shown in previous studies with substance P (245). Similarly, Schlosser and colleagues (246) showed a small (12%) increase in CBF of human cilia with substance P that involved the synthesis and release of prostaglandins and nitric oxide.

Leukotrienes

Leukotrienes (LTC_4 and LTD_4) are potent bronchoconstrictors and have been shown to act as inflammatory mediators in asthma and allergic reactions. There have been several contradictory studies on the effects of these mediators on mucociliary function (247–251). Tamaoki and colleagues (248) found that LTD_4 (10^{-7} M) stimulated CBF of dog tracheal cilia (29%) in vitro at 37°C. Similarly, Wanner et al. (252) showed that LTD_4 (10^{-7}–10^{-9} M) stimulated the CBF of sheep bronchial cilia (13–16%) at 39°C. In contrast, Bisgaard and Pedersen (250) found that 10^{-7} M decreased CBF (~10%) of cultured human cilia at 25°C. Similarly, Ganbo and colleagues (249) found that concentrations in the range of 10^{-6}–10^{-8} M inhibited human eustachian tube cilia at 37°C. Finally, Dolata and coworkers showed that intravenous administration of 0.01–10 nmol/kg did not alter mucociliary activity in rabbit maxillary sinus in vivo (251).

The variations in response described by these studies may be attributable to the different experimental conditions used (particularly temperature and hence baseline CBF) and also to variations in responsiveness between species. A recent study by Joki and coworkers (253) showed that guinea pig, rat, and human cilia show dose-dependent stimulation of CBF in all species but different sensitivity to LTD_4. Maximal stimulation occurred at 10^{-9} M in guinea pig (75% increase), 10^{-7} M in rat (119%), and 10^{-6} M in human (86%). Their observations by scanning electron microscopy indicated that LTD_4 also stimulated mucus secretion and impaired the orientation of cilia. The same group showed that the response to LTD_4 is age-dependent in guinea pigs, with older animals, which have a lower baseline CBF, showing a greater response than younger animals (254).

Leukotriene C_4 increased activity of sheep tracheal cilia in vitro (247), decreased activity of chicken tracheal cilia (255), but had no effect on human adenoid cilia (356).

Prostaglandins

Prostaglandins are metabolites of arachadonic acid, produced in the cyclooxygenase pathway, that act as inflammatory mediators, particularly in Type 1 (IgE-mediated) allergic reactions. The effects of several prostaglandins on ciliary activity have been studied.

Prostaglandin E_2 has been shown to increase CBF or MCA of rabbit oviduct (257), rabbit maxillary sinus (258), hamster ependyma (259), sheep trachea (247), and human nasal (260,262) and adenoid (262) cilia. In human adenoid cilia it has been shown that prostaglandin E_2 causes a significant dose-dependent stimulation of CBF, with a maximum increase of 37% (262). However, prostaglandins E_2 and $F_{2\alpha}$ had only mild stimulatory effects (11–18%) on CBF of hamster tracheal cilia and ependymal cilia in vitro (259). In rabbit oviducts, the stimulatory effect of prostaglandin E_2 on ciliary activity appears to be mediated by release of intracellular calcium (257). Prostaglandin E_2 has also been implicated as a mediator in the ciliostimulatory effects of bradykinin (263).

Prostaglandin D_2, on the other hand, seems to have no effect on ciliary motility (261,262).

Fewer studies have been conducted on prostaglandin F_2. Prostaglandin F_2 caused a 75% increase in CBF of cultured oviduct cilia (257) and a 24% increase in MCA of rabbit sinus (258) in vivo. In human ependymal and tracheal cilia prostaglandin F_2, at concentrations of 10^{-8}–10^{-5} M, it caused a dose-independent increase in CBF of 7% and 13%, respectively (259). Slater and colleagues investigated the effect of nasal polyp fluid, histamine, and prostaglandins D_2, E_2, and $F_{2\alpha}$ on the CBF of cilia from patients with nasal polyps. Polyp fluid increased CBF, as did prostaglandin E_2 and $F_{2\alpha}$. Histamine and prostaglandin D_2 had no effect (261).

Prostacyclin is a metabolite of arachadonic acid and a precursor to prostaglandin $F_{1\alpha}$. Both prostacyclin and its more stable analogue, beraprost, stimulate CBF in a dose-dependent manner over a similar concentration range (10^{-8}–10^{-5} M) (264). However, the magnitude and time course of the effect differed: prostacyclin had a transient effect with a maximal increase in CBF of 13.3% at 0.5×10^{-6} M that returned to baseline after 15 minutes. Beraprost, on the other hand, induced a maximal increase of 30% at the same concentration, and this level of ciliostimulation was maintained for at least 30 minutes (264).

Hydrogen Peroxide

Inflammatory lung injury involves the sequestration and activation of polymorphonuclear leukocytes (PMNs). Activated PMNs produce a wide range of metabolites including degradative enzymes, arachadonic acid metabolites, and reactive oxygen species (265).

The effects of reactive oxygen species, generated from activated PMNs, on human cilia have been studied and shown to cause a reduction in human CBF (265). Catalase and ascorbic acid inhibition suggested that this was attributable partially to H_2O_2 and partially to free radicals. Other PMN products may also be involved.

H_2O_2 has been shown to directly cause a dose-dependent decrease in CBF at low concentrations ($<10^{-6}$ M) (266). The cilioinhibition was reversible and not associated with cytotoxicity. At concentrations less than 10^{-6} M recovery of CBF was incomplete or irreversible, and there were significant morphological lesions of the epithelium. This study also showed that cilioinhibition at the lower concentrations involved protein kinase C activation.

Serotonin

Although there are numerous studies in the literature that document the effects of serotonin (5-hydroxytryptamine, 5-HT) on cilia from mussels (see, for example, Ref. 267), very few studies have addressed the effects of serotonin on mammalian cilia. In the ciliated epithelium of the frog palate, serotonin (10^{-6} M) accelerated mucociliary transport (268). Serotonin has been demonstrated histochemically to be present in the mucosa and is probably synthesized by the epithelial cells (268). It is likely, based on studies of mussel cilia, that serotonin acts to stimulate CBF via activation of adenylate cyclase and increased cAMP. However, in the one study of mammalian cilia (rat trachea) it appears that serotonin does not change CBF significantly (197).

P. Inhaled Substances

A wide variety of inhaled substances have been shown in animals and in humans to reduce MCC and ciliary activity. These include sulfuric acid (225), aerosol hairspray (226), formaldehyde (227), and sulfur dioxide (228).

MCC in rabbits exposed to sulfuric acid mist (250 μg/m^3) for 1 hour a day was significantly reduced within the first month of exposure. MCC was further decreased over a 1-year period of continued exposure (225).

Exposure of rabbit tracheal cilia to sulfur dioxide (SO_2) at concentrations of 200 ppm in vivo caused significant reductions in CBF and TMV (228). However, much lower concentrations (10 ppm) caused ciliostasis when applied directly to ciliated epithelium in vitro (228).

Formaldehyde (10 ppm) applied directly to rabbit trachea in vitro caused ciliostasis (228). More recently, formaldehyde has been reported to cause a concentration-dependent but reversible reduction in CBF of rabbit and pig tracheal ciliary explants after exposure to formaldehyde (16–66 μg/mL) (226).

Studies of the acute effects of aerosol hairspray on TMV in healthy nonsmokers indicate that aerosol hair preparations can cause a significant but transient reduction in TMV of 57% 1 hour after a 20-second exposure. No changes were reported in controls exposed to the propellant alone (227).

Smoking

Cigarette smoke consists of a complex group of substances that can affect MCC and CBF. In general, long-term cigarette smoking impairs MCC. However, in a study of healthy smokers, nonsmokers, and ex-smokers, we found no significant difference in CBF (229).

Impairment of human TMV has been reported in smokers to precede abnormalities in spirometry (71,230). Similarly, a reduction in MCC, measured by IRAT, has been reported in young smokers with normal spirometry (83). In a survey of smokers it was found that MCC in patients with bronchitis was decreased and that there was a significant correlation between the extent of smoking (pack-years) and the reduction in MCC (231). This work suggests that decreased MCC is an early functional abnormality in smokers that may precede both the development of symptoms of bronchitis and detectable airway obstruction.

In general, cigarette smoke causes cilioinhibition, but the role of individual constituents has not been fully elucidated. Nicotine alone caused a transient stimulation of CBF measured in ferret tracheal epithelial strips in vitro which were free of mucus (232). Nicotine bitartrate (0.5–10 µg/kg) has also been shown to cause acute transient stimulation of mucociliary wave frequency in rabbit maxillary sinus in vivo in a dose-dependent manner (233).

Several different aldehydes have been identified in the vapor phase of cigarette smoke. Acetaldehyde is present in greater concentrations than any other aldehyde and has been shown to bind covalently to several proteins, resulting in cellular dysfunction (209). Acetaldehyde slowed CBF in cultures of ciliated bovine bronchial epithelium in a concentration-dependent pattern at concentrations as low as 15–30 µM, and ciliostasis was seen at 250 µM. Acetaldehyde also inhibited ciliary ATPase activity in a concentration- and time-dependent manner at >30 µM. Similar findings were reported with other aldehydes, but not with ethanol.

In an in vitro study in which rabbit tracheal explants were exposed to cigarette smoke, it was shown histochemically that there was continued production of hydrogen peroxide and superoxide anion at the apical cell membrane with evidence of cell separation, focal membrane blebbing, cell disintegration, and loss of cilia (234). These effects were seen at even low doses of smoke and were dose-dependent. Sisson and colleagues (235) quantified similar changes in a bovine model. They reported a marked exfoliation of ciliated cells and concomitant increase in bronchial fluid dynein arm concentration after only very brief smoke exposure (smoke from a single cigarette). There was also evidence that, in smoke-exposed airways, the cilia were thinner and shorter than cilia exposed only to air (235).

Q. Mucolytics and Expectorants

Mucolytics are in wide clinical use with conflicting evidence of clinical efficacy. There is little evidence in the literature for a significant effect on ciliary function or MCC. Many studies report "trends and tendencies" rather than presenting findings with statistical significance.

N-Acetylcysteine (NAC) has been one of the most studied. Iravani and colleagues (269) studied the effects of NAC on mucus transport velocity and CBF in rabbits and rats, both healthy and with induced bronchitis. Their results indicated an increase in mucus velocity and CBF at low concentrations such as

$10^{-12}-10^{-10}$ g/mL with a fall in mucus velocity and CBF at higher concentrations (10^{-6} g/mL).

Similar effects have been reported in studies of canine tracheal CBF in vitro (270). In this model NAC caused an increase in CBF at 10^{-7} and 10^{-6} M with reductions at 10^{-4} and 10^{-3} M. In dogs, NAC induced a statistically significant ($p < 0.001$) increase in TMV after inhalation of a 20% aerosol (271). A modified form of NAC (*N*-acetylcysteine L-lysinate, L-NAC), administered as an aerosol (6 mg), has also been shown to increase TMV compared to placebo in dog trachea (273).

It has been demonstrated that in the general population there are normal subjects that have slightly "slowed" pulmonary MCC rates. Todisco and colleagues (272), in a double-blind, randomized crossover study with a selected group of "slow clearers," showed that NAC, given orally at a dose of 600 mg daily for 60 days, resulted in a statistically significant increase in MCC compared to baseline values. They postulated that there may be a subpopulation of patients who would benefit more from NAC treatment than others.

Olivieri and colleagues (274) conducted a double-blind crossover study comparing the effect of *N*-acetylcysteine (600 mg/day for 30 days) with placebo and demonstrated a significant increase in TMV in patients with chronic bronchitis. In this study, ambroxol produced a similar effect (see below).

Bromhexine has been studied in patients with bronchitis and shown to cause a small increase in MCC compared to baseline (275). In this study the improvement may have been due to shallower lung penetration of the aerosol than in the control subjects. However, no effect of bromhexine was demonstrated on rabbit mucociliary waves in vivo (276). In vitro studies indicated that bromhexine caused ciliostimulation of tracheal cilia only when the drug was perfused slowly (at $10^{-7}-10^{-5}$ M) (270).

Pavia and coworkers (117) reviewed several studies of bromhexine, which suggested that MCC was increased.

Ambroxol is a metabolite of bromhexine. Iravani and Melville demonstrated that ambroxol increased rat CBF in vitro (277). Further studies on guinea pig tracheal cells in vitro demonstrated that ambroxol (1–100 µmol/L) caused a small but statistically significant increase in CBF above control levels (278). The biological significance of these changes is open to question. In the same study, salbutamol (0.2–3.0 µmol/L) produced twice as much cilioexcitation, and another study (276) found no effect of ambroxol on rabbit mucociliary waves in vivo.

In studies on patients with chronic lung disease, treatment with ambroxol (30–120 mg orally/day for 3–14 days) did not lead to any improvement in MCC when measured by IRAT (279–281).

In a double-blind, crossover study comparing the effect of ambroxol (90 mg/day for 30 days) and *N*-acetylcysteine (600 mg/day for 30 days) in patients with chronic bronchitis, both drugs produced a similar significant increase in TMV compared to placebo (275).

Glycerol guaiacolate (guaiphenesin 600 mg in a single dose) was demonstrated in one study to have no effect on MCC in normal subjects but improved MCC in patients with chronic bronchitis (80). However, Clarke and Pavia quoted two studies in which guaiphenesin was given orally (single doses of 600 mg and 400 mg) without any effect on lung MCC (282).

S-Carboxymethylcysteine (S-CMC), at a dose of 4 g/day for 1 week, had no effect on MCC in patients with chronic obstructive bronchitis (283). Similarly S-CMC (0.35 g/kg) did not improve MCC in explanted rabbit trachea treated with elastase as a model for COPD (284).

Although S-CMC (0.05–0.5%) had no effect on in vitro CBF from healthy rabbit sinus and human nasal cilia, it did produce a dose-dependent increase in CBF of nasal cilia from patients with chronic sinusitis. This suggests that treatment with S-CMC may have no effect on normal mucociliary systems but may improve CBF that is pathologically slowed in chronic sinusitis (285).

R. Narcotics

Morphine and codeine are widely prescribed narcotic analgesics. Codeine impaired ciliary activity in a rat airway preparation at concentrations ranging from 10^{-7} g/mL (8% impairment) to 10^{-3} g/mL (28% impairment) (178). A similar impairment has been demonstrated in rat and guinea pig tracheal CBF in vitro (286). Concentrations of 1–10 mg/mL caused a 25% inhibition of CBF in rat tracheal explants in vitro. However, when codeine was given intravenously to rats (10 and 15 mg/kg) or subcutaneously to guinea pigs (3–30 mg/kg/day), ciliary activity was not affected significantly (286).

Morphine (10 μmol/L) had no significant effect on CBF of human nasal ciliated epithelium in vitro (287). However, at doses of 6 mg/kg, morphine depressed TMV in dogs during anesthesia with nitrous oxide (122). Similarly, in a very early study of feline clearance of insufflated barium sulfate, morphine at doses (0.5 mg/kg) below those required for an antitussive action (2 mg/kg) impaired clearance. Codeine had a similar effect (288).

Dextromethorphan, a semi-synthetic morphine derivative used widely as an antitussive agent, caused a decrease in CBF in a rat tracheal preparation at 1.0 mg/mL (17% impairment at 40 min) and at 10 mg/mL (21% impairment) (129).

S. Nonsteroidal Anti-inflammatory Drugs

Aspirin is a commonly used analgesic, antipyretic, and nonsteroidal anti-inflammatory agent that inhibits prostaglandin synthesis. The effect of aspirin on cultured nasal ciliary samples from patients with the clinical triad of asthma, aspirin intolerance, and nasal polyps has been investigated and shown not to influence CBF at doses up to 200 μg/mL (289). However, a moderate dose of aspirin (16 mg/kg, which resulted in serum levels of approximately 80 ± 2 µg/mL) induced a small (21%) but significant inhibition of TMV in nonsmokers when measured by IRAT (290).

Indomethacin is another nonsteroidal anti-inflammatory agent that inhibits the cyclooxygenase pathway and also stimulates the synthesis and release of lipoxygenase products. In rabbit tracheal rings, indomethacin induced a dose-dependent increase in CBF to a maximum of 36.5% at a concentration of 0.5×10^{-7} M. An inhibitor of the lipoxygenase pathway abolished this indomethacin-induced ciliostimulation (291). The effect of several arachadonic acid metabolites on human nasal CBF in vitro has also been studied. Iloprost, a prostacyclin analogue, significantly increased CBF by 12% at 10^{-8} M. This ciliostimulatory effect was blocked by indomethacin (260).

T. Osmotic Agents

Mannitol can provide an osmotic stimulus to the airways and in dry powder preparation has been shown to increase MCC measured by IRAT for healthy subjects and patients with asthma (293) and for patients with bronchiectasis (294). Hypertonic saline has been shown to have similar effects and to increase MCC in patients with chronic bronchitis (295), asthma (296), and cystic fibrosis (203). The mechanism of action is thought to be via altered mucus rheology and not by a direct action on ciliary function. There are no published studies on the effect of mannitol on CBF. It has been demonstrated that physiological saline (0.9%) reduces mean CBF to 46% within 10 minutes, whereas hypertonic saline led to ciliostasis: complete but reversible at 7% and irreversible at 14.4% (297).

U. Preservatives

Topical respiratory medications can result in ciliary paresis. Sometimes it is the preservative rather than the active pharmaceutical that causes this effect.

The effect of two preservatives (chlorbutol and benzalkonium chloride + EDTA) on the in vitro CBF of chicken embryo trachea and human adenoid tissue has been investigated. Exposure for 20 minutes with benzalkonium chloride at 0.006% was reported to cause decreases in CBF of 35% and 50% in human and chicken tissues, respectively. Chlorbutol 0.5% arrested CBF in both tissues at 5 minutes, but motion was restored after washing. Chlorbutol is a lipophilic preservative with rapid onset but reversible effect on CBF. Benzalkonium chloride combined with EDTA is a polar preservative, with slow but irreversible effects on ciliary motion (298).

The effect of methylparaben on ciliary activity has been studied on ferret tracheal rings in vitro. Concentrations as low as 0.06 mg/mL paralyzed cilia; at concentrations of 0.5 mg/mL, this effect was not fully reversible. When combined with lidocaine, as is the case in commercially available preparations, the ciliotoxic effects were additive (125).

Propylene glycol is a preservative that is present in aqueous preparations of two corticosteroid aerosols—BDP and flunisolide. It has been shown to cause a dose-dependent decrease in human nasal CBF in vitro after perfusion with 20 and 200 mg/mL (197).

V. Purines

Purines are nucleotide triphosphates that have been shown to be stimulators of ciliary activity.

ATP and Adenosine

In vitro studies of human (299,300) and animal cilia (301) have demonstrated that high concentrations of ATP (up to 10 mg/mL) can stimulate CBF.

In mucosal explants from healthy subjects and patients with chronic sinusitis, ATP (1–10 mg/mL) induced a small but statistically significant rise in CBF at 1 mg/mL (2.7% in chronic sinusitis group, 5% in normal subjects), with a more pronounced effect (19.6%) at 10 mg/mL (299). In a later study the same authors showed that exposure of rat tracheal cilia to ATP (0.01–1 mg/mL) in vitro increased CBF up to 10.5%. In vivo studies of ATP (1 mg/kg) infused intravenously increased CBF of guinea pig trachea by 29% (301).

The ciliostimulatory effects of ATP are inversely related to the baseline CBF. Using ATP concentrations of 10^{-5}–10^{-3} M, increases in CBF of up to 60% were seen in cilia that had a baseline of less than 9 Hz. The CBF of cilia with a baseline of less than 14 Hz increased by 40%, whereas cilia with a baseline greater than 14 Hz did not accelerate but appeared to normalize their beat pattern after administration of ATP (300). These results are consistent with earlier findings, which showed that ATP-induced increases in human nasal MCC occur mostly in patients with a lower than average baseline MCC (302).

In vivo studies on dogs (303) demonstrated that nucleotides and nucleosides modulate CBF through specific purinergic (P2) receptors on the luminal surface of dog trachea. In these experiments the dog tracheal mucosa was exposed, in vivo, to aerosolized purines and analogues. All the nucleotides studied (ATP, GTP, AMP-PNP, and GMP-PNP) were equipotent in stimulating CBF (~300%), and the stimulation was reversed within 30 minutes of cessation of exposure. As described above (see Sec. I), the ciliostimulatory effects of ATP are mediated by rises in intracellular calcium (34,304). In a recent study of the effects of ATP and UTP on rabbit tracheal cilia, it was suggested that ATP acts via two mechanisms that stimulate CBF maximally through a positive feedback loop. Extracellular ATP induces an initial rise in intracellular Ca^{2+} that activates the NO pathway and leads to activation of protein kinase G (PKG). Activated PKG (in the presence of elevated Ca^{2+}) leads to further enhancement of CBF and also induces, possibly via a cation-selective channel (34), an influx of Ca^{2+} (304).

In contrast to ATP, adenosine causes cilioinhibition. In rabbit tracheal cilia, adenosine ($10^{-5}1$–10^{-3} M) dose-dependently inhibited CBF up to 32% (45). It was further shown that this effect was mediated by a specific cell surface (A1) receptor that results in inhibition of adenylate cyclase and reduced intracellular cAMP (45). Similarly, in the dog trachea in vivo, aerosolized adenosine (10^{-5} M) reduced CBF, probably through specific P1 purinergic receptors on the luminal surface of cells (303).

UTP

Extracellular ATP and UTP mediate ciliary activity via extracellular nucleotide receptors (P2) on airway epithelia leading to an increase in intracellular calcium and, potentially, an increase in CBF (see Sec. I). Extracellular UTP has been shown to induce rapid increases in both intracellular Ca^{2+} and CBF (304).

The effects on MCC of aerosolized UTP (10^{-2} M), alone and in combination with amiloride (1.3×10^{-3} M), have been measured by the inhaled radiolabeled aerosol technique (IRAT) in healthy normal subjects. It was reported that UTP and UTP/amiloride significantly increased MCC (up to 250%) over the aerosolized vehicle or amiloride alone. It is uncertain whether the effects of UTP on MCC are due to direct effects on cilia or indirect ionic effects and altered mucus properties (201,305).

W. Xanthines

Methylxanthines affect MCC at several different levels. Theophylline-induced stimulation of MCC may be due to several mechanisms. It stimulates ciliary motility, probably mediated by inhibition of the enzyme phosphodiesterase, resulting in a decrease in the breakdown of cAMP. This is likely to have an effect on the intracellular supply of ATP (306). Theophylline increases secretion from bronchial glands (both directly and indirectly) and stimulates chloride secretion into the respiratory lumen, both of which result in an increase in water flux toward the airway lumen. As a bronchodilator it improves airway patency (306). The net result is enhancement of MCC. These effects have been reviewed extensively by Wanner (307).

Theophylline may also assist MCC indirectly by inhibiting airway inflammation and associated bronchial responsiveness, by inhibiting histamine release from mast cells and basophils, by stabilizing a variety of inflammatory cells, and by suppressing polymorphonuclear leukocyte activation (308).

Aminophylline is metabolized to theophylline, and their effects are similar. In rat airways, aminophylline increased CBF (268), a finding confirmed in human ciliated epithelium studied in vitro (309). Similarly, an analogue of theophylline, reproterol (7-[3-(β, 3,5-trihydroxyphenethylamino)-propyl]-theophylline), increased ciliary beat frequency of tracheal and bronchial cilia in vitro (310).

A number of studies have demonstrated an increase in MCC by aminophylline/theophylline. Canine tracheal transport rate was markedly increased

(311). Matthys and Kohler (87) measured clearance of radiolabeled red cells and found that theophylline increased MCC in some patients. These workers also studied infertile males and found that theophylline improved their clearance rate. On the other hand, no significant change in clearance could be demonstrated in normal subjects. However, an increase in MCC was inferred as a greater penetration of inhaled aerosol was observed after oral theophylline (4 mg/kg twice daily for 3 days) (312). Several studies in patients with obstructive airways disease have shown an improvement in clearance with theophylline (89,117,282,313,314). It has been suggested that theophylline stimulates mucus transport rate to a greater degree in central than in peripheral airways of patients with chronic obstructive airways disease (311).

V. Disease States

Ciliary function and MCC may be impaired in many disease states. MCC, measured either by IRAT or as tracheal mucus velocity (TMV), has been much more intensively studied than has ciliary function. Reports in the literature of the latter are sparse, mainly describing diseases where there is a primary abnormality of ciliary structure or function (e.g., PCD). Secondary abnormalities of ciliary function or structure have also been described (143,315–318).

Many of the drugs that have an effect on ciliary function or on clearance also cause bronchodilation, and where there is clinical improvement, differentiation between effects on airway caliber and the components of lung clearance can be difficult. As further information becomes available it may be helpful for clinical investigations of patients to include measurements of MCC and its components as well as airway function.

A. Asthma

MCC is decreased in stable asthma, and more so during acute attacks and during sleep (282,319–321). This appears to be related to abnormalities of mucus rather than impairment of ciliary function, which, measured in vitro as CBF, we have found to be within normal limits in asthmatics in remission (unpublished data).

Asthma is commonly treated with many drugs that are known to have an effect on cilia and MCC. These include β-adrenergic agonists, theophylline, as well as steroids (both inhaled and systemic).

Drug Effects in Asthma

Terbutaline (0.25 mg subcutaneously) has been shown to improve MCC (measured by IRAT) in asthmatics, although the increase in MCC was less than that found in normal subjects (322). A similar improvement was demonstrated when terbutaline was administered by metered dose inhaler, but no change in MCC was seen with use of a dry powder inhaler—the difference possibly being related to drug deposition (323). The possibility has been raised that terbutaline may inhibit the capacity of the mucociliary system to respond to increased mucus loads and that inhibition of calcium-induced ciliostimulation may be associated with β-agonist–related asthma deaths (see below) (109).

Salbutamol (albuterol) did not affect the reduced MCC (measured by IRAT) shown in sleeping asthmatic patients (320). A similar lack of improvement has been reported with theophylline (320,324). In contrast, there is one report in which aminophylline improved MCC in asthmatics (313).

Budesonide had no effect on TMV (324).

Ipratropium bromide (40 μg) did not affect MCC (measured by IRAT) in patients with reversible airways obstruction at a dose that caused bronchodilation (325).

Histamine increased MCC (measured by IRAT and TMV) in patients with asymptomatic asthma (321). In most studies of the effects of antigen inhalation in asthma, impaired MCC has been reported (326). This is thought to be due to release of chemical mediators and may be blocked by leukotriene antagonists and other drugs that inhibit these mediators.

Two osmotic agents have been shown to increase MCC in patients with asthma: mannitol (293) and hypertonic saline (296).

B. COPD: Chronic Bronchitis and Emphysema

Studies of the effect of COPD on MCC and ciliary function may be complicated by the effect(s) of cigarette smoking. Inhaled tobacco smoke may irritate and increase MCC and CBF initially (see above), or there may be no overall effect. However, in long-standing smokers who develop COPD, there is an impairment of MCC. Evidence for impaired CBF measured in vitro is much less strong than the evidence for an effect on MCC.

An impairment of MCC or its components may precede any other objective measure of pulmonary dysfunction (71). This suggests that, in some patients at least, reduced TMV may be one of the earliest objective manifestations. Tracheobronchial clearance was slowed in smokers with mild bronchitis and slowed further in patients with chronic bronchitis (83,230).

Ciliary beating in rats with chronic bronchitis appears discoordinated (327). We have found intrinsic ciliary beat frequency measured in samples of both nasal and tracheobronchial epithelium in vitro to be no different from that found in normal subjects who had never smoked and smokers who had abstained from smoking for 12 hours (unpublished data).

Patients with chronic bronchitis have slowed MCC compared to a control group of healthy non-smokers (81,281,328).

Clearance has been reported to be normal in patients with emphysema associated with α_1-antitrypsin deficiency and with no history of chronic bronchitis (329), suggesting that in COPD chronic bronchitis is more strongly associated with impaired MCC than is emphysema.

In patients with COPD who have bronchoconstriction, inhaled aerosols are deposited more centrally. This may lead to reports of a falsely elevated MCC (275). Whenever the inhaled radiolabeled aerosol method is used, it is important for penetration of the aerosol to be equivalent between study groups or for allowances to be made for any differences in aerosol penetration.

Chronic Bronchitis—Drug Effects

Terbutaline has been shown to increase TMV in patients with COPD, but not in normal subjects (330). However, terbutaline did not improve MCC measured by TMV in patients with chronic bronchitis (331) or measured by IRAT (328). In healthy subjects, but not in patients with chronic bronchitis, terbutaline caused ciliostimulation (22). However, recent work has suggested that terbutaline inhibits the increases in CBF caused by mechanical loads (see above) (109). This raises concerns that in patients where mucus load is increased (such as in exacerbations of chronic bronchitis or where patients with asthma have mucus plugging), terbutaline might impair ciliary beating. These studies need to be extended to other β agonists.

Salbutamol (albuterol) improved MCC (measured by IRAT) in both chronic bronchitis and normal subjects (332), as did clembuterol (279), another β-adrenergic agonist.

Formoterol, given by aerosol for 6 days, increased MCC in patients with chronic bronchitis (108).

Aminophylline improved MCC (measured by IRAT) in patients with chronic bronchitis (313,333).

Ipratropium bromide did not affect MCC (measured by IRAT) in chronic bronchitic patients (192,329).

A number of mucolytic agents have been studied in chronic bronchitis. Ambroxol (90 mg/day for 30 days) increased TMV in chronic bronchitis patients (274), but this was not supported by several other studies (279,281). N-Acetylcysteine improved clearance in chronic bronchitic patients (274). Several workers have reported that bromhexine increases clearance in chronic bronchitis (117,275). Glycerol guaiacolate has been reported to increase MCC in chronic bronchitis in one study (80) but not in others (109). S-Carboxymethylcysteine, in one study of chronic bronchitic patients, did not improve clearance (283). Hypertonic saline increased MCC in patients with chronic bronchitis (295).

C. Bronchiectasis

Several studies have demonstrated impaired MCC in patients with bronchiectasis regardless of the underlying cause.

Bronchiectasis Due to Cystic Fibrosis

Some investigators of airway clearance in cystic fibrosis (CF) have measured removal of aerosolized particles from the lung and concluded that mucus clearance was normal in CF (110,334). However, a later study demonstrated impaired MCC in patients with CF; the initial reports of an increased clearance may have been due to a failure to compensate for central deposition of aerosol in an IRAT study (335).

Both intrinsic CBF (97) and ciliary ultrastructure (336) are normal in CF.

In 1967 a ciliary dyskinesia factor thought to be present in the serum of patients with CF was described (337). It was suggested that this factor caused the respiratory manifestations of CF by disrupting ciliary beating and impairing MCC. This has subsequently been disproved (338).

Drug Effects in CF

Terbutaline caused a marked increase in TMV in patients with CF (110). Hypertonic saline increases MCC in CF (203).

Bronchiectasis Due to PCD

There have been many reports of impaired MCC in PCD (81,339–342). Comparison of MCC in CF and PCD showed that both groups had impaired MCC, but for a given degree of clinical impairment, MCC was slower in PCD than in CF (137). In PCD CBF is grossly abnormal, and it is well established that ultrastructural defects in cilia are the basis for this impaired ciliary motility, with dynein arm defects being the most common (229,343). It is known that dynein arms contain ATPase. There is a correlation between intrinsic CBF and dynein arm areas (344) and dynein arm numbers (229) measured on electron micrographs. There is currently interest in the use of purine analogues in patients with PCD, but this has not yet reached clinical use.

Bronchiectasis due to Young's Syndrome

Young's syndrome consists of obstructive zoosperm together with recurrent sinobronchial disease (345). MCC is reduced (346, 347), but there is no significant abnormality of CBF, ciliary beat patterns, or ciliary ultrastructure (348).

Drug Effects in Young's Syndrome

Ambroxol, bromhexine, *N*-acetylcysteine, and carbocysteine have been studied in Young's syndrome, but none were shown to improve MCC (349).

Bronchiectasis of Unknown Cause

MCC is reduced in bronchiectasis of unknown cause to the same degree as in patients with chronic bronchitis (135). CBF in these patients was normal (229).

Secretions from patients with purulent bronchiectasis cause slowed CBF in vitro, and it is postulated that this slowing might be due to elastase (145). When elastase activity was inhibited with human α_1-antitrypsin, the slowing was reversed. Sputum from bronchiectasis patients treated with amoxycillin for 2 weeks had no detectable elastase activity and little effect on CBF (145).

Mannitol has been shown to improve MCC in patients with bronchiectasis (294).

D.   Acute Respiratory Infections

MCC is impaired in many acute respiratory tract infections. Microorganisms may affect ciliary function, structure, or the mucus component of MCC.

Influenza A virus destroys ciliated epithelium and has been shown to lead to acute impairment of aerosol clearance, which improved to normal after 2–3 months, by which time turnover of the epithelium was complete (350). These workers found that aerosol clearance was reduced in patients 10–15 days after the onset of *Mycoplasma pneumoniae* infection (which also disrupts ciliated epithelium). Three weeks, 3 months, and 1 year later the MCC had improved progressively but was still abnormal (351).

A number of organisms produce ciliotoxins (see Sec. IV.E). For example, human CBF is slowed when challenged by *H. influenzae* and *P. aeruginosa* (165). *Bordetella pertussis* damages respiratory epithelium with consequent loss of ciliated cells. For those ciliated cells still present, CBF has been found to remain within the normal range (169). *Streptococcus pneumoniae* also produces a ciliotoxin, pneumolysin, which causes epithelial disruption and impaired CBF (171).

A reduction has been reported in both nasal mucociliary clearance time (NMCT) and CBF in subjects suffering from naturally occurring common cold as well as those that result from a controlled exposure to a single rhinovirus. This reduction in CBF and NMCT persisted for up to 2 months after symptoms of a cold first appeared (141). Patients with acute viral infections showed delayed aerosol clearance, which persisted for up to 6 weeks after the disappearance of symptoms (135).

Drug Effects

Antibiotics may limit impairment of MCC in acute respiratory infections by reducing the time over which the infecting agent damages cilia, by limiting the effect of ciliotoxins, or by a direct effect on ciliary beating. For example, roxithromycin has been shown to improve CBF. Salmeterol has been shown to limit the effect of ciliotoxins, and this may apply to other β-adrenergic agonists.

Antimicrobial agents may be studied by following the effect of drug treatment on impaired MCC or ciliary function. For example, the broad-spectrum antiviral agent ribavirin, when added in vitro to samples of ciliated epithelium from patients with symptoms of a "cold," resulted in improved CBF (352). This needs to be studied further in vivo.

VI. Conclusions

This chapter has reviewed the effects of drugs and other agents on ciliary function. Although much information about drug effects on ciliary activity and MCC has been learned over the last century, information of clinical usefulness is limited. At present there is no clinical situation in conventional disease management where drugs are given primarily with the aim of improving ciliary function or MCC, although these may well be an effect of drugs given for other reasons. For example, β-adrenergic agonists given with the aim of reversing airways obstruction may improve ciliary function and clearance. It has been suggested that patients with airways obstruction treated with β agonists improve symptomatically, without evidence of an improvement in airways function, because of an improvement in clearance.

Further advances in this area have been limited by lack of knowledge at several levels. These include limited understanding of the intracellular molecular signaling pathways that are involved in modulating ciliary activity and the relationships between impaired ciliary and mucociliary function and human respiratory disease and how these might be affected by pharmacological agents.

Similarly, there are limitations in techniques for measurement of ciliary and mucociliary function in humans. Ciliary beat frequency is measured most commonly, but this is only one aspect of ciliary motility. Furthermore, it is usually measured in vitro. Techniques for in vivo measurements are coming into use and can be anticipated to provide information that may be of greater relevance. At present, measurements of ciliary and mucociliary function are carried out in specialized centers in research situations. The wider availability of reliable measurement techniques that can be utilized in everyday clinical management of patients who have impaired MCC may lead to identification and development of treatment modalities, as has occurred over the last 50 years with diseases causing airways obstruction (e.g., bronchodilator and anti-inflammatory drugs).

Advances in molecular genetics can be anticipated to provide significant insights into molecular mechanisms that regulate ciliary activity and to allow the development of more specific and effective therapies in the future.

References

1. Sleigh MA. The nature and action of respiratory tract cilia. In: Brain JD, Proctor DF, Reid LM, eds. Respiratory Defense Mechanisms. Part I. New York: Marcel Dekker, 1977:247–288.

2. Sleigh MA. Ciliary adaptations for the propulsion of mucus. Biorheology 1990; 27:527–532.

3. Foliguet B, Puchelle E. Apical structures of human respiratory cilia. Bull Eur Physiopathol Respir 1986; 22:43–47.

4. de Iongh R, Rutland J. Orientation of respiratory tract cilia in patients with primary ciliary dyskinesia, bronchiectasis, and in normal subjects. J Clin Pathol 1989; 42:613–619.

5. Rautiainen M, Collan Y, Nuutinen J. A method for measuring the orientation ("beat direction") of respiratory cilia. Arch Otorhinolaryngol 1986; 243:265–268.

6. Holley MC, Afzelius BA. Alignment of cilia in immotile-cilia syndrome. Tissue Cell 1986; 18:521–529.

7. Gaillard DA, Lallement AV, Petit AF, Puchelle ES. In vivo ciliogenesis in human fetal tracheal epithelium. Am J Anat 1989; 185:415–428.

8. Boisvieux-Ulrich E, Lainé MC, Sandoz D. The orientation of basal bodies in quail oviduct is related to the ciliary beating cycle commencement. Biol Cell 1985; 55: 147–150.

9. Mogami Y, Pernberg J, Machemer H. Ciliary beating in three dimensions: steps of a quantitative description. J Math Biol 1992; 30:215–249.

10. Satir P, Hamasaki T, Holwill M. Modeling outer dynein arm activity and its relation to the beat cycle. In: Baum GL, Priel Z, Roth Y, Liron N, Ostfel EJ, eds. Cilia, Mucus, and Mucociliary Interactions. New York: Marcel Dekker, 1997: 13–19.

11. Afzelius BA, Camner AM, Mossberg B. Acquired defects compared to those seen in the immotile-cilia syndrome. Eur J Respir Dis 1983; 64(suppl 127):5–10.

12. Satir P. Studies on cilia. 3. Further studies on the cilium tip and a "sliding filament" model of ciliary motility. J Cell Biol 1968; 39:77–94.

13. Johnson KA. Pathway of the microtubule-dynein ATPase and the structure of dynein: a comparison with actomyosin. Ann Rev Biophys Chem 1985; 14:161–188.

14. Satir P. The role of axonemal components in ciliary motility. Comp Biochem Physiol 1989; 94A:351–357.

15. Sleigh MA. Coordination of the rhythm of beat in some ciliary systems. Int Rev Cytol 1969; 25:31–54.

16. Gheber L, Priel Z. Synchronization between beating cilia. Biophys J 1989; 55: 183–191.

17. Gueron S, Levit-Gurevich K, Liron N, Blum JJ. Cilia internal mechanism and metachronal coordination as the result of hydrodynamical coupling. Proc Natl Acad Sci USA 1997; 94:6001–6006.

18. Gueron S, Levit-Gurevich K, Liron N, Blum JJ. Metachronal coordination as the result of hydrodynamical coupling. In: Baum GL, Priel Z, Roth Y, Liron N, Ostfel EJ, eds. Cilia, Mucus, and Mucociliary Interactions. New York: Marcel Dekker, 1997:97–102.

19. Kim KC, McCracken K, Lee BC, Shin CY, Jo MJ, Lee CJ, Ko KH. Airway goblet cell mucin: its structure and regulation of secretion. Eur Respir J 1997; 10: 2644–2649.

20. Puchelle E, de Bentzmann S, Zahm JM. Physical and functional properties of airway secretions in cystic fibrosis—therapeutic approaches. Respiration 1995; 62(suppl 1):2–12.

21. Yeates DB. Inhibitory and excitatory neural regulation of the mucociliary transport system. In: In: Baum GL, Priel Z, Roth Y, Liron N, Ostfel EJ, eds. Cilia, Mucus, and Mucociliary Interactions. New York: Marcel Dekker, 1997:27–38.

22. Thomas A, Petro W, Konietzko N. Untersuchungen zur zirkadianen Rhythmik der Schlagfrequenz menschlicher Nasenzilien bei Lungengesunden und Patienten mit chronisch obstruktiver Lungenerkrankung einschliesslich der adrenergen Stimulation durch Terbutalin. Pneumologie 1993; 47:526–530.

23. Johnson NT, Villalon M, Roycec FH, Hard R, Verdugo P. Autoregulation of beat frequency in respiratory ciliated cells. Am Rev Respir Dis 1991; 144:1091–1094.

24. Sanderson MJ, Dirksen ER. Mechanosensitivity of cultured ciliated cells from the mammalian respiratory tract: implications for the regulation of mucociliary transport. Proc Natl Acad Sci U S A 1986; 83:7302–7306.

25. Sanderson MJ, Dirksen ER. Mechanosensitive and beta-adrenergic control of the ciliary beat frequency of mammalian respiratory tract cells in culture. Am Rev Respir Dis 1989; 139:432–440.

26. Dirksen ER, Sanderson MJ. Regulation of ciliary activity in the mammalian respiratory tract. Biorheology 1990; 27:533–545.

27. Dirksen ER. Intercellular communication in mammalian airway-ciliated epithelia. In: Baum GL, Priel Z, Roth Y, Liron N, Ostfel EJ, eds. Cilia, Mucus, and Mucociliary Interactions. New York: Marcel Dekker, 1997:59–78.

28. Salathe M, Bookman RJ. Coupling of $[Ca^{2+}]i$ and ciliary beating in cultured tracheal epithelial cells. J Cell Sci 1995; 108:431–440.

29. Salathe M, Lipson EJ, Ivonnet PI, Bookman RJ. Muscarinic signaling in ciliated tracheal epithelial cells: dual effects on Ca^{2+} and ciliary beating. Am J Physiol 1997; 272:L301–L310.

30. Hansen M, Boitano S, Dirksen ER, Sanderson MJ. Intercellular calcium signaling induced by extracellular adenosine 5-triphosphate and mechanical stimulation in airway epithelial cells. J Cell Sci 1993; 106:995–1004.

31. Levin R, Braiman A, Priel Z. Protein kinase C-induced calcium influx and sustained enhancement of ciliary beating by extracellular ATP. Cell Calcium 1997; 21:103–113.

32. Yang B, Schlosser RJ, McCaffrey TV. Signal transduction pathways in modulation of ciliary beat frequency by methacholine. Ann Otol Rhinol Laryngol 1997; 106:230–236.

33. Villalon M, Hinds TR, Verdugo P. Stimulus-response coupling in mammalian ciliated cells; demonstration of two mechanisms of control of cytosolic $[Ca^{2+}]$. Biophys J 1989; 56:1255–1258.

34. Korngreen A, Priel Z. Purinergic stimulation of rabbit ciliated airway epithelia: control by multiple calcium sources. J Physiol 1996; 497:53–66.

35. Korngreen A, Ma W, Priel Z, Silberberg SD. Extracellular ATP directly gates a cation-selective channel in rabbit airway ciliated epithelial cells. J Physiol 1998; 508:703–720.

36. Salathe M, Pratt MM, Wanner A. Protein kinase C-dependent phosphorylation of a ciliary membrane protein and inhibition of ciliary beating. J Cell Sci 1993; 106: 1211–1220.

37. Di Benedetto G, Magnus CJ, Gray PTA, Mehta A. Calcium regulation of ciliary beat frequency in human respiratory epithelium in vitro. J Physiol 1991; 439: 103–113.

38. Girard PR, Kennedy JR. Calcium regulation of ciliary activity in rabbit tracheal epithelial explants and outgrowth. Eur J Cell Biol 1986; 40:203–209.

39. Verdugo P, Raess BV, Villalon M. The role of calmodulin in the regulation of ciliary movement in mammalian epithelial cilia. J Submicrosc Cytol 1983; 15: 95–96.

40. Wanner A, Salathe M, O'Riordan TG. Mucociliary clearance in the airways. Am J Respir Crit Care Med 1996; 154:1868–1902.

41. Gordon RE, Williams KB, Puszkin S. Immune localization of calmodulin in the ciliated cells of hamster tracheal epithelium. J Cell Biol 1982; 95:57–63.

42. Tamaoki J, Kondo M, Takizawa T. Effect of cyclic AMP on ciliary function in rabbit tracheal epithelial cells. J Appl Physiol 1989; 66:1035–1039.

43. Verdugo P, Johnson NT, Tamm PY. Beta-adrenergic stimulation of respiratory ciliary activity. J Appl Physiol. 1980; 48:868–871.

44. Lansley AB, Sanderson MJ, Dirksen ER. Control of the beat cycle of respiratory tract cilia by Ca^{2+} and cAMP. Am J Physiol 1992; 263:L232–L242.

45. Tamaoki J, Kondo M, Takizawa T. Adenosine-mediated cyclic AMP-dependent inhibition of ciliary activity in rabbit tracheal epithelium. Am Rev Respir Dis 1989; 139:441–445.

46. Hamasaki T, Barkalow K, Richmond J, Satir P. cAMP-stimulated phosphorylation of an axonemal polypeptide that copurifies with the 22S dynein arm regulates microtubule translocation velocity and swimming speed in *Paramecium*. Proc Natl Acad Sci U S A 1991; 88:7918–7922.

47. Salathe M, Pratt MM, Wanner A. Cyclic AMP-dependent phosphorylation of a 26kD axonemal protein in ovine cilia isolated from small tissue pieces. Am J Respir Cell Molec Biol 1993; 9:306–314.

48. Braiman A, Zagoory O, Priel Z. PKA enhances Ca^{2+} release and enhances ciliary beat frequency in a Ca^{2+}-dependent and -independent manner. Am J Physiol 1998; 275:C790–C797.

49. Rutland J, Cole PJ. Non-invasive sampling of nasal cilia for the measurement of beat frequency and ultrastructure. Lancet 1980; 2:564–565.

50. Rutland J, Griffin WM, Cole PJ. Human ciliary beat frequency in epithelium from intrathoracic and extrathoracic airways. Am Rev Respir Dis 1982; 125:100–105.

51. Sanderson MJ, Sleigh MA. Ciliary activity of cultured rabbit tracheal epithelium: beat pattern and metachrony. J Cell Sci 1981; 47:331–347.

52. Cheung ATW, Jahn TL. High speed cine-micrographic studies on rabbit tracheal (ciliated) epithelia: determination of the beat pattern of tracheal cilia. Pediatr Res 1976; 10:140–144.

53. Rossman CM, Lee RMKW, Forrest JB, Newhouse MT. Nasal cilia in normal man, primary ciliary dyskinesia and other respiratory diseases: analysis of motility and ultrastructure. Eur J Respir Dis 1983; 64(suppl 127):64–70.

54. Lee WI, Verdugo P. Laser light-scattering spectroscopy: a new application in the study of ciliary activity. Biophys J 1976; 16:1115–1119.
55. Lee WI, Verdugo P. Ciliary activity by laser light spectroscopy. Ann Biomed Eng 1977; 5:248–59.
56. Dalhamn T, Rylander R. Frequency of ciliary beat measured with a photo-sensitive cell. Nature 1962; 196:592–593.
57. Mercke U, Håkansson CH, Toremalm NG. A method for standardized studies of mucociliary activity. Acta Otolaryngol (Stockh) 1974; 78:118–123.
58. Yager JA, Chen TM, Dulfano MJ. Measurement of ciliary beat frequency on human respiratory epithelium. Chest 1978; 73:627–633.
59. Sanderson MJ, Dirksen ER. A versatile and quantitative computer-assisted photoelectronic technique used for the analysis of ciliary beat cycles. Cell Motility 1985; 5:267–292.
60. Phillips PP, McCaffery TV, Kern EB. Measurement of human nasal ciliary motility using computerized microphotometry. Otolaryngol Head Neck Surg 1990; 103: 420–426.
61. Priel Z. Direct measurement of the velocity of the metachronal wave in beating cilia. Biorheology 1987; 24:599–603.
62. Mercke U, Hybbinette JC, Lindberg S. Parasympathetic and sympathetic influences on mucociliary activity in vivo. Rhinology 1982; 20:201–204.
63. Chandra T, Yeates DB, Miller IF, Wong LB. Stationary and non-stationary correlation frequency analysis of heterodyne mode laser light scattering: magnitude and periodicity of canine tracheal ciliary beat frequency in vivo. Biophys J 1994; 66: 878–890.
64. Reimer A, Toremalm NG. The mucociliary activity of the upper respiratory tract. II. A method for in vivo studies on maxillary sinus mucosa of animals and human beings. Acta Oto-Laryngol 1978; 86:283–288.
65. Reimer A, von Mecklenberg C, Toremalm NG. The mucociliary activity of the upper respiratory tract, III. A functional and morphological study on human and animal material with special reference to maxillary sinus disease. Acta Otolaryngol (Stockh) 1978; 355(suppl):1–20.
66. Hybbinette JC, Mercke U. A method for evaluating the effect of pharmacological substances on mucociliary activity in vivo. Acta Oto-Laryngol 1982; 93:151–159.
67. Lindberg S, Runer T. Method for in vivo measurement of mucociliary activity in the human nose. Ann Otol Rhinol Laryngol 1994; 103:558–566.
68. Sackner MA, Rosen MJ, Wanner A. Estimation of tracheal mucus velocity by bronchofiberscopy. J Appl Physiol 1973; 34:495–499.
69. Friedman M, Stott FD, Poole DO, Dougherty R, Chapman GA, Watson H, Sackner MA. A new roentgenographic method for estimating mucous velocity in airways. Am Rev Resp Dis 1977; 115:67–72.
70. Toomes H, Vogt-Moykopf I, Heller WD, Ostertag H. Measurement of mucociliary clearance in smokers and non-smokers using a bronchoscopic video-technical method. Lung 1981; 159:27–34.
71. Goodman RM, Yergin BM, Landa JF, Golinvaux MH, Sackner MA. Relationship of smoking history and pulmonary function test to tracheal mucus velocity in

nonsmokers, young smokers, ex-smokers and patients with chronic bronchitis. Am
Rev Respir Dis 1978; 117:205–214.

72. Chopra SK, Taplin GV, Elam D, Carson SA, Golde D. Measurement of tracheal
mucociliary transport velocity in human smokers versus nonsmokers. Am Rev
Respir Dis 1979; 119(suppl):205.

73. Zwas ST, Katz I, Belfer B, Baum GL, Aharonson E. Scintigraphic monitoring
of mucociliary tracheo-bronchial clearance of technetium-99m macroaggregated
albumin aerosol. J Nucl Med 1987; 28:161–167.

74. Albert RE, Arnett LC. Clearance of radioactivity dust from the lung. Arch Environ
Health 1955; 12:99–106.

75. Morrow PE, Gibb FR, Gazioglu KM. A study of particulate clearance from the
human lungs. Am Rev Respir Dis 1967; 96:1209–1221.

76. Morrow PE. An evaluation of the physical properties of monodisperse and heterodisperse aerosols used in the assessment of bronchial function. Chest 1981; 80:
809–813.

77. Lippmann M, Leikauf G, Spektor D, Schlesinger RB, Albert RE. The effects of
irritant aerosols on mucus clearance from large and small conductive airways.
Chest 1981; 80(suppl):873–877.

78. Albert RE, Lippmann M, Briscoe W. The characteristics of bronchial clearance
in humans and the effects of cigarette smoking. Arch Environ Health 1969; 18:
738–55.

79. Thompson ML, Short MD. Mucociliary function in health, chronic obstructive
airway disease, and asbestosis. J Appl Physiol 1969; 26:535–539.

80. Thomson ML, Pavia D, McNicol MW. A preliminary study of the effect of guaiphenesin on mucociliary clearance from the human lung. Thorax 1973; 28:742–
747.

81. Pavia D, Sutton PP, Agnew JE, Lopez-Vidriero MT, Newman SP, Clarke SW.
Measurement of bronchial mucociliary clearance. Eur J Respir Dis 1983; 127
(suppl):41–56.

82. Bertrand A, Puchelle E. Mesure de la clearance muco-ciliaire des bronches proxi-
males chez le bronchitique chronique. Pathol Biol 1977; 25:623–627.

83. Lourenco RV, Klimek MF, Borowski CJ. Deposition and clearance of 2 micron
particles in the tracheobronchial tree of normal subjects: smokers and non-smokers. J Clin Invest 1971; 50:1411–1420.

84. Hass FJ, Lee PS, Lourenco RV. Tagging of iron oxide particles with Tc99m for
use in the study of deposition and clearance of inhaled particles. J Nucl Med
1976; 17:122–125.

85. Wales KA, Petrow HG, Yeates DB. Production of Tc99m labeled iron oxide aerosols for human lung deposition and clearance studies. Int J Appl Radiat Isotopes
1980; 31:689–694.

86. Camner P, Philipson K, Linnman L. A simple method for nuclidic tagging of
monodisperse fluorocabon resin particles. Int J Appl Radiat Isotopes 1971; 22:
731–734.

87. Matthys H, Kohler D. Affect of theophylline on mucociliary clearance in man.
Eur J Respir Dis 1980; 61(suppl 109):98–102.

88. Robson AM, Smallman LA, Drake-Lee AB. Factors affecting ciliary function in vivo: a preliminary study. Clin Otolaryngol 1992; 17:125–9.
89. Dorow P, Weiss T, Felix R, Schmutzler H, Schiess W. Influence of propranolol, metoprolol, and pindolol on mucociliary clearance in patients with coronary heart disease. Respiration 1984; 45:286–290.
90. Mortensen J, Lange P, Nyboe J, Groth S. Lung mucociliary clearance. Eur J Nucl Med 1994; 21:953–961.
91. Yeates DB, Aspin N, Levison H, Jones MT, Bryan AC. Mucociliary tracheal transport rates in man. J Appl Physiol 1975; 39:487–495.
92. Quinlan MF, Salman SD, Swift DL, Wagner HN Jr, Proctor DF. Measurement of mucociliary function in man. Am Rev Respir Dis 1969; 99:13–23.
93. Proctor D, Wagner H. Clearance of the particles from the human nose. Arch Environ Health 1965; 11:366–371.
94. Anderson I, Lundquist G, Proctor DK. Human nasal mucosal function in a controlled climate. Arch Environ Health 1971; 23:408–420.
95. Yergin B, Saketkhoo K, Michoelson E, Serafini S, Kovitz K, Sackner M. A roentgenographic method for measuring nasal mucus velocity. J Appl Physiol Respir Environ Exerc Physiol 1978; 44:964–968.
96. Anderson I, Camner P, Jensen PL, Philipson K, Proctor DF. A comparison of nasal and tracheobronchial clearance. Arch Environ Health 1974; 29:290–293.
97. Rutland J, Cole PJ. Nasal mucociliary clearance and ciliary beat frequency in cystic fibrosis compared with sinusitis and bronchiectasis. Thorax 1981; 36:654–658.
98. Stanley P, MacWilliam L, Greenstone M, Mackay I, Cole P. Efficacy of a saccharin test for screening to detect abnormal mucociliary clearance. Br J Dis Chest 1984; 78:62–65.
99. Anderson I, Proctor DF. Measurement of nasal mucociliary clearance. Eur J Respir Dis 1983; 64(suppl 127):37–40.
100. Melville GN, Horstmann G, Iravani J. Adrenergic compounds and the respiratory tract. A physiological and electron-microscopical study. Respiration 1976: 33: 261–269.
101. Foster WM, Bergofsky EH, Bohning DE, Lippmann M, Albert RE. Effect of adrenergic agents and their mode of action on mucociliary clearance in man. J Appl Physiol 1976; 41:146–152.
102. Phillips PP, McCaffrey TV, Kern EB. The in vivo and in vitro effect of phenylephrine (Neo Synephrine) on nasal ciliary beat frequency and mucociliary transport. Otolaryngol Head Neck Surg 1990; 103:558–565.
103. Hybbinette JC, Mercke U. Effects of sympathomimetic agonists and antagonists on mucociliary activity. Acta Otolaryngol (Stockh) 1982; 94:121–130.
104. Curtis LN, Carson JL. Computer-assisted video measurement of inhibition of ciliary beat frequency of human nasal epithelium in vitro by xylometazoline. J Pharmacol Toxicol Meth 1992; 28:1–7.
105. Simon H, Drettner B, Jung B. Messung des Schleimhauttransportes in menschlichen Nase mit 51Cr markierten Harzkugelchen. Acta Otolaryngol (Stockh) 1977; 83:379–390.

106. Van As A. The role of selective β₂-adrenoceptor stimulants in the control of ciliary activity. Respiration 1974; 31:146–151.
107. Devalia JL, Sapsford RJ, Rusnak C, Toumbis MJ, Davies RJ. The effects of salmeterol and salbutamol on ciliary beat frequency of cultured human bronchial epithelial cells in vitro. Pulm Pharmacol 1992; 5:257–263.
108. Lindberg S, Khan R, Runer T. The effects of formoterol, a long-acting β₂-edrenoceptor agonist, on mucociliary activity. Eur J Pharmacol 1995; 285:275–280.
109. Honeyman G, Kemp PJ, Cobain C, Mehta A, Dhillon DP, Winter JH. β2 agonist terbutaline makes the ciliary beat frequency of freshly isolated human airway cells refractory to calcium signaling. In: Baum GL, Priel Z, Roth Y, Liron N, Ostfel EJ, eds. Cilia, Mucus, and Mucociliary Interactions. New York: Marcel Dekker, 1997:71–78.
110. Wood RE, Warner A, Hirsch J, Farrell PM. Tracheal mucociliary transport in patients with cystic fibrosis and its stimulation by terbutaline. Am Rev Respir Dis 1975; 111:733–738.
111. Mortensen J, Hansen A, Falk M, Nielsen IK, Groth S. Reduced effect of inhaled beta 2-adrenergic agonists on lung mucociliary clearance in patients with cystic fibrosis. Chest 1993; 103:805–811.
112. Yeates DB, Spektor DM, Pitt BR. Effect of orally administered orciprenaline on tracheobronchial mucociliary clearance. Eur J Respir Dis 1986; 69:100–108.
113. Isawa T, Teshima T, Hirano T, Anazawa Y, Miki M, Konno K, Motomiya M. Does a beta 2-stimulator really facilitate mucociliary transport in the human lungs in vivo? A study with procaterol. Am Rev Respir Dis 1990; 141:715–720.
114. Kanthakumar K, Cundell DR, Johnson M, Wills PJ, Taylor GW, Cole PJ, Wilson R. Effect of salmeterol on human nasal epithelial cell ciliary beating: inhibition of the ciliotoxin, pyocyanin. Br J Pharmacol 1994; 112:493–498.
115. Melloni B, Germouty J. Influence sur la fonction muco-ciliaire d'un nouveau beta-agoniste: formoterol. Rev Malad Respir 1992; 9:503–507.
116. Van de Donk HJM, Merkus FWHN. Decreases in ciliary beat frequency due to intranasal administration of propranolol. J Pharmaceut Sci 1982; 71:595–596.
117. Pavia D, Sutton PP, Lopez-Vidriero MT, Agnew JE, Clarke SW. Drug effects on mucociliary clearance. Eur J Respir Dis 1983; 64(suppl 128):304–317.
118. Chopra SK, Carson SA, Tashkin DP, Taplin GV, Elam D. Effect of terbutaline and inderal on tracheal transport velocity in anesthetized dogs. Am Rev Respir Dis 1979; 119(suppl):206.
119. Gyi A, O'Callaghan C, Langton JA. Effect of halothane on cilia beat frequency of ciliated human respiratory epithelium in vitro. Br J Anaesthesiol 1994; 73:507–510.
120. Lee KS, Park SS. Effect of halothane, enflurane, and nitrous oxide on tracheal ciliary activity in vitro. Anesth Analg 1980; 59:426–439.
121. Manawadu BR, Mostow SR, LaForce FM. Impairment of tracheal ring ciliary activity by halothane. Anesth Analg 1979; 58:500–504.
122. Forbes EAR, Horrigan RW. Mucociliary flow in the trachea during anesthesia with enflurane, ether, nitrous oxide, and morphine. Anesthesiol 1977; 46:319–321.
123. Konrad F, Marx T, Schraag M, Kilian J. Kombinationsanasthesie und BTG. Effekt

einer Anasthesie mit Isofluran, Fentanyl, Vecuronium und Sauerstoff-Lachgas-Beatmung auf den bronchialen Schleimtransport. Anaesthetist 1997; 46:403–407.

124. Pizov R, Takahashi M, Hirshman CA, Croxton T. Halothane inhibition of ion transport of the tracheal epithelium. A possible mechanism for anesthetic-induced impairment of mucociliary clearance. Anesthesiol 1992; 76:985–989.

125. Mostow SR, Dreisin RB, Manawadu BR, LaForce FM. Adverse effects of lidocaine and methylparaben on tracheal ciliary activity. Laryngoscope 1979; 89: 1697–1701.

126. Rutland J, Griffin W, Cole PJ. An in vitro model for studying the effects of pharmacological agents on human ciliary beat frequency: effects of lignocaine. Br J Clin Pharmacol 1982; 13:679–683.

127. Verra F, Escudier E, Pinchon MC, Fleury J, Bignon J, Bernaudin JF. Effects of local anaesthetics (lidocaine) on the structure and function of ciliated respiratory epithelial cells. Biol Cell 1990; 69:99–105.

128. Ingels KJAO, Nijziel MR, Graamans K, Huizing EH. Influence of cocaine and lidocaine on human nasal cilia. Beat frequency and harmony in vitro. Arch Otolaryngol Head Neck Surg 1994; 120:197–201.

129. Karttunen P, Silvasti M, Virta P, Saano V, Nuutinen J. The effects of vadocaine, dextromethorphan, diphenhydramine and hydroxyzine on the ciliary beat frequency in rats in vitro. Pharmacol Toxicol 1990; 67:159–161.

130. Tamaoki J, Chiyotani A, Sakai N, Takeyama K, Takizawa T. Effect of erythromycin on ciliary motility in rabbit airway epithelium in vitro. J Antimicrob Chemother 1992; 29:173–178.

131. Takeyama K, Tamaoki J, Chiyotani A, Tagaya E, Konno K. Effect of macrolide antibiotics on ciliary motility in rabbit airway epithelium in-vitro. J Pharm Pharmacol 1993; 45:756–758.

132. Sugiura Y, Ohashi Y, Nakai Y. Roxythromycin stimulates the mucociliary activity of the eustachian tube and modulates neutrophil activity in the healthy guinea pig. Acta Oto-Laryngol 1997; 531(suppl):34–38.

133. Sugiura Y, Ohashi Y, Nakai Y. Roxythromycin prevents endotoxin-induced otitis media with effusion in the guinea pig. Acta Oto-Laryngol 1997; 531(suppl): 39–51.

134. Wanner A. Clinical aspects of mucociliary transport. Am Rev Respir Dis 1977; 116:73–125.

135. Lourenco RV, Loddenkemper, Carlton RW. Patterns of distribution and clearance of aerosols inpatients with bronchiectasis. Am Rev Respir Dis 1972; 106:857–866.

136. Wilson R, Sykes DA, Currie D, Cole PJ. Beat frequency of cilia from sites of purulent infection. Thorax 1986; 41:453–458.

137. Kollberg H, Mossberg B, Afzelius BA, Philipson K, Camner P. Cystic fibrosis compared with the immotile-cilia syndrome: a study of mucociliary clearance, ciliary ultrastructure, clinical picture and ventilatory function. Scand J Respir Dis 1978; 59:297–306.

138. Stanley PJ, Wilson R, Greenstone MA, Mackay IS, Cole PJ. Abnormal nasal mucociliary clearance in patients with rhinitis and its relationship to concomitant chest disease. Br J Dis Chest 1985; 79:77–82.

139. Sakakura Y. Changes of mucociliary function during colds. Eur J Respir Dis 1983; 112:341–347.

140. Hers JFP. Disturbance of the ciliated epithelium due to influenza virus. Am Rev Respir Dis 1966; 93:162–171.

141. Pedersen M, Sakakura Y, Winther B, Brofeldt S, Mygind N. Nasal mucociliary transport, number of ciliated cells and beating pattern in naturally acquired colds. Eur J Respir Dis 1983; 64(suppl 128):355–365.

142. Wilson R, Alton E, Rutman A. Upper respiratory tract viral infection and mucociliary clearance. Eur J Respir Dis 1987; 70:272–279.

143. Carson JL, Collier AM, Hu SCS. Acquired ciliary defects in nasal epithelium of children with acute viral upper respiratory infections. N Engl J Med 1985; 312: 463–468.

144. Wilson R, Cole PJ. The effect of bacterial products on ciliary function. Am Rev Respir Dis 1988; 138:S49–S53.

145. Smallman LA, Hill SL, Stockley RA. Reduction of ciliary beat frequency in vitro by sputum from patients with bronchiectasis: a serine proteinase effect. Thorax. 1984; 39:663–667.

146. Gray L, Kreger A. Microscopic characterization of rabbit lungs damage produced by *Pseudomonas aeruginosa* proteases. Infect Immun 1979; 23:150–159.

147. Hingley ST, Hastie AT, Kueppers F. Disruption of respiratory cilia by proteases including those of *Pseudomonas aeruginosa*. Infect Immun 1986; 54:379–385.

148. Hingley ST, Hastie AT, Kueppers F, Higgins ML, Weinbaum G, Shyrock T. Effect of ciliostatic factors from *Pseudomonas aeruginosa* on rabbit respiratory cilia. Infect Immun 1986; 51:254–262.

149. Wilson R, Pitt T, Taylor G, Watson D, MacDermot J, Sykes D, Roberts D, Cole PJ. Pyocyanin and 1-hydroxyphenazine produced by *Pseudomonas aeruginosa* inhibit the beating of human respiratory cilia in vitro. J Clin Invest 1987; 79:221–229.

150. Amitani R, Wilson R, Rutman A, Read R, Ward C, Burnett D, Stockley RA, Cole PJ. Effects of neutrophil elastase and *Pseudomonas aeruginosa* proteinases on human respiratory epithelium. Am J Respir Cell Mol Biol 1991; 4:26–31.

151. Reimer A, Klementsson K, Ursing J, Wretlind B. The mucociliary activity of the respiratory tract, I. Inhibitory effects of products of *Pseudomonas aeruginosa* on rabbit trachea in vitro. Acta Otolaryngol (Stockh) 1980; 90:462–469.

152. Munro NC, Barker A, Rutman A, Taylor G, Watson D, McDonal-Gibson WJ, Towart R, Taylor WA, Wilson R, Cole PJ. Effect of pyocyanin and 1-hydroxyphenazine on in vivo tracheal mucus velocity. J Appl Physiol 1989; 67:316–323.

153. Jackowski JT, Szepfalusi Z, Wanner DA Seybold Z, Sielczak MW, Lauredo IT, Adams T, Abraham WM, Wanner A. Effects of *Pseudomonas aeruginosa* derived bacterial products on tracheal ciliary function: role of oxygen radicals. Am J Physiol 1991; 4:L61–L67.

154. Seybold ZV, Abraham WM, Gazeroglu H, Wanner A. Impairment of airway mucociliary transport by *Pseudomonas aeruginosa* products. Am Rev Respir Dis 1991; 146:1173–1176.

155. Read RC, Roberts P, Munro N, Rutman A, Hastie A, Shyrock T, Hall R, McDonald-Gibson W, Lund V, Taylor G, Cole PJ, Wilson R. Effects of *Pseudomonas*

aeruginosa rhamnolipids on mucociliary transport and ciliary beating. J Appl Physiol 1992; 72:2271–2277.

156. Somerville M, Taylor GW, Watson D, Rendell NB, Rutman A, Todd H, Davies JR, Wilson R, Cole P, Richardson PS. Release of mucus glycoconjugates by *Pseudomonas aeruginosa* rhamnolipids into feline trachea in vivo and human bronchus in vitro. Am J Respir Cell Mol Biol 1992; 6:116–122.

157. Graham A, Steel DM, Wilson R, Cole PJ, Alton EW, Geddes DM. Effects of purified *Pseudomonas* rhamnolipids on bioelectric properties of sheep tracheal epithelium. Exp Lung Res 1993; 19:77–89.

158. Kanthakumar K, Taylor G, Tsang KWT, Cundell DR, Rutman A, Smith S, Jeffrey PK, Cole PJ, Wilson R. Mechanisms of action of *P. aeruginosa* pyocyanin on human ciliary beat frequency in vitro. Infect Immun 1993; 61:2848–2853.

159. Kanthakumar K, Taylor G, Cundell DR, Dowling RB, Cole PJ, Wilson R. The effects of bacterial toxins on levels of intracellular adenosine nucleotides and human ciliary beat frequency. Pulm Pharmacol 1996; 9:223–230.

160. Rautiainen M, Yoshitsugu M, Matsune S, Nuutinen J, Happonen P, Ohyama M. Effect of exogenous ATP and physical stimulation on ciliary function impaired by bacterial endotoxin. Acta Otolaryngol (Stockh) 1994; 114:337–340.

161. Dowling RB, Rayner CFJ, Rutman A, Jackson AD, Kanthakumar K, Dewar A, Taylor GW, Cole PJ, Johnson M, Wilson R. Effect of salmeterol on *Pseudomonas aeruginosa* infection of respiratory mucosa. Am J Respir Crit Care Med 1997; 155:327–336.

162. Hoorn B, Lofkist T. The effects of staphylococcal alpha toxin and preparations of staphylococcal antigens on ciliated respiratory epithelium. Acta Otolaryngol (Stockh) 1965; 60:452–460.

163. Denny FW. Effect of a toxin produced by *Haemophilus influenzae* on ciliated respiratory epithelium. J Infect Dis 1974; 129:93–100.

164. Johnson AP, Inzana TJ. Loss of ciliary activity in organ cultures of rat trachea treated with lipooligosaccharide isolated from *Haemophilus influenzae*. J Med Microbiol 1986; 22:265–268.

165. Wilson R, Roberts D, Cole PJ. Effect of bacterial products on human ciliary function in vitro. Thorax 1985; 40:125–131.

166. Tsang KW, Rutman A, Kantahkumar K, Belcher J, Lund V, Roberts DE, Read RC, Cole PJ, Wilson R. *Haemophilus influenzae* infection of human respiratory mucosa in low concentrations of antibiotics. Am Rev Respir Dis 1993; 148:201–207.

167. Rutman A, Dowling R, Wills P, Feldman C, Cole PJ, Wilson R. Effect of dirithromycin on *Haemophilus influenzae* infection of the respiratory mucosa. Antimicrob Agents Chemother 1998; 42:772–778.

168. Dowling RB, Johnson M, Cole PJ, Wilson R. Effect of salmeterol on *Haemophilus influenzae* infection of respiratory mucosa in vitro. Eur Respir J 1998; 11:86–90.

169. Wilson R, Read R, Thomas M, Rutman A, Harrison K, Lund V, Cookson B, Goldman W, Lambert H, Cole PJ. Effects of *Bordetella pertussis* infection on human respiratory epithelium in vivo and in vitro. Infect Immun 1991; 59:337–345.

170. Rosenthal RS, Nogami W, Cookson BP, Goldman WE, Falkening WJ. Major

fragment of soluble peptidoglycan released from growing *Bordetella pertussis* is tracheal cytotoxin. Infect Immun 1987; 55:2117–2120.

171. Steinfort C, Wilson R, Mitchell T, Feldman C, Rutman A, Todd H, Sykes D, Walker J, Saunders K, Andrew PW, Boulnois GJ, Cole PJ. Effect of *Streptococcus pneumoniae* on human respiratory epithelium in vitro. Infect Immun 1989; 57: 2006–2013.

172. Rayner CFJ Jackson AD, Rutman A, Dewar A, Mitchell TJ, Andrew PW, Cole PJ, Wilson R. Interaction of pneumolysin-sufficient and -deficient isogenic variants of *Streptococcus pneumoniae* with human respiratory mucosa. Infect Immun 1995; 63:442–447.

173. Jarstrand C, Camner P, Philipson K. *Mycoplasma pneumoniae* and tracheobronchial clearance. Am Rev Respir Dis 1977; 110:415–419.

174. Collier AM, Clyde WA. Relationships between *Mycoplasma pneumoniae* and human respiratory epithelium. Infect Immun 1971; 3:694–701.

175. Chandler DKF, Barile MF. Ciliostatic, hemagglutinating, and proteolytic activities in a cell extract of *Mycoplasma pneumoniae*. Infect Immun 1980; 29:1111–1116.

176. Kordik P, Beulbring E, Burn JH. Ciliary movement and acetylcholine. Br J Pharmacol 1952; 7:67.

177. Corssen G, Allen CR. Acetylcholine: its significance in controlling ciliary activity of human respiratory epithelium in vitro. J Appl Physiol 1959; 14:901–904.

178. Melville GN, Iravani J. Factors affecting ciliary beat frequency in the intrapulmonary airways of rats. Can J Physiol Pharmacol 1974; 53: 1122–1128.

179. Hybbinette JC, Mercke U. Effects of the parasympathomimetic drug methacholine and its antagonist atropine on mucociliary activity. Acta Otolaryngol (Stockh) 1982; 93:465–473.

180. Wong LB, Miller IF, Yeates DB. Regulation of ciliary beat frequency by autonomic mechanisms in vitro. J Appl Physiol 1988; 65:1895–1901.

181. Wong LB, Miller IF, Yeates DB. Stimulation of ciliary beat frequency by autonomic agonists: in vivo. J Appl Physiol 1988; 65:971–981.

182. Gatto LA. Cholinergic and adrenergic stimulation of mucociliary transport in the rat trachea. Respir Physiol 1993; 92:209–217.

183. Annis P, Landa J, Lichtiger M. Effects of atropine on velocity of tracheal mucus in anesthetized patients. Anesthesiology 1976; 44:74–77.

184. Chopra SK. Effect of atropine on mucociliary transport velocity in anesthetized dogs. Am Rev Respir Dis 1978; 118:367–371.

185. Whiteside ME, Lauredo I, Chapman GA, Ratzan KR, Abraham WM, Wanner A. Effect of atropine on tracheal mucociliary clearance and bacterial counts. Bull Eur Physiopathol Respir 1984; 20:347–351.

186. Camner P, Strandberg K, Philipson K. Increased mucociliary transport by cholinergic stimulation. Arch Environ Health 1974; 29:220–224.

187. Pavia D, Thomson ML. Inhibition of mucociliary clearance from the human lung by hyoscine. Lancet 1971; 1:449–450.

188. Miyata T, Matsumoto N, Yuki H, Oda Y, Takahama K, Kai H. Effects of anticholinergic bronchodilators on mucociliary transport and airway secretion. Jpn J Pharmacol 1989; 51:11–15.

189. Wanner A. Effect of ipratropium bromide on airway mucociliary function. Am J Med 1986; 81:23–27.

190. Francis RA, Thompson ML, Pavia D, Douglas RB. Ipratropium bromide: mucociliary clearance rate and airway resistance in normal subjects. Br J Dis Chest 1977; 71:173–178.

191. Sackner MA, Chapman GA, Dougherty RD. Effects of nebulized ipratropium bromide and atropine sulphate on tracheal mucus velocity and lung mechanics in anesthetized dogs. Respiration 1977; 34:181–185.

192. Foster WM, Bergofsky EH. Airway mucus membrane: effects of β-adrenergic and anticholinergic stimulation. Am J Med 1986; 81:28–35.

193. Sugiura Y, Ohashi Y, Nakai Y, The herbal medicine, Sairei-to, enhances the mucociliary activity of the tubotympanum in the healthy guinea pig. Acta Otolaryngol (Stockh) 1997; 531(suppl):17–20.

194. Sugiura Y, Ohashi Y, Nakai Y. The herbal medicine, Sairei-to, prevents endotoxin induced otitis media with effusion in the guinea pig. Acta Otolaryngol (Stockh) 1997; 531(suppl): 21–33.

195. Riechelmann H, Brommer C, Hinni M, Martin C. Response of human ciliated respiratory cells to a mixture of menthol, eucalypyus oil and pine needle oil. Arzneimittelforschung 1997; 47:1035–1039.

196. Stafanger G. In vitro effect of beclomethasone dipropionate and flunisolide on the mobility of human nasal cilia. Eur J Allergy Clin Immunol 1987; 42:507–511.

197. Iravani J, Melville GN. Effects of drugs and environmental factors on ciliary movement. Respiration 1975; 32:157–164.

198. Kai H, Yamamoto S, Takahama K, Miyata T. Influence of corticosterone on tracheal mucociliary transport in pigeons. Jpn J Pharmacol 1990; 52:496–499.

199. Lindqvist N, Holmberg K, Pipkorn U. Intranasally administered budesonide, a glucocorticoid, does not exert its clinical effect through vasoconstriction. Clin Otolaryngol 1989; 14:519–523.

200. Hasani A, Pavia D, Spiteri MA, Yeo CT, Agnew JE, Clarke SW, Chung KF. Inhaled frusemide does not affect lung mucociliary clearance in healthy and asthmatic subjects. Eur Respir J 1994; 7:1497–1500.

201. Daviskas E, Anderson SD, Gonda I, Bailey D, Bautovich G, Seale JP. Mucociliary clearance during and after isocapnic hyperventilation with dry air in the presence of frusemide. Eur Respir J 1996; 9:716–724.

202. Di Benedetto G, Lopez-Vidriero MT, Carratu, Clarke SW. Effect of amiloride on human bronchial ciliary activity in vitro. Respiration 1990; 57:37–39.

203. Robinson M, Regnis JA, Bailey DL, King M, Bautovich GJ, Bye PT. Effect of hypertonic saline, amiloride, and cough on mucociliary clearance in patients with cystic fibrosis. Am J Respir Crit Care Med 1996; 153:1503–1509.

204. Graham A, Hasani A, Alton EW, Martin GP, Marriott C, Hodson ME, Clarke SW, Geddes DM. No added benefit from nebulized amiloride in patients with cystic fibrosis. Eur Respir J 1993; 6:1243–1248.

205. Middleton PG, Geddes DM, Alton EW. Effect of amiloride and saline on nasal mucociliary clearance and potential difference in cystic fibrosis and normal subjects. Thorax 1993; 48:812–816.

206. Olivier KN, Bennett WD, Hohneker KW, Zeman KL, Edwards LJ, Boucher RC, Knowles MR. Acute safety and effects on mucociliary clearance of aerosolized uridine 5′-triphosphate ± amiloride in normal human adults. Am J Respir Crit Care Med 1996; 154:217–223.

207. Maurer D, Liebman J. Effects of ethanol on in vitro ciliary motility. J Appl Physiol 1988; 65:1617–1620.

208. Sisson JH. Ethanol stimulates apparent nitric oxide-dependent ciliary beat frequency in bovine airway epithelial cells. Am J Physiol 1995; 268:L596–L600.

209. Sisson JH, Tuma DJ, Rennard SI. Acetaldehyde-mediated cilia dysfunction in bovine bronchial epithelial cells. Am J Physiol 1991; 260:L29–L36.

210. Venizelos PC, Gerrity TR, Yeates DB. Response of human mucociliary clearance to acute alcohol administration. Arch Environ Health 1981; 36:194–201.

211. Kobayashi K, Tamaoki J, Sakai N, Kanemura T, Horii S, Takizawa T. Angiotensin II stimulates airway ciliary motility in rabbit cultured tracheal epithelium. Acta Physiol Scand 1990; 138:497–502.

212. Tamaoki J, Kobayashi K, Sakai K, Kanemura T, Horii S, Isono K, Takeuchi S, Chiyotani A, Yamawaka I, Takizawa T. Atrial natriuretic factor inhibits ciliary motility in cultured rabbit tracheal epithelium. Am J Physiol 1991; 260:C201–C205.

213. Sakamoto O, Iwama A, Amitani R, Takehara T, Yamaguchi N, Yamamoto T, Masuyama K, Yamanaka T, Ando M, Suda T. Role of macrophage-stimulating protein and its receptor, RON tyrosine kinase, in ciliary motility. J Clin Invest 1997; 99:701–709.

214. Schuil PJ, Rosmalen JG, Graamans K, Huizing EH. Calcitonin gene-related peptide in vitro stimulation of ciliary beat in human upper respiratory cilia. Eur Arch Oto-Rhino-Laryngol 1995; 252:462–464.

215. Kobayashi K, Tamaoki J, Sakai N, Kanemura T, Chiyotani A, Shibasaki T, Takizawa T. Corticotropin-releasing factor and adrenocorticotrophin stimulate ciliary motility in rabbit tracheal epithelium. Life Sci 1989; 45:2043–2049.

216. Sabater JR, Otero R, Abraham WM, Wanner A, O'Riordan TG. Endothelin-1 depresses tracheal mucus velocity in ovine airways via ET-A receptors. Am J Respir Crit Care Med 1996; 154:341–345.

217. Tamaoki J, Kanemura T, Sakai N, Kobayashi K, Takizawa T. Endothelin stimulates ciliary beat frequency and chloride secretion in canine tracheal epithelium. Am J Respir Cell Mol Biol 1991; 4:426–431.

218. Amble FR, Lindberg SO, McCaffrey TV, Runer T. Mucociliary function and endothelins 1, 2 and 3. Otolaryngol Head Neck Surg 1993; 109:634–645.

219. Sakai N, Tamaoki J, Kobayashi K, Kanemura T, Isono K, Takeyama K, Takeuchi S, Takizawa T. Vasoactive intestinal peptide stimulates ciliary motility in rabbit tracheal epithelium: modulation by neutral endopeptidase. Reg Pep 1991; 34:33–41.

220. Tamaoki J, Chiyotani A, Sakai N, Takeyama K, Konno K. Effect of azelastine on sulphur dioxide induced impairment of ciliary motility in airway epithelium. Thorax 1993; 48:542–546.

221. Su XY, Li A. The effect of some commercially available antihistamine and decongestant intranasal formulations on ciliary beat frequency. J Clin Pharm Ther 1993; 18:219–222.

222. Carson SA, Chopra SK, Tashkin DP. Effect of intravenous cimetidine on mucociliary transport in anesthetized dogs. Eur J Respir Dis 1982; 63:310–315.

223. Esaki Y, Ohashi Y, Furuya H, Sugiura Y, Ohno Y, Okamoto H, Nakai Y. Histamine-induced mucociliary dysfunction and otitis media with effusion. Acta Oto-Laryngologica 1991; 486(suppl):116–134.

224. Sykes DA, Wilson R, Chan KL, Mackay IS, Cole PJ. Relative importance of antibiotic and improved clearance in topical treatment of chronic mucopurulent rhinosinusitis: a controlled study. Lancet 1986; 16:359–360.

225. Gearhart JM, Schlesinger RB. Response of the tracheobronchial mucociliary clearance system to repeated irritant exposure: effect of sulfuric acid mist on function and structure. Exp Lung Res 1988; 14:587–605.

226. Hastie AT, Patrick H, Fish JE. Inhibition and recovery of mammalian respiratory ciliary function after formaldehyde exposure. Toxicol Appl Pharmacol 1990; 102: 282–291.

227. Friedman M, Dougherty R, Nelson SR., White RP, Sackner MA, Wanner A. Acute effects of an aerosol hair spray on tracheal mucociliary transport. Am Rev Respir Dis 1977; 116:281–286.

228. Dalhman T. Studies on the effect of sulfur dioxide on ciliary activity in rabbit trachea in vivo and in vitro and on the resorptional capacity of the nasal cavity. Am Rev Respir Dis 1961; 83:566–567.

229. de Iongh R, Rutland J. Ciliary defects in healthy subjects, bronchiectasis and primary ciliary dyskinesia. Am J Respir Dis Crit Care Med 1995; 151:1559–1567.

230. Camner P, Philipson K, Arvidsson T. Withdrawal of cigarette smoking: a study on tracheobronchial clearance. Arch Environ Health 1973; 26:90–92.

231. Vastag E, Matthys H, Zsamboki G, Kohler D, Daikeler G. Mucociliary clearance in smokers. Eur J Respir Dis 1986 ; 68:107–113.

232. Hahn HL, Kleinschrot D, Hansen D. Nicotine increases ciliary beat frequency by a direct effect on respiratory cilia. Clin Invest 1992; 70:244–251.

233. Lindberg S. Reflex-induced acceleration of mucociliary activity in rabbit after exposure to cigarette smoke. Bull Eur Physiopathol Respir 1986; 22:273–279.

234. Hobson J, Wright J, Churg A. Histological evidence for generation of active oxygen species on the apical surface of cigarette smoke-exposed tracheal explants. Am J Pathol 1991; 139:573–580.

235. Sisson J, Papi A, Beckmann J, Leise K, Wisecarver J, Brodersen BW, Kelling CL, Spurzem JR, Rennard SI. Smoke and viral infection cause cilia loss detectable by bronchoalveolar lavage cytology and dynein ELISA. Am J Respir Crit Care Med 1994; 149:205–213.

236. Hameister WM, Wong LB, Yeates DB. Tracheal ciliary beat frequency in baboons: effects of peripheral histamine and capsaicin. Agents Actions 1992; 35(3–4):200–207.

237. de Iongh R, Rutland J. Random ciliary orientation. N Engl J Med 1990; 323: 1681–1684.

238. Cervin A, Lindberg S, Mercke U. The effect of neuropeptide Y on mucociliary activity in the maxillary sinus. Acta Otolaryngol (Stockh) 1991; 111:960–966.

239. Cervin A, Lindberg S, Mercke U, Uddman R. Neuropeptide Y in the rabbit maxil-

lary sinus modulates cholinergic acceleration of mucociliary activity. Acta Otolaryngol (Stockh) 1992; 112:872–881.

240. Wong LB, Park CL, Yeates DB. Neuropeptide Y inhibits ciliary beat frequency in human ciliated cells via nPKC, independently of PKA. Am J Physiol 1998; 275:C440–C448.

241. Lindberg S, Hybbinette JC, Mercke U. Effects of neuropeptides on mucociliary activity. Ann Otol Rhinol Laryngol 1986; 95:94–100.

242. Wong LB, Miller IF, Yeates DB. Pathways of substance-P stimulation of canine tracheal ciliary beat frequency. J Appl Physiol 1991; 70:267–273.

243. Schuil PJ, Ten Berge M, Van Gelder JM, Graamans K, Huizing EH. Substance-P and ciliary beat of human upper respiratory cilia in vitro. Ann Otol Rhinol Laryngol 1995; 104:798–802.

244. Khan AR, Bengtsson B, Lindberg S. Influence of substance P on ciliary beat frequency in airway isolated preparations. Eur J Pharmacol 1986; 130:91–96.

245. Smith RP, Shellard R, Di Benedetto G, Magnus CJ, Mehta A. Interaction between calcium, neural endopeptidase and the substance-P mediated ciliary response in human respiratory epithelium. Eur Respir J 1996; 9:86–92.

246. Schlosser RJ, Czaja JM, Yang B, McCaffrey TV. Signal transduction mechanisms in substance P-mediated ciliostimulation. Otolaryngol Head Neck Surg 1995: 113: 582–588.

247. Wanner A, Maurer D, Abraham WM, Szepfalusi Z, Sielczak M. Effects of chemical mediators of anaphylaxis on ciliary function. J Allergy Clin Immunol 1983; 72:663–667.

248. Tamaoki J, Sakai N, Kobayashi K, Kanemura T, Takizawa T. Stimulation of airway ciliary motility by immunologically activated canine pulmonary macrophages: role of leukotrienes. Acta Physiol Scand 1991; 141:415–420.

249. Ganbo T, Hisamatsu KI, Shimomura SI, Nakajima T, Inoue H, Murakami Y. Inhibition of mucociliary clearance of the eustachian tube by leukotrienes C4 and D4. Ann Otol Rhinol Laryngol 1995; 104:231–236.

250. Bisgaard H, Pedersen M. SRS-A leukotrienes decrease the activity of human respiratory cilia. Clin Allergy 1987; 17:95–103.

251. Dolata J, Lindberg S, Mercke U. The influence of leukotriene and platelet activating factor on mucociliary activity in the rabbit maxillary sinus. Acta Otolaryngol 1990; 109:149–154.

252. Wanner A, Sielczak M, Mella JF, Abraham WM. Ciliary responsiveness in allergic and nonallergic airways. J Appl Physiol 1986; 60:1967–1971.

253. Joki S, Saano V, Koskela T, Toskala E, Bray MA, Nuutinen J. Effect of leukotriene D4 on ciliary activity in human, guinea pig and rat respiratory mucosa. Pul Pharmacol 1996; 9:231–238.

254. Joki S, Saano V. Influence of ageing on ciliary beat frequency and on ciliary response to leukotriene D4 in guinea-pig tracheal epithelium. Clin Exp Pharmacol Physiol 1997; 24:166–169.

255. Weisman Z, Fink A, Alon A, Poliak Z, Tabachnik E, Priscu L, Bentwich Z. Leukotriene C4 decreases the activity of respiratory cilia in vitro. Clin Exp Allergy 1990; 20:389–393.

256. Schuil PJ, van Golder JM, Ten Berg M, Graamans K, Huizing EH. Histamine and leukotriene C4 effects on in vitro ciliary beat frequency of human upper respiratory tract cilia. Eur Arch Otorhinolaryngol 1994; 251:325–328.

257. Verdugo P. Ca^{2+}-dependent hormonal stimulation of ciliary activity. Nature 1980; 283(5749):764–765.

258. Dolata J, Lindberg S, Mercke U. The effects of prostaglandins E1, E2 and F2 alpha on mucociliary activity in the rabbit maxillary sinus. Acta Oto-Laryngol 1989; 108:290–297.

259. Roth Y, Kronenberg J. The effect of prostaglandins E_2 and F_{2a} on brain and tracheal ciliary activity. Laryngoscope 1994; 104:856–859.

260. Bonin SR, Phillips PP, McCaffrey TV. The effect of arachadonic acid metabolites on the ciliary beat frequency of human nasal mucosa in vitro. Acta Otolaryngol (Stockh) 1992; 112:697–702.

261. Slater A, Smallman LA, Logan AC, Drake-Lee AB. Mucociliary function in patients with nasal polyps. Clin Otolaryngol 1996; 21:343–347.

262. Schuil PJ, Ten Berge M, Van Gelder JM, Graamans K, Huizing EH. Effects of prostaglandins D2 and E2 on ciliary beat frequency of human upper respiratory cilia in vitro. Acta Oto-Laryngol 1995; 115:438–442.

263. Tamaoki J, Kobayashi K, Sakai N, Chiyotani A, Kanemura T, Takizawa T. Effect of bradykinin on airway ciliary motility and its modulation by neutral endopeptidase. Am Rev Respir Dis 1989; 140:430–435.

264. Tamaoki J, Sakai S, Chiyotani A, Takeyama K, Tagaya E, Konno K. Effects of prostacyclin and beraprost on ciliary motility of rabbit airway epithelium. Pharmacology 1994; 48:194–200.

265. Kantar A, Oggiano N, Giorgi PL, Braga PC, Fiorini R. Polymorphonuclear leukocyte-generated oxygen metabolites decrease beat frequency of human respiratory cilia. Lung 1994; 172:215–222.

266. Kobayashi K, Salathe M, Pratt MM, Cartagena NJ, Soloni F, Seybold ZV, Wanner A. Mechanism of hydrogen peroxide-induced inhibition of sheep airway cilia. Am J Respir Cell Mol Biol 1992; 6:667–673.

267. Stephens RE, Prior G. Dynein from serotonin-activated cilia and flagella: extraction characteristics and distinct sites for cAMP-dependent protein phosphorylation. J Cell Sci 1992; 103:999–1012.

268. Maruyama I, Inagaki M, Momose K. The role of serotonin in mucociliary transport system in the ciliated epithelium of frog palatine mucosa. Eur J Pharmacol 1984; 106:499–506.

269. Iravani J, Melville GN, Horstmann G. N-Acetylcysteine and mucociliary activity in mammalian airways. Arzneimittelforschung 1978, 28:250–255.

270. Yanaura S, Imamura N, Misawa M. Effects of expectorants on the canine tracheal ciliated cells. Jpn J Pharmacol 1981; 31:957–965.

271. Giordano A, Holsclaw D, Litt M. Effects of various drugs on canine tracheal mucociliary transport. Ann Otol 1978; 87:484–490.

272. Todisco T, Polidori R, Rossi F, Iannacci L, Bruni B, Fedeli L, Palumbo R. Effect of N-acetylcysteine in subjects with slow pulmonary mucociliary clearance. Eur J Respir Dis 1985, 139(suppl):136–141.

273. Tomkiewicz RP, App EM, De Sanctis GT, Coffiner M, Maes P, Rubin BK, King M. A comparison of a new mucolytic N-acetylcysteine L-lysinate with N-acetylcysteine: airway epithelial function and mucus changes in dog. Pulm Pharmacol 1995; 8:259–265.

274. Olivieri D, Marsico SA, Del Donno M. Improvement of mucociliary transport in smokers by mucolytics. Eur J Respir Dis 1985; 139(suppl):142–145.

275. Thomson ML, Pavia D, Gregg I, Stark JE. Bromhexine and mucociliary clearance in chronic bronchitis. Br J Dis Chest 1974; 68:21–27.

276. Gunnarson M, Hybbinette JC, Mercke U. Mucolytic agents and mucociliary activity. Rhinology 1984; 22:223–231.

277. Iravani J, Melville GN. Mucociliary function of the respiratory tract as influenced by drugs. Respiration 1974; 31:350–357.

278. Disse BG, Ziegler HW. Pharmacodynamic mechanism and therapeutic activity of ambroxol in animal experiments. Respiration 1987; 51:15–22.

279. Weiss T, Dorow P, Felix R. Effects of a beta adrenergic drug and a secretolytic agent on regional mucocilary clearance in patients with COLD. Chest 1981, 80: 881–885.

280. Ericsson CH, Juhasz J, Mossberg B, Philipson K, Svartengren M, Camner P. Influence of ambroxol on tracheobronchial clearance in simple chronic bronchitis. Eur J Respir Dis 1987; 70:163–170.

281. Dirksen H, Hermansen F, Groth S, Molgaard F. Mucociliary clearance in early simple chronic bronchitis. Eur J Respir Dis 1987; 153:145–149.

282. Clarke SW, Pavia D, eds. Aerosols and the Lung: Clinical and Experimental Aspects. London: Butterworths, 1984.

283. Thomson ML, Pavia D, Jones CJ, McQuiston TAC. No demonstrable effect of S-carboxymethylcysteine on the clearance of secretions from the human lung. Thorax 1975; 30:669–673.

284. Daffonchio L, De Santi MM, Gardi C, Lungarella G, Omini C. Effect of S-carboxymethylcysteine lysine salt on mucociliary clearance in rabbits with secretory cell metaplasia. Res Commun Mol Pathol Pharmacol 1994; 86:59–74.

285. Ohashi Y, Nakai Y, Sugiura Y, Ohno Y, Okamoto H, Hayashi M. Effect of S-carboxymethylcysteine on ciliary activity in chronic sinusitis. Rhinology 1993; 31:107–111.

286. Karttunen P, Silvasti M, Saano V, Nuutinen J, Joki S, Muranen A, Virta P. Effect of codeine on rat and guinea pig tracheal ciliary beat frequency. Arzneimittelforschung 1991; 41:1095–1097.

287. Selwyn DA, Raphael JH, Lambert DG, Langton JA. Effects of morphine on human nasal cilia beat frequency in vitro. Br J Anaesth 1996; 76:274–277.

288. Van Dongen K, Leusink H. The actions of opium alkaloids and expectorants on the ciliary movements in the air passages. Arch Int Pharmacodyn 1953; 93:261–277.

289. Lewis FH, Beals TF, Carey TE, Baker SR, Mathews KP. Ultrastructural and functional studies of cilia from patients with asthma, aspirin intolerance, and nasal polyps. Chest 1983; 83:487–490.

290. Gerrity TR, Cotromanes E, Garrard CS, Yeates DB, Lourenco RV. The effect of aspirin on lung mucociliary clearance. N Engl J Med 1983; 308:139–141.

291. Tamaoki J, Kondo M, Takizawa T. Stimulation of ciliary activity by indomethacin in rabbit tracheal epithelial organ culture. Respiration 1988; 54:127–131.

293. Daviskas E, Anderson SD, Brannan JD, Chan HK, Eberl S, Bautovich G. Inhalation of dry-powder mannitol increases mucociliary clearance. Eur Respir J 1997; 10:2449–2454.

294. Daviskas E, Anderson SD, Eberl S, Meikle S, Chan HK, Bautovich GJ. Inhalation of dry powder mannitol improves clearance of mucus in patients with bronchiectasis. Am J Respir Crit Care Med 1999; 159:1843–1848.

295. Pavia D, Thomson M, Clarke S. Enhanced clearance of secretions from the human lung after administration of hypertonic saline aerosol. Am Rev Respir Dis 1978; 117:199–203.

296. Daviskas E, Anderson SD, Gonda I, Eberl S, Meikle S, Seale JP, Bautovich GJ. Inhalation of hypertonic saline aerosol enhances mucociliary clearance in asthmatic and healthy subjects. Eur Respir J 1996; 9:725–732.

297. Boek WM, Keles N, Graamans K, Huizing EH. Physiologic and hypertonic saline solutions impair ciliary activity in vitro. Laryngoscope 1999; 109:396–399.

298. Van de Donk HJ, Zuidema J, Merkus FW. Correlation between the sensitivity of the ciliary beat frequency of human adenoid tissue and chicken embryo tracheas for some drugs. Rhinology 1982; 20:81–87.

299. Saano V, Nuutinen J, Virta P, Joki S, Karttunen P, Silvasti M. The effect of ATP on the ciliary activity of normal and pathological human respiratory mucosa in vitro. Acta Oto-Laryngol 1991; 111:130–134.

300. Yoshitsugu M, Rautiainen M, Matsune S, Nuutinen J, Ohyama M. Effect of exogenous ATP on ciliary beat of human ciliated cells studied with differential interference microscope equipped with high speed vide. Acta Otolaryngol (Stockh) 1993; 113:655–659.

301. Saano V, Virta P, Joki S, Nuutinen J, Kartutunen P, Silvasti M. ATP induces respiratory ciliostimulation in rat and guinea pig in vitro and in vivo. Rhinology 1992; 30;33–40.

302. Nuutinen J. Activation of the nasal cilia. Preliminary study in healthy subjects. Rhinology 1985; 23:3–10.

303. Wong LB, Yeates DB. Luminal purinergic regulatory mechanisms of tracheal ciliary beat frequency. Am J Respir Cell Mol Biol 1992; 7:447–454.

304. Uzlaner N, Priel Z. Title interplay between the NO pathway and elevated $[Ca^{2+}]i$ enhances ciliary activity in rabbit trachea. J Physiol 1999; 516:179–190.

305. Bennett WD, Olivier KN, Zeman KL, Hohneker KW, Boucher RC, Knowles MR. Effect of uridine 5'-triphosphate plus amiloride on mucociliary clearance in adult cystic fibrosis. Am J Respir Crit Care Med 1996; 153(6 pt 1):1796–1801.

306. Ziment I. Theophylline and mucociliary clearance. Chest 1987; 92:38S–43S.

307. Wanner A. Effects of methylxanthines on airway mucociliary function. Am J Med 1985; 79:16–21.

308. Pauwels RA. New aspects of the therapeutic potential of theophylline in asthma. J Allergy Clin Immunol 1989; 83:548–553.

309. Konietzko N, Kasparek R, Kellner U, Petro J. Effect of bronchospasmolytics on ciliary beat frequency in vitro. Prax Klin Pneumol 1983; 37(suppl 1):904–906.

310. Hesse BH, Kasparek R, Mizera W, Unterholzner C, Konietzko N. Influence of

reproterol on ciliary beat frequency of human bronchial epithelium in vitro. Arzneimittelforschung 1981; 31:716–718.

311. Serafini SM, Wanner A, Michaelson ED. Mucociliary transport in central and intermediate size airways: effect of aminophyllin. Bull Eur Physiopathol Respir 1976; 12:415–422.

312. Cotromanes E, Gerrity TR, Garrard CS, Harshbarger RD, Yeates DB, Kendzierski DL, Lourenco RV. Aerosol penetration and mucociliary transport in the healthy human lung. Effect of low serum theophylline levels. Chest 1985; 88:194–200.

313. Sutton PP, Pavia D, Bateman JRM, Clarke SW. The effect of oral aminophylline on lung mucociliary clearance in man. Chest 1981; 80:889–891.

314. Pavia D. Effects of pharmacological agents on the clearance of airway secretions. Semin Respir Med 1984; 5:345–352.

315. Afzelius BA. Ultrastructural basis for ciliary motility. Eur J Respir Dis 1983; 128(suppl 1):280–286.

316. Carson JL, Collier AM, Fernald GW, Hu SS. Microtubular discontinuities as acquired defects in airway epithelium of patients with chronic respiratory diseases. Ultrastruct Pathol 1994; 18:327–332.

317. Lurie M, Rennert, G, Goldenberg S, Rivlin J, Greenberg E, Katz I. Ciliary ultrastructure in primary ciliary dyskinesia and other chronic respiratory conditions: the relevance of microtubular abnormalities. Ultrastruct Pathol 1992; 16:547–553.

318. Rutland J, Cox T, Dewar A, Cole PJ, Warner JO. Transitory ultrastructural abnormalities of cilia. Br J Dis Chest 1982; 76:185–188.

319. Pavia D, Lopez-Vidriero MT, Clarke SW. Mediators and mucociliary clearance in asthma. Bull Eur Physiopathol Respir 1987; 23(suppl 10):89s–94s.

320. Hasani A, Agnew JE, Pavia D, Vora H, Clarke SW. Effect of oral bronchodilators on lung mucociliary clearance during sleep in patients with asthma. Thorax 1993; 48:287–289.

321. Garrard CS, Mussartto DJ, Lourenco RV. Lung mucociliary transport in asymptomatic asthma: effects of inhaled histamine. J Lab Clin Med 1989;113:190–195.

322. Mossberg B, Strandberg K, Philipson K, Camner P. Tracheobronchial clearance in bronchial asthma: response to beta-adrenoceptor stimulation. Scand J Respir Dis 1976; 57:119–128.

323. Mortensen J, Groth S, Lange P, Hermansen F. Effect of terbutaline on mucociliary clearance in asthmatic and healthy subjects after inhalation from a pressurised inhaler and a dry powder. Thorax 1991; 46:817–823.

324. Matthys H, Muller S, Herceg R. Theophylline versus budesonide in the treatment of mild-to-moderate bronchial asthma. Respiration 1994; 61:241–248.

325. Pavia D, Bateman JR, Sheahan NF, Clarke SW. Effect of ipratropium bromide on mucociliary clearance and pulmonary function in reversible airways obstruction. Thorax 1979; 34:501–507.

326. Wanner A, Sielczak M, Mella JF. Abraham WM. Ciliary responsiveness in allergic and nonallergic airways. J Appl Physiol 1986; 60:1967–1971.

327. Iravani J, As van A. Mucus transport in the tracheobronchial tree of normal and bronchitic rats. J Pathol 1972; 106:81–93.

328. Pavia D, Bateman JR, Sheahan NF, Clarke SW. Clearance of lung secretions in

patients with chronic bronchitis: effect of terbutaline and ipratropium bromide aerosols. Eur J Respir Dis 1980; 61:245–253.

329. Mossberg B, Strandberg K, Philipson K, Camner P. Tracheobronchoial clearance in patients with emphysema associated with alpha1-antitrypsin deficiency. Scand J Respir Dis 1978; 59:1–7.

330. Santa Cruz R, Landa J, Hirsch J, Sackner MA. Tracheal mucous velocity in normal man and patients with obstructive lung disease: effects of terbutaline. Am Rev Respir Dis 1974; 109:458–463.

331. Sadoul P, Puchelle E, Zahm JM, Jacquot J, Aug F, Polu JM. Effect of terbutaline on mucociliary transport and sputum properties in chronic bronchitis. Chest 1981; 80(suppl 6):885–889.

332. Lafortuna CL, Fazio F. Acute effect of inhaled salbutamol on mucociliary clearance in health and chronic bronchitis. Respiration 1984; 45:111–123.

333. Matthys H, Vastag E, Kohler D, Daikeler G, Fischer J. Mucociliary clearance in patients with chronic bronchitis and bronchial carcinoma. Respiration 1983; 44: 392–337.

334. Sanchis J, Dolovich M, Rossman C, Wilson W, Newhouse M. Pulmonary mucociliary clearance in cystic fibrosis. N Engl J Med 1973; 288:651–654.

335. Yeates DB, Sturgess JM, Kahn SR, Levison H, Aspin N. Mucociliary transport in trachea of patients with cystic fibrosis. Arch Dis Child 1976; 51:28–33.

336. Tegner H, Ceder O, Roomans GM, Kollberg H, Toremalm NG. Effects of cystic fibrosis serum and cell culture medium on the mucociliary activity of the respiratory tract. Acta Paediatr Scand 1981; 70:629–633.

337. Spock A, Heick HMC, Cress H, Logan WS. Abnormal serum factor in patients with cystic fibrosis of the pancreas. Pediatr Res 1967; 1:173–177.

338. Rutland J, Penketh A, Griffin WM, Hodson ME, Batten JC, Cole PJ. Cystic fibrosis serum does not inhibit human ciliary beat frequency. Am Rev Respir Dis 1983; 128:1030–1034.

339. Camner P, Mossberg B, Afzelius BA. Measurements of tracheobronchial clearance in patients with immotile-cilia syndrome and its value in differential diagnosis. Eur J Respir Dis 1983; 127(suppl):57–63.

340. Baum GL, Zwas ST, Katz I, Roth Y. Mucociliary clearance from central airways in patients with excessive sputum production with and without primary ciliary dyskinesia. Chest 1990; 98:608–662.

341. van der Baan S, Veerman AJ, Heidendahl GA, den Hollander W, Feenstra L. Primary ciliary dyskinesia and nasal mucociliary clearance. Respiration 1987; 52: 69–75.

342. Mossberg B, Camner P, Afzelius BA. The immotile-cilia syndrome compared to other obstructive lung diseases: a clue to their pathogenesis. Eur J Respir Dis 1983; 127(suppl):129–136.

343. Rutland J, Morgan L, Waters KA, van Asperen P, de Iongh RU. Diagnosis of primary ciliary dyskinesia. In: Baum G, Priel Z, Roth Y, Liron N, Ostfeld EJ, eds. Cilia, Mucus, and Mucociliary Interactions. New York: Marcel Dekker, 1998: 407–428.

344. Rutland J, Cox T, Dewar A, Rehahn M, Cole P. Relationship between dynein

arms and ciliary motility in Kartagener's syndrome. Eur J Respir Dis 1983; 128(suppl):470–472.

345. Hendry WF, Knight RK, Whitfield HN, et al. Obstructive azospermia: respiratory function tests, electron microscopy and the results of surgery. Br J Urol 1978; 50: 598–604.

346. Pavia D, Agnew JE, Bateman JR, Sheahan NF, Knight RK, Hendry WF, Clarke SW. Lung mucociliary clearance in patients with Young's syndrome. Chest 1981; 80(6 suppl):892–895.

347. Greenstone MA, Rutman A, Hendry WF, Cole PJ. Ciliary function in Young's syndrome. Thorax 1988; 43:153–154.

348. de Iongh R, Ing A, Rutland J. Mucociliary function, ciliary ultrastructure and ciliary orientation in Young's syndrome. Thorax 1992; 47:184–187.

349. Currie DC, Greenstone M, Pavia D, Agnew JE, Pellow P, Clarke SW, Hendry WF, Cole PJ. Efficacy of mucoregulatory agents in Young's syndrome. Thorax 1988; 43:480–481.

350. Camner P, Jarstrand C, Philipson K. Tracheobronchial clearance in patients with influenza. Am Rev Respir Dis 1973; 108:131–135.

351. Camner P, Jarstrand C, Philipson K. Tracheobronchial clearance 5–15 months after infection with *Mycoplasma pneumoniae*. Scand J Infect Dis 1978; 10:33–35.

352. Dolovich MB, Eng P, Mahony JB, Chambers C, Newhouse M, Chernesky MA. Ciliary function, cell viability and in vitro effect of ribavirin on nasal epithelial cells in acute rhinorrhoea. Chest 1992; 102:284–287.

11

Mucokinetic Agents and Surfactant

ANTONIO ANZUETO

University of Texas Health Science
    Center
San Antonio, Texas, U.S.A.

BRUCE K. RUBIN

Wake Forest University School of Medicine
Winston-Salem, North Carolina, U.S.A.

I. Introduction

In healthy individuals, airway secretions constitute a bi-layer with a periciliary fluid interposed between the epithelium and the mucous gel. In the airways, mucus is usually cleared by the airflow and ciliary interaction. Effective cough clearance requires high flow velocity to detach the sputum from the epithelium and to mobilize secretions so that they can be expectorated. For the mucus to slide on top of the epithelium, there is a need for a complex of phospholipid-protein compound—similar to the alveolar surfactant to be present (1). Mucokinetic agents improve the cough clearance of mucus by increasing airflow or by altering the sputum/epithelium interface by reducing mucus adhesiveness. In this chapter we discuss the role of surfactant in sputum clearance, its anti-inflammatory activity, and the role of surfactant supplementation in improving mucus clearance in some conditions, i.e., chronic bronchitis and cystic fibrosis. We will also review the effect of bronchodilators, β_2 agonists, and methylxanthines in mucus clearance.

II. Surfactant Composition and Metabolism

Pulmonary surfactant is a complex mixture of phospholipids and proteins that creates a unique interface separating gas and liquids at the alveolar cell surface, reducing surface tension and maintaining lung volumes at end expiration. Surfactant has effects on surface tension, not only in the alveolus, where it is produced by Type II cells, but also in the bronchi and probably in the entire airway (1,2). Airway surfactant consists of phospholipids that represent 80–90% of the mass (3). In the lung, phosphatidylcholine (70–80%) and phosphatidylglycerol (10%) are the most common phospholipid constituents. Lesser amounts of phosphatidylserine, neutral lipids, and glycolipids are also detected in surfactant. Proteins account for approximately 5–15% of the mass of pulmonary surfactant and include serum proteins and proteins produced by respiratory epithelial cells. To date, four surfactant apoproteins have been identified. Surfactant protein (SP)-A, SP-B, SP-C, and SP-D (named in order of discovery) are produced primarily by respiratory epithelial cells and play a role in surfactant homeostasis and host defense (4,5). These proteins are synthesized by the alveolar Type II cell and are secreted into the alveolar air space, where they influence the structure, metabolism, and function of surfactant. Two classes of proteins have been distinguished on the basis of their structure. SP-A is also expressed in serous cells of the human bronchial and tracheal glands. SP-B is also expressed in bronchial cells, and SP-C is restricted to alveolar Type II cells (9). SP-A and SP-D are relatively abundant, hydrophilic, structurally related proteins that are members of the calcium-dependent lectin family of proteins. These molecules have relatively weak "surfactant-like" qualities but are able to bind complex carbohydrates, including those on the surface of bacteria, virus, and other lung pathogens. These proteins also act as opsonins and activate alveolar macrophages, and therefore are likely to play important roles in host defense in the lung (6). In contrast, SP-B and SP-C are small, hydrophobic proteins that play critical roles in enhancing the rate of spreading and stability of phospholipids (7).

Surfactant is primarily synthesized by Type II pneumocytes, but it is also secreted in other parts of the upper respiratory tract including the nose, Eustachian tube, trachea, and bronchial tree (1). Initially it was thought that the surfactant present in the lower airway was a runoff of the surfactant secreted by the alveoli epithelium. Recently several investigators have shown that there is active surfactant secretion in the bronchus by submucous glands in proximal airway and Clara cells in the distal airway (1). It has been suggested that a relative deficiency or an altered production of Eustachian tube surfactant plays a role in the accumulation of fluid in the middle ear (8). Surfactant apo-protein A, B, and D mRNA is expressed in bronchiolar and alveolar type II cells, SP-A is expressed in the serous cells of the human bronchial and tracheal glands, but SP-C is expressed only in alveolar Type II epithelial cells (9).

Surfactant production is enhanced by glucocorticoids, epidermal growth factor, and cyclic adenosine monophosphate (cAMP), and inhibited by tumor necrosis factor alpha (TNF-α), transforming growth factor beta (TGF-β), and insulin (10). Pulmonary surfactant is taken up rapidly in the lung, and much of the lipid is reutilized. Measurements of the efficiency of recycling of phosphatidylcholine (PC) in animal experiments suggest that up to 90% of PC is reutilized. Thus, only 10–15% of surfactant lipids are cleared by catabolism by alveolar macrophages.

The pulmonary surfactant provides the gas/liquid interface in the alveolar compartment of the lung. This lipid-protein complex increases lung compliance by reducing surface tension and stabilizes the lung airway. The variations in surface tension are related to changes in surfactant component at various lung capacities. Dipalmitoyl-phosphatidylcholine (DPPC) (16:0, 16:0) comprises 50% of the surfactant phospholipids at rest, but this increases to more than 90% during strenuous exercise and at residual volume (11). This monomolecular layer will pass back and forth through a phase transition from liquid crystalline stage at high lung volumes to gel state at low volume (12). Some authors have suggested that the composition of alveolar surfactant will vary rapidly in response to exercise (13). Other factors that affect surfactant composition include changes in temperature. These changes in surfactant composition play an important role in providing alveoli and airway stability.

Surfactant can reduce sputum adhesiveness and increase efficiency of energy transfer from the cilia to the mucus layer. Several investigators have shown that surfactant forms a monolayer above the cilia in order to facilitate mucus clearance. Girod and colleagues (14) have studied the composition and surface activity of conductive airway phospholipids. These investigators analyzed the phospholipid composition, protein content, and surface activity of surfactant isolated from tracheal aspirates, bronchoalveolar lavage (BAL) fluid, and lung parenchyma. The composition of phosphatidylcholine molecular species of tracheal aspirates was similar to that of lung parenchyma and BAL. Analysis of surfactant apo-proteins A, B, and C (SP-A, SP-B, and SP-C) revealed that SP-A was decreased and SP-B and SP-C were absent, whereas total protein was increased in surfactant from tracheal aspirates. These investigators concluded that, as compared with alveolar surfactant, the phospholipid composition of tracheal surfactant is similar but the surface tension function is impaired and the protein concentration is decreased.

III. Role of Surfactant in Airway Patency

Pulmonary surfactant also has the significant function of maintaining airway stability and patency. This concept is based on studies by Clements (15) and Pattle (16), showing that when a film of pulmonary surfactant is compressed as during exhalation, the surface tension will drop to almost zero. Pulmonary surfactant covers both the alveolar wall and the small conducting airways surface (1,8,17,18), thus helping to maintain the patency of small cylindrical airways.

It was hypothesized that if surfactant is inadequate in quantity or quality, there is a risk that liquid will accumulate in the most narrow section of the airway and form a blocking column (19). In order to study this hypothesis, these investigators studied airflow through a narrow glass tube. In the lumen of the capillary tube, a volume of liquid was deposited, which formed a blocking column. If the liquid column consisted of calf lung surfactant and the pressure was raised on one side of the column, the air could pass through the capillary tube and a new liquid column did not form. If the liquid column consisted of saline solution or a diluted surfactant solution containing inhibiting protein, the column of fluid repeatedly reformed as soon as the air was pressed out of the capillary narrow section. These experiments have been corroborated through ex vivo studies by other investigators. In extirpated lungs, Enhorning and colleagues (20) showed that resistance to airflow through the small conducting airways is normally reduced by the action of endogenous surfactant. When surfactant was depleted by a saline lavage, airway resistance increased. The airway resistance was reduced again by installation of exogenous surfactant (Fig. 1). This showed that the conducting airway remains patent when it is coated with surfactant and surrounded by negative pressure. In vivo, this pressure difference between airway lumen and surrounding tissue is provided by the negative intrapleural pressure.

IV. Role of Surfactant in Lung Defense Mechanisms

In conditions characterized by airway inflammation, surfactant dysfunction may play an important role. In asthma it has been demonstrated that there is edema

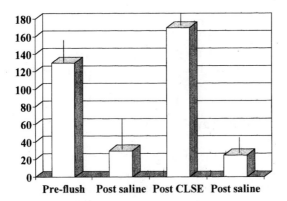

Figure 1 Time of airway openness in an excised rat lung model after calf lung surfactant extract (CLSE) or saline instillation. There was a statistically significant increase in airway openness after CLSE flush compared with saline flush ($p \leq 0.0001$). (From Ref 13.)

in the wall of the airway, increased inflammatory cells, and diminished airway surfactant function (21). Several investigators have suggested that airway inflammation may result in surfactant dysfunction (22). Plasma protein that leaks into the lumen of conducting airways has been suggested to contribute to surfactant dysfunction (23). Hydrolysis of surfactant-associated phospholipids by secretory phospholipases A_2 (sPLA2) is another potential mechanism for surfactant dysfunction in inflammatory lung diseases. In these conditions, airway sPLA2 activity is increased, but the type of sPLA2 and its impact on surface function are not well understood. The effect of different secretory phospholipases A_2 on surfactant hydrolysis was evaluated in vitro by measuring the release of free fatty acids, lysophospholipids, and increase in the minimum surface tension (24). Porcine surfactant and Survanta (calf surfactant preparation) were exposed to mammalian group I (porcine pancreatic) and group II (recombinant human) sPLA2. Mammalian group I sPLA2 readily hydrolyzed phosphatidylcholine, producing free fatty acids and lysophosphatidylcholine and increasing surface tension. In contrast, mammalian group II sPLA2 produced minimal hydrolysis of phosphatidylcholine and did not increase the surface tension. Therefore, sPLA2 present during inflammation may contribute to surfactant dysfunction.

Surfactant has an important role in the immune defense mechanisms of the lung. Thomassen and colleagues (25) studied in vitro cytokine secretion of human macrophages that were exposed to bacterial endotoxin (lipopolysaccharide, LPS) and an artificial surfactant (Exosurf®). These investigators showed that Exosurf suppresses LPS-induced secretion of TNF, interleukin-1 (IL-1), and IL-6 (Fig. 2). IL-8 secretion was suppressed only by giving higher concentrations of artificial surfactant. These in vitro studies demonstrated that Exosurf modulates cytokine secretion for LPS-stimulated human macrophages. The

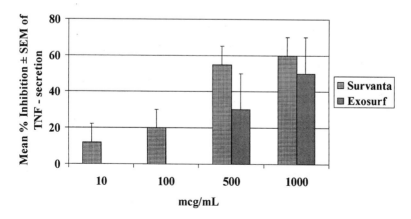

Figure 2 Effect of Exosurf on alveolar macrophage cytokine secretion. (From Ref 26.)

mechanisms involved in these effects may be complex, and further studies are needed to define the nature of this relationship. The same investigators showed that an animal-derived surfactant preparation that contains native bovine surfactant proteins B and C showed the same suppressive effects as with Exosurf (26) (Fig. 3). Earlier experiments using only the lipid component of surfactant (DPPC) showed no effect on cytokine secretion (27). This suggests that the inhibitory effects of surfactant require the combination of DPPC with other agents, such as alcohols or surfactant-associated proteins, that facilitate the spreading of the phospholipids. Other investigators have reported that surfactant has bacteriostatic and opsonic properties against some microorganisms (28). Some of the lipid components are bacteriostatic to many gram-positive organisms. Thus, surfactant may enhance bacterial opsonization and uptake by macrophages.

V. Mucociliary Transport

Mucus is secreted into the epithelial surface of the respiratory tract. The airway secretions form a biphasic fluid composed of an aqueous phase (epithelial lining fluid), in which the cilia beat and relax, and a gel phase located above the tips of the cilia. The latter is propelled by the tips of the cilia and mechanically eliminated by means of mucociliary clearance (29,30). Mucociliary transport is the most important defense mechanism in the respiratory tract and is dependent on the physical properties of mucus as well as interactions between mucus and airflow or mucus and cilia (31). Mucus is essential for particle transport, and cilia alone are unable to transfer particles in the absence of mucus (32). Mucus adheres to the cilia and epithelium. A surfactant layer between the periciliary fluid and the mucus allows the efficient transfer of energy from beating cilia to the mucus, preventing entanglement of the cilia or attachment of the sputum to the epithelium like sticky gum to a carpet. Some mucus adhesiveness is probably necessary to prevent the mucus from sliding down the airway and to entrap particulate matter. Several investigators have shown that the balance between mucus adhesiveness and adhesiveness is largely determined by airway surfactant.

Phospholipid preparations that are present in the alveolar surfactant have been identified in secretions from the central airways, nasal cavity, and eustachian tube (33). These phospholipids influence mucociliary transport (Fig. 4). Sputum tenacity (the product of adhesivity and cohesivity) has the greatest influence on the ability to expectorate sputum by cough. Decreasing tenacity effectively increases the cough transportability of secretions. Surfactant has been shown to reduce mucus adhesivity, resulting in both a reduction in tenacity and an increase in the ability of the cilia to transport mucus. This effect of surfactant

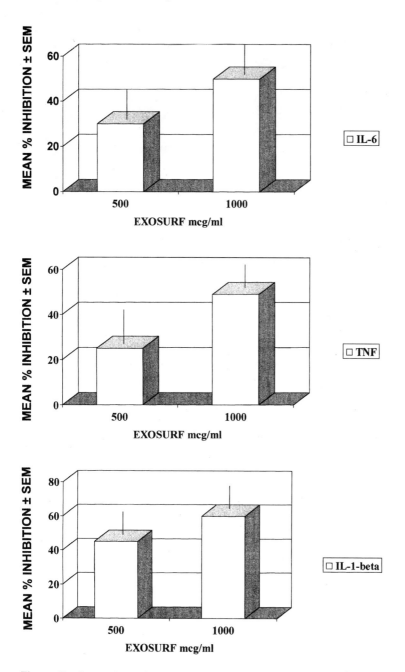

Figure 3 Comparison of Survanta- and Exosurf-mediated inhibition of LPS-stimulated TNF secretion from alveolar macrophages. (From Ref 26.)

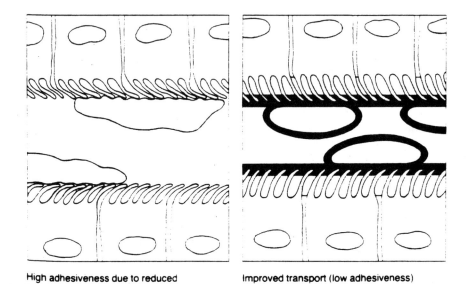

Figure 4 Schematic representation of the antiadhesiveness of surfactants on the ciliary epithelium and improvement in mucociliary transport. (A) High adhesiveness due to reduced surfactant. (B) Improved transport (low adhesiveness) due to surfactant material. Surfactant material may be localized in the periciliary fluid/gel interface along the airways and facilitate the displacement of mucus secretions.

on mucociliary transport in vitro has been studied using an excised frog palate depleted of mucus. The palate was sprayed with porcine surfactant or normal saline, and mucociliary transport was then measured (1). Saline solution induced a constant decrease in transport rate ($p < 0.001$), while the surfactant-treated palate had an increased mucus transport of approximately 16 (NS). The difference between the two treatments was highly significant ($p \leq 0.001$). Surfactant treatment increased canine tracheal mucociliary clearance without significant changes in mucus viscoelastic properties (34). These investigators showed that in vivo aministration of surfactant (Curosurf®) produced a 400% increase in tracheal mucus velocity (Fig. 5). These effects could be due to the surfactant's increasing the efficiency of energy transfer from the beating cilia to the mucus layer by reducing mucociliary frictional energy loss.

A surfactant layer between the cilia and mucus gel phases can facilitate the efficient transfer of energy from the beating cilia to the mucus by decreasing the loss of ciliary kinetic energy and preventing entrapment of the cilia in the

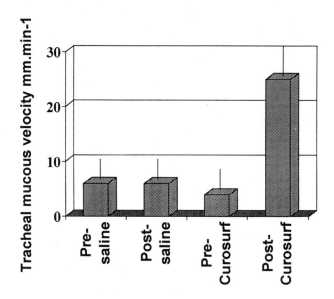

Figure 5 Canine tracheal mucus velocity (TMV) (mm-min^{-1}) 5 days before and after treatment with either saline or surfactant (Curosurf). The increase in TMV with Curosurf was significant as compared to pre-Curosurf and both saline groups. Data presented as mean ±SD. (Data from Ref 34.)

mucous gel (35). Ciliary beat frequency on excised airways decreases continuously in the absence of surfactant, but exogenous surfactant restores the beat frequency. The difference between the ciliary beat frequency in the presence and absence of surfactant is significant, and the effect of surfactant is dose dependent (36). This may be a direct effect of the surfactant on ciliary beating or secondary to surfactant acting as a barrier to water loss from the excised tissue.

No systematic studies of the pulmonary surfactant system in healthy adults are available. However, some of the experimental observations in animals have been confirmed in humans. In BAL supernatant obtained from healthy adults, phosphatidylcholine comprises approximately 80% of the total phospholipid, and surfactant apo-proteins represent <10% of the total proteins (37). Concentrations of SP-A and total phospholipids appear to be age dependent (38).

Thus, morphological, physiological, and biochemical studies show that surfactant has an important function in bronchoalveolar and bronchial mucociliary clearance. Surfactant acts as a lubricant and augments the efficiency transfer of energy from the cilia to the mucus layer.

VI. Surfactant and Chronic Lung Disease

A. Respiratory Distress Syndrome of the Newborn

Prematurely born newborns are at risk for respiratory distress syndrome (RDS) resulting from deficient production of alveolar surfactant by Type II cells. In those infants who die as a result of RDS, there are characteristic hyaline membranes in the alveolar air spaces and generalized obstruction of small airways by tenacious material. In early clinical trials of surfactant therapy for RDS, it was often observed that surfactant therapy was associated with secretion mobilization requiring frequent endotracheal tube suctioning. Rubin and colleagues hypothesized that surfactant deficiency impaired mucus clearance in these neonates, leading to airway obstruction. They tested this hypothesis by collecting airway secretions from newborns with RDS who were treated with either artificial surfactant (Exosurf) or saline and demonstrated that the mucociliary transportability of secretions collected from infants with RDS was significantly increased after surfactant installation (39).

B. Cigarette Smokers

The reported concentration and activity of surfactant in smokers vary widely. In one study, BAL fluid from smokers had a reduced concentration of total surfactant and individual phospholipids (40). Other investigators have shown an abnormal sputum phospholipid composition in chronic tobacco smokers (41,42). Higenbottan (43) had suggested that the proposed mechanism for the decreased surfactant in smokers is increased removal by phagocytes. The ratio of phospholipids to protein in BAL is decreased compared with that in nonsmokers (14,44). The BAL phosphatidylglycerol-cardiolipin fraction is significantly increased in patients with chronic obstructive pulmonary disease (COPD) without a significant difference in the total protein content (Table 1) (45). Furthermore, there is a significant decrease in SP-A and SP-D in cigarette smokers (46). The total phospholipid in BAL from healthy smokers is reported to be normal (47) or

Table 1 Total Alveolar Phospholipids in Bronchoalveolar Lavage (BAL) Supernatants in COPD Patients and Normal Subjects

	N	BAL-phospholipids[a]	Range
Smoker—COPD patient	20	18.97 ± 12.67	4.66–50.63
Nonsmoker controls	5	144 ± 55.8	79.0–194.8

Data: Mean ± SD.
[a]mg of phospholipids % ml of BAL fluid.
Source: Ref. 45.

even increased (48). These differences may be related to the BAL sampling technique, surfactant isolation, or surfactant analytical techniques.

C. Cystic Fibrosis

There are few data on the surface activity and biochemical composition of surfactant in cystic fibrosis (CF) patients. Several investigators have reported alterations in the phospholipid composition and SP-A content of CF tracheobronchial secretions (49,50). CF bronchial lavage fluid has been reported to have an extremely depressed fraction of phosphatidylcholine (3% of phospholipids) compared to controls, associated with increased fluid surface tension (51).

In vitro experiments have shown that the addition of surfactants to cystic fibrotic sputum reduces tenacity and increases mucus clearance (52). In BAL obtained from 20 CF patients (6–20 years) while clinically stable and from 17 healthy children and adults, there was a significantly reduced percentage of surface-active phospholipids and SP-A in CF BAL fluid (53). This was associated with decreased surface activity in CF BAL fluid.

D. Asthma

Surfactant probably contributes to small airway stabilization and prevents collapse (17). Thus, surfactant may have an important role in the therapy of asthma. Studies in vitro have shown that surfactant deficiency may lead to closure of small airways (18,19). Surfactant also appears to have a smooth muscle relaxant effect (54). Surfactant can also suppress the immune lung injury response to inhaled antigen in laboratory animals (22) and in cell culture after antigen exposure (55).

VII. Clinical Trials of Surfactant in Chronic Lung Disease

A. Chronic Bronchitis

In vitro studies on the role of surfactant in chronic bronchitis are controversial. Robertson (56) showed that exogenous surfactant decreases the adhesiveness of mucus and increases mucus transport on a ciliated epithelium using either CF or chronic bronchitis sputum. On the other hand, Rubin (57) analyzed sputum from patients with stable bronchitis. In vitro assessment of dynamic viscoelasticity, surface mechanical impedance, cohesiveness, wettability, and mucociliary transportability of sputum was determined. When exogenous surfactant (Exosurf, GlaxoSmithKline) was added to the sputum, there was a reduction in elasticity and decreased surface mechanical impedance (frictional adhesiveness) compared with untreated sputum. However, there were no differences, including mucociliary transport. The authors concluded that surfactant and other potential mucoactive agents can alter the transportability properties of sputum by acting directly on the secretions, but these data suggest that in vitro assessment cannot be a substitute for clinical trials to evaluate the effectiveness of these compounds.

Our group (58) reported the effects of aerosolized surfactant on sputum surface properties, mucus transportability, pulmonary function (spirometry and lung volumes), and respiratory symptoms in patients with stable COPD. This study was a prospective, multicenter, randomized, double-blind, placebo-controlled comparison of the effects of 2 weeks of treatment with three doses of aerosolized surfactant (DPPC—Exosurf) or saline (placebo). A total of 87 patients diagnosed with COPD were studied. Sixty-six patients were randomized to surfactant treatment and 21 patients to saline treatment. The patients' demographic characteristics between groups were similar at baseline. The mean age was 53 years and baseline forced expiratory volume in 1 second (FEV_1) was 1.23 ± 0.09 ($43 \pm 3\%$ of predictive). The same number of patients in both treatment groups received concomitant medications, including short- and long-acting β_2-agonist, anticholinergic, and corticosteroid inhalers. In patients who received a DPPC dose of 607.5 mg/day for 2 weeks, prebronchodilator, FEV_1 increased from 1.22 ± 0.08 liters to 1.33 ± 0.09 L on day 21 ($p = 0.05$), an improvement of 11.4%. Postbronchodilator FEV_1 improved 10.4% by day 14 and day 21 ($p < 0.02$) (Fig. 6). Lung volumes were also measured, and the ratio of residual volume to total lung capacity—a measure of thoracic gas trapping—decreased 6.2% by day 21 ($p = 0.009$).

Post hoc analysis showed that the effect of aerosolized surfactant was more significant in patients who had lower baseline FEV_1. The patients with a baseline FEV_1 of less than 55% of predicted and who received aerosolized surfactant (607.5 mg/d) had an improvement of 10% and 13.4% on days 14 and 21, respectively ($p \leq 0.05$). An analysis based on the patients' bronchial hyperresponsiveness showed that patients who received a DPPC dose of 607.5 mg/d, but did not have a significant bronchodilator response at baseline, had a more significant increase in posttreatment FEV_1 by days 14 and 21. In the surfactant group there was also a dose-dependent in vitro decrease in sputum tenacity and increase in ciliary transportability of sputum (Fig. 7). These findings confirm that the improvement in pulmonary function seen in patients with COPD after exogenous surfactant administration was due, in part, to improvement in sputum clearance.

B. Asthma

A randomized, masked, and placebo-controlled pilot study using aerosol therapy with Surfactant TA (Tanebe, Tokyo) showed a significant increase in FVC (11.7%), FEV_1 (27.3%), and maximal midexpiratory flow (33.2%) during an acute asthmatic attack inpatients receiving surfactant (59). However, nebulization of a similar surfactant preparation (Alveofact, Boehringer Ingelheim, Germany) did not improve airflow obstruction or bronchial responsiveness to hista-

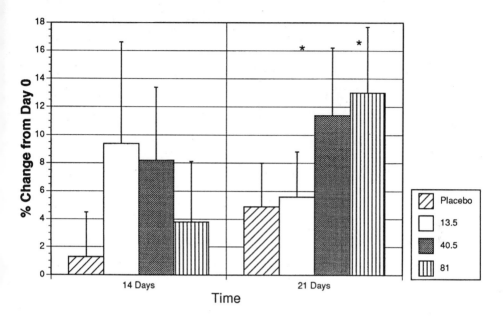

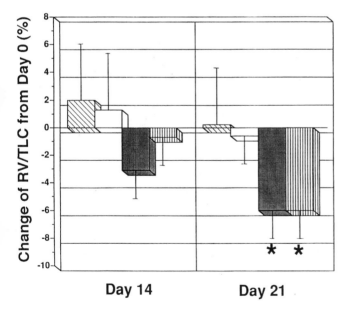

Figure 6 FEV₁ (A) and RV/TLC (B) in patients who received different doses of aero-solized surfactant or placebo after 2 weeks of treatment and 1 week later. The data presented are percentage change from baseline (*p < 0.05). (From Ref 42.)

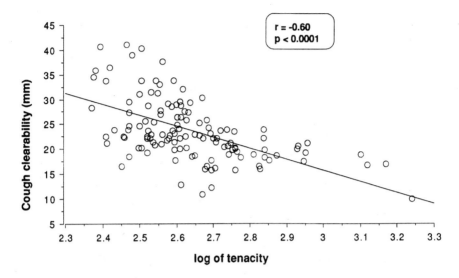

Figure 7 Linear regression analysis between the log of sputum tenacity and transport-ability in surfactant-treated groups ($p < 0.001$; $R = -0.60$). (From Ref 42.)

mine in clinically stable children with asthma (60). These studies differ in that adult patients were studied during an asthma attack and children during the stable phase of the disease. Some of the differences in results may be explained by the fact that part of the airflow obstruction during an asthma attack is caused by mucus plugging and exogenous surfactant may promote removal of these plugs. sPLA2 are generated during an acute asthma attack, leading to the production of highly reactive lipid mediators resulting from arachidonic acid metabolism. Exogenous surfactant could serve as a substrate for sPLA2 (24), preventing the generation of ecosanoids such as leukotrienes and lipid mediators such as platelet-activating factor. These studies also used different surfactant preparations with different concentrations of lipids. Finally, the surfactant dose and delivery systems used were different. Further studies are needed to characterize the role of surfactant in asthma.

C. Cystic Fibrosis

A double-blind, placebo-controlled trial reported the effects of bovine surfactant (Alveofact) in patients with moderate to severe cystic fibrosis (61). Patients received 120 mg of bovine surfactant or placebo aerosolized over a period of 30 minutes for 5 consecutive days. No differences in FVC and FEV_1 were found before or 30 or 90 minutes after the inhalation. Similar results were reported by Rubin and colleagues (49) using aerosolized artificial surfactant (Exosurf).

VIII. Ambroxol

Ambroxol (Mucosolvan™) is widely used in Europe as an antioxidant and possibly as a mucoactive agent. Ambroxol may increase the number and activity of Type II pneumocytes (56,62), thus increasing surfactant production (63). Although some studies have shown that mucociliary transport improved with ambroxol (64,65), clinical benefit has been controversial. Ambroxol has also been shown to increase bronchial tissue antibiotic concentration (66) and reduce the TNF-α and IL-2 content of sputum from patients with chronic bronchitis (66).

It has been reported that ambroxol can reconstitute alveolar phosphatidylcholine in smokers (67), but these results were challenged by Lusuardi and colleagues (67), who studied two groups of 10 COPD patients who received a 14-day trial with ambroxol 150 mg a day or placebo. BAL was performed the day before treatment and at the end of the 2 weeks. There was no significant increase in BAL phospholipids in either ambroxol- or placebo-treated patients. These results are consistent with clinical trial results. In a double-blind, randomized, placebo-controlled trial of ambroxol compared with placebo in 90 patients with chronic bronchitis, the use of ambroxol did not result in any improvement in pulmonary function or clinical symptoms (55). Given the relatively small sample size, there is a need for large, multicenter studies to assess the effect of ambroxol in patients with COPD.

IX. Agents that Increase Air Flow

Bronchodilators can be considered as mucokinetic agents, but only in patients who demonstrate significant improvement in airflow with bronchodilator therapy. β2 agonists are bronchodilators that improve mucus clearance by reducing gas trapping and increasing airflow-dependent clearance. β2 agonists have been shown to increase ciliary beat frequency (70,71) and are mucin secretagogues (72), but their effectiveness in promoting mucociliary transport is conflicting (73,74). This ciliotropic activity would be of limited value in patients with chronic airway inflammation and extensive ciliary damage. Xanthines can also increase ciliary beat frequency, but these medications have not been clearly demonstrated to improve mucus clearance (75).

X. Summary

Bronchial surfactant plays an important role in mucus clearance. Preliminary results using aerosolized exogenous surfactant in patients with stable COPD showed an improvement in sputum clearance associated with a significant improvement in pulmonary function. Data suggest that there are also functional and biochemical surfactant abnormalities in patients with cystic fibrosis and asthma. Further studies are necessary to further characterize these findings.

Acknowledgments

We are grateful to Helle Brown for her secretarial support. Funded in part by a grant from the Cystic Fibrosis Foundation RUBIN96P0. Dr. Rubin is co-holder of US Patent 5,925,334, "Use of Surface Active Agents to Promote Mucus Clearance."

References

1. Allegra L, Bossi R, Braga P. Influence of surfactant on mucociliary transport. Prog Respir Dis 1985; 19:441–460.
2. Yoneda K. Mucus blanket of bronchus. Am Rev Respir Dis 1976; 114:837–842.
3. Whitsett JA. Composition of pulmonary surfactant lipids and proteins. In: Polin RA, Fox WW, eds. Fetal and Neonatal Physiology. Vol 2. Philadelphia: Saunders, 1991:941–949.
4. Baatz JE, Elledge B, Whitsett JA. Surfactant protein SP-B induces ordering at the surface of model membrane bilayers. Biochemistry 1990; 29:6714–6720.
5. Baritussio A, Alberti A, Quaglino D, et al. SP-A, SP-B, and SP-C in surfactant subtypes around birth: reexamination of the alveolar life cycle of surfactant. Am J Physiol 1994; 266(Lung Cell Mol Physiol 20), L436-L447.
6. Curstedt T, Jornvall H, Robertson B, et al. Two hydrophobic molecular mass protein fractions of pulmonary surfactant: characterization and biophysical activity. Eur J Biochem 1987; 168:255.
7. Curstedt T, Johansson J, Persson P, et al. Hydrophobic surfactant-associated peptides: SP-C is a lipopeptide with two-palmitoylated cysteine resides, whereas SP-B lacks covalently linked fatty acyl group. Proc Natl Acad Sci USA 1990; 87: 2985–2989.
8. Mira E, Benazzo M, De Paoli F, Casasco A, Calligaro A. Surfactants of the airways: critical review and personal research. Acta Otorhinolaryngol Ital 1997; 17(1 suppl 56):3–16.
9. Whitsett JA, Korfhagen TR. Regulation of gene transcription in respiratory epithelial cells. Am J Respir Cell Mol Biol 1996; 14:118–120.
10. Whitsett JA, Nogee LM, Weaver TE, Horowitz AD. Human surfactant protein B: structure, function, regulation and genetic disease. Physiol Rev 1995; 75:749–757.
11. Hildebran JN, Goerke J, Clements JA. Pulmonary surface film stability and composition. J Appl Physiol 1979; 47:604–611.
12. Goerke J, Clements JA. Alveolar surface tension and lung surfactant. In: Fishman AP, ed. Handbook of Physiology: The Respiratory System. Vol. 3. Washington, DC: American Physiological Society, 1985:247–261.
13. Doyle IR, Jones ME, Barr HA, Orgeig S, Crockett AJ, McDonald CF, Nicholas

TE. Composition of human pulmonary surfactant varies with exercise and level of fitness. Am J Respir Crit Care Med 1994; 149:1619–1627.

14. Girod S, Calabert C, Lecuire A, Zahm JM, Puchelle E. Phospholipid composition and surface-active properties of tracheobronchial secretions from patients with cystic fibrosis and chronic obstructive pulmonary diseases. Pediatr Pulmonol 1992; 13: 22–27.

15. Clements JA. Surface tension of lung extracts. Proc Soc Exp Biol Med 1957; 95: 170–172.

16. Pattle RE. Properties, function, and origin of alveolar lining layer. Proc R Soc Lond B Biol Sci 1958; 148B:217–240.

17. Macklem PT, Proctor DF, Hogg JC. The stability of peripheral airways. Respir Physiol 1970; 8:191–203.

18. Enhorning G, Holm BA. Disruption of pulmonary surfactant's ability to maintain openness of a narrow tube. J Appl Physiol 1993; 74:2922–2927.

19. Liu M, Wang L, Li E, Enhorning G. Pulmonary surfactant will secure free airflow through a narrow tube. J Appl Physiol 1991; 71:742–748.

20. Enhorning G, Duffy LC, Welliver RC. Pulmonary surfactant maintains patency of conducting airways in the rat. Am J Respir Crit Care Med 1995; 151:554–556.

21. Kay AB. Asthma and inflammation. J Allergy Clin Immunol 1987; 87:892–910.

22. Richman PS, Batcher S, Catanzaro A. Pulmonary surfactant suppresses the immune lung injury response to inhaled antigen in guinea pigs. J Lab Clin Med 1990; 116: 18–26.

23. Persson CGA. Leakage of macromolecules from the tracheo-bronchial microcirculation. Am Rev Respir Dis 1987; 135:S71–S75.

24. Hite RD, Seeds MC, Jacinto RB, Balasubramanian R, White M, Bass D. Hydrolysis of surfactant-associated phosphatidylcholine by mammalian secretory phospholipases A2. Am J Physiol 1998; 275:L740–L747.

25. Thomassen MJ, Meeker DP, Antal JM, Connors MJ, Wiedemann HP. Synthetic surfactant (Exosurf) inhibits endotoxin-stimulated cytokine secretion by human alveolar macrophages. Am J Respir Cell Mol Biol 1992; 1:257–260.

26. Thomassen MJ, Antal JM, Connors MJ, Meeker DP, Widemann HP. Characterization of Exosurf (surfactant)-mediated suppression of stimulated human alveolar macrophage cytokine responses. Am J Respir Cell Mol Biol 1994; 10:399–404.

27. Antal JM, Connors MJ, Meeker DP, Wiedemann HP, Thomassen MJ. Dipalmitoylphosphatidylcholine (DPPC) alone does not mimic the inhibitory effect of surfactant on human alveolar macrophage cytokine secretion. J Immunol 1993; 150:211A.

28. Baughman RP, Gunter KL, Reshkin MC, et al. Changes in the inflammatory response of the lung during acute respiratory distress syndrome with prognostic indicators. Am J Respir Crit Care Med 1996; 154:76–81.

29. Phipps RJ. The airway mucociliary system. Int Rev Physiol 1981; 23:213–260.

30. Puchelle E. Airway secretions: new concepts and functions. Eur Respir J 1992; 5: 3–4.

31. Silberberg A, Meyer FA, Gilboa A, Gelman RA. Function and properties of epithelial mucus. Adv Exp Med Biol 1977; 89:171–180.

32. Birken EA, Brookler KH. Surface tension lowering substance of canine eustachian tube. Ann Otol Rhinol Laryngol 1972; 81:268–277.

33. Rubin BK Therapeutic aerosols and airway secretions. J Aerosol Med 1996; 9: 212–128.
34. De Sanctis GT, Tomkiewicz RP, Rubin BK, Schürch S, King M. Exogenous surfactant enhances mucociliary clearance in the anaesthetized dog. Eur Respir J 1994; 7:1616–1621.
35. Morgenroth K, Bolz J. Morphological features of the interaction between mucus and surfactant on the bronchial mucosa. Respiration 1985; 47:225–231.
36. Hohlfeld J, Fabel H, Hamm H. The role of pulmonary surfactant in obstructive airways disease. Eur Respir J 1997; 10:482–491.
37. Griese M. Pulmonary surfactant in health and human lung diseases: state of the art. Eur Respir J 1999; 13:1455–1476.
38. Ratjen F, Rehn B, Costabel U, Brunch J. Age-dependency of surfactant phospholipids and surfactant protein A in bronchoalveolar lavage fluid of children without bronchopulmonary disease. Eur Respir J 1996; 9:328–333.
39. Rubin BK, Ramirez O, King M. Mucus rheology and transport in neonatal respiratory distress syndrome and the effect of surfactant therapy. Chest 1992; 101:1080–1085.
40. Finley TN, Ladman A. Low yield of pulmonary surfactant in cigarette smokers. N Engl J Med 1972; 286:223–227.
41. Finley TN. Smoking and lung surfactant. In: Cosmi EV, Scarpelli EM, eds. Pulmonary Surfactant System. Amsterdam: Elsevier Science Publishers, 1983:297–310.
42. De Blasio F, Diodato F, Napoletano G, Pezza A. Surfactant phospholipids in BAL fluid of laryngectomy patients suffering from chronic bronchitis. Chest 1993; 104: 16S.
43. Higenbottan T. Pulmonary surfactant and chronic lung disease. Eur J Respir Dis 1987; 71:222–228.
44. Low RB, Davis GS, Giancola MS. Biochemical analysis of bronchoalveolar lavage fluids of healthy human volunteer smokers and non-smokers. Am Rev Respir Dis 1978; 118:863–875.
45. Lusuardi M, Capelli A, Carli S, Tacconi MT, Salmona M, Donner CF. Role of surfactant in chronic obstructive pulmonary disease: therapeutic implications. Respiration 1992; 59(suppl 1):28–32.
46. Honda Y, Takahashi H, Kuroki Y, Aktino T, Abe S. Decreased contents of surfactant proteins A and D in BAL fluid from healthy smokers. Chest 1996; 109:1006–1009.
47. Mancini NM, Bene MC, Gerard H, Chabot F. Early effects of short-time cigarette smoking on the human lung: a study of bronchoalveolar lavage fluids. Lung 1993; 171:277–291.
48. Hughes DA, Haslam PL. Effect of smoking on the lipid composition of lung lining fluid and relationship between immuno stimulatory lipids, inflammatory cells and foamy macrophages in extrinsic allergic alveolitis. Eur Respir J 1990; 3:1128–1139.
49. Rubin BK, Albers GM, Smith E, Browning I III, Colombo J, Kanga, J, Eid N, Regelman W, Anzueto A, Barrett J, et al. Results of a phase II trial of aerosolized Exosurf for the therapy of cystic fibrosis lung disease. Ninth Annual North American Cystic Fibrosis Conference, Dallas, TX, 1995, LB32.

50. Sharma A, Meyer K, Zimmerman J. Surfactant protein A depletion in patients with cystic fibrosis. Am J Respir Crit Care Med 1994; 149:A670.
51. Gillman H, Andresson O, Ellin A, Robertson B, Strandvik B. Composition and surface properties of the bronchial lipids in adult patients with cystic fibrosis. Clin Chim Acta 1988; 176:229–238.
52. Girod S, Pierrat D, Fuchey C, et al. Distearoyl phosphatidylglycerol liposomes improve surface and transport properties of CF mucus. Eur Respir J 1993; 6:1156–1161.
53. Griese M, Birrer P, Demisoy A. Pulmonary surfactant in cystic fibrosis. Eur Respir J 1997; 10:1983–1988.
54. Bergmann JS, Schnitzler S, Seide M, Lachman S. Suppression of angiotensin II induced contraction of the isolated guinea pig ileum by alveolar surfactants. Z Erkrank Atm Org 1997; 149:328–330.
55. Wilsher ML, Hughes DA, Haslam P. Immunomodulatory effects of pulmonary surfactant on natural killer cell and antibody-dependent cytotoxicity. Clin Exp Immunol 1988; 74:465–470.
56. Robertson B. Pharmacological stimulation of surfactant secretion and surfactant replacement. Eur J Respir Dis 1985; 67:63–70.
57. Rubin BK. An in vitro comparison of the mucoactive properties of guaifenesin, iodinated, glycerol, surfactant, and albuterol. Chest 1999; 116:195–200.
58. Anzueto A, Jubran A, Ohar JA, Piquette CA, Rennard SI, Colice G, Pattishall EN, Barrrett J, Engle M, Perrett KA, Rubin BK. Effects of aerosolized surfactant in patients with stable chronic bronchitis: a prospective randomized controlled trial. JAMA 1997; 278:1426–1431.
59. Kurashima K, Ogawa H, Ohka T, Fujimura M, Matsuda T, Kobayashi T. A pilot study of surfactant inhalation for the treatment of asthmatic attack. Jpn J Allergol 1991; 40:160–163.
60. Oetomo SB, Dorrepaal C, Bos H, Gerritsen J, van der Mark TW, Koeter GH, van Aalderen WMC. Surfactant nebulization does not alter airflow obstruction and bronchial responsiveness to histamine in asthmatic children. Am J Respir Crit Care Med 1996; 153:1148–1152.
61. Griese M, Bufler P, Teller J, Reinhardt. Nebulization of a bovine surfactant in cystic fibrosis: a pilot study. Eur Respir J 1997; 10:1989–1994.
62. Seefeld HV, Weiss JM, Eberhards H. Stimulation of lung maturity: investigation of ambroxol in various animal models. Acta Physiol Hungarica 1985; 65:305–312.
63. Egberts J, Fontijne P, Wamsteker K. Indication of increase of the lecithin/sphingomyelin (L/S) ratio in lung fluid in lambs maternally treated with metabolite VIII of Bisolvon. Biol Neonate 1976; 29:315–322.
64. Pfeifer S, Zissel G, Kienast K, Muller-Quernheim J. Reduction of cytokine release of blood and bronchoalveolar mononuclear cells by ambroxol. Eur J Med Res 1997; 2:129–132.
65. Gillissen A, Nowak D. Characterization of N-acetylcysteine and ambroxol in antioxidant therapy. Respir Med 1998; 92:609–623.
66. Paganin F, Bouvet O, Chanez P, Fabre D, Galtier M., Godard P, Michel FB, Bressolle F. Evaluation of the effects of ambroxol on the ofloxacin concentrations in

bronchial tissues in COPD patients with infectious exacerbation. Biopharm Drug Dispos 1995; 16:393–401.

67. Lusuardi M, Capelli A, Salmona M, Tacconi MT, Cerutti CG, Donner CF. Intraluminal inflammation in the airways of patients with chronic bronchitis after treatment with ambroxol. Monaldi Arch Chest Dis 1995; 50:346–351.

68. Zavattini G, Leproux GB, Dagiotti S. Ambroxol. In: Braga PC, Allegra L, eds. Drugs in Bronchial Mucology. New York: Raven Press, 1989:263–291.

69. Guyatt GH, Townsend M, Kazim F, Newhouse MT. A controlled trial of ambroxol in chronic bronchitis. Chest 1987; 92:618–620.

70. Mossberg B, Strandberg K, Philipson K, Camner P. Tracheobronchial clearance in bronchial asthma: response to beta-adrenoreceptor stimulation. Scand J Respir Dis 1976; 57:119–128.

71. Isawa T, Teshima T, Hirano T, et al. Effect of oral salbutamol on mucociliary clearance mechanisms in the lung. Tohoku J Exp Med 1986; 150:51–61.

72. Webber SE, Widdicombre JG. The actions of methacholine, phenylephrine, salbutamol and histamine on mucus secretion from the ferret in-vivo trachea. Agents Actions 1987; 22:82–85.

73. Pavia D, Bateman JR, Sheahan NF, Clarke SW. Clearance of lung secretions in patients with chronic bronchitis: effect of terbutaline and ipratropium bromide aerosols. Eur J Respir Dis 1980; 61:245–253.

74. Roberts DN, Birchall MA, East CA, Scadding G. Intranasal salbutamol has no effect on mucociliary clearance in normal subjects. Clin Otolaryngol 1995; 20:246–248.

75. Wanner A. Effects of methylxanthines on airway mucociliary function. Am J Med 1985; 79:16–21.

12

Mucoregulatory Medications

JUN TAMAOKI, MITSUKO KONDO, and ATSUSHI NAGAI

Tokyo Women's Medical University School of Medicine
Tokyo, Japan

I. Introduction

Mucociliary clearance is an important lung defense mechanism, trapping inhaled bacteria, particles, and cellular debris deposited on the mucosal surface and clearing them from the tracheobronchial tree. This transport function is dependent on several factors, including the beat frequency and coordination of cilia, rheological properties of airway surface liquid, and mucus production (1). The airway epithelium is covered by a surface liquid throughout its length. Lucas and Douglas (2) proposed a two-layer principle of the surface liquid. The upper layer of the fluid is assumed to be a viscoelastic gel, consisting principally of cross-linked glycoproteins forming a tangled network. The lower serous layer, which bathes the cilia, is an ideal liquid. The mucus flows on the sol layer and is transported toward the oropharynx by the ciliary action.

It has been established that airway hypersecretion can be caused by a wide variety of physical and chemical stimuli and is one of the characteristic features of various airway diseases, such as chronic bronchitis, asthma, bronchiectasis, and cystic fibrosis (CF). Mucus hypersecretion and alterations in the biophysical properties of mucus can produce mucociliary dysfunction, which may result in airway infection and further decrease airflow. Patients who have excessive sputum and difficulty in expectoration often complain of impairment of their quality of life. Therefore, it is important to understand the pathophysiology of airway secretion and develop mucoregulators, the compounds that regulate airway secretory responses.

II. Mucoregulators

A. Drugs Acting on the Autonomic Nervous System

Autonomic nerve fibers innervate submucosal glands and airway epithelial cells and regulate airway secretory responses, including mucin secretion and water transport. Thus, the drugs that modify autonomic nerve function might be used as mucoregulating agents.

Anticholinergic Agents

Histological studies using a specific anticholinesterase stain indicate the presence of cholinergic innervation to submucosal glands of monkeys (3), dogs (4), and sheep (5), and electron microscopic studies have shown the localization of cholinergic axon varicosities to submucosal glandular serous and mucous cells of ferrets (6), cats (7), and humans (8). There appears to be general agreement that mucus secretion by submucosal glands is stimulated by cholinergic agonists. Stimulation of efferent postganglionic nerve fibers causes a marked increase in the volume of secretion (9,10) and the output of radiolabeled glycoproteins from submucosal glands (11). Because the both effects are prevented by muscarinic antagonists (9–11), these secretory responses are mediated by cholinergic nerves via muscarinic receptors. Moreover, acetylcholine and methacholine may also increase water movement from the submucosa toward the airway lumen through a stimulation of Cl secretion by airway epithelial cells (12) and submucosal glands (13). These results suggest that stimulation of airway cholinergic muscarinic receptors produces secretion of both mucus glycoprotein and water, and anticholinergic agents may thus reduce airway secretion that is associated with increased cholinergic tone.

Lopez-Vidriero and colleagues (14) have shown that the anticholinergic agent atropine, a tertiary ammonium compound, decreases sputum volume in patients with asthma, chronic bronchitis, and bronchiectasis by inhibiting bronchial mucous gland secretion without apparent changes in mucus viscoelastic properties. However, Pavia et al. (15) reported that the quarternary ammonium compound oxitropium bromide, an anticholinergic drug that has been widely used in the treatment of asthma and chronic obstructive pulmonary disease (COPD), did not alter sputum production or rheology during a 4-week course of treatment. More recently, to assess the long-term effect of oxitropium bromide as a mucoregulator, Tamaoki et al. (16) conducted a parallel, double-blind, placebo-controlled study in patients with chronic bronchitis and diffuse panbronchiolitis. They measured the volume and physical properties of sputum and found that regular inhalation of oxitropium bromide (600 μg daily) for 8 weeks decreased the sputum production by 31% (Fig. 1), with a slight increase in solid composition (the ratio of wet to dry weight) and elastic modulus and no change in dynamic viscosity of the sputum (Table 1). The increases in percentage solid composition and elasticity suggest less hydration of the sputum or increased mucus glycoprotein secretion, but the latter possibility is unlikely, as calculated values of total solids (sputum wet weight × percentage of solid composition) decreased by 17% after treatment. Therefore, inhalation of oxitropium bromide decreases sputum production, presumably through the inhibition of both mucus secretion and fluid transport, the latter component being predominant. These results suggest that long-term use of inhaled anticholinergic agents may be of value in the treatment of patients with COPD and other lung diseases involving airway hypersecretion.

Adrenergic Receptor Agonists

Anatomical studies show the presence of catecholamine-containing nerve fibers in the vicinity of the tracheal and bronchial submucosal glans of ferrets (6), cats (7), and humans (17), and physiological evidence indicates that α-adrenergic

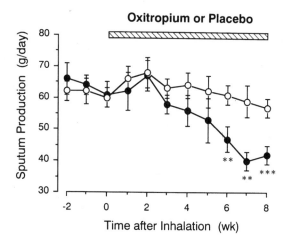

Figure 1 Time course of the volume of sputum expectorated by patients with chronic bronchitis and diffuse panbronchiolitis. Oxitropium bromide (closed circles) or placebo (open circles) was inhaled for 8 weeks after a 2-week observation period. Bar lines indicate 1 SEM ($n = 17$ for oxitropium group and $n = 16$ for placebo group). ** $p < 0.01$, *** $p < 0.001$, significantly different from values for placebo.

Table 1   Values Before and After 8 Weeks of Treatment with Oxitropium Bromide or Placebo

	Oxitropium group			Placebo group		
	Before	After	Difference	Before	After	Difference
Sputum						
Wet weight, g/day	61 (4)	42 (3)	$p < 0.001$	60 (3)	57 (3)	NS
SC, %	2.52 (0.43)	3.02 (0.34)	$p < 0.05$	2.43 (0.72)	2.37 (0.60)	NS
G', dyne/cm^2	68 (12)	97 (20)	$p < 0.05$	57 (23)	63 (18)	NS
η', poise	32 (14)	40 (22)	NS	38 (17)	33 (21)	NS
Log_{10} CFU bacteria/g	4.7 (0.7)	3.9 (1.0)	NS	3.7 (0.8)	3.2 (0.6)	NS
FEV$_1$, %pred	67.6 (4.0)	75.3 (3.2)	$p < 0.05$	71.3 (2.8)	73.7 (4.5)	NS
VC, %pred	84.4 (3.5)	84.7 (2.5)	NS	81.0 (3.3)	83.1 (2.8)	NS

SC, solid composition; G', elastic modulus; η', dynamic viscosity; CFU, colony-forming units; NS, not significant. $n = 17$ for oxitropium group, $n = 16$ for placebo group.

nerves (9) and receptors (10) mediate glandular fluid secretion in some species, but β-adrenergic mechanisms may be less potent in causing fluid secretion (9). On the other hand, mucus secretion is potently stimulated by α- and β-adrenergic [mechanisms (18). Previous studies have shown that norepinephrine and phenylephrine (α-adrenergic), dobutamine (β$_1$-adrenergic), albuterol and terbutaline (β$_2$-adrenergic), and isoproterenol (β$_1$- and β$_2$-adrenergic) increase the output of secretory glycoproteins in many species including humans (19,20). However, there seems to be a selective stimulation of serous and mucous cells of submucosal glands by adrenergic mechanism. For example, stimulation of α-adrenergic receptors with phenylephrine depletes the secretory granules of serous cells in the ferret trachea, whereas β$_2$-adrenergic stimulation with terbutaline is without effect (6). Similarly, a loss of mucous cell granules occurs with terbutaline but not with phenylephrine.

Mucociliary clearance in the respiratory tract is generally impaired in patients with asthma (21,22), and the use of β$_2$-adrenergic agonists might produce favorable effects because they not only cause bronchodilation but also potently stimulate ciliary motility (23), which in turn accelerates mucociliary transport (24,25). However, based on the in vitro findings as mentioned above, stimulation of β$_2$-adrenergic receptor also increases glycoprotein production, thereby causing mucus accumulation in the airway lumen. To date, there are no clinical studies on the effects of β$_2$-agonists on sputum production and its rheological properties, and it remains uncertain whether β$_2$-adrenergic agents are effective as mucoregulating agents in humans.

B. Peptide and Peptide Antagonists

Electrical stimulation of nerves both in vitro and in vivo induces mucus secretion in the airways of a number of animal species, and a proportion of the secretion persists despite adrenoceptor and cholinoceptor blockade (11,26), where the latter nonadrenergic, noncholinergic (NANC) component of neurogenic secretion is mediated by two principal neural pathways. The first pathway comprises an orthodromic system of adrenergic and cholinergic nerves, which contain neuropeptides colocalized with neurotransmitters including vasoactive intestinal peptide (VIP) and neuropeptide Y (NPY), both of which may alter mucus secretion or modulate stimulus-evoked secretion, depending on how this is studied. The effects of VIP on airway mucus secretion are conflicting (27,28). VIP inhibits the release of radiolabeled glycoprotein from human bronchial mucosa but increases its output from the dog trachea; it has little action on basal volume secretion into the ferret trachea. There could be either species difference or different receptors for VIP. Since VIP may be released with acetylcholine, the interaction between the two is potentially important. Webber and Widdicombe (29) have shown that VIP enhances mucus output and lysozyme secretion (as a marker for serous cell secretion) produced by phenylephrine, suggesting an activation of serous cells, but it decreases the volume output of mucus produced by methacholine without affecting lysozyme secretion, suggesting an inhibition of mucous cells. NPY has a distribution in the airways similar to that of sympathetic nerves and is found close to submucosal glands. Like other motor neuropeptides, NPY has little effect on resting output of mucus. However, when mucus secretion is stimulated by phenylephrine, mimicking sympathetic activation, NPY enhances the total volume output from mucous cells, an effect that is opposite to that of VIP. Recently, Lacroix and Mosimann (30) tested the effect of NPY on allergen-evoked nasal responses in patients with allergic rhinitis. They found that intranasal administration of NPY caused a great reduction of mucus secretion induced by nasal challenge with grass pollen allergen.

The second pathway of NANC regulation comprises a system of capsaicin-sensitive nerves, which subserve a motor function and may be termed "sensory-efferent" nerves. The neurotransmitters of this neural system are collectively termed sensory neuropeptides and include calcitonin gene–related peptide (CGRP) and the tachykinins substance P (SP) and neurokinin A (NKA) and NKB. Of these, SP elicits mucus secretion, whereas CGRP is a weak secretagogue (31). SP strongly increases the output of radiolabeled macromolecules from explants of ferret trachea (32) and also depletes the granules of airway goblet cells in guinea pigs (33), indicating that SP stimulates mucus production by goblet cells. Furthermore, SP acts by contracting myoepithelial cells in the secretory duct of submucosal glands, thereby squeezing the mucus already in the duct into the airway lumen. Gentry (34) studied the relative potency of various tachykinins to stimulate the release of high molecular weight glycocon-jugate from ferret trachea and found a rank order of potency of SP > physalae-min ≥ eledoisin ≥ NKA > NKB, which is most consistent with the tachykinin receptor type NK_1.

In addition, tachykinins stimulate Cl secretion and, hence, increase water secretion across airway epithelium. Rangachari and McWade (35) showed that SP caused a transient increase in short-circuit current of dog tracheal epithelium. Using similar preparations, Tamaoki et al. (36) examined the effects of NKA and NKB on the bioelectric and ion transport properties and found that both of these peptides induced a dose-related increase in short-circuit current; the re-sponse to NKA exceeded that of NKB. The investigators concluded that this change was related to an increase in Cl secretion toward the tracheal lumen associated with an increase in intracellular cAMP. In contrast to the finding in submucosal glands, the tachykinin receptor involved in epithelial ion transport may be of the NK_2 subtype.

In recent years, several tachykinin receptor antagonists have been devel-oped (37), which include the selective NK_1 receptor antagonists FK888 (38) and CP 96345 (39), the NK2 receptor antagonist SR 48968 (40), and the dual NK_1/NK_2 receptor antagonist FK224 (41). Ramnarine et al. (42) examined the effects of tachykinin antagonists on mucus secretion from the ferret tracheal submuco-sal glands in vitro. Pretreatment with FK888 inhibited the NANC-mediated re-lease of $^{35}SO_4$-labeled macromolecules by 47%, whereas SR 48968 had no ef-fect. These observations indicate that "sensory-efferent" neurogenic mucus secretion in the ferret airway is mediated by tachykinin NK_1 receptors with no involvement of NK_2 receptors and suggest that potent and selective tachykinin antagonists may have therapeutic potential in airway diseases such as asthma and chronic bronchitis in which neurogenic mucus hypersecretion might be etio-logically important.

C. Antimicrobial Agents

Macrolides

There is increasing evidence that long-term administration of macrolide antibiot-ics is effective in the treatment of chronic airway inflammatory diseases, proba-bly through actions other than their antimicrobial properties. Erythromycin re-duces the volume of airway secretions in some patients with asthma (43), bronchorrhea (44), chronic bronchitis, and diffuse panbronchiolitis (45,46), but the mechanism of action is not clear. One explanation would be that macrolides exert their effects through anti-inflammatory activities. For instance, erythromy-cin inhibits cytokine production by airway epithelial cells and modulates im-mune responses of inflammatory cells, such as neutrophils, lymphocytes, and macrophages (47). On the other hand, there are data suggesting that erythromycin has a direct effect on secretory cells. Goswami et al. (48) studied nasal mucus glycoconjugate secretion from healthy nonsmoking adults before and after treatment with erythromycin base, penicillin, ampicillin, tetracycline, or cephalosporins. Erythromycin at a concentration of 10 μM reduced nasal secretion by 35% both in the resting state and when the nose was stimulated with methacholine or histamine. The other antibiotics had no effect on glycoconjugate secretion. Additionally, in the experiment with electrical properties of cultured canine tracheal epithelium (49), erythromycin added to the submucosal side at concentrations of 10 μM and higher dose-dependently decreased short-circuit current, and this effect was not altered by the Na channel blocker amiloride but abolished by the Cl channel blocker diphenylamine-2-carboxylate or substitution of Cl in the bathing medium with gluconate, an anion that cannot be transported by airway epithelium. These in vitro findings suggest that erythromycin may reduce both mucus and water secretion via mechanisms other than the control of infection. A discrepancy seems to exist in the concentrations of erythromycin required to produce its in vitro and in vivo effects. The mean serum concentration following the ingestion of 500 mg erythromycin by adult volunteers has been reported to be 1.6 μM (50), whereas in vitro experiments showed that at least 10 μM erythromycin was required to decrease mucus production and Cl transport. However, because of species differences, the findings may not necessarily be clinically contradictory. In addition, the serum concentration of erythromycin does not accurately reflect the local concentration, since this drug has been shown to concentrate intracellularly more than 10-fold (51).

Other studies suggest that erythromycin has anti-inflammatory properties with direct effects on neutrophil migration and function and secondary effects on mucus secretion. Several studies show that erythromycin reduces neutrophil chemotaxis (45,52) and the generation of oxygen radicals (53), but other studies have failed to show a direct effect of erythromycin on neutrophil function or motility (54). It has recently been shown that inhalation of lipopolysaccharide from *Escherichia coli* in guinea pigs increases neutrophil accumulation into the tracheal mucosa and stimulates goblet cell secretion, as assessed histologically by mucus score, which is inversely related to the magnitude of mucus discharge (55) (Fig. 2), and that these effects are dose-dependently inhibited by orally administered macrolide antibiotics, including erythromycin and clarithromycin, but not by amoxicillin or cefaclor (56). Similarly, erythromycin and roxithromycin inhibit interleukin-8–induced recruitment of neutrophils and the associated goblet secretion in the guinea pig trachea (57) (Fig. 3). However, whether macrolides exert their antisecretory effect by solely inhibiting neutrophil function or by acting on goblet cells and neutrophils independently remains uncertain.

In clinical studies, Tamaoki et al. (46) examined the effect of clarithromycin on sputum production and its rheological properties in patients with

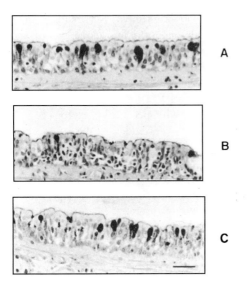

Figure 2 Photomicrographs of the airway epithelium in guinea pig tracheal mucosa stained with alcian blue pH 2.5 and periodic acid Schiff. Scale bar = 10 mm. The guinea pigs were given inhaled saline (A), LPS (5 mg/kg) alone (B), or were treated pretreated with oral clarithromycin at a daily dose of 10 mg/kg for 1 week and then given inhaled LPS (C). Tracheal tissues were prepared 3 hours after inhalation of saline or LPS.

chronic lower respiratory tract infections. Clarithromycin was given at 100 mg twice daily for 8 weeks and compared with placebo. We showed that clarithromycin decreased sputum volume from 51 to 24 g/day and that the percent solids of the sputum increased from 2.44 to 3.01%, with no effect of placebo. Elastic modulus (G′) increased from 66 to 87 dyne/cm^2 (at 10 Hz), whereas dynamic viscosity (η′) remained unchanged (Fig. 4). More recently, Rubin et al. (58)

FACING PAGE

Figure 3 Dose-dependent effects of macrolide antibiotics on IL-8–induced goblet cell secretion (upper panel) and neutrophil recruitment (lower panel) in guinea pig trachea. The guinea pigs orally received roxithromycin (▨) or erythromycin (▦) at a daily dose of 1, 3, 5, or 10 mg/kg for 1 week, or amoxicillin (▤) or cefaclor (▨) at a daily dose of 30 mg/kg for 1 week, and the responses were determined 6 hours after inhalation of IL-8 (1.7 μg/kg). Values are expressed as mucus score, a histologically assessed parameter that inversely relates to the degree of goblet cell discharge. Data are means ± SE; $n = 10$ guinea pigs for each column. * $p < 0.05$, ** $p < 0.01$, significantly different from values for IL-8 alone.

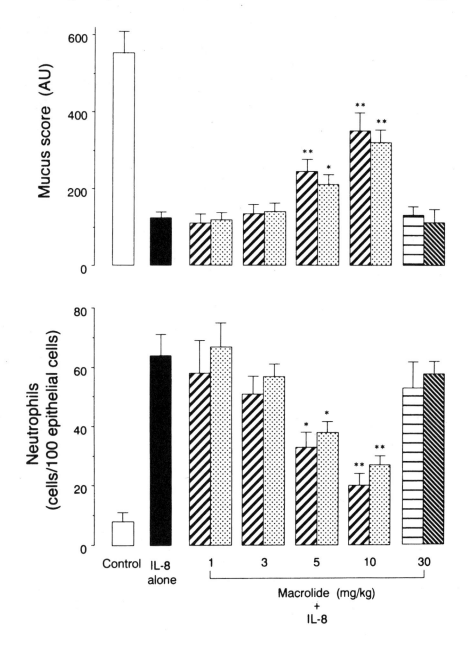

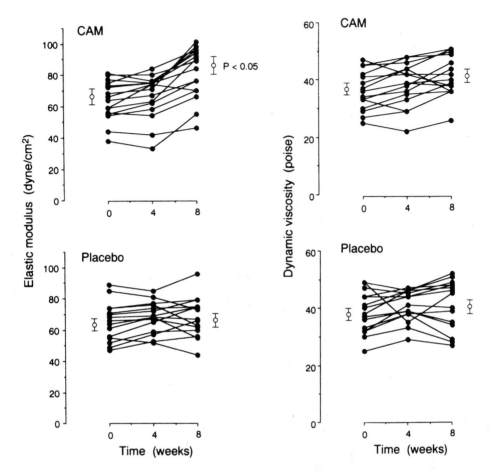

Figure 4 Individual values (closed circles) for elastic modulus and dynamic viscosity of the sputum in patients with chronic bronchitis, bronchiectasis, or diffuse panbronchiolitis obtained before (0 week), during (4 weeks), and after (8 weeks) the treatment with clarithromycin (CAM) or placebo. Open circles indicate means ± SE values at 0 and 8 weeks of treatment.

showed that in patients with purulent rhinitis clarithromycin (500 mg twice daily) for 2 weeks did not significantly alter sputum viscoelasticity but decreased secretion volume from 500.1 to 28.3 mg/day and increased mucociliary transportability by 30%. The increased transportability of mucus may be attributed to diminished secretion adhesiveness (59) and/or direct stimulation of airway ciliary motility (60).

Other Antibiotics

Middleton et al. (61) showed that trimethoprim and tetracycline induced a rapid decrease in electrogenic ion transport in sheep tracheal epithelium in vitro. The responses were mediated through the mucosal surface and reduced by treatment with amiloride, suggesting inhibition of Na absorption. Ampicillin, ceftazidime, colistin, chloramphenicol, gentamicin, and sulfamethoxazole had no significant effects. They also demonstrated that trimethoprim and tetracycline decreased nasal potential difference in healthy human volunteers in vivo, which was atten- uated by amiloride pretreatment. In subjects with CF who exhibited increased Na absorption across respiratory epithelia, the responses to trimethoprim and tetracycline were enhanced, providing further evidence that these drugs inhibit Na absorption. These drugs may thus prevent dehydration of airway surface and potentially offer combined effects for the management of CF patients.

An antifungal agent, ketoconazole, has been reported to alter epithelial ion transport. Kersting et al. (62) showed that ketoconazole inhibited the conduc- tance of apical cell membrane to Na and K and induced a striking stimulation of the conductance to Cl in cultured CF cells (CEPAC-1) through a cAMP- independent pathway. These findings suggest that ketoconazole could also be of value in the treatment of CF.

The usual clinical features of bronchiectasis include hypersecretion of mu- copurulent sputum and chronic or recurrent pulmonary infections with accumu- lation of neutrophils. Recruitment or sequestration of neutrophils increases the inflammatory burden, which is exaggerated during airway infection. Neutrophils in the bronchial lumen are capable of releasing toxic oxygen radical species and proteolytic enzymes, which may lead to goblet cell hyperplasia (63), impairment of mucociliary clearance, cleavage of immunoglobulins or complement (64), and increasing mucus secretion. Therefore, inhibition of neutrophil recruitment and/or activation in patients with bronchiectasis may be of therapeutic signifi- cance. Gentamicin and other aminoglycosides have been shown to decrease my- eloperoxidase activity in vitro (65) in addition to their bactericidal effects, and Lin et al. (66) recently studied whether gentamicin prevents mucus hypersecre- tion in bronchiectasis. A short course of aerosol therapy with gentamicin (40 mg, twice daily) decreased the amount of daily sputum without affecting wet/ dry ratio, viscosity, or protein content of mucus. Because the change in the sputum volume was related to that in the sputum myeloperoxidase level, they conclude that the gentamicin-induced suppression of mucus hypersecretion may be due at least in part to the inhibition of myeloperoxidase activity.

D. Drugs That Modify Arachidonic Acid Metabolism

There is ample evidence that lung is one of the major sites of arachidonic acid metabolism and that cyclooxygenase and lipoxygenase products of arachidonic acid may play a role in the pathogenesis of various airway diseases. In 1981, Marom and coworkers (67) demonstrated that arachidonic acid caused an increase in mucous glycoprotein release from human airways in vitro. The sputum from patients with COPD contains many different cell types, including pulmonary macrophages, neutrophils, and eosinophils, and these cells are capable of synthesizing and releasing phospholipid-derived mediators via cyclooxygenase and lipoxygenase pathways (68,69). These results suggest that prostaglandins (PGs) and/or leukotrienes (LTs) may be involved in mucus hypersecretion.

Modification of Cyclooxygenase Pathway

It has been known that inhaled $PGF_{2\alpha}$ increases the amount of sputum expectorated in normal human subjects (70), and Rich et al. (71) showed that $PGF_{2\alpha}$ at 0.1 µg/mL stimulated mucus secretion from excised human airways. In contrast, the results of PGE_2 action are conflicting: PGE_2 has been reported to have no effect (71) or an inhibitory effect (67) on the output of radiolabeled macromolecules. However, cyclooxygenase products as a whole appear to stimulate gland secretions since Na salicylate, an inhibitor of cyclooxygenase, can reduce the incorporation of $[^3H]$-glucose and $[^3H]$-glucosamine into the mucus and serous cells of human submucosal glands (70,72). Regarding airway epithelial ion transport, both PGE_2 and $PGF_{2\alpha}$ stimulate Cl secretion toward the lumen and promote water accumulation (73). Inoue and colleagues (74) showed that indomethacin suppository and aspirin inhalation reduced the amount of sputum in patients with bronchiectasis and chronic bronchitis, respectively, but indomethacin had no effect on excessive sputum in asthmatic subjects. In a double-blind, placebo-controlled study (75), the effect of indomethacin on bronchorrhea was investigated in patients with chronic bronchitis, diffuse panbronchiolitis, and bronchiectasis. Patients who received 2 mL of inhaled indomethacin (1.2 µg/ mL) three times a day for 14 days showed a decrease in sputum production from 189 to 95 g/day (Fig. 5) and an increase in the solid composition of sputum without alterations in sputum microbiology or measures of systemic inflammatory responses such as circulating white blood cells and erythrocyte sedimentation rate. The reduction of sputum was accompanied by a significant decrease in the concentrations of PGE_2, $PGF_{2\alpha}$, thromboxane (Tx) B_2, and 6-oxo-$PGF_{1\alpha}$ in the sputum (Fig. 6). These results suggest that indomethacin inhalation is effective in reducing bronchorrhea sputum, probably through the inhibition of PG-dependent airway secretions. In another double-blind, placebo-controlled study, Sofia et al. (76) evaluated the effect of a 3-week treatment course of the nonsteroidal anti-inflammatory drug nimesulide (100 mg, twice daily) on both clinical parameters and rheological properties of sputum in patients with chronic bronchitis and varying degrees of airway obstruction. They found that, in comparison with placebo, nimesulide significantly reduced the volume of daily spu-

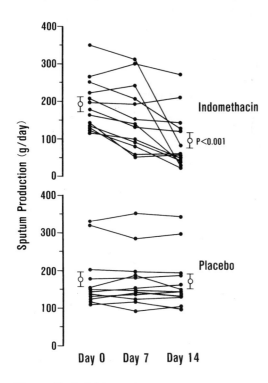

Figure 5 Individual values (closed circles) for daily sputum production before (day 0) and during (day 7 and day 14) inhalation of indomethacin or placebo in patients with chronic bronchitis (solid line), diffuse panbronchiolitis (dot/dash line), and bronchiectasis (dashed line). Open circles indicate means ± SE values on days 0 and 14 after the treatment.

tum expectoration and decreased sputum viscosity by an average of 10% after 7 days and 30% at the end of treatment. These effects correlated with the degree of clinical improvement. The investigators concluded that nimesulide might have exerted its effect by modulating neutrophil function and by inhibiting the production of inflammatory mediators, and that the decrease in sputum viscosity might be accomplished by decreasing plasma exudation into the airway lumen.

The cyclooxygenase product TxA_2 is a potent bronchoconstrictor but may not possess a direct action on mucus production by submucosal glands and goblet cells or water secretion by airway epithelial cells. On the other hand, Yanni et al. (77) have shown that an orally administered TxA_2 analog increases the thickness of the mucous gel layer in rats. This effect is probably associated with the increased plasma exudation into the airway lumen. In fact, U-46619, a

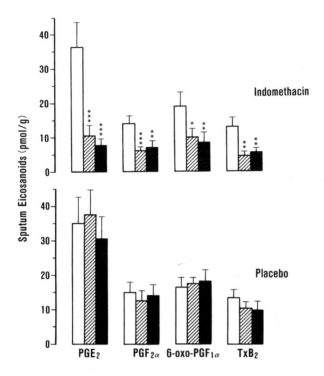

Figure 6 Concentrations of cyclooxygenase products in the sputum obtained before (day 0, open bars) and during (day 7, shaded bars; day 14, solid bars) inhalation of indomethacin or placebo. Values are means ± SE, $n = 13$ for indomethacin group, and $n = 12$ for placebo group. * $p < 0.05$, ** $p < 0.01$, *** $p < 0.001$, significantly different from values on day 0.

TxA_2 mimetic, has been shown to cause airway microvascular leakage in guinea pigs (78). OKY-046 is a selective inhibitor of TxA_2 synthase in various species, including humans (79), and Kurashima and colleagues (80) studied the effect of OKY-046 on mucociliary clearance in asthmatic subjects. Oral administration of OKY-046 (400 mg/day) for 4 weeks decreased the amount of sputum expectorated by 45% and increased mucociliary transport rate by 120%, as assessed by nasal clearance time (81). The same investigators also reported, in a double-blind, placebo-controlled study, that patients with chronic bronchitis and diffuse panbronchiolitis receiving OKY-046 showed a 22% decrease in sputum production after 4 weeks and a 39% decrease after 12 weeks (82). Although the bio-physical properties of the sputum, including viscosity and spinnability (adhe-siveness), and the concentrations of fucose and immunoglobulin A in the sputum remained unchanged, significant decreases were noted in the concentrations of total protein, albumin, sialic acid, and phospholipid. Since albumin and fucose are chemical markers of plasma exudation and mucus secretion, respectively, while sialic acid is derived from both serum and mucus, these results indicate that the inhibition of TxA2 synthesis by OKY-046 may attenuate airway microvascular leakage and consequently reduce sputum production.

Modification of Lipoxygenase Pathway

The 5-lipoxygenase products of arachidonic acid (LTs, 5-hydroperoxyeicosatetraenoic acid [5-HPETE] and 5-hydroxyeicosatetraenoic acid [5-HETE]) are potent inflammatory mediators relevant to pathophysiology of asthma. In addition to their potent bronchoconstrictor effects, LTC_4 and LTD_4 have strong mucus releasing actions in human airways in vitro. Coles and colleagues (83) showed that these LTs induced a concentration-dependent increase in the release of radiolabeled glycoprotein but not of lysozyme from human lung fragments. This secretagogue effect was selective for high molecular weight glycoproteins of about $2-5 \times 106$ daltons and 100-fold more potent than the cholinergic agonist methacholine. Similar findings were reported by Marom et al. (84). Hoffstein et al. (85) conducted in vivo experiments and showed that aerosolized LTD4 produced a dose-related decrease in the content of alcian blue–periodic acid Schiff positive granules in the epithelium of guinea pig bronchi. This stimulatory effect was inhibited by pretreatment with the specific LTD_4 receptor antagonist SK&F 104353 (86). Although this suggests that LT antagonists may be useful to treat mucus hypersecretion, there are no clinical studies on the mucoregulating effects of such agents. LTC_4 and LTD_4 can stimulate Cl secretion from canine tracheal epithelium in vitro, thereby causing an increase in water movement across the airway mucosa (87). However, the effects of LTs on ion transport in human airways has not been studied.

Apart from 5-lipoxygenase products, substantial amounts of the 15-lipoxygenase product 5-HETE is produced in human airways (88,89). In the canine model of mucus secretion, Johnson et al. (90) showed that 15-HETE caused elevations (hillocks) in the tantalum layers on the tracheal mucosa when given by arterial injection or when aerosolized directly into the lung, indicating an increased mucus secretion from submucosal glands. These investigators also found that, after hypoxia or arachidonic acid loading, the levels of 15-HETE extracted from tracheal mucus correlated well with hillocks and weight of secreted mucus and that the effects were abolished by a 15-lipoxygenase inhibitor (91). Thus, blockade of 15-lipoxygenase pathway might be another possibility for the treatment of mucus hypersecretion.

E. Glucocorticosteroids

Despite the clinical impression that glucocorticosteroids reduce bronchorrhea in patients with asthma, there have been few reports concerning the effect on mucus secretion. Previous in vitro reports have shown that steroid causes a dose-related reduction in glycoconjugate release from cat tracheal submucosal glands (92) and human airway explants (93). The mechanism of action is explained by the induction of lipocortin, a phospholipase inhibitor, which prevents the cleavage of arachidonic acid from cell membranes and the initiation of cyclooxygenase and lipoxygenase metabolic pathways (94).

The accumulation of mucus in airways has long been recognized as a major factor contributing to the morbidity and mortality of asthma (95,96). The cause of mucus hypersecretion that leads progressively to the plugging of airways and respiratory insufficiency is not completely understood. An increase in the synthesis and rate of secretion and/or changes in the biophysical properties of the secreted mucous glycoprotein would obviously affect the balance between secretion and mucociliary clearance, thereby allowing a buildup of airway mucus to occur. Glucocorticoids have been widely used in the treatment of asthma, and, from clinical experience, these drugs appear to be the most effective among the few useful compounds in reducing airway secretion. Savoie and coworkers (97) reported that dexamethasone decreased antigen-induced high molecular weight glycoconjugate secretion in allergic guinea pigs. Blyth et al. (98) showed that dexamethasone inhibited airway goblet hyperplasia following repeated intratracheal antigen challenge in mice and accelerated the recovery from established goblet hyperplasia. Although the mechanism of goblet cell hyperplasia in asthma is unknown, mediators such as platelet-activating factor (99) and Th2 cytokines, such as interleukin-4 (110), are reported to induce goblet cell hyperplasia and MUC5AC gene expression. It is thus possible that suppression of these mediators and cytokines could result in the improvement of goblet cell hyperplasia. Dexamethasone can also inhibit agonist-induced ion transport in canine and feline airway epithelial cells and submucosal glands (101), but the mechanism of action is uncertain.

In contrast to ample findings in animal models, there are very few studies documenting the benefits of glucocorticoid therapy on airway hypersecretion in humans. Boothman-Burrell et al. (102) recently reported that treatment with either oral steroid or inhaled steroid caused a reduction in sputum production in patients with chronic airflow obstruction. On the other hand, the use of inhaled steroid showed no significant benefit in mucus hypersecretion in CF patients (103).

F. Other Mucoactive Agents

Nitric oxide (NO), a gaseous molecule synthesized from L-arginine, plays a role in a variety of physiological and pathophysiological processes in the airways (104). Indeed, NO is the dominant NANC neurotransmitter of airway bronchodilator nerves, as well as being a regulator of pulmonary blood flow and bronchial plasma exudation. However, there are conflicting reports regarding the effects of NO on mucus secretion. In the in vitro experiment with ferret trachea in

Ussing chambers (105), the NO synthase inhibitor L-N^G-monomethyl-L-arginine (L-NMMA) increased both basal and neurogenic secretion of $^{35}SO_4$-labeled macromolecules, which was reversed by L-arginine. Conversely, both basal and neurogenic mucus secretion were inhibited by the NO donor FK409 (106). Thus, NO may be an endogenous inhibitor of mucus glycoprotein secretion. In contrast, Nagaki and coworkers (107) showed, in isolated submucosal glands from feline and human trachea, that L-NMMA had no effect on basal output of [^{3}H]-glycoconjugate but inhibited the secretory responses to the subsequent addition of methacholine and bradykinin. The NO generator isosorbide dinitrate induced a significant increase in the secretion. These findings indicate that endogenous NO has a stimulatory action in submucosal gland secretion. The reason for the discrepancy between these results might be species difference and/or differences in experimental conditions. Nevertheless, NO has been shown to increase ciliary motility (108,109) and probably Cl secretion in airway epithelium (110), suggesting that NO can alter physicochemical properties of mucus and stimulate mucociliary transport.

Histamine is one of the most important chemical mediators in the initiation and development of antigen-induced immediate asthmatic responses, including airway smooth muscle contraction and microvascular leakage. It is known that histamine stimulates airway secretory responses. Previous studies showed that histamine increased transepithelial Cl secretion and decreased Na absorption via stimulation of H_1-receptors (111), which may result in the increase in water content in the mucous sol phase. Histamine also increases mucus glycoprotein release from human bronchial preparations (112) and from goblet cells of guinea pig trachea (113), both effects being mediated by H_2-receptors. Taken together, it can be speculated that stimulation of airway H_1-receptors could increase mucus viscosity while stimulation of H_2-receptors might decrease viscosity. The clinical effectiveness of a specific histamine receptor antagonist as a potential mucoregulating medication needs to be clarified.

Protease-antiprotease imbalance is involved in a variety of inflammatory lung diseases, such as COPD, bronchiectasis, CF, and adult respiratory distress syndrome. Among several proteases released from inflammatory cells, human neutrophil elastase causes epithelial damage (114), vascular hyperpermeability (115), mucus gland metaplasia (116), mucus hypersecretion (117,118), and a reduction in mucociliary clearance (119,120). In fact, the threshold concentration of this enzyme to cause mucus secretion from bovine airway gland serous cells is lower by two orders of magnitude than other agonists (e.g., histamine, β-adrenergic agonists) (121). As a protective mechanism against proteases, there are antiprotease proteins, namely α_1-antitrypsin and secretory leukoprotease inhibitor (SLPI). Thus, antiprotease therapy for chronic pulmonary inflammation associated with neutrophils may be a useful adjunct in controlling mucus hypersecretion. Addition of exogenous α_1-antitrypsin to CF sputum in vitro results in a dose-dependent inhibition of neutrophil elastase activity and a reduction of CF sputum's ability to induce mucus secretion. Clinical trial with aerosols of α_1-antitrypsin indicated that inhaled α_1-antitrypsin increased α_1-antitrypsin levels and decreased neutrophil elastase activity in airway epithelial lining fluid in CF (122).

SLPI is a 12 kDa nonglycosylated, single-chain, 107-residue serine antiprotease produced by the cells of mucosal surface and may play an important role in antielastase protection in the human airways (123). It consists of two inhibitory domains, and the elastase inhibitory site is in the COOH-terminal domain (124). Recombinant human SLPI (rhSLPI) administration via aerosol has been evaluated in the treatment of CF patients (125). As with α_1-antitrypsin, inhaled rhSLPI reduces neutrophil elastase activity and, furthermore, IL-8 levels in CF epithelial lining fluid (126). Recent studies have also shown that neutrophil elastase inhibitors, such as ICI 200,355 (127), MR 889 (128) and L-658,758 (129), can potently block elastinolytic activity of CF sputum and reduce the secretory response of airway submucosal gland to CF sputum supernatant. Thus, the use of selective inhibitors of human neutrophil elastase and rhSLPI might provide a novel strategy for intervention in inflammatory diseases with airway hypersecretion (118,130).

Acknowledgments

The authors thank Harumi Satoh for excellent secretarial assistance. This study was supported in part by a Scientific Grant-in-Aid (No. 06670632, 08670681, 10671563) from the Ministry of Education, Science and Culture, Japan.

References

1. Wanner A, Salathé M, O'Riordan TG. Mucociliary clearance in the airways. Am J Respir Crit Care Med 1996; 154:1868–1902.
2. Lucas AM, Douglas LC. Principles underlying ciliary activity in the respiratory tract. II. A comparison of nasal clearance in man, monkey and other mammals. Arch Otolaryngol 1934; 20:518–541.
3. El-Bermani A-W, Grant M. Acetylcholinesterase-positive nerves of the rhesus monkey bronchial tree. Thorax 1975; 30:162–170.
4. Wardell JR Jr, Chakrin LW, Payne BJ. The canine tracheal pouch. A model for use in respiratory mucus research. Am Rev Respir Dis 1970; 101:741–754.
5. Mann SP. The innervation of mammalian bronchial smooth muscle: the localization of catecholamines and cholinesterases. Histochem J 1971; 3:319–331.
6. Basbaum CB, Ueki I, Brezina L, Nadel JA. Tracheal submucosal gland serous cells stimulated in vitro with adrenergic and cholinergic agonists: a morphometric study. Cell Tissue Res 1981; 220:481–498.

7. Murlas C, Nadel JA, Basbaum CB. A morphometric analysis of the autonomic innervation of cat tracheal glands. J Autonom Nerv Syst 1980; 2:23–37.

8. Meyrick B, Reid L. Ultrastructure of cells in the human bronchial submucosal glands. J Anat 1970; 107:281–299.

9. Borson DB, Chinn RA, Davis B, Nadel JA. Adrenergic and cholinergic nerves mediate fluid secretion from tracheal glands of ferrets. J Appl Physiol 1980; 49: 1027–1031.

10. Ueki I, German VF, Nadel JA. Micropipitte measurement of airway submucosal gland secretion. Autonomic effects. Am Rev Respir Dis 1980; 121:351–357.

11. Borson DB, Charlin M, Gold BD, Nadel JA. Neural regulation of 35SO4-macromolecule secretion from tracheal glands of ferrets. J Appl Physiol 1984; 57:457–466.

12. Marin MG, Davis B, Nadel JA. Effect of acetylcholine on Cl^- and Na^+ fluxes across dog tracheal epithelium in vitro. Am J Physiol 1976; 231:1546–1549.

13. Yamaya M. Finkbeiner WE, Widdicombe JH. Ion transport by cultures of human tracheobronchial submucosal glands. Am J Physiol 1991; 261:L485-L490.

14. Lopez-Vidriero MT, Costello J, Clarke TJH, Das I, Keal EE, Reid L. Effect of atropine on sputum production. Thorax 1975; 30:543–547.

15. Pavia D et al. Effect of four-week treatment with oxitropium bromide on lung mucociliary clearance in patients with chronic bronchitis or asthma. Respiration 1989; 55:33–43.

16. Tamaoki J, Chiyotani A, Tagaya E, Sakai N, Konno K. Effect of long term treatment with oxitropium bromide on airway secretion in chronic bronchitis and diffuse panbronchiolitis. Thorax 1994; 49:545–548.

17. Pack RJ, Richardson PS, Smith ICH, Webb SR. The functional significance of the sympathetic innervation of mucous glands in the bronchi of man. J Physiol 1988; 403:211–219.

18. Phipps RJ, Nadel JA. Davis B. Effect of alpha-adrenergic stimulation on mucus secretion and on ion transport in cat trachea in vitro. Am Rev Respir Dis 1980; 121:359–365.

19. Phipps RJ, Williams JP, Richardson PS, Pell J, Pack RJ, Wright N. Sympathomimetic drugs stimulate the output of secretory glycoproteins from human bronchi in vitro. Clin Sci 1982; 63:23–28.

20. Pack RJ, Richardson PS, Smith ICH, Webb SR. The functional significance of the sympathetic innervation of mucous glands in the bronchi of man. J Physiol 1988; 403:211–219.

21. Bateman JRM, Pavia D, Sheahan NF, Agnew JE, Clarke SW. Impaired tracheobronchial clearance in patients with mild stable asthma. Thorax 1983; 38:463–467.

22. Messina MS, O'Riordan TG, Smaldone GC. Changes in mucociliary clearance during acute exacerbations of asthma. Am Rev Respir Dis 1991; 143:993–997.

23. Devalia JL, Sapsford RJ, Rusznak C, Toumbis MJ, Davies RJ. The effects of salmeterol and salbutamol on ciliary beat frequency of cultured human bronchial epithelial cells, in vitro. Pulm Pharmacol 1992; 5:257–263.

24. Mossberg B, Strandberg K, Philipson K, Camner P. Tracheobronchial clearance in bronchial asthma: response to beta-adrenoceptor stimulation. Scand J Respir Dis 1976; 57:119–128.

25. Lafortuna CL, Fazio F. Acute effect of inhaled salbutamol on mucociliary clearance in health and chronic bronchitis. Respiration 1984; 45:111–123.

26. Fung DCK, Allenby MI, Richardson PS. NANC nerve pathways controlling mucus glycoconjugate secretion into feline trachea. J Appl Physiol 1992; 73:625–630.

27. Coles SJ, Bhaskar KR, O'Sullivan DD, Neill KH, Reid LM. Airway mucus: composition and regulation of its secretion by neuropeptides in vitro. Ciba Found Symp 1984; 109:40–60.

28. Richardson PS, Webber SE. The control of mucous secretion in the airways by peptidergic mechanisms. Am Rev Respir Dis 1987; 136(suppl):S72–S76.

29. Webber SE, Widdicombe JG. The effects of vasoactive intestinal peptide on smooth muscle tone and mucus secretion from the ferret trachea. Br J Pharmacol 1987; 91:139–148.

30. Lacroix JS, Mosimann BL. Attenuation of allergen-evoked nasal responses by local pretreatment with exogenous neuropeptide Y in atopic patients. J Allergy Clin Immunol 1996; 98:611–616.

31. Webber SE, Lim JCS, Widdicombe JG. The effects of calcitonin gene-related peptide on submucosal gland secretion and epithelial albumin transport in the ferret trachea in vivo. Br J Pharmacol 1991; 102:79–84.

32. Borson DB, Corrales R, Varsano S, Gold M, Viro N, Caughey G, Ramachandran J, Nadel JA. Enkephalinase inhibitors potentiate substance P-induced secretion of 35SO4-macromolecules from ferret trachea. Exp Lung Res 1987; 12:21–36.

33. Kuo H-P, Rohde JAL, Tokuyama K, Barnes PJ, Rogers DF. Capsaicin and sensory neuropeptide stimulation of goblet cell secretion in guinea-pig trachea. J Physiol 1990; 431:629–641.

34. Gentry SE. Tachykinin receptors mediating airway macromolecular secretion. Life Sci 1991; 48:1609–1618.

35. Rangachari PK, McWade D. Peptides increase anion conductance of canine trachea: an effect on tight junctions. Biochem Biophys Acta 1986; 863:305–308.

36. Tamaoki J, Ueki IF, Widdicombe JH, Nadel JA. Stimulation of Cl secretion by neurokinin A and neurokinin B in canine tracheal epithelium. Am Rev Respir Dis 1988; 137:899–902.

37. Joos GF, Kips JC, Peleman RA, Pauwels RA. Tachykinin antagonists and the airways. Arch Int Pharmacodyn 1995; 329:205–219.

38. Fujii T, Murai M, Morimoto H, Maeda Y, Yamaoka M, Hagiwara D, Miyake H, Ikari N, Matsuo M. Pharmacological profile of a high affinity dipeptide NK1 receptor antagonist, FK888. Br J Pharmacol 1992; 107:785–789.

39. Snider MR, Constantine JW, Lowe JA III, Longo KP, Lebel WS, Woody HA, Dronzda SE, Desai MC, Vinick FJ, Spencer RW, Hess H. A potent nonpeptide antagonist of the substance P (NK1) receptor. Science 1991; 251:435–437.

40. Advenier C, Rouissi N, Nguyen QT, Edmonds-Alt X, Breliere J-C, Neliat G, Naline E, Regoli D. Neurokinin A (NK2) receptor revisited with SR 48968, a potent non-peptide antagonist. Biochem Biophys Res Commun 1992; 184:1418–1424.

41. Morimoto H, Murai M, Maeda Y, Yamaoka M, Nishikawa M, Kiyotoh M, Fujii T. FK224, a novel cyclopeptide substance P antagonist with NK1 and NK2 receptor selectivity. J Pharmacol Exp Ther 1992; 262:398–402.

42. Ramnarine SI, Hirayama Y, Barnes PJ, Rogers DF. "Sensory-efferent" neural control of mucus secretion: characterization using tachykinin receptor antagonists in ferret trachea in vitro. Br J Pharmacol 1994; 113:1183–1190.

43. Suez D, Szefler SJ. Excessive accumulation of mucus in children with asthma: a potential role for erythromycin? A case discussion. J Allergy Clin Immunol 1986; 77:330–334.

44. Marom ZM, Goswami SK. Respiratory mucus hypersecretion (bronchorrhea): a case discussion. Possible mechanism(s) and treatment. J Allergy Clin Immunol 1991; 87:1050–1055.

45. Kadota J, Sakito O, Kohno S, Sawa H, Mukae H, Oda H, Kawakami K, Fukushima K, Hiratani K, Hara K. A mechanism of erythromycin treatment in patients with diffuse panbronchiolitis. Am Rev Respir Dis 1993; 147:153–159.

46. Tamaoki J, Yakeyama K, Tagaya E, Konno K. Effect of clarithromycin on sputum production and its rheological properties in chronic respiratory tract infections. Antimicrob Agent Chemother 1995; 39:1688–1690.

47. Roche Y, Gougerot-Pocidalo MA, Fay M, Forest N, Pocidalo JJ. Macrolide and immunity: effects of erythromycin and spiramycin on human mononuclear cell proliferation. J Antimicrob Chemother 1986; 17:195–203.

48. Goswami SK, Kivity S, Marom Z. Erythromycin inhibits respiratory glycoconjugate secretion from human airways in vitro. Am Rev Respir Dis 1990; 141:72–78.

49. Tamaoki J, Isono K, Sakai N, Kanemura T, Konno K. Erythromycin inhibits Cl secretion across canine tracheal epithelial cells. Eur Respir J 1992; 5:234–238.

50. Anderson R, Fernandes AC, Eftychis HE. Studies on the effects of ingestion of a single 500 mg oral dose of erythromycin stearate on leucocyte motility and transformation and on release in vitro of prostaglandin E2 by stimulated leucocytes. J Antimicrob Chemother 1984; 14:41–50.

51. Johnson JD, Hand WL, Francis JB, King-Thompson N, Corwin RW. Antibiotic uptake by alveolar macrophages. J Lab Clin Med 1980; 95:429–439.

52. Oda H, Kadota J, Kohno S, Hara K. Erythromycin inhibits neutrophil chemotaxis in bronchoalveoli of diffuse panbronchiolitis. Chest 1994; 106:1116–1123.

53. Umeki S. Anti-inflammatory action of erythromycin. Its inhibitory effect on neutrophil NADPH oxidase activity. Chest 1993; 104:1191–1193.

54. Hojo M, Fujita I, Hamasaki Y, Miyazaki M, Miyazaki S. Erythromycin does not directly affect neutrophil functions. Chest 1994; 105:520–523.

55. Tokuyama K, Kuo HP, Rohde JAL, Barnes PJ, Rogers DF. Neural control of goblet cell secretion in guinea pig airways. Am J Physiol 1990; 259:L108–L115.

56. Tamaoki J, Takeyama K, Yamawaki I, Kondo M, Konno K. Lipopolysaccharide-induced goblet cell hypersecretion in the guinea-pig trachea: inhibition by macrolides. Am J Physiol 1997; 272:L15–L19.

57. Tamaoki J, Nakata J, Tagaya E, Konno K. Effects of roxithromycin and erythromycin on interleukin 8-induced neutrophil recruitment and goblet cell secfetion in guinea pig tracheas. Antimicrob Agent Chemother 1996; 40:1726–1728.

58. Rubin BK, Druce H, Ramirez OE, Palmer R. Effect of clarithromycin on nasal mucus properties in healthy subjects and in patients with purulent rhinitis. Am J Respir Crit Care Med 1997; 155:2018–2023.

59. Mikami M. Clinical and pathophysiological significance of neutrophil elastase in

sputum and the effect of erythromycin in chronic respiratory diseases. Jpn J Thorac Dis 1991; 29:72–83.

60. Tamaoki J, Chiyotani A, Sakai N, Takeyama K, Takizawa T. Effect of erythromycin on ciliary motility in rabbit airway epithelium in vitro. J Antimicrob Chemother 1992; 29:173–178.

61. Middleton PG, Geddes DM, Alton EWFW. Trimethoprim and tetracycline inhibit airway epithelial sodium absorption. Am J Respir Crit Care Med 1996; 154: 18–23.

62. Kersting U, Kersting D, Spring KR. Ketoconazole activates Cl⁻ conductance and blocks Cl⁻ and fluid absorption by culture cystic fibrosis (CFPAC-1) cells. Proc Natl Acad Sci U S A 1993; 90:4047–4051.

63. Lundgren JD, Kaliner M, Logun C, Shelhamer JH. Dexamethasone reduces rat tracheal goblet cell hyperplasia produced by human neutrophil products. Exp Lung Res 1988; 14:853–863.

64. Sibille Y, Reynolds Y. Macrophages and polymorphonuclear neutrophils in lung defense and injury. Am Rev Respir Dis 1990; 141:471–501.

65. Cantin A, Woods DE. Protection by antibiotics against myeloperoxidase-dependent cytotoxicity to lung epithelial cells in vitro. J Clin Invest 1993; 91:38–45.

66. Lin H-C, Cheng H-F, Wang C-H, Liu C-Y, Yu C-T, Kuo H-P. Inhaled gentamicin reduces airway neutrophil activity and mucus secretion in bronchiectasis. Am J Respir Crit Care Med 1997; 155:2024–2029.

67. Marom Z, Shelhamer JH, Kaliner M. Effects of arachidonic acid, monohydroxyeicosatetraenoic acid and prostaglandins on the release of mucous glycoproteins from human airways in vitro. J Clin Invest 1981; 67:1695–1702.

68. Moncada S, Vane JR. Pharmacology and endogenous roles of prostaglandins, endoperoxides, thromboxane A2 and prostacyclin. Pharmacol Rev 1979; 30:293–331.

69. Samuelsson B. The leukotrienes: a novel group of compounds including SRS-A and mediators of inflammation. In: Piper PJ, ed. SRS-A and Leukotrienes. New York: Research Studies Press, Wiley, 1981:45–64.

70. Lopez-Vidriero MT, Das I, Smith AP, Picot R, Reid L. Bronchial secretion from normal human airways after inhalation of prostaglandin F2a, acetylcholine, histamine, and citric acid. Thorax 1977; 32:734–739.

71. Rich B, Peatfield AC, Williams IP, Richardson PS. Effects of prostaglandin E1, E2, and F2a on mucin secretion from human bronchi in vitro. Thorax 1984; 39: 420–423.

72. Sturgess J, Reid L. An organ study of the effect of drugs on the secretory activity of the human bronchial submucosal gland. Clin Sci 1972; 43:533–543.

73. Al-Bazzaz F, Yadava VP, Westenfelder C. Modification of Na and Cl transport in canine tracheal mucosa by prostaglandins. Am J Physiol 1981; 240:F101–F105.

74. Inoue H, Aizawa H, Koto H, Miyagawa Y, Ikeda T, Shigematsu N. Effect of cyclooxygenase inhibitor on excessive sputum. Fukuoka Acta Med 1991; 82:177–180.

75. Tamaoki J, Chiyotani A, Kobayashi K, Sakai N, Kanemura T, Takizawa T. Effect of inhaled indomethacin on bronchorrhea in patients with chronic bronchitis, diffuse panbronchiolitis or bronchiectasis. Am Rev Respir Dis 1992; 145:548–552.

76. Sofia M, Molino A, Mormile M, Stanziola A, De Simone F. Modificaziono dei parametri clinici e delle proprieta reologiche dell'espettorato durante il trattamento con nimesulide in pazienti affetti da bronchite cronica. Studio controllato verso placebo. G Ital Mal Torace 1991; 45:24–28.

77. Yanni JM, Smith WL, Foxwell MH. U46619 and carbocyclic thromboxane A2-induced increases in tracheal mucus gel layer thickness. Prostaglandins Leukotr Essent Fatty Acids 1988; 32:45–49.

78. Lotvall J, Elwood W, Tokuyama K, Sakamoto T, Barnes PJ, Chung KF. A thromboxane mimetic, U-46619, produces plasma exudation in airways of the guinea-pig. J Appl Physiol 1992; 72:2415–2419.

79. Hiraku S, Taniguchi K, Wakitani K, Omawari N, Kita H, Miyamoto T, Okegawa T, Kawasaki A, Ujiie A. Pharmacological studies on the TxA2 synthetase inhibitor: (E)-3-[p-(1H-imidazol-l-yl) methyl-) phenyl]-2-propenoic acid (OKY-046). Jpn J Pharmacol 1986; 41:396.

80. Kurashima K, Ogawa H, Ohka T, Fujimura M, Matsuda T. Thromboxane A2 synthetase inhibitor (OKY-046) improves abnormal mucociliary transport in asthmatic patients. Ann Allergy 68:53–56, 1992.

81. Rutland J, Cole PJ. Nasal mucociliary clearance and ciliary beat frequency in cystic fibrosis compared to sinusitis and bronchiectasis. Thorax 1981; 36:654–658.

82. Kurashima K, Fujimura M, Hoyano Y, Takemura K, Mtsuda T. Effect of thromboxane A2 synthetase inhibitor, OKY-046, on sputum in chronic bronchitis and diffuse panbronchiolitis. Eur Respir J 1995; 8:1705–1711.

83. Cole SJ, Neill KH, Reid LM, Austen KF, Nii Y, Corey EJ, Lewis RA. Effects of leukotrienes C4 and D4 on glycoprotein and lysozyme secretion by human bronchial mucosa. Prostaglandins 1983; 25:155–170.

84. Marom Z, Shelhamer JH, Bach MK, Morton DR, Kaliner M. Slow reacting substances LTC4 and D4 increase the release of mucus from human airways in vitro. Am Rev Respir Dis 1982; 126:449–451.

85. Hoffstein ST, Malo PE, Bugelski P, Wheeldon EB. Leukotriene D4 (LTD4) induces mucus secretion from goblet cells in the guinea pig respiratory epithelium. Exp Lung Res 1990; 16:711–725.

86. Wasserman MA, Torphy TJ, Hay DWP, Muccitelli RM, Tucker SS, Wilson KA, Osborn RR, Vickory-Clark L, Hall RF, Erhard KF, Gleason JG. Pharmacologic profile of SK&F 104353, a novel, highly potent and selective peptide leukotriene antagonist. In: Samuelsson B, Paoletti R, Ramwell P, eds. Advances in Prostaglandins, Thromboxane and Leukotriene Research. Vol. 17. New York: Raven Press, 1987:532–535.

87. Widdicombe JH, Coleman DL, Finkbeiner WE, Friend DS. Primary cultures of the dog's tracheal epithelium: fine structure, fluid, and electrolyte transport. Cell Tissue Res 1987; 247:95–103.

88. Borgeat P, Sirois P. Leukotrienes: a major step in the understanding of immediate hypersensitivity reactions. J Med Chem 1981; 24:121–126.

89. Hamberg M, Hedqvist P, Radegran K. Identification of 15-hydroxy-5,8,11,13-eicosatetraenoic acid (15-HETE) as a major metabolite of arachidonic acid in human lung. Acta Physiol Scand 1980; 110:219–221.

90. Johnson HG, McNee ML, Sun FF. 15-Hydroxyeicosatetraenoic acid is a potent inflammatory mediator and agonist of canine tracheal mucus secretion. Am Rev Respir Dis 1985; 131:917–922.

91. Johnson HG, McNee ML. Regulation of canine mucus secretion by a novel leukotriene synthesis inhibitor (U-60257). Int Arch Allergy Appl Immunol 1984; 75: 97–101.

92. Shimura S, Sasaki T, Ikeda K, Yamauchi K, Sasaki H, Takishima T. Direct inhibitory action of glycoconjugate secretion from airway submucosal glands. Am Rev Respir Dis 1990; 141:1044–1049.

93. Marom Z, Shelhamer J, Alling D, Kaliner M. The effect of corticosteroids on mucous glycoprotein secretion from human airways in vitro. Am Rev Respir Dis 1984; 129:62–65.

94. Lundgren J, Hirata F, Marom Z, Logun C, Steel L, Kaliner M, Shelhamer J. Dexamethasone inhibits respiratory glycoconjugate secretion from feline airways in vitro by the induction of lipocortin (lipomudulin) synthesis. Am Rev Respir Dis 1988; 137:353–357.

95. Aikawa T, Shimura S, Sasaki H, Ebina M, Takishima T. Marked goblet cell hyperplasia with mucus accumulation in the airways of patients who died of severe acute asthma attack. Chest 1992; 101:916–921.

96. Lundgren JD. Pathogenesis of airway mucus hypersecretion. J Allergy Clin Immunol 1990; 30:257–262.

97. Savoie C, Plant M, Zwikker M, van Staden C, Boulet L, Chan C, Rodger I, Pon D. Effect of dexamethasone on allergen-induced high molecular weight glycoconjugate secretion in allergic guinea pigs. Am J Respir Cell Mol Biol 1995; 13: 133–143.

98. Blyth D, Pedrick M, Savage T, Bright H, Beesley J, Sanjar S. Induction, duration, and resolution of airway goblet cell hyperplasia in a murine model of atopic asthma: effect of concurrent infection with respiratory syncytial virus and response to dexamethasone. Am J Respir Cell Mol Biol 1998; 19:38–54.

99. Lou Y, Takeyama K, Grattan K, Lausier J, Ueki I, Agusti C, Nadel J. Platelet activating factor induces goblet cell hyperplasia and mucin gene expression in airways. Am J Respir Crit Care Med 1998; 157:1927–1934.

100. Temann U, Prasad B, Gallup M, Basbaum C, Ho S, Flavell R, Rankin J. A novel role for murine IL-4 in vivo: induction of MUC5AC gene expression and mucin hypersecretion. Am J Respir Cell Mol Biol 1997; 16:471–478.

101. Satoh M, Shimura S, Ishihara H, Yamada K, Masuda T, Sasaki T, Sasaki H, Takishima T. Dexamethasone modulation of ion transport and fluid movement across airway secretion. Am J Physiol 1993; 264:L376–L381.

102. Boothman-Burrell D, Delany SG, Flannery EM, Hancox RJ, Taylor DR. The efficacy of inhaled corticosteroids in the management of non asthmatic chronic airflow obstruction. N Z Med J 1997; 110:370–373.

103. Balfour-Lynn IM, Klein NJ, Dinweddie R. Randomised controlled trial of inhaled corticosteroids (fluticasone propionate) in cystic fibrosis. Arch Dis Child 1997; 77:124–130.

104. Barnes PJ, Belvisi MG. Nitric oxide and lung disease. Thorax 1993; 48:1034–1043.

105. Ramnarine SI, Khawaja AM, Barnes PJ, Rogers DF. Nitric oxide inhibition of basal and neurogenic mucus secretion in ferret trachea in vitro. Br J Pharmacol 1996; 118:998–1002.

106. Kita Y, Hirasawa Y, Maeda K, Nishio M, Toshida K. Spontaneous nitric oxide release accounts for the potent pharmacological actions of FK409. Eur J Pharmacol 1994; 257:123–130.

107. Nagaki M, Shimura S, Irokawa T, Sasaki T, Shirato K. Nitric oxide regulation of glycoconjugate secretion from feline and human airways in vitro. Respir Physiol 1995; 102:89–95.

108. Jain B, Lubinstein I, Robbinson RA, Leise KL, Sisson JH. Modulation of airway epithelial cell ciliary beat frequency by nitric oxide. Biochem Biophys Res Commun 1993; 191:83–88.

109. Tamaoki J, Chiyotani A, Kondo M, Konno K. Role of nitric oxide generation in β-adrenoceptor-mediated stimulation of rabbit airway ciliary motility. Am J Physiol 1995; 268:C1342–C1347.

110. Takemura H, Tamaoki J, Tagaya E, Chiyotani A, Konno K. Isoproterenol increases Cl diffusion potential difference of rabbit trachea through nitric oxide generation. J Pharmacol Exp Ther 1995; 274:584–588.

111. Marin MG, Davis B, Nadel JA. Effect of histamine on electrical and ion transport properties of tracheal epithelium. J Appl Physiol 1977; 42:735–738.

112. Shelhamer JH, Marom Z, Kaliner M. Immunologic and neuropharmacologic stimulation of mucus glycoprotein release from human airways in vitro. J Clin Invest 1980; 66:1400–1408.

113. Tamaoki J, Nakata J, Takeyama K, Chiyotani A, Konno K. Histamine H2 receptor-mediated airway goblet cell secretion and its modulation by histamine-degrading enzymes. J Allergy Clin Immunol 1997; 99:233–238.

114. Amitani R, Wilson R, Rutman A, Read R, Ward C, Burnett D, Stockley RA, Cole PJ. Effect of human neutrophil elastase and Pseudomonas aeruginosa proteinases on human respiratory epithelium. Am J Respir Cell Mol Biol 1991; 4:26–32.

115. Goldman G, Welbourn R, Kobzik L, Valeri C, Shepro D, Hechtman HB. Reactive oxygen species and elastase mediate lung permeability after acid aspiration. J Appl Physiol 1992; 73:571–575.

116. Snider GL, Lucey EC, Christensen TG, Stone PJ, Calore JD, Catanese A, Franzblau C. Emphysema and bronchial secretory cell metaplasia induced in hamsters by human neutrophil products. Am Rev Respir Dis 1984; 129:155–160.

117. Fahy JV, Schuster A, Ueki I, Boushey HA, Nadel JA. Mucus hypersecretion in bronchiectasis. The role of neutrophil elastase. Am Rev Respir Dis 1992; 146:1430–1433.

118. Schuster A, Ueki I, Nadel JA. Neutrophil elastase stimulates tracheal submucosal gland secretion that is inhibited by ICI 200,355. Am J Physiol 1992; 262:L86–L91.

119. Tegner H, Ohlsson K, Toremalm NG, Mecklenburg C. Effect of human leukocyte enzymes on tracheal mucosa and its mucociliary activity. Rhinology 1979; 17:199–206.

120. Smallman LA, Hill SL, Stockley RA. Reduction of ciliary beat frequency in vitro by sputum from patients with bronchiectasis: a serine protease effect. Thorax 1984; 39:663–667.

121. Nadel JA. Role of mast cell and neutrophil proteases in airway secretion. Am Rev Respir Dis 1991; 144:S48–S51.
122. McElvanery NG, Hubbard RC, Birrer P, Chernick MS, Caplan DB, Frank MM, Crystal RG. Aerosol a1-antitrypsin treatment for cystic fibrosis. Lancet 1991; 337: 392–394.
123. Mooren HWD, Kramps JA, Franken C, Meijer CJLM, Dijkman JA. Localization of a low-molecular-weight bronchial protease inhibitor in the peripheral human lung. Thorax 1983; 38:180–183.
124. Kramps JA, Twisk C, Appelhans H, Meckelein B, Nikiforov T, Dijkman JH. Proteinase inhibitory activities of antileukoprotease are represented by its second COOH-terminal domain. Biochem Biophys Acta 1990; 1038:178–185.
125. McElvaney NG, Nakamura H, Birrer P, Hébert CA, Wong WL, Alphonso M, Baker JB, Catalano MA, Crystal RG. Modulation of airway inflammation in cystic fibrosis: in vivo suppression of interleukin-8 levels on the respiratory epithelial surface by aerosolization of recombinant secretory leukoprotease inhibitor. J Clin Invest 1992; 90:1296–1301.
126. Allen ED. Opportunities for the use of aerosolized a1-antitrypsin for the treatment of cystic fibrosis. Chest 1996; 110:256S–260S.
127. Schuster A, Fahy JV, Ueki I, Nadel JA. Cystic fibrosis sputum induces a secretory response from airway gland serous cells that can be prevented by neutrophil protease inhibitors. Eur Respir J 1995; 8:10–14.
128. Moretti M, Gorrini M, Donnetta AM, Baldini EV, Venturini R, Marchioni CF, Iadarola P, Luisetti M. Effects of MR 889, a cyclic thilic neutrophil elastase inhibitor, on rheologic properties of mucus. Life Sci 1994; 54:463–469.
129. Rees DD, Brain JD, Wohl ME, Humes JL, Mumford RA. Inhibition of neutrophil elastase in CF sputum by L-658,758. J Pharmacol Exp Ther 1997; 283:1201–1206.
130. Van-Seuningen I, Aubert J-P, Davril M. Interaction between secretory leucocyte proteinase inhibitor and bronchial mucins or glycopeptides. Biochem J 1992; 281: 761–766.

13

Hyperosmolar Solutions and Ion Channel Modifiers

CHIKAKO KISHIOKA

Mie University School of Medicine
Mie, Japan

I. Introduction

Mucus covers the airway epithelium, and its volume and composition affects the efficiency of airway clearance. Mucus secretion is regulated by a complex of various pathways. Mucins are responsible for the primary structure of mucus. These are secreted from submucosal glands and epithelial goblet cells and hydrated rapidly after secretion. The hydration process is one of the major determinants of the mucus volume and rheological properties, and thus hydration has a large effect on mucociliary clearance. Hydration depends on the salt concentration and pH of the airway liquid (1), which is determined, in part, by epithelial ion transport.

Active ion transport and associated transepithelial water flux can modulate periciliary fluid viscosity and depth (2). Mucus that is too viscous or too thin may lead to a reduction of clearance rate. Also, if the periciliary fluid is too deep or shallow, the clearance will be inefficient.

Epithelia are composed of polarized cells organized as monocellular or multicellular layers. These epithelial cells perform vectorial transport of solutes, and this is the principal means of ion transport in the airways. There are two major routes for solute movement across epithelia: by passive diffusion through the paracellular pathways and by transport through the cells (transcellular pathway), with the apical and the basolateral membrane arranged in series (3).

Submucosal glands are thought to be major source of respiratory (mucous) secretions, but less is known about ion transport and its regulation in these glands. Possible modes of glandular secretion include an osmotic secretory mechanism that is driven by mucin secretion, a chloride secretory mechanism in serous cells, perhaps similar to that which is present in the surface epithelia (4).

We review here the effect of hyperosmolar solutions and ion channel modifiers on mucin secretion and ion transport.

II. Hyperosmolar Solutions

A. Mucin Secretion

Sputum induction using hypertonic saline inhalation has been used to obtain sputum specimens for diagnosing airway infection (5) and for collecting secretions for research in patients with asthma (6,7). It has been demonstrated that when patients with chronic bronchitis or cystic fibrosis inhale a hypertonic saline aerosol, whole lung mucociliary clearance (MCC) measured using a radiolabeled aerosol increased in the first 90 minutes over the MCC after inhalation of isotonic (0.9%) saline (8–10).

The increase in MCC noted in these studies could be due to an increase in mucus secretion and ion transport. Instillation of hyperosmolar solution, such as sucrose or hypertonic saline, induces an osmolarity-dependent increase in mucus secretion in the cat trachea (11).

Hyperosmolar solutions have been reported to induce plasma exudation through neurogenic inflammation in the rat trachea (12). Neurogenic inflammation, due to the release of neuropeptides from sensory nerves, has been demonstrated in airways (13,14) and tachykinins, including substance P and neurokinin A, cause mucus secretion as well as plasma exudation (15). It has also been shown that hyperosmolarity can induce leukotriene and prostaglandin production (16,17), and these arachidonic acid metabolites can directly stimulate mucin secretion. It is possible that hyperosmolar solutions induce mucin secretion, in part, through these pathways.

Secretion can also be induced by epithelial damage after osmotic challenge (18), although there is no histologically visible injury to the epithelial or endothelial barriers of the lung after inhalation of hypertonic (3%) saline (19), which can profoundly stimulate mucus secretion (20).

B. Ion Transport and Water Movement

Hypertonic saline has been thought to promote mucus clearance by osmotically extracting fluid from the respiratory epithelium, thereby increasing the volume and water content of mucus (21,22). Upon administration of hypertonic saline by means of a nebulizer, water from the tissues may be shifted across the epithelial membrane to dilute the saline by osmotic pressure.

Price et al. reported that hypo- or hyperosmolar fluid caused water and ion fluxes in the directions of increasing or decreasing luminal osmolarity (23). They suggested that ion transport across the airway epithelium occured first and water movement followed. Cooling the airway decreased this osmotic flux due to nonisomolar solutions, presumably by inhibiting the active ion pumping (23). Thus, hyperosmolar solution may promote active ion transport, leading to chloride secretion and water flux, as well as extracting water directly by osmotic gradient.

Yankaskas et al. reported that increased tracheal surface liquid osmolarity caused an increase in paracellular permeability and an inhibition of active ion transport (24). These data suggest that responses to hyperosmolarity may occur in both the cellular and the paracellular compartments of the mucosa.

C. Clinical Aspects

Hypertonic saline has been reported to enhance the clearance of lung secretions in patients with cystic fibrosis (9,25). Other hyperosmolar drugs, such as mannitol, heparin, and low molecular weight dextran, have been reported to increase MCC (26–28).

Hyperosmolar drugs can be divided into two groups: ionic and nonionic. Ionic agents are believed to be mucoactive by breaking the ionic bonds and shielding the fixed charges along the macromolecular core of the mucin polymer, making it less stiff and less extended and thus reducing the number of entanglement crosslinks with neighboring macromolecules (29). In purulent mucus, these agents also separate the DNA molecules from the mucoprotein, making the mucoprotein susceptible to proteolytic enzyme digestion (30).

Nonionic agents such as sugars that increase osmolarity can also reduce the crosslink density of sputum. Although they could share a common mechanism with low molecular weight salts, it is more likely that they act by disrupting the hydrogen bonds between mucin molecules (31). In these ways, hyperosmolar drugs make mucus more easily transportable, leading to increased MCC.

There are concerns about the inactivation of tracheal antibacterial peptides such as human β-defensin-1 at the airway surface in the presence of high salt concentration (32), which might increase the risk of airway infection. It has also been shown that hyperosmolar solution inhalation can produce bronchospasm (33). Thus, hyperosmolar aerosols may be a useful therapeutic approach to enhance secretion clearance in airway diseases such as chronic bronchitis, bronchiectasis, asthma, and cystic fibrosis, but long-term safety and efficacy must be demonstrated in larger clinical trials.

III. Ion Channnels

Ion transport is regulated by a variety of neurohormonal agents and metabolites. The ion transport function of the epithelium is primarily altered in diseases such as cystic fibrosis. It has also been suggested that abnormalities of ion transport may play an important role in the pathogenesis of airway disease associated with smoking and in asthma (34).

A. General Characteristics of Ion Transport by Airway Mucosa

Melon showed that the rabbit nasal epithelia maintains a bioelectric potential difference and actively absorbs sodium (35). Gatzy reported that the bullfrog lung actively secrets chloride (36,37). Fluid formation in the lung of the fetal lamb is controlled by active chloride secretion (38). Olver et al. demonstrated chloride secretion and sodium absorption in the dog tracheal mucosa (39). Since then, many additional studies have been done in various mammalian airway epithelia. It has been documented that the trachea and bronchi of all species studied, including humans, have a negatively charged luminal mucosa with reference to the submucosal surface (40). This negative charge is maintained by active ion transport.

It is now generally agreed that several airway regions are capable of both active electrolyte absorption and secretion and that the net balance between these absorptive and secretory ion transport processes regulate the direction of transepithelial water flow by osmotic forces (41).

Epithelial cells have two different cell membranes. Figure 1 shows the polarity. The apical membrane faces the luminal surface, and the other (the basolateral) membrane faces the submucosal side. These two membranes have a different function in ion transport.

It is the segregation of specific ion-transport proteins to one or the other of the two membranes that allows vectorical (polarity-directed) ion transport. In

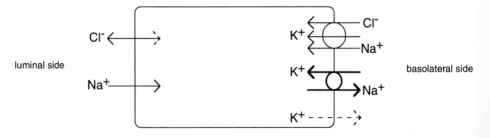

Figure 1   Diagram showing polarity of the two cell membranes in epithelial cells.

general, ions enter the cell at one membrane through one set of transport proteins and exit the cell across the other membrane by a different set of ion transport proteins.

The NaK-ATPase sodium pump is located in the basolateral portion of the cell membrane (42). This enzyme plays a primary role in active ion transport and maintains a gradient of sodium and potassium concentration (lower sodium inside of cells and higher sodium outside). This osmotic gradient and the segregation of channels lead to unidirectional sodium movement, influx from the lumen, and efflux to the serosal side. The NaK-ATPase may not be directly regulated by second messengers but responds to changes in $[Na^+]_i$. Intracellular sodium concentration is kept low by the NaK-ATPase.

Active chloride secretion is regulated through changes in the kinetics of several channels (43,44), as described in the following section. Net movement of chloride into the cells across the basolateral membrane is via a $NaKCl_2$ cotransporter. Net chloride efflux across the apical membrane is down an electrochemical gradient via chloride channels.

The potassium that enters by cotransport with chloride and sodium recycles to the basolateral space via potassium channels. Other ions also move with these under the influence of the concentration and charge gradient and channel conductance. The active transport of salts and/or solutes from one side to the other side of the epithelium can induce net fluid transport by the development of osmotic gradients.

B. Intracellular Regulation of Channels

Cells can rapidly and reversibly alter solute transport rates by changing the kinetics of transport proteins within the plasma membrane. Many ion channels are subject to modulation by reversible phosphorylation. A variety of protein kinase signaling pathways can participate in the regulation of ion channel activity, and it is not unusual to find that a particular channel is modulated by several different protein kinases, each influencing channel activity in a unique way (45).

Acute regulation of plasma membrane transport rates can also be brought about by the exocytic insertion of transport proteins from intracellular vesicles into the plasma membrane and their subsequent endocytic retrieval (46). For example, apical membrane chloride channels mainly control the rate of transepithelial chloride secretion in airway epithelia (47). Sustained increases in chloride secretion require increases in the turnover of chloride channels in the apical membrane and the NaK-ATPase, NaK_2Cl cotransporter and potassium channels in the basolateral membrane.

The chloride channels are the most throughly investigated channels. Phosphorylation of chloride channels or associated regulatory proteins by cAMP-dependent protein kinase in excised patches of membrane activates chloride channels (48,49). Cyclic-AMP–dependent opening of the apical chloride channel can be triggered by the phosphorylation of the cystic fibrosis transmembrane ion conductance regulator (CFTR) at one of six protein kinase A domains (50). The CFTR is a large (170 kDa; 1480 amino acid) membrane-bound chloride channel.

Activation of protein kinase C (PKC) by phorbol ester either stimulates or inhibits chloride secretion, depending on the physiological status of the cell (51). In cell-free membrane patches, PKC also has a dual effect: at a high internal calcium concentration PKC inactivates chloride channels, while at a low calcium concentration PKC activates chloride channels (51).

Chloride channels can also be activated by other maneuvers, including an increase in the cytosolic calcium $[Ca^{2+}]$, changes in cell volume, sustained membrane depolarization, an increase in temperature, proteolysis, and changes in osmolarity (48).

$[Ca^{2+}]$ can be increased by receptor activation. Serous gland cells contain IP3 receptors in their apical poles (52), and in response to methacholine, calcium rises in the apical region and chloride currents increase. Chloride channel activation by $[Ca^{2+}]$ can be mediated by multifunctional calcium/calmodulin-dependent protein kinase. Wagner et al. reported that intracellular application of activated kinase and ATP activates a chloride current similar to that activated by a calcium ionophore, that peptide inhibitors of either the kinase or calmodulin blocks $[Ca^{2+}]$-dependent activation of chloride channels, and that a peptide inhibitor of protein kinase C does not block $[Ca^{2+}]$-dependent activation (53). Calcium-activated chloride channels can also be activated directly by calcium without the involvement of protein kinases (54).

One channel can be modulated by several different pathways. Also, one pathway can modulate different channels; for example, calcium and cAMP activate different chloride channels in the apical membrane (55).

P-glycoprotein (relative molecular mass 170,000) is an ATP-dependent, active transporter that pumps hydrophobic drugs out of cells, but its normal physiological role is unknown. The expression of P-glycoprotein generates volume-regulated, ATP-dependent, chloride-selective channels (56,57).

Other important signaling systems involve arachidonic acid and G-protein. Arachidonic acid is released from cell membranes during receptor-mediated stimulation, and arachidonic acid itself, not a cyclooxygenase or lipoxygenase metabolite, reversibly inhibits apical membrane chloride channels in cell-free patches of membrane (47). Heterotrimeric G proteins also inhibit cAMP-activated chloride currents in airway epithelial cells (58).

Other channels are also regulated through multiple pathways. Basolateral K channels and NaK_2Cl cotransport are stimulated both by cAMP via activation of protein kinase A and by calcium (44).

IV. Ion Channel Modifiers

A. Pharmacological Agents

Several pharmacological agents have been demonstrated to alter ion transport. Tracheal chloride secretion is inhibited by loop diuretics, such as furosemide (59). Ouabine has been shown to inhibit sodium absorption in bovine, rabbit, and cat trachea (60–63). Sodium absorption is also blocked by luminal application of the potassium-sparing diuretic amiloride (64), without altering net chloride secretion in the dog trachea (65). However, amiloride inhibits sodium absorption and increases chloride secretion in sheep and rabbit trachea (66,67). Also in the rabbit trachea, blockade of sodium influx by amiloride causes a parallel decrease in chloride influx from the lumen to the serosa. The persistence of the oppositely directed chloride influx leads to a net chloride secretion (68).

B. Paracellular Pathway

Ropke et al. suggested the presence of separate routes for paracellular chloride and sodium flux and a significant anion selectivity of a low-resistance paracellular pathway (69). A short-chain phospholipid didecanoyl-L-α-phosphatidylcholine (DDPC) increased epithelial conductance, probably due to formation of a paracellular shunt conductance in parallel with unaffected anion-selective tight junction channels (70). DDPC may cause structural changes in tight junctions. Oxidant stress also altered the permeability of the tracheal epithelium and the increased paracellular permeability was cation selective (71).

Histamine increases nasal epithelial permeability to macromolecules in guinea pigs (72), and this may lead to increased water movement by osmotic gradient. Exposure to nitrogen dioxide increased transepithelial permeability in vitro. This may be secondary to damage to the passive airway epithelial barrier leading to leaky tight junctions (73). Respiratory syncytial virus infection increases tissue resistance in cotton rats (74). This is associated with significant restriction to sodium and chloride movement through the paracellular pathway.

C. Water Movement

Water can be transported by both passive and active means in airway epithelia. In epithelia in general it has long been established that active transepithelial fluid movement is brought about by active solute transport. Transport of solutes across epithelial tissue causes alterations in transepithelial ion concentration and therefore creates a gradient in osmotic pressure across the epithelial tissue. Due to the gradient in osmotic pressure, water will move from the solution of lower to one of higher solute concentration.

Water-selective channels, or aquaporins, have been discovered and characterized. Aquaporins are a family of intrinsic membrane proteins that function as water-selective channels, and facilitate cell membrane water transport. Aquaporin (AQP) 1 is present in apical and basolateral membranes of bronchial, tracheal, and nasopharyngeal vascular endothelium and fibroblasts (75). It is involved in airway hydration (76), but little is known about AQP 1 function in diseased airway.

AQP 3 is present in basal cells of tracheal and nasopharyngeal epithelium and is abundant in basolateral membranes of surface epithelial cells in the nasal concha. Schreiber et al. suggested that CFTR is a regulator of AQP 3 in airway epithelial cells (77), and Tanaka and colleagues reported that dexamethasone upregulated the expression of AQP 3 (78).

AQP 4 resides in the basolateral membranes of columnar cells of bronchial, tracheal, and nasopharyngeal epithelium. In the nasal conchus AQP 4 is restricted to basolateral membranes of a subset of intra- and subepithelial glands. AQP 5 is localized to the apical plasma membrane of type I pneumocytes and the apical plasma membranes of secretory epithelium in the upper airway and salivary glands. Thus, AQP 5 is coupled with water secretion in exocrine tissues (76).

These aquaporins may play important roles in water movement across airway epithelia and airway hydration.

D. Effect of Adrenergic Agents

β-Agonists increase chloride secretion in fetal lamb, canine, bovine, cat, and ferret trachea (62,79–81) but have no apparent effect in maternal sheep and rabbit trachea (64,79,82) (Table 1). The lack of effect could be because maternal sheep or rabbit trachea are primarily sodium absorbers and not chloride secretors (68,79,82). In bovine and cat airway epithelia, there is an associated decrease in sodium absorption (62,81). α-Adrenergic agents (e.g., phenylephrine) increase the flux of radioactive sodium and chloride towards the lumen of cat tracheal sheets, equivalent to a flow of isotonic saline solution (83–85). However, α-adrenergic agonists have no effect on ion transport in canine or rabbit trachea (82,86). In canine trachea, epinephrine also induces calcium secretion (86) and adrenergic agonists open calcium-activated potassium channels in cystic fibrosis epithelia (87).

α-Adrenergic and β-adrenergic stimulation increases tracheal glycoprotein secretion in the cat trachea (88,89). β-Adrenergic modulation of mucus secretion would seem to be effected by cAMP and involve the activation of cAMP-dependent protein kinase in cat gland cells (90). α_2-Adrenergic agents inhibit this stimulation of mucus secretion by β-adrenergic agents (91). This effect may be due to inhibition of membrane-bound adenylate cyclase (92). On the other hand, phenylephrine increased intracellular calcium ($[Ca^{2+}]_i$) in cat glands (93) and

Table 1 Effects of Ion Channel Modifiers in Tracheal Epithelium

Agent	Ion	Dog	Cow	Cat	Ferret	Rabbit	Maternal sheep	Fetal sheep
Cholinergic agents	Na	+—		+—	+—	NE		
	Cl	+—		+—	+—	NE		
α-Adrenergic agents	Na	NE		+—		NE		
	Cl	NE		+—		NE		
β-Adrenergic agents	Na	NE	−	+—	−	NE	NE	NE
	Cl	+	+	+	+	NE	NE	+
Prostaglandin E₁	Na	−						
	Cl	+	+		+			
Substance P and VIP	Na	NE				NE		
	Cl	+				NE		
Adenosine	Cl	+						
cAMP	Na	−	NE			NE		
	Cl	+	NE			NE		

+ or −: increase or decrease in comparison with the direction of resting flux (sodium flux is absorptive and chloride flux is secretory). +—: the net movement of sodium changed to secretion with an associated increase in chloride secretion due to mucin secretion.

calcium may play a role in α-adrenergic stimulation of mucin secretion. α-Adrenergic stimulation also increases cGMP levels, and 8-bromo-cGMP increases mucin secretion (94). Thus, α-adrenergic stimulation of mucin secretion might be mediated also through a G-protein (cGMP-dependent) pathway.

E. Effect of Cholinergic Agents

Acetylcholine and methacholine do not appear to affect chloride or sodium transport by tracheal surface epithelial cells in some studies (95), but it has been reported that acetylcholine increases the net movement of chloride and sodium towards the canine tracheal lumen in vitro (96,97). This might be because there is net ion movement that is driven by mucin secretion without active ion transport. Cholinergic stimulation of mucin release has been demonstrated in human airway gland and explants of human bronchus (98), and sodium and chloride secretion may accompany this.

Calcium influx from outside of the cells and calcium release from intracellular stores are both involved in the stimulation of mucus secretion by cholinergic agents (99–101). The same secretagogues that increase $[Ca^{2+}]_i$ also increase intracellular levels of IP_3 (102). The change in $[Ca^{2+}]_i$ in response to methacholine is biphasic with a large, transient, 10-fold increase followed by a smaller, sustained increase. The former may reflect release from stores, the latter influx from outside the cell (93). In human airway explants, Shelhamer et al. (94) reported that cholinergic stimulation increases cGMP levels, so mucin secretion might also be mediated, in part, through G-protein–activated pathways.

F. Arachidonic Acid Metabolites

$PGF_{2\alpha}$ and PGE_1, metabolites of the cyclooxygenase pathway of arachidonic acid metabolism, stimulate chloride secretion. PGE_1 also depresses sodium absorption (95). This is supported by data that indomethacin, a cyclooxygenase inhibitor, decreases net chloride secretion and increases net sodium absorption in bovine trachea (81). Sheep trachea responds to leukotriene D_4, a lipoxygenase pathway metabolite, by an increase in chloride, sodium, water, and glycoprotein secretion (103). Leukotriene C_4, LTD_4, prostaglandin E_1, PGE_2, and $PGF_{2\alpha}$ stimulate ion transport (104,105). Lazarus and colleagues reported that mast cell–derived mediators other than histamine produced an increase in net chloride secretion without a significant effect on net sodium absorption in canine trachea, and this effect was thought to be dependent on the cyclooxygenase pathways (106). These data suggest that endogenous arachidonic acid metabolites increase cell membrane chloride permeability.

Immunocytochemistry has shown that prostaglandins increase cAMP in gland cells (107), and PGE_2 has been reported to stimulate adenylcyclase, leading to protein kinase A activation (108). The cAMP pathway may be involved in the response to PGs.

$PGF_{2\alpha}$, LTC_4, and LTD_4 increase mucin secretion (109–111), and these metabolites may play an important role in mucin secretion regulation.

G. Neurotransmitters and Hormones

Substance P and vasoactive intestinal peptide (VIP) stimulate net chloride secretion by dog tracheal mucosa (112,113), while substance P does not significantly change net sodium absorption (112). Platelet-activating factor causes the release of substance P and can stimulate net chloride secretion in the rat trachea (114). Tamaoki reported a rapid and dose-dependent increase in NO concentration caused by the addition of neurokinins and substance P, suggesting that NO generation may contribute to chloride ion secretion mediated by tachykinin NK_2 receptors (115).

Substance P increases mucin secretion in human nasal and bronchial explants (116,117) and increases mucus secretion in the ferret trachea (118). Substance P increased $[Ca^{2+}]_i$ in cat glands (83), suggesting that a calcium-dependent pathway may be involved in this response. VIP decreased mucus secretion in human tracheal explants (119), while it increased secretion in human nasal explants (117). VIP may act differently in different regions of the airway depending upon the secretory cells present.

Bradykinin also stimulates chloride (and mucin) secretion in the canine trachea, and its action may be mediated by the release of prostaglandins (120, 121), because the effect on short circuit current is greatly diminished by indomethacin. This modification of chloride conductance by bradykinin in epithelial cells has been attributed to an activation of protein kinase A by arachidonic acid cyclooxygenase products (PGE$_2$) (108). Bradykinin also increases [Ca^{2+}]$_i$ in gland cells (93), which suggests that the calcium-dependent pathway might also be involved in this response.

Adenosine stimulates chloride secretion in the canine trachea, especially when added to the luminal side (122). The P$_2$Y$_2$ (purinoceptor) receptor system has been shown to have a role in regulating both ion transport and mucus secretion. Extracellular nucleotides are agonists of this receptor system. In the airway epithelium, extracellular nucleotides activate chloride conductance, induce goblet cell mucin secretion, and stimulate ciliary beat frequency (123,124).

Thus, chloride secretion is mediated through both [Ca^{2+}]$_i$-dependent and [Ca^{2+}]$_i$-independent signaling pathways, resulting in opening outwardly rectifying chloride channels (ORCC), the CFTR chloride channels, and [Ca^{2+}]$_i$-dependent chloride channels (125). ATP increases cAMP levels and [Ca^{2+}]$_i$ (93), and cAMP stimulates several pathways of chloride conductance, consistent with simultaneous activation of both CFTR and ORCC (125). Thus, ATP or UTP stimulates chloride secretion via multiple signal transduction pathways and activation of at least three types of channels. Because it is reported that an increase in cAMP and [Ca^{2+}]$_i$ stimulated mucin secretion (126), ATP may also stimulate mucin secretion through these pathways.

It is suggested that antidiuretic hormone blocks apical membrane chloride channels and that angiotensin II reverses this effect by increasing apical membrane permeability to chloride (127). Neurotensin, somatostatin, bombesin, leucine enkephalin, etorphine, and aldosterone have all been shown to have no effect on the bioelectric properties of the dog tracheal mucosae. Rabbit trachea did not respond to vasopressin or aldosterone.

H. Macrolides

Erythromycin has been shown to inhibit chloride secretion across cultured canine tracheal epithelial cells (128). This may be of benefit to some patients with inflammatory airway diseases.

I. Nitric Oxide

Chloride secretion is inhibited by an inducible nitric oxide synthase (iNOS) inhibitor in murine nasal mucosae. Thus, constitutive NO production likely plays some role in the downregulation of sodium absorption and leads to an increase in transepithelial chloride secretion (129).

J. Therapeutic Use of Ion Channel Modifiers

Airway epithelial ion transport, particularly that of sodium and chloride, influences the volume and composition of airway surface liquid (130). Defects in ion transport play an important role in the pathogenesis of some chronic airway diseases characterized by accumulation of airway secretions, such as bronchitis, asthma, and cystic fibrosis. In cystic fibrosis, lack of functional CFTR in the apical membrane of serous gland cells (131) leads to failure of gland water secretion (132), making it more difficult to clear these secretions. Development of therapies for disorders of mucus clearance needs to consider not only the direct action of mucoactive agents, but also the stimulation or suppression of secretion and the postsecretory adjustment of mucus properties by transepithelial salt and water transport.

Therapy using amiloride and UTP to block the excess absorption of sodium and stimulate secretion of chloride ion can acutely improve airway mucociliary clearance in patients with cystic fibrosis (133,134), but this has not yet been shown to be clinically effective.

Other channel modifiers could be used in therapy for respiratory diseases if safety and efficacy can be demonstrated clinically. Potassium channel openers, by stimulating transepithelial chloride transport, may represent an innovative approach. Calcium/calmodulin activation of chloride channels also presents a pathway with therapeutic potential for circumventing defective regulation of chloride channels in cystic fibrosis, and modulation of the inhibitory G protein signaling pathway may have the therapeutic potential for improving cAMP-activated chloride secretion in CF.

References

1. Verdugo P. Hydration kinetics of exocytosed mucins in cultured secretory cells of the rabbit trachea: a new model. Ciba Found Symp 1984; 109:212–225.
2. Boucher RC. State of the art: human airway ion transport. Am J Respir Crit Care Med 1994; 150:271–281, 581–593.
3. Rechkemmer GR. The molecular biology of chloride secretion in epithelia. Am Rev Respir Dis 1988; 138:S7–S9.
4. Knowles MR, Clark CE, Fischer ND, et al. Nasal secretions: role of epithelial ion transport.
5. Foot AB, Caul EO, Roome AP, et al. An assessment of sputum induction as an aid to diagnosis of respiratory infections in the immunocompromised child. J Infect 1992; 24:49–54.
6. Pin I, Gibson PG, Kolendowicz R, et al. Use of induced sputum cell counts to investigate airway inflammation in asthma. Thorax 1992; 47:25–29.
7. Popov TA, Pizzichini MMM, Pizzichini E, et al. Some technical factors influencing the induction of sputum for cell analysis. Eur Respir J 1995; 8:559–565.

8. Pavia D, Thomson ML, Clarke SW. Enhanced clearance of secretions from the human lung after the administration of hypertonic saline aerosol. Am Rev Respir Dis 1978; 117:199–203.

9. Robinson M, Regnis JA, Bailey DL, et al. Effect of hypertonic saline, amiloride, and cough on mucociliary clearance in patients with cystic fibrosis. Am J Respir Crit Care Med 1996; 153:1503–1509.

10. Eng PA, Morton J, Douglass JA, et al. Short term efficacy of ultrasonically nebulized hypertonic saline in cystic fibrosis. Pediatr Pulmon 1996; 21:77–83.

11. Peatfield AC, Richardson PS, Wells UM. The effect of airflow on mucus secretion into the trachea of the cat. J Physiol 1986; 380:429–439.

12. Umeno E, MacDonald DM, Nadel JA. Hypertonic saline increases vascular permeability in the rat trachea by producing neurogenic inflammation. J Clin Invest 1990; 85:1905–1908.

13. Solway J, Leff AR. Sensory neuropeptides and airway function. J Appl Physiol 1991; 71:2077–2087.

14. Kowalski ML, Didier A, Kaliner MA. Neurogenic inflammation in the airways. I. Neurogenic stimulation induces plasma protein extravasation into rat airway lumen. Am Rev Respir Dis 1989; 140:101–109.

15. Barnes PJ. Neurogenic inflammation in airways. Int Arch Allergy Appl Immunol 1991; 94:303–309.

16. Assouline G, Leibson V, Danon A. Stimulation of prostaglandin output from rat stomach by hypertonic solutions. Eur J Pharmacol 1977; 44:271–273.

17. Gravelyn TR, Pan PM, Eschenbacher WL. Mediator release in an isolated segment in subjects with asthma. Am Rev Respir Dis 1988; 137:641–646.

18. Holt WV, North RD. Effects of temperature and restoration of osmotic equilibrium during thawing on the induction of plasma membrane damage in cryopreserved ram spermatozoa. Biol Reprod 1994; 51:414–424.

19. Folkesson HG, Kheradmand F, Matthay M. The effect of saltwater on alveolar epithelial barrier function. Am J Respir Crit Care Med 1994; 150:1555–1563.

20. Peatfield AC, Richardson PS, Wells UM. The effect of airflow on mucus secretion into the trachea of the cat. J Physiol 1986; 380:429–439.

21. Winters SL, Yeates DB. Role of hydration, sodium, and chloride in regulation of canine mucociliary transport system. J Appl Physiol 1997; 83:1360–1369.

22. Ziment I. Hypertonic solutions, urea, and ascorbic acid. In: Braga PC, Allegra L, eds. Drugs in Bronchial Mucology. New York: Raven Press, 1989:137–143.

23. Price AM, Webber SE, Widdicombe JG. Osmolarity affects ion and water fluxes and secretion in the ferret trachea. J Appl Physiol 1993; 74:2788–2794.

24. Yankaskas JR, Gatzy JT, Boucher RC. Effects of raised osmolarity on canine tracheal epithelial ion transport function. J Appl Physiol 1987; 62:2241–2245.

25. Robinson M, Hemming AL, Regnis JA, et al. Effect of increasing doses of hypertonic saline on mucociliary clearance in patients with cystic fibrosis. Thorax 1997; 52:900–903.

26. Anderson SD, Daviskas E, Brannan JD, et al. Inhalation of dry powder mannitol increases mucociliary clearance. Eur Respir J 1997; 10:256s.

27. Lee MM, King M. Effect of low molecular weight heparin on the elasticity of dog mucus. Clin Invest Med 1998; 21:S102.

28. Feng W, Garrett H, Speert DP, et al. Improved clearability of cystic fibrosis sputum with dextran treatment in vitro. Am J Respir Crit Care Med 1998; 157:710–714.
29. Wills PJ, Hall RL, Chan WM, et al. Sodium chloride increases the ciliary transportability of cystic fibrosis and bronchiectasis sputum on the mucus-depleted bovine trachea. J Clin Invest 1997; 99:9–13.
30. Lieberman J, McGaughey C, Trimmer BM, Kurnick NB. Inhibition of trypsin by deoxyribonucleic acid. Arch Biochem Biophys 1965; 110:601–610.
31. Feng W, Nakamura S, Sudo E, et al. Effects of dextran on dog mucus in vivo. Am J Respir Crit Care Med 1998; 157:A127.
32. Selsted ME, Tang YQ, Morris WL, et al. Purification, primary structures, and antibacterial activities of beta-defensins, a new family of antimicrobial peptides from bovine neutrophils. J Biol Chem 1993; 268:6641–6648.
33. Boulet LP, Turcotte H, Tennina S. Comparative efficacy of salbutamol, ipratropium, and cromoglycate in the prevention of bronchospasm induced by exercise and hyperosmolar challenges. J Allergy Clin Immunol 1989; 83:882–887.
34. Welsh MJ. Mechanisms of airway epithelial ion transport. Clin Chest Med 1986; 273–283.
35. Melon J. Contribution à L'étude de l'activité secretoire de la muqueuse nasale. Acta Otolaryngol Belg 1968; 22:5–216.
36. Gatzy JT. Bioelectric properties of the isolated amphibian lung. Am J Physiol 1967; 213:425–431.
37. Gatzy JT. Ion transport across the excised bullfrog lung. Am J Physiol 1975; 228:1162–1171.
38. Olver RE, Strang LB. Ion fluxes across the pulmonary epithelia and secretion of lung liquid in the foetal lamb. J Physiol (Lond) 1974; 241:327–357.
39. Olver RE, Davis B, Marin MG, et al. Active transport of Na and Cl across the canine tracheal epithelium in vitro. Am Rev Respir Dis 1975; 112:811–815.
40. Boucher RC, Brombrg PA, Gatzy JT. Airway transepithelial electric potential in vivo: species and regional differences. J Appl Physiol 1980; 48:169–176.
41. Frizzell RA. Molecular biology. Role of absorptive and secretory processes in hydration of the airway surface. Am Rev Respir Dis 1988; 138:S3–S6.
42. Widdicombe JH, Basbaum CB, Yee JY. Localization of Na pumps in the tracheal epithelium of the dog. J Cell Biol 1979; 82:380–390.
43. Welsh MJ. Electrolyte transport by airway epithelia. Physiol Rev 1987; 67:1143–1184.
44. Widdicombe JH. Ion transport by airway epithelia. In: Crystal RG, West JB, Weibel E, Barnes PJ, eds. The Lung: Scientific Foundations. New York: Raven Press, 1996:39.1–39.12.
45. Levitan IB. Modulation of ion channels by protein phosphorylation and dephosphorylation. Annu Rev Physiol 1994; 56:193–212.
46. Bradbury NA, Bridges RJ. Role of membrane trafficking in plasma membrane solute transport. Am J Physiol 1994; 267:C1–C24.
47. Anderson MP, Welsh MJ. Fatty acids inhibit apical membrane chloride channels in airway epithelia. Proc Natl Acad Sci U S A 1990; 87:7334–7338.
48. Welsh MJ. Abnormal regulation of ion channels in cystic fibrosis epithelia. FASEB J 1990; 4:2718–2725.

49. Chang XB, Tabcharani JA, Hou YX, et al. Protein kinase A (PKA) still activates CFTR chloride channel after mutagenesis of all 10 PKA consensus phosphorylation sites. J Biol Chem 1993; 268:11,304–11,311.
50. Rich DP, Berger HA, Cheng SH, et al. Regulation of the cystic fibrosis transmembrane conductance regulator Cl⁻ channel by negative charge in the R domain. J Biol Chem 1993; 268:20,259–20,267.
51. Li M, McCann JD, Anderson MP, et al. Regulation of chloride channels by protein kinase C in normal and cystic fibrosis airway epithelia [see comments]. Science 1989; 244:1353–1356.
52. Sasaki T, Shimura S, Wakui M, et al. Apically localized IP3 receptors control chloride current in airway gland acinar cells. Am J Physiol 1994; 267:L152–L158.
53. Wagner JA, Cozens AL, Schulman H, et al. Activation of chloride channels in normal and cystic fibrosis airway epithelial cells by multifunctional calcium/calmodulin-dependent protein kinase. Nature 1991; 349:793–796.
54. Clancy JP, McCann JD, Welsh MJ. Evidence that calcium-dependent activation of airway epithelial chloride channels is not dependent on phosphorylation. Am J Physiol 1990; 259:L410–L414.
55. Anderson MP, Welsh MJ. Calcium and cAMP activate different chloride channels in the apical membrane of normal and cystic fibrosis epithelia. Proc Natl Acad Sci U S A 1991; 88:6003–6007.
56. Gill DR, Hyde SC, Higgins CF, et al. Separation of drug transport and chloride channel functions of the human multidrug resistance P-glycoprotein. Cell 1992; 71:23–32.
57. Valverde MA, Diaz M, Sepulveda FV, et al. Volume-regulated chloride channels associated with the human multidrug-resistance P-glycoprotein. Nature 1992; 355: 830–833.
58. Schwiebert EM, Kizer N, Gruenert DC, et al. GTP-binding proteins inhibit cAMP activation of chloride channels in cystic fibrosis airway epithelial cells. Proc Natl Acad Sci U S A 1992; 89:10,623–10,627.
59. Welsh MJ. Inhibition of chloride secretion by furosemide in canine tracheal epithelium. J Membr Biol 1983; 71:219–226.
60. Vulliemin P, Durand-Arczyrska W, Durand J. Electrical properties and electrolyte transport in bovine tracheal epithelium: effects of ion substitution, transport inhibitors and histamine. Pflugers Arch 1983; 12:54–59.
61. Bolton JE, Field M. Ca ionophore stimulated ion secretion in rabbit ileal mucosa: relation to actions of cyclic 3', 5'-AMP and carbamylcholine. J Membr Biol 1977; 35:159–173.
62. Corrales RJ, Leikauf GD, Coleman DL, et al. Ion transport across cat and ferret tracheal epithelia [abstract]. Am Rev Respir Dis 1985; 131:A362.
63. Widdicombe JH, Ueki IF, Bruderman I, et al. The effects of sodium substitution and ouabain on ion transport by dog tracheal epithelium. Am Rev Respir Dis 1979; 120:385–392.
64. Widdicombe JH, Welsh MJ. Ion transport by dog tracheal epithelium. Fed Proc 1980; 39:3060–3066.
65. Al-Bazzaz FJ, Zevin R. Ion transport and metabolic effects of amiloride in canine tracheal mucosa. Lung 1984; 162:357–367.

66. Cotton CU, Lawson EE, Boucher RC, et al. Bioelectric properties and ion transport of airways excised from adult and fetal sheep. J Appl Physiol Respir Environ Exerc Physiol 1983; 55:1542–1549.
67. Van Scott MR, Davis W, Boucher RC. Na$^+$ and Cl$^-$ transport across rabbit nonciliated bronchiolar epithelial (clara) cells. Am J Physiol 1989; 256:C893–C901.
68. Boucher RC, Gatzy JT. Characteristics of sodium transport by excised rabbit trachea. J Appl Physiol 1980; 48:169–176.
69. Ropke M, Hansen M, Carstens S, et al. Effects of a short-chain phospholipid on ion transport pathways in rabbit nasal airway epithelium. Am J Physiol 1996; 271: L646–L655.
70. Ropke M, Carstens S, Holm M, et al. Ion transport mechanisms in native rabbit nasal airway epithelium. Am J Physiol 1996; 271:L637–L645.
71. Mc Bride RK, Stone KK, Marin MG. Oxidant injury alters barrier function of ferret tracheal epithelium. Am J Physiol 1993; 264:L165–L174.
72. Kawaguchi S, Ukai K, Jin CS, et al. Effect of histamine on nasal epithelial permeability to horseradish peroxidase in allergic guinea pigs. Annal Otol Rhinol Laryngol 1995; 104:394–398.
73. Robinson TW, Kim KJ. Dual effect of nitrogen dioxide on barrier properties of guinea pig tracheobronchial epithelial monolayers cultured in air interface. J Toxicol Environ Health 1995; 44:57–71.
74. Cloutier MM, Wong D, Ogra PL. Respiratory syncytial virus alters electrophysiologic properties in cotton rat airway epithelium. Pediatr Pulmonol 1989; 6:164–168.
75. Nielsen S, King LS, Christensen BM, et al. Aquaporins in complex tissues. II. Subcellular distribution in respiratory and glandular tissues of rat. Am J Physiol 1997; 273:C1549–C1561.
76. Dibas AI, Mia AJ, Yorio T. Aquaporins (water channels)' role in vasopressin-activated water transport. Proc Soc Exp Biol Med 1998; 219:183–199.
77. Schreiber R, Nitschke R, Greger R, et al. The cystic fibrosis transmembrane conductance regulator activates aquaporin 3 in airway epithelial cells. J Biol Chem 1999; 274:11,811–11,816.
78. Tanaka M, Inase N, Fushimi K, et al. Induction of aquaporin 3 by corticosteroid in a human airway epithelial cell line. Am J Physiol 1997; 273:L1090–L1095.
79. Cotton CU, Lawson EE, Boucher RC, et al. Bioelectric properties and ion transport of airways excised from adult and fetal sheep. J Appl Physiol 1983; 55:1542–1549.
80. Davis B, Marin MG, Yee JW, et al. Effect of terbutaline on movement of Cl and Na across the trachea of the dog in vitro. Am Rev Respir Dis 1979; 120:547–552.
81. Langridge-Smith, JE, Rao MC, Field M. Chloride and sodium transport across bovine tracheal epithelium: effects of secretagogues and indomethacin. Pflugers Arch 1984; 402:42–47.
82. Jarnigan F, Davis JD, Bromberg PA, et al. Bioelectric properties and ion transport of excised rabbit trachea. J Appl Physiol 1983; 55:1884–1892.
83. Phipps RJ, Nadel JA, Davis B. Effect of alpha-adrenergic stimulation on mucus secretion and on ion transport in cat trachea in vitro. Am Rev Respir Dis 1980; 121:359–365.

84. Corrales R, Widdecombe JH Nadel JA. Relationship between mucus output and active chloride secretion in cat tracheal epithelium. Chest 1982; 81(suppl):7S–9S.

85. Al-Bazzaz FJ. Role of cyclic AMP in regulation of chloride secretion by canine tracheal mucosa. Am Rev Respir Dis 1981; 123:295–298.

86. Al-Bazzaz FJ, Cheng E. Effect of catecholamines on ion transport in dog tracheal epithelium. J Appl Physiol 1979; 47:397–403.

87. Welsh MJ, Liedtke CM. Chloride and potassium channels in cystic fibrosis airway epithelia. Nature 1986; 322:467–470.

88. Peatfield AC, Richardson PS. The control of mucin secretion into the lumen of the cat trachea by α- and β-adrenoreceptors, and their relative involvement during sympathetic nerve stimulation. Eur J Pharmacol 1982; 81:617–626.

89. Phipps RJ, Nadel JA, Davis B. Effect of alpha-adrenergic stimulation on mucus secretion and on ion transport in cat trachea in vitro. Am Rev Respir Dis 1980; 121:359–365.

90. Sasaki T, Shimura S, Sasaki H, et al. Effect of epithelium on mucus secretion from feline tracheal submucosal glands. J Applied Physiol 1989; 66:764–770.

91. Culp DJ, McBride RK, Graham LA, et al. Alpha-adrenergic regulation of secretion by tracheal glands. Am J Physiol 1990; 259:L198–L205.

92. Gierschik P, Jakobs KH. Mechanisms for inhibition of adenylate cyclase by alpha-2 adrenergic receptors. In: Limbird LE, ed. The Alpha 2 Adrenergic Receptors. Clifton, NJ: Humana, 1988:75–114.

93. Ishihara H, Shimura S, Sato M, et al. Intracellular calcium concentration of acinar cells in feline tracheal submucosal glands. Am J Physiol 1990; 259:L345–L350.

94. Shelhamer JH, Marom Z, Kaliner M. Immunologic and neuropharmacologic stimulation of mucous glycoprotein release from human airways in vitro. J Clin Invest 1980; 66:1400–1408.

95. Al-Bazzaz FJ. Regulation of salt and water transport across airway mucosa. Clin Chest Med 1986; 7:259–272.

96. Nadel JA, Davis B, Phipps RJ. Control of mucus secretion and ion transport in airways. Am Rev Physiol 1979; 41:369–381.

97. Marin MG, Davis B, Nadel JA. Effect of acetylcholine on Cl and Na fluxes across dog tracheal epithelium in vitro. Am J Physiol 1977; 42:735–738.

98. Logun C, Mullol J, Rieves D, et al. Use of a monoclonal antibody enzyme-linked immunosorbent assay to measure human respiratory glycoprotein production in vitro. Am J Respir Cell Mol Biol 1991; 5:71–79.

99. Shimura S, Sasaki T, Ikeda K, et al. VIP augments cholinergic-induced glycoconjugate secretion in tracheal submucosal glands. J Appl Physiol 1988; 65:2537–2544.

100. Barsigian C, Barbieri EJ. The effects of indomethacin and prostaglandins E2 and F2α on canine tracheal mucus generation. Agents Actions 1982; 12:320–327.

101. Colcs SJ, Judge J, Reid L. Differential effects of calcium ions on glycoconjugate secretion by canine tracheal explants. Chest 1982; 81:34S.

102. Hall IP. Agonist-induced inositol response in bovine airway submucosal glands. Am J Physiol 1992; 262:L257–L262.

103. Phipps RJ, Denas S, Wanner A. Effects of indomethacin on leukotriene D4-

induced secretion of ions, water, and glycoproteins in sheep trachea [abstract].
Fed Proc 1985; 44:641.

104. Al-Bazzaz FJ, Yadava VP, Westenfelder C. Modification of Na and Cl transport
in canine tracheal mucosa by prostaglandins. Am J Physiol 1981; 240; Renal Fluid
Electrolyte Physiol 9:F101–F105.

105. Leikauf GD, Ueki IF, Widdicombe JH, et al. Effects of leukotrienes B4, C4, and
E4 on electrical properties and prostaglandin release from tracheal epithelium [abstract]. Fed Proc 1984; 43:829.

106. Lazarus SC, McCabe LJ, Nadel JA, et al. Effects of mast cell-derived mediators
on epithelial cells in canine trachea. Am J Physiol 1986; 251:C387–C394.

107. Lazarus SC, Basbaum CB, Gold WM. Prostaglandins and intracellular cyclic
AMP in respiratory secretory cells. Am Rev Respir Dis 1984; 130:262–266.

108. Levistre R, Lemnaouar M, Rybkine T, et al. Increase of bradykinin-stimulated
arachidonic acid release in a delta F508 cystic fibrosis epithelial cell line. Biochim
Biophys Acta 1993; 1181:233–239.

109. Marom Z, Shellhamer JH, Bach MK, et al. Slow-reacting substances, leukotrienes
C4 and D4, increase the release of mucus from human airways in vitro. Am Rev
Respir Dis 1982; 126:449–451.

110. Peatfield AC, Piper JC, Richardson PS. The effect of leukotriene C4 on mucin
release into the cat trachea in vivo and in vitro. 1982; 77:391–393.

111. Hoffstein ST, Malo PE, Bugelski P, et al. Leukotriene D4 (LTD4) induces mucus
secretion from goblet cells in the guinea pig respiratory epithelium. Exp Lung Res
1990; 16:711–725.

112. Al-Bazzaz FJ, Kelsey JG, Kaage WD. Substance P stimulation of chloride secretion by canine tracheal mucosa. Am Rev Respir Dis 1985; 131:86–89.

113. Nathanson I, Widdicombe JH, Barnes PJ. Effect of vasoactive intestinal peptide
on ion transport across dog tracheal epithelium. J Appl Physiol Respir Environ
Exerc Physiol 1983; 55:1844–1848.

114. Sestini P, Bienenstock J, Crowe SE, et al. Ion transport in rat tracheal epithelium
in vitro. Role of capsaicin-sensitive nerves in allergic reactions. Am Rev Respir
Dis 1990; 141:393–397.

115. Tamaoki J. Airway epithelium and nitric oxide. Nihon Kyobu Shikkan Gakkai
Zasshi 1995; 33(suppl):204–211.

116. Rogers DF, Aursudkij B, Barnes PJ. Effects of tachykinins on mucus secretion in
human bronchi in vitro. Eur J Pharmacol 1989; 174:283–286.

117. Mullol J, Rieves RD, Baraniuk JN, et al. The effects of neuropeptides on mucous
glycoprotein secretion from human nasal mucosa in vivo. Neuropeptides 1992;
21:231–238.

118. De Sanctis GT, Rubin BK, Ramirez O, et al. Ferret tracheal mucus rheology,
clearability and volume following administration of substance P or methacholine.
Eur Res J 1993; 6:76–82.

119. Amin DN, Goswami S, Klein T, et al. functional antagonism between hormone
receptor systems: modulation of glycoprotein secretion in secretory epithelial
cells. Am J Respir Cell Mol Biol 1991; 4:135–139.

120. Leikauf GD, Ueki IF, Nadel JA, et al. Bradykinin stimulates Cl secretion and

prostaglandin E2 release by canine tracheal epithelium. Am J Physiol 1985; 248: F48–F55.

121. Davis B, Roberts AM, Coleridge HM, et al. Reflex tracheal gland secretion evoked by stimulation of bronchial C-fibers in dogs. J Appl Physiol 1982; 53: 985–991.

122. Pratt AD, Welsh MJ. Adenosine stimulates chloride secretion in canine tracheal epithelium [abstract]. Am Rev Respir Dis 1985; 131:A368.

123. Kim KC, Lee BC. P2 purinoceptor regulation of mucin release by airway goblet cells in primary culture. Br J Pharmacol 1991; 103:1053–1056.

124. Tamaoki J, Kondo M, Takizawa T. Adenosine-mediated cyclic AMP-dependent inhibition of ciliary activity in rabbit tracheal epithelium. Am Rev Respir Dis 1989; 139:441–445.

125. Hwang TH, Schwiebert EM, Guggino WB. Apical and basolateral ATP stimulates tracheal epithelial chloride secretion via multiple purinergic receptors. Am J Physiol 1996; 270:C1611–C1623.

126. Whimster WF, Reid L. The influence of dibutyrylcyclic adenosine monophosphate and other substances on human bronchial mucous gland discharge. Exp Mol Pathol 1973; 18:234–240.

127. Palacios SM, Contreras GM, Norris BC, et al. Effects of antidiuretic hormone on the electrical properties of canine tracheal epithelium. Pharmacology 1987; 35: 327–332.

128. Tamaoki J, Isono K, Sakai N, et al. Erythromycin inhibits Cl secretion across canine tracheal epithelial cells. Eur Respir J 1992; 234–238.

129. Elmer HL, Brady KG, Drumm ML, et al. Nitric oxide-mediated regulation of transepithelial sodium and chloride transport in murine nasal epithelium. Am J Physiol 1999; 276:L466–L473.

130. Noone PG, Knowles MR. Trends in therapy of abnormal airway epithelial ion and liquid transport. Monaldi Arch Chest Dis 1993; 48:140–143.

131. Engelhardt JF, Yankaskas JR, Ernst S, et al. Submucosal glands are the predominant site of CFTR expression in the human bronchus. Nat Genet 1992; 2:240–247.

132. Jiang C, Finkbeiner WE, Widdicombe JH, et al. Fluid transport across cultures of human tracheal glands is altered in cystic fibrosis. J Physiol 1997; 501:637–648.

133. Knowles, MR, Church NL, Waltner WE, et al. A pilot study of aerosolized amiloride for the treatment of lung disease in cystic fibrosis. N Eng J Med 1990; 322: 1189–1194.

134. Tomkiewicz, RP, App EM, Zayas JG, et al. Amiloride inhalation therapy in cystic fibrosis. Am J Respir Crit Care Med 1993; 148:1002–1007.

135. Finkbeiner WE, Shen BQ, Widdicombe JH. Chloride secretion and function of serous and mucous cells of human airway glands. Am J Physiol 1994; 267:L206–L210.

14

Mucoactive Agents and the Upper Airway

YASUO SAKAKURA, YUICHI MAJIMA, and KOSUKE OKAMOTO
Mie University School of Medicine
Mie, Japan

JOHN W. GEORGITIS
Wake Forest University School of Medicine
Winston-Salem, North Carolina, U.S.A.

I. Respiratory Mucosa Structures in the Upper Airways

A. Nose and Paranasal Sinuses

Behind the vestibular region of the human nose, the epithelial lining of the nasal cavity is divided into a large respiratory region and a small olfactory region. The respiratory region is covered by a typical airway epithelal layer, which is pseudostratified, ciliated, and columnar. The epithelial cell types found in the human nose include basal cells, goblet cells, and columnar ciliated or nonciliated cells. Unlike in the tracheobronchial epithelium, brush cells and Clara cells are not present. The mucous membrane of the paranasal sinuses has a pseudostratified, ciliated, and columnar epithelium.

Goblet cells are irregularly distributed in the nasal and paranasal mucosa. Quantitative studies of goblet cells have shown that the cell density in the frontal, ethmoid, and sphenoid sinuses is very similar to that in the nasal septum (5700 cells/mm^2), but considerably higher in the maxillary mucosa, where it comes close to the density in the inferior nasal turbinate ($11,000$ cells/mm^2) (1). The goblet cell density in the trachea is higher than that in the nasal septum and in most sinuses, and somewhat lower than that in the inferior turbinate (1).

The nasal glands are tubuloalveolar and seromucous and are found throughout the respiratory region of the nose. Nasal gland density is 8.2–8.8 glands/mm^2. In paranasal sinuses the density of the glands is very much lower than in the nose varying between 0.06 glands/mm^2 in the sphenoid sinus and 0.47 glands/mm^2 in the ethmoid sinus (1). The nasal glands produce the major portion of nasal secretions under normal conditions.

The epithelial mucosa of the nose and the paranasal sinuses is covered by a secretion that, according to the classical description by Lucas and Douglas (2), consists of a periciliary fluid layer and outer mucous layer, riding on the top of the cilia. Although the origin of the periciliary fluid layer is not known, water transport across the respiratory epithelium may have an important role. The outer mucous layer originates in the seromucous glands and goblet cells. Mucociliary clearance involves the outer mucous layer, ciliary activity, and interactions between mucus and cilia (3). The direction of mucociliary clearance of the nose is from anterior to posterior (4). In the paranasal sinuses, mucociliary clearance moves to the sinus ostium, and after leaving the ostium it joins the nasal mucociliary flow (5).

B. Middle Ear and Eustachian Tube

The middle ear cavity is connected to the nasopharynx through the eustachian tube. The eustachian tube is composed of pseudostratified columnar cells, and interspersed between these cells are goblet cells. Away from the opening of the eustachian tube, the number of ciliated cells becomes small in the middle ear cavity, and very few ciliated cells are present in the mastoid air cells (6). The density of goblet cells in the pharyngeal ostium of the eustachian tube is almost the same as in the inferior turbinate or maxillary sinus, but it decreases sharply toward the tympanic ostium (1). There are few goblet cells in the middle ear cavity: 11–135 cells/mm^2 (7).

The submucous, seromucous, and tubuloalveolar glands are present only in the cartilaginous part of the eustachian tube, not in the bony part or in the middle ear cavity under normal conditions (7). The normal middle ear mucosa can actively clear foreign material toward and into the eustachian tube by mucociliary clearance (8). Thus, the clearance in the middle ear and the eustachian tube is called tubotympanal clearance (9).

II. Upper Respiratory Mucosa Under Pathological Conditions

In the upper airways, the administration of mucoactive agents is usually indicated for treatment of hypersecretory diseases, such as chronic sinusitis (CS) and otitis media with effusion (OME). Therefore, we have summarized the available information on such diseases.

A. Nose and Paranasal Sinuses

CS is one of the most common airway diseases in the world. The U.S. Department of Health and Human Services estimated that in 1981, 31 million people suffered from sinusitis (10). In Japan, the Ministry of Health and Welfare reported the rate of CS to be 273 per 100,000 people in 1995 (11). CS has been generally accepted as an inflammation of the nasal and sinus mucosa with persistent mucous or mucopurulent nasal discharge for longer than 8 or 12 weeks that is resistant to medical therapy without intervening acute infection (12).

In chronic maxillary sinusitis, the surface of the maxillary sinus mucosa is covered by cilia in $60.7 \pm 28.8\%$ (mean $\pm$ SD), ranging from 33.2 to 95.8% (13). This is in contrast to the normal maxillary sinus mucosa, where more than 90% of the surface is covered by cilia (14). These reports suggest that the cilia of the maxillary mucosa are well preserved or damaged to various degrees under pathological conditions. The decrease in ciliated area is a result of the increase in nonciliated cells and squamous metaplasia of the mucosa (13). The beat frequency of cilia obtained by cytology brush from maxillary sinus mucosa is significantly reduced in severe maxillary lesions compared with that in mild maxillary lesions (15). The goblet cell density of the maxillary mucosa is reduced in CS, whereas the gland density is obviously increased (16). The mucociliary clearance of maxillary sinus is often impaired in CS (17). The pathological changes of maxillary mucosa may contribute to the impairment of the mucociliary clearance.

In CS, the cilia of the nasal mucosa is well preserved, and $90.2 \pm 9.9\%$ of the mucosal surface is covered by cilia (3). The ciliary beat frequency of CS nasal mucosa is normal (15,18). The number of goblet cells on the nasal mucosa in CS is not different from that in normal subjects, but the number of gland cells is significantly increased (19) (Fig. 1). These reports indicate that hypersecreted nasal mucus in CS may originate not only from pathological sinus mucosa but also from nasal mucosa, and the source of hypersecretion is gland cells rather than goblet cells. Nasal mucociliary clearance in CS will be discussed below.

B. The Middle Ear and the Eustachian Tube

The principal symptom of OME is conductive hearing loss due to the accumulation of serous or mucoid effusion in the middle ear. Most patients affected by OME are children. In pediatric OME, the number of goblet cells in the middle ear mucosa is 20–300 times normal (20), and gland density is also increased (7.1 glands/mm^2) (7). Because of the difficulties in obtaining histological specimens, secretory cells and ciliated cells are rarely studied in the eustachian tube under pathological conditions.

Two eliminative functions, muscular and ciliary, make up the clearance

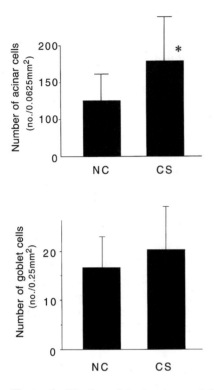

Figure 1 Number of (top) acinar and (bottom) goblet cells in normal control (NC) and in chronic sinusitis (CS). Asterisk indicates significantly high number compared with NC at $p < 0.01$. (From Ref. 19.)

of effusions from the middle ear cavity through the eustachian tube. Although a larger amount of effusion is eliminated from the middle ear by muscular clearance than by ciliary clearance, muscular clearance does not take place under negative pressure in the middle ear cavity such as occurs in OME (21). In other words, mucociliary clearance is important for removing effusions in patients with OME. However, the mucociliary function of the middle ear is reduced in the pediatric patients with OME (9).

III. Rheological Properties of Mucus in the Upper Airways

A. Measurement of Viscoelasticity

Viscosity and elasticity are fundamental rheological properties of mucus. The importance of measuring viscoelasticity is described in Chapter 1. We measured the dynamic viscosity (η') and elastic modulus (G') of respiratory mucus by using an oscillating sphere magnetic rheometer (22,23). In this rheometer, a small amount of test material (about 4 μL) together with a small iron sphere with a radius of 100 μm is placed into the sample cell, which is set in the space between the upper and the lower magnetic poles. The iron sphere is oscillated in a vertical direction applying sinusoidally varying magnetic field gradients. The motion of the iron sphere is followed through a light microscope and transduced to an electrical signal by an optoelectric tracker. Both η' and G' were calculated using the amplitude of the displacement of the iron sphere and the phase lag of the sphere with respect to the oscillatory magnetic driving force (22,23). η' is a measure of viscous behavior, and G' is indicative of the elastic behavior of the sample.

B. Viscoelasticity and Mucociliary Clearance

Although middle ear effusions (MEE) from pediatric OME exhibit macroscopic consistency ranging from watery to sticky, the viscoelasticity of freshly harvested MEE has rarely been described because of the small amount of sample available for analysis. However, our oscillating sphere magnetic rheometer was able to determine the viscoelasticity of MEE. We also measured the transportability of the same sample on mucus-depleted frog palate. The frog palate epithelium has many characteristics in common with mammalian airway epithelia, and the mucus-depleted model has proved a useful model for the study of transport of exogenous mucus by frog cilia (24). Figure 2 shows the mucociliary

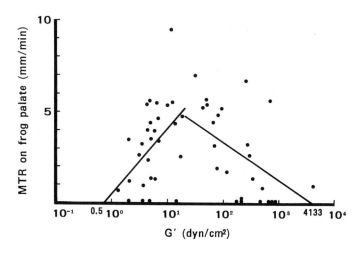

Figure 2 Mucociliary transport rate on mucus-depleted frog palate versus elastic modulus (G') of mucus. Measurements were performed at frequency of 1 Hz and 25°C. (From Ref. 23.)

transportability of MEE on mucus-depleted frog palate as a function of elasticity
(G′) at a frequency of 1 Hz (25°C). A maximal transport rate was observed at
G′ of about 20 dyne/cm^2, and below this value there was a significant positive
correlation between the transport rate and logarithm of G′. Above 20 dyne/cm^2,
the negative correlation between the transport rate and G′ was significant (23).
The maximum transport rate was achieved at η′ of 2 poise (1 Hz, 25°C), and
similar significant correlations were observed between the mucociliary transport
rate (MTR) and η′ values lower or higher than at optimal viscosity (23). These
results are consistent with the results obtained by Shih et al. in reconstituted
canine tracheal mucus (25). They studied the transportability of the reconstituted
mucus samples on the frog palate and found that maximum MTR was obtained
at an optimal concentration of nondialyzable solid concentration of 1.5–2.0%.
Our and their results clearly indicate that the transportability of mucus, by cilia
largely depends on the viscoelasticity of mucus, and there is an optimal viscoelasticity for mucociliary transport.

C. Viscoelasticity of Upper Airway Mucus

Normal Nasal Mucus

We measured G′ and η′ of 29 normal nasal mucus from healthy human adults.
The normal nasal mucus was obtained with the Juhn-Tym Tap®, a disposable
instrument for collecting MEE (Xomed, Jacksonville, FL). The volume of nasal
mucus collected from each nasal cavity ranged from 5 to 100 μL,with a mean
value of 51 μL. The mean values of G′ and η′ of the normal nasal mucus were
35 dyne/cm^2 and 1.8 poise, with a SD of 0.46 and 0.47 log units, respectively (1
Hz, 25°C) (26). In Figure 3, the mean G′ value and a SD of normal nasal mucus
are shown on the line indicating the relationship between MTR and G′ shown in
Figure 2. The G′ values of normal nasal mucus exist in the optimal range for
mucociliary transport. The distribution of η′ of normal nasal mucus was also
within the optimal range. These results suggest that the normal human body may
produce nasal mucus with optimal viscoelasticity for mucociliary clearance.

Nasal Mucus from Chronic Sinusitis

Figure 4 shows the distribution of nasal mucus from 42 adult patients with CS.
The G′ and η′ values are much higher than the optimal value for mucociliary
transport. When the nasal mucus was classified as either mucoid or mucopurulent according to its macroscopic appearance, mucopurulent nasal mucus showed
significantly higher viscoelasticity (G′, 638 ± 520 dyne/cm^2; η′, 32.1 ± 27.9
poise) than mucoid nasal mucus (G′, 105 ± 84 dyne/cm^2; η′, 6.8 ± 4.1 poise)
(27). These observations indicate that mucopurulent nasal mucus is not transported by cilia effectively, and that mucoid mucus is transported more easily but
its viscoelasticity is still higher than the optimal value for mucociliary transport.

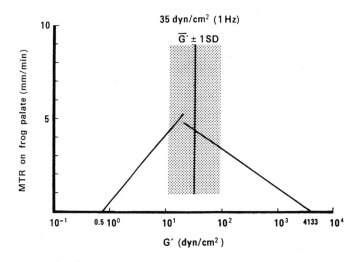

Figure 3 Elastic modulus (G′) of nasal mucus from normal subjects. Measurements of G′ were performed at frequency of 1 Hz and 25°C. The distribution of G′ for normal nasal mucus is shown on the line indicating the relationship between mucociliary transport rate and G′ that appears in Figure 2. (From Ref. 87.)

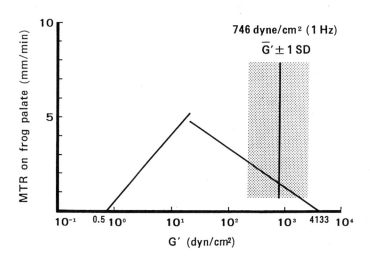

Figure 4 Elastic modulus (G′) of nasal mucus from patients with chronic sinusitis. G′ values were determined at frequency of 1 Hz and 25°C. (From Ref. 87.)

The nasal mucociliary clearance of adult CS patients was significantly reduced compared with that of adult normal subjects (Fig. 5) (28). Moreover, no clearance was observed in about 50% of patients (29). However, reduced nasal mucociliary clearance in CS was recovered by repeated antral lavage or the oral administration of S-carboxymethylcysteine (SCMC) (30). This indicates that malfunction of nasal mucociliary clearance is not the cause of CS, but a result of chronic inflammation of respiratory mucosa. The high viscoelasticity of nasal mucus could be one of the causes of reduced nasal mucociliary clearance in CS.

Nasal Mucus from Allergic Rhinitis

The nasal mucus from patients with perennial allergic rhinitis to house dust mite was studied before and after allergen challenge. Before allergen challenge, G' and η' of nasal mucus were 193 ± 117 dyne/cm^2 and 12.0 ± 7.4 pose, respectively (1 Hz, 25°C). These viscoelastic values are similar to the values of mucoid nasal mucus from CS. After allergen challenge to the nose, both G' and η' of nasal mucus were significantly reduced (G', 89 ± 46 dyne/cm^2; η', 4.1 ± 3.7 poise) (31). Results indicate that allergen exposure decreases the viscoelasticity of nasal mucus in allergic patients, and the resulting viscoelastic values distribute around the optimal values for mucociliary clearance.

Middle Ear Effusions from Pediatric OME

In contrast to nasal mucus, the viscoelasticity of MEE showed a broad distribution: $G' = 1.92\text{--}5890$ dyne/cm^2 and $\eta' = 0.16\text{--}460$ poise (1 Hz, 25°C) (23). In

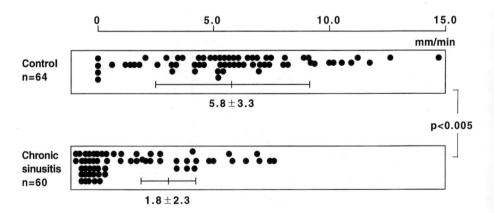

Figure 5 Nasal mucociliary transport rate in normal adults and adult patients with chronic sinusitis. (From Ref. 28.)

order to clarify the relationship between the viscoelastic properties of MEE and the probability of fluid retention in the middle ear, both G' and η' values of MEE at an initial visit were classified into four groups: group 2 shows the optimal G' value for mucociliary clearance, group 1 shows G' values below the optimal value, and G' values in groups 3 and 4 were above the optimal value. In this study, 84% of patients from group 2 were free of ear effusions within 4 months. The incidence of good prognosis for patients in group 2, where the duration of fluid retention was less than 4 months, was significantly higher than for patients from the other three groups (32). These results suggest that MEEs in group 2 patients could be effectively transported by cilia of the eustachian tube and middle ear and hence easily cleared from the middle ear.

D. Mucus Glycoproteins and Viscoelasticity

The contributions of the biochemical constituents of CS nasal mucus to viscosity and elasticity have been studied. A multiple stepwise regression was performed to predict viscoelasticity as a function of the biochemical parameters (33).The results indicate that fucose is the most important determinant of both G' and η' of CS nasal mucus. IgG is the next most important determinant of G' and η'. The results indicate that fucose together with IgG accounted for about 73% of the variance in viscoelasticity of nasal mucus in CS (33).

Fucose is present in purified respiratory mucus glycoproteins (MGs) and is virtually absent in serum glycoproteins. Thus, fucose is a marker for MGs. Because respiratory MGs are produced by goblet cells and submucosal gland cells, locally produced MGs from such secretory cells largely contribute to the high viscoelasticity of nasal mucus in CS. In respiratory mucus, IgG is mainly derived from serum and partly derived from local production. Although the exact mechanism of the contribution of IgG to viscoelasticity is not known, subsidence of inflammation may decrease the viscoelasticity of mucus as a result of a reduction in mucus IgG level.

Subunits of MGs can be identified following two peptide regions. The first is a polypeptide containing oligosaccharide groups attached to serine and threonine and resistant to proteolytic digestion. The second region is a polypeptide devoid of sugars that is sensitive to proteolytic attack, called the naked peptide region. The MGs are formed by an end-to-end association of subunits via disulfide bonds and become very large macromolecules (34). Other intermolecular bonds such as ionic bonds, hydrogen bonds, and van der Waals forces may contribute to the entanglement of large molecules to form network-like structures. Strands of DNA molecules from inflammatory cells also attach to glycoprotein with such bonds. Thus, the viscoelasticity of mucus is dependent not only on the quantities of MGs, but also on the mucous structures containing disulfide and the other intermolecular bonds (35).

IV. Mucoactive Agents and Upper Airway Diseases

A. Thiols with Free Sulfhydryl Group

N-*Acetyl-L-Cysteine*

N-Acetyl-L-cysteine (NAC) is the most popular proprietary mucokinetic agent administered to loosen respiratory tract secretions. The free sulfhydryl group of NAC interacts with the disulfide bonds of mucoprotein, breaking the protein network into less viscous strands. Evidence suggests that NAC is an effective mucolytic for mucoid secretions but less so for other types of sputum, because there is no evidence that NAC can break down DNA (35). However, in vitro administration of 10% NAC tremendously decreased the viscoelasticity of mucopurulent nasal mucus (36). As already shown, the viscoelasticity of CS nasal mucus, especially mucopurulent nasal mucus, is much higher than optimal. The nasal administration of NAC may bring viscoelastic levels closer to optimal values.

NAC is usually used as a 10% solution by diluting with saline or sodium bicarbonate or even sterile water (35). NAC is most effective when directly instilled into the nasal cavity in a dose of 0.5–1.0 mL to each nostril. It can also be administered via jet nebulizer, but use of an ultrasonic nebulizer is not recommended (37). When air is allowed into the solution, NAC breaks down and a marked loss of effectiveness occurs after a few days. It is incompatible with tetracycline, ampicilin, erythromycin, amphotericin, and chymotripsin (38). Untoward effects of topical administration of NAC include a burning sensation in the airways and sulfurous taste and odor.

2-Mercaptoethane sulfonate (MESNA), another drug containing a free sulfhydryl group, has no irritating or bronchodilating activity. In placebo-controlled studies, MESNA nasal splay was similar to NAC and more effective than bromhexine (39). Sputum weight was significantly lower with MESNA in a crossover placebo-controlled study (39).

Other drugs containing free sulfhydryl group, such as L-cysteine and dithiothreitol, has never been reported in the treatment of CS and OME. Toxicity studies in the inner ear has never been performed.

L-*Cysteine Ethyl Ester Hydrochloride (CEE)*

CEE is a sulfhydryl oral mucolytic agent that has been used in patients with obstructive lung diseases, especially in Japan. In one study the drug was administered orally at a dose of 300 mg/day for 4 weeks to adult patients with CS, and 20 paired nasal mucus samples were collected both before and 4 weeks after administration. Significant reductions in both G' and η' of nasal mucus were observed after CEE administration (Fig. 6) (40). However, the post-treatment viscoelastic value was still higher than the optimal value for mucociliary clearance (40). It is known that orally and intravenously administered CEE dem-

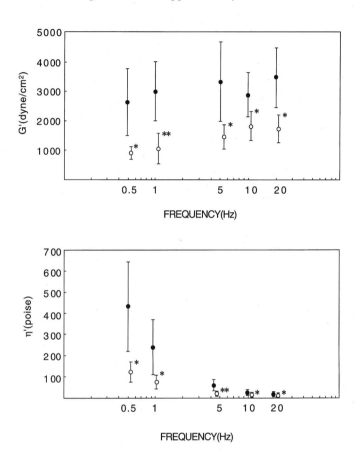

Figure 6 Effects of L-cysteine ethyl ester hydrochloride (CEE) on (top) elastic modulus (G′) and (bottom) dynamic viscosity (η′) of nasal mucus in chronic sinusitis. Oral administration of CEE significantly reduced both G′ and η′ at all frequencies examined (38). CEE was administered at a dose of 300 mg/day for 4 weeks. Closed circle indicates before and open circle indicates after drug administration. $*p < 0.05$; $**p < 0.01$. (From Ref. 40.)

onstrated similar biotransformation to NAC (41). Because NAC is first metabolized to cysteine (42) and increases tissue sulfhydryl groups (43), in vivo administration of CEE may change the conformation of a protein substance or cleave the covalent bonds of nasal mucus, leading to a reduction in viscoelasticity.

B. Thiols with a Blocked Sulfhydryl Group

Some thiol drugs without a free sulfhydryl group do not break mucin disulfide bonds, but may act via alternative mechanisms (39).

S-Carboxymethylcysteine (SCMC or carbocysteine) is an oral mucokinetic agent commonly used as an expectorant. Its sulfur is blocked by a carboxymethyl group. Thus, in vitro administration of SCMC did not change the viscoelasticity of respiratory mucus (44). Conflicting results have been reported as to its effect on mucus in the human lower respiratory tract. It is said to reduce the apparent viscosity of sputum in patients with chronic obstructive lung diseases (45), but another report showed no significant change in the viscoelasticity of sputum after SCMC administration (46). When SCMC was administered to CS patients at a dose of 1500 mg/day for 4 weeks, the drug did not change either the viscosity or the elasticity of nasal mucus (40). On the other hand, the reduced nasal mucociliary clearance of CS patients was significantly improved by the oral administration of SCMC during 4 weeks of treatment (30). However, no demonstrable effect of SCMC on lung mucociliary clearance has been reported in chronic bronchitis (47,48). The different effects of SCMC on mucociliary clearance of the upper and lower respiratory tracts may be due, in part, to different methodologies employed (e.g., different administration periods).

Although there are several reported trials of SCMC in OME (49–51), there is a lack of agreement on its beneficial effects. In our clinical and rheological studies of pediatric OME, 21 patients received SCMC at a daily dosage of 30 mg/kg, and another 21 patients were administered Kampo medicine, a Japanese traditional herbal medicine, for 4 weeks following myringotomy (51). At the end of the 4-week treatment period, 47% of the ears of the SCMC group and 41% in the Kampo group were regarded as being free from MEE, and this difference was not significant. For rheologically thick MEE, where pretreatment η' and G' values were much greater than the optimal values, the posttreatment value of η' for the SCMC group decreased significantly, but the value of G' did not, in comparison with pretreatment values. No such change in either η' or G' was observed in the Kampo group. The results suggest that combined therapy for myringotomy and oral SCMC is effective in improving the rheological properties of thick MEE in children.

C. Proteolytic Enzymes

Recombinant Human Deoxyribonuclease

In vitro administration of recombinant human deoxyribonuclease (rhNDase) has been demonstrated to reduce viscosity and to improve the transport capacity of purulent lower respiratory mucus in cystic fibrosis (52). Extensive clinical data have established the efficacy and safety of nebulized rhDNase, and it has become widely incorporated into standard therapy for cystic fibrosis (53). The beneficial in vitro effect of rhDNase on rheological and transport properties was reported in purulent sputum of chronic bronchitis (54). However, the administration of rhDNase by nebulizer did not change the sputum transportability in patients with bronchiectasis (55). rhDNase is an enzyme with a specific action on

DNA; a recent report suggests that the mucolytic effect of DNase might be due to actin disaggregation rather than DNA hydrosis (56). Both DNA and actin are mainly released from host neutrophils (57,56), and the number of neutrophils was tremendously increased in mucopurulent nasal mucus of CS (44992 ± 9792 cells/mm^3) compared with mucoid CS mucus (5791 ± 969) and normal nasal mucus (388 ± 199) (58). Thus, nasal administration of this drug seems to be useful for the treatment of mucopurulent nasal mucus. However, the efficacy of rhDNase in CS has never been investigated.

Other Proteolytic Enzymes

Topical Administration

Trypsin, chymotrypsin, streptodornase, and streptokinase are digestive proteolytic enzymes that break down mucus glycoproteins and other proteins. There is no definite evidence that enzymes attack living tissue (35). Proteolytic enzymes have been advocated as a useful adjunct to myringotomy in the management of glue ear, chymotrypsin being the one most frequently used (59).

Oral Administration

Orally administered proteolytic enzyme may break down complex protein substances at a pathological site. A proteolytic enzyme derived from strain E_{15} of the genus *Serratia*, serratiopeptidase (SER), was given orally at a dose of 30 mg/day for 4 weeks to CS patients. SER administration reduced η' but not G', leading to a reduction in the η/G value (40,60). It was reported that the ratio of viscosity to elasticity (η/G) is an important determinant of mucociliary transport (61,62). Since an inverse correlation between the η/G value and the mucociliary transport rate has been reported (62), the was posited that nasal mucus could be transported more effectively by cilia after SER administration. This speculation is in fair agreement with the study reported by Braga et al. (63). They administered SER at the same dose to patients with chronic bronchitis and compared the mucociliary transportability of sputum on mucus-depleted frog palate before and after the administration. Seven days of treatment with SER significantly increased mucociliary transportability. SER was absorbed from intestinal mucosa into the blood stream, and its absorbed form was enzymatically active (64). Under pathological conditions, orally administered SER may be excreted in the nasal or tracheobronchial mucus in a active form and may break down mucus structures with its proteolytic action.

D. Antibiotics

Norfloxacin

Antimicrobial drugs are used in upper respiratory medicine to prevent infection from developing as well as to treat established disease. Norfloxacin (NFLX) is a pyridone carboxylic acid derivative effective against common pathogens observed in the nasal and sinus mucus of CS patients. It has been reported that antibiotic therapy decreases the inflammatory process and the permeability of the epithelium to serum proteins, leading to a decrease in the amount of DNA and a fall in the production and exudation of serum and local proteins (65). Oral administration of NFLX to adult CS patients at a dose of 600 mg/day for 2 weeks significantly reduced the elasticity but not the viscosity of nasal mucus (40). This significant reduction in the elasticity might be due to the reduction in DNA and in serum-derived and locally produced proteins.

Macrolide Antibiotics

There is increasing evidence that long-term oral administration of the 14-membered macrolide antibiotic erythromycin (EM) is effective in the treatment of chronic lower respiratory infections, probably through actions other than its antimicrobial properties (66). In the upper respiratory tract, however, conflicting results have been reported. Moriyama et al. (67) reported long-term administration of low-dose EM after endoscopic sinus surgery in chronic pansinusitis with nasal polyposis. Better improvement was achieved in subjective symptoms and objective findings in the EM-treated group than the non–EM-treated group. Iino et al. administered EM at a dose of 600 mg/day for more than 4 months to patients with sinobronchial syndrome with OME and found EM therapy to be effective in the treatment of such patients (68). Husfeldt et al. administered ofloxacin or EM to patients with acute or chronic sinusitis for 7–14 days. EM was not superior to ofloxacin as to clinical efficacy (69). Moller and Dingsor reported that EM did not increase the frequency of air-filled middle ear after one month's administration in children with OME (70). The effects of EM on upper respiratory diseases must be clarified in further clinical studies.

Although the mechanism of the efficacy of macrolide antibiotics is still uncertain, several hypotheses have been advanced, such as immunomodulatory action on inflammatory cells (71,72), inhibition of glycoconjugate secretion from cultured human respiratory epithelial cells (73), and inhibition of airway epithelial chloride transport and the concomitant secretion of water across the airway mucosa toward the luminal surface (74). In patients with chronic obstructive lung diseases (COLD), Tamaoki et al. reported that clarithromycin (CAM), a newly developed 14-member macrolide, decreased sputum production and increased both solid composition and G′, but did not change η′ of sputum (75). They suggested that CAM may reduce both mucus and water secretion in the lower respiratory airway. When CAM was administered to CS patients at a dose of 500 mg/day for 4 weeks, CAM increased both spinability and solid composition and decreased η/G of nasal mucus (76). In patients with acute purulent rhinitis, 2 weeks of CAM treatment decreased the volume of nasal secretion and increased mucociliary transportability of nasal mucus (77). A positive correlation between the spinability and mucociliary transportability in sputum of COLD has been reported (78). Moreover, a decrease in η/G may result in an increase in mucociliary transport (62). The results obtained from upper and lower respiratory tracts suggest that CAM administration may reduce hypersecreted respiratory mucus and could improve mucociliary clearance of respiratory tracts. Since EM inhibits activation of NF-κB and activator protein-1 (AP-1) (79), 14-member macrolide antibiotics may regulate MG production by the inhibitory effects of mRNA expression of MGs and/or proinflammatory cytokines.

E. Corticosteroids

Corticosteroids reduce mucus secretion in vivo (80) and in vitro (81). The proposed mechanism for this mucus-suppressive effect is thought to be the generation of the phospholipase inhibitor lipocortin, which inhibited arachinoic acid release and eicosanoid formation (80,81). Glucocorticoids induce the transcription of IκBα synthesis, resulting in the inactivation of NF-κB (82). Since the transcription of certain mucin genes, such as MUC2 and MUC5AC, is activated by the activation of NF-κB (83), glucocorticoids may suppress MG production via inactivation of NF-κB. However, the effect of systemic or topical glucocorticoids on nasal mucus production has never been fully elucidated in CS.

Corticosteroids are the most potent medications available for the treatment of allergic rhinitis. The effect of corticosteroids on nasal symptoms is largely due to reduced synthesis of Th2-type cytokines and is probably secondary to this action (84). Topical corticosteroids remarkably reduce watery nasal secretions in the patients with allergic rhinitis.

F. Bromhexine, Ambroxol

Bromhexine is derived from vascine, an alkaloid derived from *Adhatoda vasica nees*. A number of investigators have found that oral bromhexine results in an increase in expectoration of sputum in chronic bronchitis (35). A double-blind trial of the drug in OME showed that it was ineffective in reinstating ventilation and did not influence clearance of the effusion (85).

Ambroxol is related to bromhexine and appears to stimulate mucus secretion, yet promotes a normalization of mucus viscosity in viscid secretions (39). However, oral administration of ambroxol at a dose of 45 mg/day for 4 weeks did not alter either viscoelasticity of nasal mucus or reduced nasal mucociliary clearance (Y. Majima, unpublished data).

G. Saline Solution

Normal saline (0.9% sodium chloride) is known as an isotonic or physiological saline solution. It is the most siutable salt solution for routine nebulization therapy (35). Normal saline nebulization (0.7 mL normal saline for 2 min) significantly improved nasal mucociliary clearance in patients with CS, but did not alter clearance in normal subjects (86). The improvement of clearance in CS might be due to hydration of nasal mucus and/or an increase in depth of the periciliary fluid layer (35).

V. Conclusions

The hypersecretion of chronic upper airway diseases originates mainly from hypertrophied and hyperfunctioning secretory cells, including gland and goblet cells. The resulting respiratory mucus, such as nasal mucus and MEE, is not rheologically normal. Such abnormal mucus may contribute to the reduced nasal or tubotympanal mucociliary clearance and may delay recovery from the disease. The effects of mucoactive drugs on the rheological and transport properties of upper airway mucus are similar to those of lower respiratory mucus, especially in CS. Scientific study of the rheological and transport properties of mucus in health and disease has given us improved tools to use in various treatments. Such studies will also help us understand the mechanisms of upper airway diseases, develop and assess new therapeutic agents, and identify the patients most likely to benefit from mucoactive therapy.

References

1. Tos M. Goblet cells and glands in the nose and paranasal sinuses. In: Proctor DF, Andersen I, eds. The Nose: Upper Airway Physiology and the Atmospheric Environment. Amsterdam: Elsevier Biomedical Press, 1982:99–144.
2. Lucas A, Douglas LC. Principles underlying ciliary activity in the respiratory tract. Arch Otolaryngol 1934; 20:518–541.
3. Majima Y, Sakakura Y, Matsubara T, Miyoshi Y. Possible mechanisms of reduction of nasal mucociliary clearance in chronic sinusitis. Clin Otolaryngol 1986; 11: 55–60.
4. Proctor DF. The mucociliary system. In: Proctor DF, Andersen I, eds. The Nose: Upper Airway Physiology and the Atmospheric Environment. Amsterdam: Elsevier Biomedical Press, 1982:245–278.
5. Messerklinger W. Über die Drainage der menschlichen Nasennebenholen unter normalen und pathologischen Bedingungen. 1. Mitteilung. Mschr Ohrenheilk Lar Rhinol 1966; 100:56–68.
6. Shimada T, Lim DJ. Distribution of ciliated cells in the human middle ear: electron and light microscopic observations. Ann Otol 1972; 81:203–211.
7. Tos M. Quantitative histology and histopathology of the mucosa of the middle ear and eustachian tube. In: Sadé J, ed. Secretory Otitis Media and Its Sequelae. New York: Churchill-Livingstone, 1979:56–88.

8. Sadé J. Ciliary activity and middle ear clearance. Arch Otolaryngol 1967; 86:128–135.
9. Takeuchi K, Majima Y, Hirata K, Hattori M, Sakakura Y. Quantitation of tubotympanal mucociliary clearance in otitis media with effusion. Ann Otol Rhinol Laryngol 1990; 99:211–214.
10. Slavin RG. Sinusitis in adults and its relation to allergic rhinitis, asthma, and nasal polyps. J Allergy Clin Immunol 1988; 82:950–956.
11. Data Book for Patients' Population in Japan by the Reports from Statistics and Information Department of Japan Ministry of Health and Welfare. Tokyo: Koseitokeikyokai, 1996.
12. Lund VJ, Kennedy DW, the Staging and Therapy Group. Quantification for staging sinusitis. Ann Otol Rhinol Laryngol 1995; 167(suppl):17–21.
13. Guo Y, Majima Y, Hattori M, Seki S, Sakakura Y. Effects of functional endoscopic sinus surgery on maxillary sinus mucosa. Arch Otolaryngol Head Neck Surg 1977; 123:1097–1100.
14. Halma AR, Decreton S, Bijloos JM, Clement PAR. Density of epithelial cells in the normal human nose and the paranasal sinus mucosa: a scanning electron microscopic study. Rhinology 1990; 28:25–32.
15. Saida S. Ciliary activity of nasal and maxillary epithelia in man. Mie Med J 1986; 36:9–18.
16. Tos M, Mogensen C. Mucus production in chronic maxillary sinusitis. A quantitative histopathological study. Acta Otolaryngol (Stockh) 1984; 97:151–159.
17. Renttila MA, Rautiainen MEP, Koskinen MO, Turjanmaa V, Laranne JE, Pukander JS. Mucociliary clearance of maxillary sinuses in patients with recurrent or chronic sinusitis. Am J Rhinol 1994; 8:285–290.
18. Rutland J, Cole PJ. Nasal mucociliary clearance and ciliary beat frequency in cystic fibrosis compared with sinusitis and bronchitis. Thorax 1981; 36:654–658.
19. Majima Y, Masuda S, Sakakura Y. Quantitative study of nasal secretory cells in normal subjects and patients with chronic sinusitis. Laryngoscope 1997; 107:13–16.
20. Tos M, Bak-Pedersen K. Goblet cell population in the pathological middle ear and eustachian tube of children and adults. Ann Otol 1977; 86:209–218.
21. Bluestone CD, Beery QC, Andrus WS. Mechanics of the eustachian tube as it influences susceptibility to and persistence of middle ear effusions in children. Ann Otol Rhinol Laryngol 1974; 83(suppl 11):27–34.
22. Hirata K. Dynamic viscoelasticity of nasal mucus from children with chronic sinusitis. Mie Med J 1985; 34:205–219.
23. Majima Y, Sakakura Y, Matsuibara T, Hamaguchi Y, Hirata K, Takeuchi K, Hiyoshi Y. Rheological properties of middle ear effusions from children with otitis media with effusion. Ann Otol Rhinol Laryngol 1986; 95(suppl 124):1–4.
24. Rubin BK, Ramirez O, King M. Mucus-depleted frog palate as a model for study of mucociliary clearance. J Appl Physiol 1990; 62:424–429.
25. Shih CK, Litt M, Khan MA, Wolf DP. Effect of nondialyzable solids concentration and viscoelasticity on ciliary transport of tracheal mucus. Am Rev Respir Dis 1977; 115:989–995.

26. Hirata K, Majima Y, Takeuchi K, Sakakura Y. Viscoelastic measurement of normal mucus in the respiratory tract [abstract]. Biorheology 1986; 23:521.
27. Majima Y, Sakakura Y, Hattori M, Hirata K. Rheologic properties of nasal mucus from patients with chronic sinusitis. Am J Rhinol 1993; 7:217–221.
28. Majima Y, Sakakura Y. Nasal mucociliary clearance in chronic sinusitis and allergic rhinitis. In: Tos M, Thomsen J, Balle V, eds. Rhinology—A State of the Arts. Amsterdam: Kugler Publications, 1995:323–325.
29. Sakakura Y, Ukai K, Majima Y, Murai S, Harada T, Miyoshi Y. Nasal mucociliary clearance under various conditions. Acta Otolaryngol 1983; 96:167–173.
30. Sakakura Y, Majima Y, Saida S, Miyoshi Y. Reversibility of reduced mucociliary clearance in chronic sinusitis. Clin Otolaryngol 1985; 10:79–83.
31. Hattori M, Majima Y, Ukai K, Sakakura Y. Effects of nasal allergen challenge on dynamic viscoelasticity of nasal mucus. Ann Otol Rhinol Laryngol 1993; 102:314–317.
32. Takeuchi K, Majima Y, Hirata K, Morishita A, Hattori M, Sakakura Y. Prognosis of secretory otitis media in relation to viscoelasticity of effusions in children. Ann Otol Rhinol Laryngol 1989; 98:443–446.
33. Majima Y, Harada T, Shimizu T, Takeuchi K, Sakakura Y, Yasuoka S, Yoshinaga S. Effect of biochemical components on rheologic properties of nasal mucus in chronic sinusitis. Am J Respir Crit Care Med 1999; 160:421–426.
34. Carlstedt I, Sheehan JK. Macromolecular properties and polymeric structure of mucus glycoproteins. In: Ciba Foundation Symposium 109. Mucus and Mucosa. London: Pitman Press, 1984:157–172.
35. Ziment I. Respiratory Pharmacology and Therapeutics. Philadelphia: W. B. Saunders Company, 1978.
36. Rhee CS, Majima Y, Cho JS, Arima S, Min YG, Sakakura Y. Effects of mucokinetic drugs on rheological properties of reconstituted human nasal mucus. Arch Otolaryngol Head Neck Surg 1999; 125:101–105.
37. Lieberman J. The appropriate use of mucolytic agents. Am J Med 1970; 49:1–4.
38. Lawson D, Saggers BA. N.A.C. and antibiotics in cystic fibrosis. Br Med J 1965; 1:317.
39. Yuta A, Baraniuk JN. Therapeutic approaches to airway mucus hypersecretion. In: Rogers DF, Lethem MI, eds. Airway Mucus: Basic Mechanisms and Clinical Perspectives. Basel, Switzerland: Birkhauser Verlag, 1997:365–383.
40. Majima Y, Hirata K, Takeuchi K, Hattori M, Sakakura Y. Effects of orally administered drugs on dynamic viscoelasticity of human nasal mucus. Am Rev Respir Dis 1990; 141:79–83.
41. Servin AL, Goulinet S, Renault H. Pharmacokinetics of cysteine ethyl ester in rat. Xenobiotica 1988; 18:839–847.
42. Sheffner AL, Medler EM, Bailey KR, Gallo DG, Mueller AJ, Sarett HP. Metabolic studies with acetylcysteine. Biochem Pharmacol 1966; 15:1523–1535.
43. Lorber A, Chang CC, Matsuoka D, Meacham I. Effect of thiols in biological systems on protein sulfhydryl content. Biochem Pharmacol 1970; 19:1551–1560.
44. Martin R, Litt M, Marriott C. The effect of mucolytic agents on the rheological and transport properties of canine tracheal mucus. Am Rev Respir Dis 1980; 121:495–500.

45. Edwards G, Steel AE, Scott JK, Jordan JW. S-Carboxymethylcysteine in the fluidification of sputum and treatment of chronic airway obstruction. Chest 1976; 70: 506–513.

46. Cox AJ, Jabbal-Gill I, Marriott C, Davis SS. Effect of S-carboxymethylcysteine on the biophysical and biochemical properties of mucus in chronic bronchitis. Adv Exp Med Biol 1982; 144:423–429.

47. Thomson ML, Pavia D, Johnes CJ, McQuiston TAC. No demonstrable effect of S-carboxymethylcysteine on clearance of secretion from human lung. Thorax 30; 1975:669–673.

48. Goodman RM, Yergin BM, Sackner MA. Effect of S-carboxymethylcysteine on tracheal mucus velocity. Chest 1978; 74:615–618.

49. Ramsden RT, Moffat DA, Gibson WPR, Jay MM. S-Carboxymethylcysteine in the treatment of glue ear: a double blind trial. J Laryngol Otol 1977; 91:847–851.

50. Khan JA, Narcus P, Cummings SW. S-Carboxymethylsysteine in otitis media with effusion (a double-blind study). J Laryngol Otol 1981; 95:995–1001.

51. Majima Y, Takeuchi K, Sakakura Y. Effects of myringotomy and orally administered drugs on viscosity and elasticity of middle ear effusions from children with otitis media with effusion. Acta Otolaryngol Suppl 1990; 471(suppl):66–72.

52. Stern M, Alton EW. Therapeutic approaches to the lung problems in cystic fibrosis. In: Rogers DF, Lethem MI, eds. Airway Mucus: Basic Mechanisms and Clinical Perspectives. Basel, Switzerland: Birkhauser Verlag, 1997:342–364.

53. Zahm JM, Girod de Bentzmann S, Deneuville E, Perrot-Minnot C, Dabadie A, Pennaforte F, Roussey M, Shak S, Puchelle E. Dose-dependent in vitro effect of recombinant human DNase on the rheological and transport properties of cystic fibrosis respiratory mucus. Eur Respir J 1995; 8:381–386.

54. Puchelle E, Zahm JM, de Bentzmann S, Grosskopf C, Shak S, Mougel D, Polu JM. Effects of rhDNase on purulent airway secretions in chronic bronchitis. Eur Respir J 1996; 9:765–769.

55. Willis PJ, Wodehouse T, Corkery K, Mallon K, Wilson R, Cole PJ. Short-term recombinant human DNase in bronchiectasis. Effect on clinical state and in vitro sputum transportability. Am J Respir Crit Care Med 1996; 154:413–417.

56. Vasconcellos CA, Allen PG, Wohl ME, Drazen JM, Janmey PA, Stossel TP. Reduction in viscosity of cystic fibrosis sputum in vitro by gelsolin. Science 1994; 263:969–971.

57. Lethem MI, James SL, Marriott C, Burke JF. The origin of DNA associated with mucus glycoproteins in cystic fibrosis sputum. Eur Respir J 1990; 3:19–23.

58. Lee HS, Majima Y, Sakakura Y, Shinogi J, Kawaguchi S, Kim BW. Quantitative cytology of nasal secretions under various conditions. Laryngoscope 1993; 103: 533–537.

59. Litton WW, McCabe BF. Chymotrypsin: a useful adjunct to the management of glue ears. Laryngoscope 1972; 72:182–187.

60. Majima Y, Inagaki M, Hirata K, Takeuchi K, Morishita A, Sakakura Y. The effect of an orally administered proteolytic enzyme on the elasticity and viscosity of nasal mucus. Arch Otorhinolaryngol 1988; 244:355–359.

61. Ross SM, Corrsin S. Results of an analytical model of mucociliary pumping. J Appl Physiol 1974; 37:333–340.

62. King M, Engel LA, Macklem PT. Effect of pentobarbital anesthesia on rheology and transport of canine tracheal mucus. J Appl Physiol 1979; 46:504–509.
63. Braga PC, Bossi R, Allegra L. Effects of serratio-peptidase on muco-ciliary clearance in patients with chronic bronchitis. Curr Ther Res 1981; 29:738–744.
64. Miyata K. Hirai S, Yashiki T, Tomoda K. Intestinal absorption of *Serratia* protease. J Appl Biochem 1980; 2:111–116.
65. Brown DT, Potsic WP, Marsh RR, Litt M. Drugs affecting clearance of middle ear secretions: a perspective for the management of otitis media with effusion. Ann Otol Rhinol Laryngol 1985; 94(suppl 117):3–15.
66. Kadota J, Sakito O, Kohno S, Sawa H, Mukae H, Oda H, Kawakami K, Fukushima K, Furushima K, Hiratani K, Hara K. A mechanism of erythromycin treatment in patients with diffuse panbronchitis. Am Rev Respir Dis 1993; 147:153–159.
67. Moriyama H, Yanagi K, Ohtori N, Fukami M. Evaluation of endoscopic sinus surgery for chronic sinusitis: post-operative erythromycin therapy. Rhinology 1995; 33:166–170.
68. Iino Y, Sugita K. Toriyama M, Kudo K. Erythromycin therapy for otitis media with effusion in sinobronchial syndrome. Arch Otolaryngol Head Neck Surg 1993; 119:648–651.
69. Husfeldt P, Egede F, Nielsen PB. Antibiotic treatment of sinusitis in general practice. A double-blind study comparing ofloxacin and erythromycin. Eur Arch Oto-rhinolaryngol 1993; 250(suppl 1):S23-S25.
70. Moller P, Dingsor G. Otitis media with effusion: can erythromycin reduce the need for ventilating tube? J Laryngol Otol 1990; 104:200–202.
71. Roche Y, Gougerot-Pocidalo MA, Fay N, Pocidalo JJ. Maclorides and immunity: effects of erythromycin and spiramycin on human mononuclear cell proliferation. J Antimicrob Chemother 1986; 17:195–203.
72. Anderson R. Erythromycin and roxithromycin potentiate human neutrophil locomotion in vitro by inhibition of leukoattractant-activated superoxide generation and auto-oxidation. J Infect Dis 1989; 159:966–973.
73. Goswami SK, Kivity S, Marom Z. Erythromycin inhibits respiratory glycoconjugate secretion from human airways in vitro. Am Rev Respir Dis 1990; 141:72–78.
74. Tamaoki J, Isono K, Sakai N, Kanemura T, Konno K. Erythromycin inhibits Cl secretion across canine tracheal epithelial cells. Eur Respir J 1992; 5:234–238.
75. Tamaoki J, Takeyama K, Tagaya E, Konno K. Effect of clarithromycin on sputum production and its rheological properties in chronic respiratory tract infections. Antimicrob Agents Chemother 1995; 39:1688–1690.
76. Rhee CS, Majima Y, Arima S, Jung HW, Jinn TH, Min YG, Sakakura Y. Effects of clarithromycin on rheological properties of nasal mucus in patients with chronic sinusitis. Ann Otol Rhinol Laryngol 200; 109:484–487.
77. Rubin BK, Druce H, Ramirez OE, Palmer R. Effect of clarithromycin on nasal mucus properties in healthy subjects and in patients with purulent rhinitis. Am J Respir Crit Care Med 1997; 155:2018–2023.
78. Puchelle E, Zahm JM, Duvivier C. Spinability of bronchial mucus. Relationship with viscoelasticity and mucous transport properties. Biorheology 1983; 20:239–249.

79. Desaki M, Takizawa H, Ohtoshi T, Kasama T, Kobayashi K, Sunazuka T, Omura S, Yamamoto K. Erythromycin suppresses nuclear factor-κB and activator protein-1 activation in human bronchial epithelial cells. Biochem Biophys Res Commun 2000; 267:124–128.

80. Takahashi Y, Shimizu T, Sakakura Y. Effects of indomethacin, dexamethasone, and erythromycin on endotoxin-induced intraepithelial mucus production of rat nasal epithelium. Ann Otol Rhinol Laryngol 1997; 106:683–687.

81. Lundgren JD, Hirata F, Marom Z, Logun C, Steel L, Kaliner M, Shelhamer J. Dexamethasone inhibits respiratory glycoconjugate secretion from feline airways in vitro by the reduction of lipocortin (lipomodulin) synthesis. Am Rev Respir Dis 1988; 137:353–357.

82. Scheinman RI, Cogswell PC, Lofquist AK, Baldwin AS. Role of transcriptional activation of IκBα in mediation of immunosuppression by glucocorticoids. Science 1995; 270:283–290.

83. Li D, Gallup M, Fan N, Szymkowski DE, Basbaum CB. Cloning of the amino-terminal and 5'-flanking region of the human MUC5AC mucin gene and transcriptional up-regulation by bacterial exoproducts. J Biol Chem 1998; 273:6812–6820.

84. Mygind N, Dahl R, Pedersen S, Thestrup-Pedersen K. Essential Allergy. 2nd ed. Oxford, UK: Blackwell Science, 1996.

85. Elcock HW, Lord IJ. Bromhexine hydrochloride in chronic secretory otitis media—a clinical trial. Br J Clin Pract 1972; 26:276–278.

86. Majima Y, Sakakura Y, Matsubara T, Murai S, Miyoshi Y. Mucociliary clearance in chronic sinusitis: related human nasal clearance and in vitro bullfrog palate clearance. Biorheology 1983; 20:251–262.

87. Majima Y, Sakakura Y. Rheological aspects of mucociliary clearance. In: Passali D, ed. Rhinology Up-to-Date. Rome: Industria Grafica Romana, 1994:127–137.

15

Issues on Regulatory Approval of Mucoactive Drugs

DONALD J. KELLERMAN

Inspire Pharmaceuticals
Durham, North Carolina, U.S.A.

**RICHARD J. MORISHIGE and
BABATUNDE A. OTULANA**

Aradigm Corporation
Hayward, California, U.S.A.

I. Introduction

In recent years, regulatory authorities appear to have paid more attention to precise delineation of the clinical indication for which a drug is approved. This trend toward narrowing disease indication for medications parallels the improvement in the understanding of disease etiology and pathophysiology as well as the mechanism of action of drugs. Prior to this, a number of drugs were approved worldwide for indications that were poorly defined, and with minimal delineation of the specific disease conditions for which they were indicated.

Many mucoactive drugs currently on the market fall in this category. They have been used in medical practice under such labels as "antitussive," "cough suppressant," "mucolytic," and so on (1,2). By implication, these medications are deemed approved for the treatment of cough in any disease in which cough is a symptom. In some respects, such claims put these drugs in a category similar to that of analgesics, which can be used to treat pain associated with any disease (3,4). However, unlike analgesics that tend to be indicated for a specified category of pain (e.g., "acute" or "chronic," "mild," or "severe"), the majority of mucoactive agents currently on the market do not carry indications for any specific type of cough or mucus-related condition.

The European and American regulatory authorities have not recently published any guidelines on how new mucoactive drugs should be studied or any changes in the way they are approved or labeled. Based on the clinical and drug development issues surrounding these products, many of which are discussed elsewhere in this book, the regulatory issues of importance for development of new therapies in this field appear to include the following:

> Specific diseases or conditions to be studied in order to establish the effectiveness of the drug
> Precise statements of indication and/or expected benefits for use of the drugs
> Clearer definition of the classes of drugs to be grouped under the term "mucoactive agents"
> Clinical endpoints by which to demonstrate efficacy and safety during development

Opinions on these issues as they relate to various mucoactive drugs individually and as a group have been expressed in many publications (5–7), including other chapters in this book. This chapter reviews the options available to drug developers and to regulatory agencies on each of the issues. Although regulatory authorities have not yet published specific guidelines on mucoactive agents, there are general strategies on clinical development of drugs that provide insights into the requirements for approval of these agents. In addition, we have attempted to incorporate our understanding of regulatory requirements in the general field of pulmonary drug development.

II. Classification of Products and Labeling Indication

The taxonomy for mucoactive agents is fully discussed in Chapter 6. From the regulatory perspective, clear and concise classification of these drugs is important as it helps define many of the parameters for clinical development of the drug, such as choice of comparators, selection of clinically relevant endpoints, and the positioning of the medication in the therapeutic armamentarium for the treatment of specific diseases.

Ideally, drug classes should be defined such that the mechanism of action for their intended use is clear. Currently, a number of products grouped together under the term "mucoactive agents" have very different therapeutic uses and modes of action. More work is required by the scientific community and the regulatory authorities to improve the categorization of these products along logical groupings.

Improvement in classification should also benefit the indication statement in the product labeling. Typically, the indication statement in the package insert of a drug product is a reflection of the specific diseases or conditions for which the drug was studied during clinical development. In the past, many approved drugs were granted generous indication statements such as "for the treatment of cough," as stated in some over-the-counter medications.

In recent years, regulatory authorities appear to be moving toward changing this trend and are requiring manufacturers of prescription mucoactive drugs to study and label them for specific types of cough and even perhaps cough associated with a disease. Thus, rhDNase (Pulmozyme®, Genentech), for which original studies were conducted in cystic fibrosis, has a package insert indicating its use "in the management of cystic fibrosis patients to improve pulmonary function." Given the trend in other therapeutic areas, manufacturers can expect that regulatory authorities will require drugs to carry label claims specific for the disease for which the drug was studied. Whether this will have an effect on off-label use of the existing products, especially the over-the-counter medications often used to treat cough of any origin, remains to be seen.

III. Specific Diseases to Study

With products used to treat symptoms or a general pathological process rather than specific diseases, many developers face a challenge in selecting the population to study. For example, a product being developed as a mucolytic may find utility in chronic bronchitis, upper respiratory tract disease, or cystic fibrosis.

From a regulatory perspective, it is important to carefully define the target patient population to be studied in clinical trials. This is particularly critical for "pivotal" clinical trials, which provide the definitive evidence of efficacy and safety on which the decisions for approval are based. In general, there are at least four large categories of patients who are obvious candidates for mucoactive agents:

1. Patients with chronic bronchitis, particularly those with a primary complaint of lung congestion
2. Patients with cystic fibrosis
3. Patients with common cold
4. Patients with allergic rhinitis

In each of these conditions, impairment of mucociliary clearance has been demonstrated (8–11) and likely contributes in varying degrees to the symptoms experienced. The characteristics of each of these populations that should be included in pivotal trials are discussed below.

A. Chronic Bronchitis

Patients with chronic bronchitis as a consequence of long-term cigarette smoking have difficulty clearing excess mucus resulting from mucus hypersecretion and impaired ciliary function. Clearly, a drug that helps these patients "clear their lungs" would be expected to provide discernible benefits to these individuals who have symptoms and impaired function because of their retained mucus. Defining this patient population, particularly those with sufficient symptoms such that they are likely to benefit from mucoactive agents in a clinical trial, is critical if one wishes to definitively demonstrate clinical efficacy. These patients may be thought of as a subset of COPD patients who have symptoms that are largely related to retained mucus.

Based on our understanding of regulatory requirements for drugs developed in the past in this therapeutic area, important inclusion criteria to consider for this group of chronic bronchitis patients should include the following:

> Age greater than 40 years
> Significant history of tobacco cigarette smoking (at least 10 pack-years)
> Diagnosis of COPD as defined by established national or international scientific criteria (e.g., American Thoracic Society, European Respiratory Society)
> History of productive cough for at least 1 year prior to study entry
> FEV_1/FVC ratio less than 0.7
> FEV_1 <70% of predicted; lower limit between 30 and 40%
> Oxyhemoglobin saturation >92% on room air
> Symptoms characteristic of chronic bronchitis, particularly cough and "chest congestion"
> History of exacerbations of COPD requiring medical intervention
> Concomitant illnesses and medications that will not interfere with the therapy being evaluated or put the patient at imminent risk of dying

These general inclusion criteria have been used in most trials of mucoactive therapies (12). Since smoking status can affect the outcome, stratification at randomization based on current smoking status is often performed (13). The level of pulmonary function impairment chosen will correlate somewhat with the symptoms reported; patients with near-normal lung function may not be symptomatic enough to show improvement on a symptom questionnaire.The choice of inclusion criteria is driven in part by the efficacy endpoint selected; impairment severe enough that improvement can be clearly demonstrated is necessary (to avoid the "ceiling effect"). The various endpoints used for evaluating mucoactive agents are discussed in Section IV.

B. Cystic Fibrosis

The pulmonary complications of cystic fibrosis are chronic and devastating. Premature death in individuals with cystic fibrosis is usually from respiratory causes (14). Treatment with recombinant rhDNase, which appears to have definite effects on respiratory mucus composition, has been shown to slow decline in lung function (15) and reduce pulmonary exacerbation rates (16) in patients with cystic fibrosis, which were the basis of the approval for recombinant human deoxyribonuclease (rhDNase, Pulmozyme®). Patients having the diagnosis of cystic fibrosis have a spectrum of disease severity, from normal lung function and relatively asymptomatic to pulmonary and functional impairment similar to that of patients with advanced chronic bronchitis.

General inclusion criteria for patients in pivotal trials in cystic fibrosis have included the following:

Age greater than 5 years
Genetic mutations consistent with cystic fibrosis or sweat sodium or chloride value of 60 meq/L or greater
FEV_1 between 40 and 90% of predicted normal for age, height, and gender
Symptoms related to pulmonary congestion
Be clinically stable at the time of study entry
An oxyhemoglobin saturation of 90% or greater
Be on stable doses of rhDNase, inhaled tobramycin, or other antibiotics

Patients included in cystic fibrosis clinical trials of new therapies (i.e., those not already approved or tested in older patients) should be old enough to reliably perform the forced vital capacity maneuver. The range of acceptable pulmonary impairment is debatable, but, as in chronic bronchitis, there is likely a relationship between pulmonary function and symptoms of chest congestion, such that patients with normal lung function are unlikely to perceive benefit from mucoactive agents. If exacerbations are an endpoint of the study, it is important that patients be stable at the time of study entry so that the time to exacerbation may be measured. A difficult issue in cystic fibrosis is avoiding confounding by concomitant medications, as these patients are often taking several medications that can make assessing the effects of mucoactive agents difficult. Unfortunately, from a clinical trial design standpoint, several of these therapies have become fairly standard treatment for cystic fibrosis patients to the point that stopping these agents before and/or during the trial period may not be feasible.

C. Allergic Rhinitis

There are well-established guidelines for patient selection for allergic rhinitis trials (FDA Draft Guidance Document on Allergic Rhinitis—http://www.fda.gov/cder/guidance/2718dft.htm). Studies of mucoactive function have generally enrolled patients meeting the standard criteria in this guidance document. Since trials published on the use of mucoactive agents for the treatment of allergic rhinitis are limited, little is known about targeting a specific population of patients who would be likely to respond to mucoactive therapies. A major decision is whether to select patients with seasonal or perennial allergic rhinitis. Although there is considerable overlap in the symptom complex of these two groups, congestion may be a more prominent feature of perennial allergic rhinitis and that may make it the preferable therapeutic target. Saccharin transport time may be a useful measure for assessing the effect of a mucoactive compound (17), but there are few data on what an appropriate baseline value should be in patients with allergic rhinitis, nor are there data that link findings on this test to clinical benefit. As with other airway diseases and even more importantly in allergic rhinitis, symptoms must be present to a sufficient degree at baseline to allow significant improvement after commencing treatment with the study drug.

D. Common Cold

Common cold—or, more precisely, viral infections of the upper airways—results in impairment of mucociliary clearance (10,18). Some studies of products such as guaifenesin have been performed (19). In recent years, products for treating symptoms and infections have been evaluated. Since colds are short-lived and almost always self-limiting, it is important that patients be enrolled soon after onset of the illness. An understanding of the usual pattern of the main symptoms of common cold—sore throat, nasal congestion, rhinorrhea, cough, and malaise—can also help ensure that patients enrolled in clinical trials have the symptoms of interest when they receive active medication.

Typical inclusion criteria for studies of patients with common cold include the following:

Age of at least 12 years
A self-reported diagnosis of "cold"
Symptom onset less than 36 hours prior to study entry
Symptoms of interest of at least moderate severity at the time of study entry
A temperature of less than 101.5 degrees Fahrenheit
Have not taken medications for treatment of common cold in the last 12 hours

Since patient-performed symptom scores are generally the primary efficacy assessment, new therapies should be first performed in patients old enough to complete diary cards and perceive when they are suffering from a common cold. Ascertaining the onset of symptoms is important, as symptoms may resolve spontaneously fairly quickly. Missing the period when patients are most symptomatic can greatly reduce the chances of observing a treatment effect. To avoid including patients with influenza or other more serious respiratory disorders, the oral temperature can help in discriminating patients likely to be suffering from more serious infections. Since patients often self-medicate to treat common cold symptoms, it is important to eliminate the use of non-study medications during the trial.Additionally, as only one pretreatment assessment is usually recorded, medications taken immediately prior to study enrollment are also potentially confounding.

E. Other Mucoactive Agents

In addition to the medications used in the diseases discussed above, a number of drugs are discussed in various chapters of this book as agents that have some mucoactive effects. In many cases, because these medications are used as adjuncts in the treatment of a variety of diseases, the regulatory requirements for their development as a mucoactive agent may not be as clearly defined as those discussed in this chapter. These drugs include antibiotics used in the treatment of airway infections, experimental gene therapy treatment (e.g., CFTR gene for cystic fibrosis), and indomethacin used experimentally for reducing mucus hypersecretion in patients with diffuse panbronchiolitis (21)

In some cases (e.g., antibiotics for treatment of airway infections), the drug is already approved for use in that condition, and its mucoactive properties are a side benefit rather than the main indication for use. In other cases, a drug such as indomethacin is approved for an entirely different indication and is used off-label and experimentally to treat chronic bronchitis.It is unlikely that these and other drugs with mucoactive side benefits would seek regulatory license as a mucoactive agent, although experimental use of even approved medications may necessitate the institution of an Investigational New Drug application in the United States.

IV. Endpoints and Comparator Selection

Many of the endpoints that could have utility for evaluating mucoactive therapies are discussed in Chapter 4 of this book, and many illustrative examples of how these endpoints have been used in clinical trials are included in other chapters. In this chapter, the discussion focuses on how these endpoints have been used as a basis for regulatory approvals or how they could potentially be used in the future to evaluate mucoactive therapies.

Along with selection of endpoints, manufacturers also have to select comparator drugs or placebo to include in their clinical trials in order to demonstrate efficacy, safety, and/or comparability to existing therapies. The selection of the appropriate comparator agent is often a difficult decision. To date, most trials have used a placebo for comparison, which seems appropriate since mucoactive agents are not generally considered standard of care for any of the diseases discussed above and therefore withholding the mucoactive agent does not raise any ethical concerns. For oral agents, use of a placebo is somewhat easier, as formulating a product that matches the trial agent is relatively simple. For inhalation studies, this may be more challenging.

In general, the most appropriate comparator for a study in which the study drug is inhaled via a nebulizer or sprayed into the nose is 0.9% saline. There will likely be some therapeutic effect from the saline/placebo, particularly with nasal administration. However, because of the subjective nature of many of the endpoints that might be used to assess these agents, the requirement of performing a blinded study should be preserved. Ideally, the comparator should be identical in appearance to the study drug (a problem for studies of agents like surfactant) and be free of preservatives or other substances that can affect mucociliary function unless the study drug contains preservatives.

A. Spirometry

Pulmonary function tests are used in the diagnosis and assessment of most diseases of the lower respiratory tract. Improvements in lung function, particularly the forced expiratory volume in one second (FEV_1), have also been the basis for approval for most drugs indicated for the treatment of asthma and COPD. Whether pulmonary function tests should have a central role in the assessment of mucoactive therapies has been debated (13). Theoretically, mucoactive drugs should improve lung function by aiding the clearance of excess sputum from distal airways, thus allowing increased airflow. The magnitude of this potential improvement is difficult to estimate from the literature.

Measurement of improvements in spirometry was used successfully in the rhDNase program. In a 12-week study of patients with advanced cystic fibrosis, an improvement of 9.4% in FEV_1 and 12.4% in FVC was observed in the subjects who received rhDNase compared with 2.1% and 7.3%, respectively, for the placebo group (22). In two large 6-month trials of 968 patients with less severe impairment of lung function (15), a smaller increase in FEV_1 of slightly greater than 5% was observed as compared with virtually no improvement in the placebo group (Figure 1). Whether changes of this magnitude are sufficient in and of themselves to be considered primary evidence of efficacy is debatable. Nonetheless, significant improvement over placebo on a well-accepted endpoint like FEV_1 is very compelling evidence of the effectiveness of a mucoactive compound, and these data were considered important evidence of the effectiveness of rhDNase by the FDA Medical Reviewer [Pulmozyme® Summary Basis of Approval (16)]. These data were corroborated by improvements in several other endpoints in the Phase 3 trials that thus provided support to the small changes observed in FEV_1.

Other trials of mucoactive agents have shown modest but statistically significant improvements in spirometry in the subjects who received mucoactive compounds. A 2-week trial in aerosolized surfactant therapy of patients with

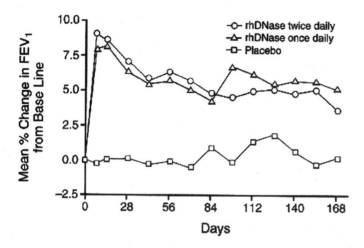

Figure 1 Improvement in FEV_1 in cystic fibrosis patients who received nebulized rhD-Nase once or twice daily over a 24-week period compared with placebo. (From Ref. 15.)

chronic bronchitis reported by Anzueto et al. (23) showed improvements greater than placebo after 2 weeks of treatment. However, other trials have not shown an effect of mucoactive therapies on pulmonary function. Although it would be desirable to have a positive effect on lung function, the absence of benefit on FEV_1 relative to placebo following initiation of mucoactive therapy should not be a reason for nonapproval of a mucoactive compound, since there are other clinical benefits that may occur regardless of any positive effect on lung function. However, a persistently negative effect on lung function compared with placebo (even if not statistically significant) would argue against the approval of a mucoactive product.

Given that a short-term improvement in lung function may not be observed, another approach is to assess whether mucoactive drugs can slow the rate of decline in lung function known to occur in patients with chronic bronchitis or cystic fibrosis. A trial evaluating the rate of decline of lung function over time likely needs to be of sufficient duration to monitor the effects of preservation of lung function relative to placebo gradual effect—at least 6 months and possibly longer.

B. Pulmonary Exacerbations

Exacerbations of chronic bronchitis and cystic fibrosis are associated with significant morbidity and frequently result in hospitalizations and antibiotic therapy to treat the exacerbations. Because the clinical relevance of reducing exacerbations is easily appreciated, this endpoint is potentially quite appropriate as the primary efficacy parameter for trials of mucoactive agents. The rationale for mucoactive therapies improving patients' susceptibility to infections that trigger the exacerbation is also quite intuitive. The results of trials that employ this measure as an endpoint are often reported as the number of exacerbations per patient per month, although patients with no exacerbations have also been used as a categorical responder analysis (12).

If this endpoint is used, it is important that patients enrolled have a history of exacerbations at a sufficient frequency such that a significant percentage of the subjects can be expected to experience exacerbation during the trial. Using this endpoint also mandates that the trial be at least 3 months in duration, preferably 6 months or 1 year, to allow a long enough observation period. When trials are less than a year long, the seasonal nature of exacerbations must be taken into account and enrollment should be instituted accordingly. It is also critical that standardized criteria be established at the start of the study as to what constitutes an exacerbation. The criteria described by Anthoniesen et al. (24) are often used and provide a useful classification system. Exacerbations can also be categorized by patient outcome (e.g., in order of increased severity):

Call or unscheduled visit to the investigator
Outpatient visit
Visit to an emergency facility
Hospitalization
Admission to intensive care unit
Death

It may also be advisable to have an independent committee evaluate exacerbations without knowledge of the treatment code and decide on the appropriate classification of the exacerbation prior to unblinding the treatment codes.

To avoid confounding factors when exacerbations are used as an endpoint, it is important to ensure that factors that might influence susceptibility to infection are equal across the treatment groups. Therefore, factors such as vaccinations for influenza and pneumococcal pneumonia should be carefully considered. Likewise, chronic use of antibiotics (such as tobramycin for cystic fibrosis) should be avoided if possible, or equalized across the treatment groups. Seasonal increases in rhinovirus infection often coincide with increases in exacerbations, but in a randomized trial this increase should affect all treatment groups equally.

A reduction in the number of pulmonary infections requiring parenteral or any other antibiotics for patients with cystic fibrosis provided strong evidence of the efficacy of rhDNase (Figure 2). Exacerbation rates were higher in patients who were 17 to 23 years of age, so an adjustment in the analysis was performed based on age. The analysis demonstrated a significant reduction in exacerbation rates for the patients who received rhDNase, as compared with the patients who received placebo. These results, combined with the modest improvement

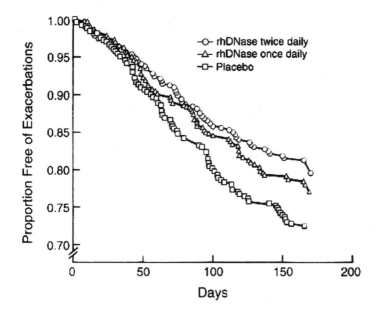

Figure 2 Improvement in the proportion of cystic fibrosis patients free of exacerbation of respiratory symptoms requiring parenteral antibiotic therapy following treatment with nebulized rhDNase once or twice daily over a 24-week period. (From Ref. 15.)

in pulmonary function mentioned previously, provided the pivotal evidence supporting the approval of Pulmozyme in the United States.

A number of studies have evaluated the effects of carbocysteine, n-acetyl-cysteine, and other agents on exacerbation rates in patients with chronic bronchitis (25,26). Although most trials have shown a modest trend toward a benefit from the therapies as compared with placebo, most individual trials have not demonstrated a clear statistical superiority of active therapy. Meta-analyses of the trials suggest that there is benefit from these therapies (27). Whether or not sufficient evidence exists of a meaningful clinical response to support more widespread approval of the individual agents is a question we hope will be answered in the near future.

C. Symptom Scores

Patients with chronic bronchitis and advanced cystic fibrosis have symptoms of chest congestion and breathlessness that bother them and impair their daily living. Therefore, reduction in symptoms should provide meaningful clinical benefit to these patients, even if not attended by an improvement in lung function. Symptomatic relief also represents an excellent target for mucoactive therapies, since inability to "clear the lungs" may be corrected by an effective mucoactive therapy.

One of the most ambitious attempts to demonstrate by use of a symptom questionnaire the effectiveness of a product widely believed to have mucoactive properties was the National Mucolytic Study (28). This 8-week study evaluated the effectiveness of iodinated glycerol in 361 patients with chronic bronchitis. Some of the questions asked of patients related to the following categories: cough frequency and severity, chest discomfort, dyspnea, and difficulty in bringing up sputum. Although other parameters such as exacerbations were also evaluated, the primary efficacy focus was on improvement in symptoms. The study demonstrated a modest but statistically significant benefit for the iodinated glycerol treatment group as compared with placebo. The regulatory outcome of this trial is uncertain, since iodinated glycerol was withdrawn from the market for apparent safety concerns. Nonetheless, the trial represented a significant effort at attempting to utilize the cardinal symptoms of chronic bronchitis to assess the effectiveness of a product thought to have mucoactive properties.

Many excellent symptom questionnaires are available that are widely used in evaluating patients with COPD, and most have been well validated using appropriate psychometric techniques. At a recent presentation before the Pulmonary Allergy Drug Advisory Committee discussing the combination product salmeterol xinafoate and fluticasone propionate (Advair®), the sponsor (GlaxoSmithKline) presented data collected using the Chronic Respiratory Disease Questionnaire (CRDQ), the Chronic Bronchitis Symptoms Questionnaire (CBSQ), and the Transitional Dyspnea Index (TDI). Although some differences were seen in favor of active treatment as compared with placebo, the results for the CBSQ were minimally affected by active treatment, which is somewhat disappointing since this questionnaire focuses directly on the main symptoms of chronic bronchitis (Meeting of the FDA Pulmonary Allergy Drug Advisory Committee on Advair®, January 15, 2002).

A reduction of symptoms remains an attractive endpoint for mucoactive therapies aimed at treating chronic bronchitis or cystic fibrosis and should be acceptable primary evidence of efficacy. Thus, the development of a well-validated questionnaire focusing specifically on symptoms would provide a valuable research tool. Critical steps in the development of this questionnaire would include the following standard questionnaire development steps to establish face validity, construct validity, and discriminant validity:

Focus groups of patients with chronic bronchitis to hear what words they use to describe their symptoms and the impact of these symptoms on their daily life

A study of healthy individuals and patients with chronic bronchitis to show that the symptoms are reported in patients but not in healthy individuals

A study to show that patients with a diagnosis of chronic bronchitis report the symptoms on the questionnaire and that the symptoms correlate with known measures, such as the FEV_1

A study showing that scores are changed during an exacerbation compared to when the patient is clinically stable (that is, if a scale has higher scores with less disease, that the patient scores lower during an exacerbation).

If symptoms are going to be assessed as a primary outcome for a clinical trial, a decision needs to be made as to whether they will be collected on a daily basis by the patients or periodically in the clinic. We believe collection of daily symptoms is preferable; however, patient compliance with diary cards is notoriously poor, particularly over the course of long-term trials.

D. Quality of Life

Assessment of health status or health-related quality of life (HRQL) is now a standard part of most large long-term clinical trials (29). Despite the widespread collection of HRQL data in clinical trials, the results are rarely used as pivotal evidence of efficacy for new therapies. The clinical relevance of changes in HRQL measures has been well established in the last 20 years, and instruments for measuring HRQL have been validated for shorter periods of time, such that they can be used for 1- to 3-month clinical trials. Historically, most assessments of HRQL were performed with non-disease-specific instruments such as the Medical Outcomes Survey Short Form 36 (SF-36); sometimes the questionnaires were completed by interviewers and sometimes by patients. However, in recent years, there has been increasing use of disease-specific HRQL questionnaires. Some of these disease-specific questionnaires have questions very similar to those on symptom questionnaires.

There are a number of instruments that are generally thought of as COPD-specific instruments, including the commonly used Chronic Respiratory Questionnaire (CRQ) and the St. George's Hospital Questionnaire (SGRQ). These questionnaires focus on items that are relevant to COPD patients in both frequency and importance. Most contain "domains" which generally contain a group of questions related to a specific aspect of their respiratory illness (for example, the impact of the disease on activity levels).

Selection of a health status instrument for a clinical trial should be based on finding an instrument that has been validated for the duration of the trial (this can be a problem for trials of less than 3 months in duration) and shown to be useful for detecting changes over time (30).A decision will need to be made as to whether the entire instrument or specific domains of the instrument will be considered evidence of primary efficacy. If specific domains of an instrument that has been validated overall are used, the use of these domains for such purposes would require its own validation. It is advisable to discuss this approach with relevant regulatory bodies prior to commencing the clinical trials, as the use of health status assessment as a primary endpoint for efficacy clinical trials is still not standard.

E. Other Endpoints for Diseases of the Lower Airways

A number of other endpoints are useful for demonstrating activity of mucoactive medications, but would be unlikely to be useful as the sole evidence for the primary demonstration of efficacy. These include: 1) measurement of sputum volume, 2) measurement of sputum characteristics, 3) measurement of mucociliary clearance, and 4) assessment of lung changes using high-resolution computerized tomography (HRCT). If changes in any of these parameters can be convincingly linked to clinical outcomes, then regulatory authorities might be willing to consider them as valuable surrogate endpoints for pivotal efficacy demonstration. Alternatively, demonstrated improvement in such measures along with an improvement in another endpoint (e.g., symptoms) may provide more convincing evidence of efficacy than changes in either endpoint alone.

Measurement of sputum volume is usually performed using a cup for collection. Patients generally collect for a fixed period of time prior to and after initiation of mucoactive therapy. Increases in sputum production are generally thought to be beneficial and likely show that the drug under study has activity. Similarly, elegant studies on the effects of various compounds on the characteristics of sputum such as viscoelasticity, cohesiveness, and percent solids can provide mechanistic support for potential mucoactive medications (31), but again the link to clinical effects at this time is uncertain.

Assessment of rates of mucociliary clearance has been carried out using technetium-labeled iron oxide particles and gamma camera imaging to provide video images of the pharmacological activity of mucokinetic agents (32). Here again, the link to clinical benefit has not been established. A newer technique that may have utility in future studies of chronic bronchitis and cystic fibrosis is evaluating changes over time via HRCT (33). Scans are scored using a grading scale by independent observers. It is anticipated that changes in air trapping, mucus plugging, or peribronchial thickening may be observed following therapy with mucoactive agents.

F. Endpoints Specific for Allergic Rhinitis

As stated above, a draft guidance document from the U.S. FDA outlines regulatory guidelines for studies in allergic rhinitis. Those design features seem appropriate for trials of mucoactive therapies, such as the use of symptoms as the primary efficacy endpoint. Focusing primarily on the nasal symptom complex of congestion, rhinorrhea, and sneezing would seem appropriate based on mechanism. Measurement of the saccharin transport time is an easily performed method to assess of mucociliary clearance rate, but a limited amount of work has been done establishing whether improving saccharin transport time improves overall symptoms of allergic rhinitis.

G. Endpoints Specific for Common Cold

Evaluating the effectiveness of mucoactive agents for the symptoms associated with a cold should obviously focus on those symptoms likely to be affected by therapy. Therefore, rhinorrhea, cough, and nasal congestion should be tracked on a frequent basis (at least twice daily) during the duration of the cold. Symptoms have traditionally been scored on a 0–3 scale, with 0 signifying no symptoms and 3 severe symptoms. Severity of rhinorrhea can also be quantified by counting the number of tissues used per hour (Picovir® FDA Advisory Committee Minutes). As mentioned previously and reviewed elsewhere in this book, expectorants have been frequently studied in cough associated with common cold.

Since the common cold is almost always self-limited in duration, the analysis of the data generally focuses on the time to resolution of symptoms. However, since the disease can wax and wane in severity, it is useful to have two or more consecutive periods of no symptoms before declaring that symptoms are "resolved." Number of nights with sleep disturbance and the amount of concomitant medication used to treat common cold symptoms may also be useful endpoints. Saccharin transport time has been shown to be impaired in patients with acute rhinovirus infection (10), and changes may be seen with a mucoactive agent. Finally, complications of common colds, such as the development of sinusitis that may be related to impairment of mucociliary function, should be monitored.

H. Safety Endpoints

The discussion so far has focused on endpoints useful for demonstrating the effectiveness of mucoactive compounds for a variety of disorders in which mucus-related impairment may be present. When discussing safety, most of the assessments recommended would be those considered standard for any new therapeutic agent. Therefore, standard monitoring including physical examinations, clinical laboratory tests, electrocardiograms, and adverse-events recording should be part of any protocol. Since it is possible that enhancement of mucociliary clearance can have acute deleterious effects on lung function, monitoring of pulmonary function and oxyhemoglobin saturation may be advisable.

Much of what is known about acute enhancement of lung clearance is from studies of sputum induction. When sputum induction is performed in patients with chronic bronchitis and significant impairment in lung function, falls in FEV$_1$ (and other spirometric indices) and oxyhemoglobin saturation can occur (34). The effect is usually transient; nonetheless, if an acute effect is expected, it is advisable to monitor the FEV$_1$ and oxyhemoglobin saturation for the period following drug administration.

The appropriate number of patients to be studied and the duration of studies should be in accordance with ICH (International Committee on Harmonization) guidelines.

V. Conclusions

Mucoactive agents cover a wide variety of class compounds, used for treating different diseases and conditions. As a result of an increase in our understanding of the mechanism of action of drugs and the pathophysiology of the diseases, the development of new drugs in this therapeutic area is likely to be more challenging in the future. More than in the past, and beyond the regulatory rigor applied to the approval of currently approved mucoactive products, manufacturers of new products may be required by regulatory authorities to pay closer attention to selection of clinical endpoints, precise definition of clinical indications, and choice of comparator in their pivotal trials. For now, regulatory authorities have not issued specific published guidelines for the clinical development of this class of drugs. Ultimately, as interest in this therapeutic area increases, it is expected that authorities will provide guidelines on the requirements for approval for new products that take into consideration the various issues discussed in this chapter.

References

1. Michelson F. Which cough mixture? Aust Fam Physician 1998; 27:1041–1046.
2. Irwin RS, Curley FJ, Bennett FM. Appropriate use of antitussives and protussives: a practical review. Drugs 1993; 46:80–91.
3. MacPherson RD. The pharmacological basis of contemporary pain management. Pharmacol Ther 2000; 88:163–185.
4. Ruoff G. Management of pain in patients with multiple health problems: a guide for the practicing physician. Am J Med 1998; 105:53S–60S.
5. Wills PJ, Cole PJ. Mucolytic and mucokinetic therapy. Pulm Pharmacol 1996; 9: 197–204.
6. Lurie A, Mestiri M, Huchon G, Marcas J, Lockhart A, Strauch G, Bergogne-Berezin E, Brignon J, Carbon C, Chwalow J. Methods for clinical assessment of expectorants: a critical review. Int J Clin Pharmacol Res 1992; 12:47–52.
7. Rubin BK. Pharmacologic management of mucus retention based on a taxonomy of mucoactive medications. In: Baum GL, Priel Z, Roth Y, Liron N, Ostfeld EJ, eds. Cilia, Mucus and Mucociliary Interactions. New York: Marcel Dekker, 1998: 383–389.

8. Van der Schans CP, Piers DA, Beekhuis H, Koeter GH, van der Mark TW, Postma DS. Effect of forced expirations on mucus clearance in patients with chronic airflow obstruction: effect of recoil pressure. Thorax 1990; 45:623–627.

9. Regnis JA, Robinson M, Bailey DL, Cook P, Hooper P, Chan HK, Gonda I, Bautovich G, Bye PT. Mucociliary clearance in patients with cystic fibrosis and in normal subjects. Am J Resp Crit Care Med 1994; 150:66–71.

10. Pedersen M, Sakakura Y, Winther B, Brofeldt S, Mygind N. Nasal mucociliary transport, number of ciliated cells, and beating pattern in naturally acquired common cold. Eur J Respir Dis 1983; 128:355–364.

11. Schuhl JF. Nasal mucociliary clearance in perennial rhinitis. J Investig Allergol Clin Immunol 1995; 5:333–336.

12. Pool PJ, Black PN. Mucolytic agents for chronic bronchitis (Cochrane Review). In: The Cochrane Library, 2001; Issue 2.

13. Task Force on Mucoactive Drugs. Recommendations for guidelines on clinical trials of mucoactive drugs in chronic bronchitis and chronic obstructive pulmonary disease. Chest 1994; 106:1532–1537.

14. Fitsimmons SC. The changing epidemiology of cystic fibrosis. J Pediatr 1993; 122: 1–9.

15. Fuchs HJ, Borowitz DS, Christiansen DH, Morris EM, Nash ML, Ramsey BW, Rosenstein BJ, Smith AL, Wohl ME. Effects of aerosolized recombinant human DNase on exacerbations of respiratory symptoms and on pulmonary function in patients with cystic fibrosis. N Engl J Med 1994; 331:637–642.

16. Pulmozyme ®: Summary Basis of Approval. Rockville, MD: U.S. Food and Drug Administration, 1993.

17. Moriarity BG, Robson AM, Smallman LA, Drake-Lee AB. Nasal mucociliary function: comparison of saccharin clearance with ciliary beat frequency. Rhinology 1991; 29:173–179.

18. Lindberg S. Morphological and functional studies of the mucociliary system during infections in the upper airways. Acta Otolaryngol 1994; 515:22–25.

19. Kuhn JJ, Hendley JO, Adams KF, Clark JW, Gwaltney JM Jr. Antitussive effect of guaifenesin in young adults with natural colds: objective and subjective assessment. Chest 1982; 82:713–718.

20. Rubin BK, Tomkiewicz RP, King M. Mucoactive agents: old and new. In: Wilmott RW, ed. The Pediatric Lung. Basel, Switzerland: Birkhauser Verlag, 1997:155–179.

21. Tamaoki J, Chiyotani A, Kobayashi K, Sakai N, Kanemura, T, Takizawa T. Effect of indomethacin on bronchorrhea in patients with chronic bronchitis, diffuse panbronchiolitis, or bronchiectasis. Am Rev Respir Dis 1992; 145:548–552.

22. McCoy K, Hamilton S, Johnson C. Pulmozyme Study Group. Effects of 12-week administration of dornase alfa in patients with advanced cystic fibrosis lung disease. Chest 1996; 110:889–895

23. Anzueto A, Jubran A, Ohar JA, Piquette CA, Rennard SI, Colice G, Pattishall EN, Barrett J, Engle M, Perret KA, Rubin BK. Effects of aerosolized surfactant in patients with stable chronic bronchitis: a prospective randomized controlled trial. JAMA 1997; 278:1426–1431.

24. Anthonisen NR, Manfreda J, Warren CP, Hershfield ES, Harding GK, Nelson NA.

Antibiotic therapy in exacerbations of chronic obstructive pulmonary disease. Ann Intern Med 1987; 106:196–204.

25. Allegra L, Cordaro CI, Grassi C. Prevention of acute exacerbations of chronic obstructive bronchitis with carbocysteine lysine salt monohydrate: a multicenter, double-blind, placebo-controlled trial. Respiration 1996; 63:174–180.

26. Stey C, Steurer J, Bachmann S, Medici TC, Tramer MR. The effect of oral N-acetylcysteine in chronic bronchitis: a quantitative systematic review. Eur Respir J 2000; 16:253–262.

27. Grandjean EM, Berthet P, Ruffmann R, Leuenberger P. Efficacy of oral long-term N-acetylcysteine in chronic bronchopulmonary disease: a meta-analysis of published double-blind, placebo-controlled clinical trials. Clin Ther 2000; 22:209–221.

28. Petty TL. The National Mucolytic Study: results of a randomized, double-blind, placebo-controlled study of iodinated glycerol in chronic obstructive bronchitis. Chest 1990; 97:75–83.

29. Jones PW. Health status measurements in chronic obstructive pulmonary disease. Thorax 2001; 56:880–887.

30. Spencer S, Anie K, Jones PW. Annual rate of health status decline in COPD patients is significantly related to frequency of exacerbation. Eur Respir J 1999; 14: 19s.

31. Rubin BK. An in vitro comparison of the mucoactive properties of guaifenesin, iodinated glycerol, surfactant, and albuterol. Chest 1999; 116:195–200.

32. Kellerman DJ, Bennett WD, Zeman KL, Foy C, Gorden JC, Shaffer CL, Johnson FL. Dose response relationship of the $P2Y_2$ agonist INS365 on mucociliary clearance in smokers [abstr]. J Allergy Clin Immunol 2001; 107:S164.

33. Brody AS, Molina PL, Klein JS, Rothman BS, Ramagopal M, Swartz DR. High-resolution computed tomography of the chest in children with cystic fibrosis: support for use as an outcome surrogate. Pediatr Radiol 1999; 29:731–735.

34. Bhowmik A, Seemungal TA, Sapsford RJ, Devalia JL, Wedzicha JA. Comparison of spontaneous and induced sputum for investigation of airway inflammation in chronic obstructive pulmonary disease. Thorax 1998; 53:953–956.

16

Airway-Clearance Techniques Individually Tailored to Each Patient

LONE OLSÉNI and
LOUISE LANNEFORS

University Hospital
Lund, Sweden

CEES P. VAN DER SCHANS

University for Professional Education
"Hanzehogeschool"
Groningen, The Netherlands

I. Introduction

Airway-clearance techniques traditionally play an important role in the treatment of patients with bronchial mucus-clearance or bronchial hypersecretion disorders (1). Many different techniques are available today, and more are coming. The choice of treatment may vary considerably between countries and centers and is often based on tradition and popularity. However, in clinical practice the decision to use a technique or combination of techniques in an individual patient should take into account the pathophysiology of the disease, the physiological mechanisms and aspects behind each technique, and the outcome of clinical trials concerning the technique like described in the concept of evidence-based medicine (2). When a certain technique is used, the clinical efficacy should be assessed regularly to adjust the treatment if necessary. However, in some techniques the physiological mechanism is unclear or there is no consensus concerning the physiological mechanisms. Therefore, the outcome variables used in several studies is often difficult to judge because some outcome variables may not or not only reflect changes in mucus transport or mucus retention (3). In short-term studies the measurement of bronchial mucus clearance using a radioactive tracer technique is probably the most reliable outcome variable.

413

The relationship between changes in mucus transport or mucus retention and pulmonary function is poor. Therefore, the use of pulmonary function to evaluate changes in mucus transport is not adequate. In long-term studies the decline in pulmonary function may be an important outcome variable. In the Cochrane Collaboration a systematic review was published on physical therapeutic measures to improve mucus transport in patients with chronic obstructive pulmonary disease (COPD) and patients with bronchiectasis (4). The reviewers concluded that there is as yet insufficient evidence in the literature to judge the effectiveness of mucus-clearance techniques in COPD/bronchiectasis patients. In another meta-analysis in patients with cystic fibrosis (CF), Thomas et al. (5) concluded that chest physical therapy clears more mucus than no treatment. Another important factor is that the effects of an airway-clearance technique may be dependent on actual use, transferred and instructed by a physical therapist. Consequently, individual difference in the practical approach may result in considerable differences of the effects achieved.

The basis for the application of mucus-clearance techniques is formed by the potential pathophysiological consequences of retention of mucus in the airways and the effects of chronic expectoration and coughs on the quality of life of patients. A potentially important pathophysiological consequence of retention of mucus is that airways gradually are being clogged, which can contribute to bronchial obstruction, impaired ventilation distribution, dyspnea, repeated or chronic pulmonary infections and perhaps injured lung tissue or airways. Thereby the impact of chronic expectoration of mucus, as a socially disabling symptom, for the individual patient should not be underestimated. Chronic expectoration of mucus and coughing may affect the patient's quality of life. Seemungal et al. (6) investigated risk factors for exacerbation severity and frequency in COPD patients. Additionally, the impact of exacerbations on quality of life was investigated in their study. The results of this study show that cough and mucus expectoration are predictors of frequent pulmonary exacerbations in COPD patients and that quality-of-life scores were worse in those patients with frequent exacerbations. Vestbo and coworkers (7,8) found in a large epidemiological study that chronic expectoration of mucus is strongly associated with an excess decline in pulmonary function, hospital admissions for pneumonia, and hospital admission because of COPD.

The specific situation of the patient may influence the goals of treatment and thus the choice of mucus-clearance techniques. Treatment of acutely ill patients differs from that of chronically stable patients. When treating severely ill patients admitted to a hospital, the immediate aim is to improve ventilation by reducing obstruction and, if possible, hyperinflation, which apart from hypersecretion can be caused by bronchoconstriction, edema, tissue damage, or a combination of them all. When retention of mucus is considered as a major problem in the acutely ill patient, mucus-clearance techniques are very important. The choice of techniques is dependent on the patient's clinical status and stability, including the status of the respiratory muscles, the familiarity of the patient with clearance techniques, and the ability to follow instructions. Another important aspect to consider is that different approaches are needed to clear mucus from central and peripheral airways. Regular short treatments are usually more appropriate than less frequent and longer treatments. When hypersecretion is not considered as the major problem in acutely ill patients, the use of mucus-clearance techniques is probably not indicated. When the clinical status of the patient is improved by medical intervention, the application of mucus-clearance techniques could be reconsidered again.

In patients with chronic mucus disorders, the aim of chest physical therapy is to achieve or maintain an optimal physical status and, more specifically, to prevent and minimize the number of exacerbations and the tissue damage. The airway-clearance technique, or combination of techniques, chosen for the patient with a chronic disease has to function on a regular basis at home, not only in the hospital. This means that the techniques should be easy to use, mostly independent of caregivers or relatives, and independent of technical devices that are difficult to use or to handle. Patients should be educated in the technique or combination of techniques chosen during stable conditions. They should be taught how to assess the need for and amount of chest physical therapy and the effect of a treatment session. Patients should realize that preventive treatment is their own responsibility. The physical therapist has a responsibility to support the patient, to assess to the quality of the treatment, to follow it up regularly, and, when necessary, to change the overall strategy or certain aspects of the treatment. However, compliance to mucus-clearance techniques is a major problem (9–13). Currie et al. (13) found in a group of 50 COPD patients that 27 did inadequate chest physical therapy despite instruction and follow-up. Passero et al. (9) showed that compliance to chest physical therapy was lower than for other treatments in patients with cystic fibrosis. Blomquist et al. (14), however, found that 6 months of self-treatment was equally effective as supervised treatment in patients with cystic fibrosis. It is possible that compliance in Blomquist's study was higher or that compliance does not influence the effects of chest physical therapy to a large extent. In a recent national questionnaire addressed to all Swedish CF patients, 63% answered that they adhere to the chest physical therapy recommended, 12% do so intermittently, and 23% do not adhere.

In this chapter the airway-clearance techniques most commonly used today are discussed. The mechanism behind each technique is explained, if possible from a physiological point of view.

II. Coughing

When mucociliary clearance is insufficient, spontaneous cough plays a compensating role as a back-up mechanism, at least in the more central airways. Coughing consists of different stages, as described by Masserey (15). A more or less deep inspiration is followed by glottis closure. With the closed glottis, an expiratory maneuver is started with more or less isometric contraction of the expiratory muscles, resulting in compression of the thorax and increased intrapulmonary pressure. Then the glottis is opened, resulting in a burst of expiratory flow.

Frequent coughing, however, may lead to side effects such as fatigue, damaged mucosa, costal fractures, and vomiting. Holland et al. (16) found in healthy subjects that coughing significantly increased energy expenditure and induced mild airway narrowing. This effect may not be clinically relevant in healthy subjects but may be extremely important in patients with severe pulmonary disease who are already tired and depleted and have severe airflow obstruction. Some of these side effects may influence the quality of the coughing maneuvers, and thereby their effect, and also the patient's social life. Another often overlooked problem with coughing is that it may also lead to urinary incontinence. It has been shown that women who cough may frequently suffer from incontinence (17–19). Patients with this problem must learn how to control the pelvic floor muscles during coughing. Teaching these patients to replace spontaneous coughing with other techniques to transport secretions is also important, e.g., huffing, as this strains the pelvic floor muscles to a lesser degree.

Many studies have shown that directed controlled coughing may be an effective intervention for clearing the airways (20–27). It has even been shown that in some patient groups cough and chest physical therapy have equal effects on pulmonary function (24) and mucus transport (25,26). The effect of coughing, but also of huffing (see below), on mucus transport may be limited to the central and intermediate zones of the lungs (22,28).

III. Forced Expirations, Huffing

This technique also starts with an inspiration like coughing, but after that a forced expiration is performed without glottis closure. This requires a dynamic contraction of the expiratory muscles. This maneuver is repeated from different lung volumes. The huffing technique, but also coughing, is based on the conception of the equal pressure point (EPP) (29). During a forced expiration, the high alveolar pressure is the driving force for the expiratory airflow, and there is a pressure decay from the alveoli to the mouth (Fig. 1). Somewhere in that pressure decay the intrabronchial pressure equals the surrounding pleural pressure. This point is called the equal pressure point (EPP). In the airways central from the EPP the intrabronchial pressure is lower than the surrounding pleural pressure and airways are dynamically compressed (29). Due to the dynamic compression of the airways central from the EPP, airflow velocity is increased at the point of airway compression. Thereby airflow may become turbulent at the

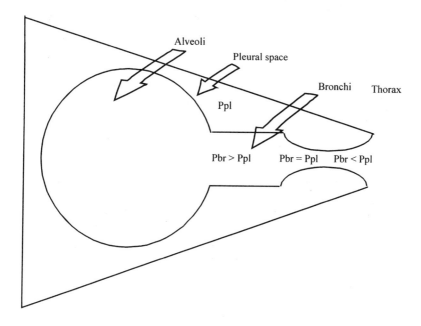

Figure 1 During a forced expiration, the high alveolar pressure is the driving force for the expiratory airflow and there is a pressure decay from the alveoli to the mouth. Somewhere along that pressure decay the intrabronchial pressure (Pbr) equals the surrounding pleural pressure (Ppl). This point is called the equal pressure point (EPP). In the airways central from the EPP the intrabronchial pressure is lower than the surrounding pleural pressure, and airways are dynamically compressed.

site of the EPP. Both the turbulent airflow and the increased airflow velocity may contribute to the transport of bronchial secretions (30). The location of the EPP can be varied by the lung volume and the expiratory force (Fig. 2). A high lung volume results in an EPP in the more central airways and a low lung volume in the more peripheral airways. A high expiratory force results in an EPP in the more peripheral airways and a low expiratory force in the more central airways.

During a forced expiration from total lung capacity to residual lung volume, the EPP shifts from the central airways toward the peripheral airways. Theoretically this would clear secretions first from central and then from peripheral airways in one forced expiratory maneuver. But such a forced expiration can be tiring and difficult to control. Therefore it is suggested that the mean linear flow in the airways be higher in case of repeated separate coughs as compared with a single cough from high to low lung volume (31). This higher airflow probably has a greater effect on mucus transport. Another aspect of

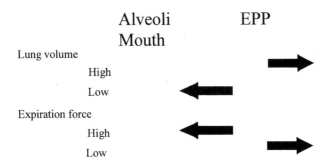

Figure 2 EPP and dynamic compression at different lung volumes and expiratory forces.

repeated huffing or coughing is that this may temporarily decrease the viscosity of mucus and thereby help mucus transport. This can be explained by the fact that mucus is a non-Newtonian fluid. This means that the viscosity is not a constant but is dependent on the shear rate. A burst of air flowing over a mucus sheet can be considered as a high shear rate that may temporarily decrease the viscosity of mucus. A subsequent second forced expiration may transport the mucus more easily due to the decreased viscosity. Repeated separate coughs or huffs are therefore considered as more effective and more comfortable and easier to control for the patient. This hypothesis is supported by the findings of an in vitro study of Zahm et al. (32). These authors found that repetitive coughing was more effective than a single cough but, more important, that the effect of repetitive coughing was even higher when the time between coughs was reduced. An explanation for this finding is that the first cough reduces the viscosity of the mucus, which is then more easily transported by subsequent coughs.

Huffs or coughs can be started at different lung volume levels with the EPP placed in different airway generations. How much muscle activity is put into each huff depends on the lung volume from which it is started and on physiological and pathophysiological factors. If a huff started from a small lung volume or is too forced, this will cause a collapse of the airways, especially in patients with unstable airways. Overall, the expiratory force should decline with the lung volume in the sense that at lower lung volume the expiratory force should also be lower to prevent airway collapse (Fig. 3). Van der Schans et al. (33) found that forced expirations and coughing were less effective in patients with pulmonary emphysema with unstable airways as compared with chronic bronchitis patients with more stable (33) airways. Airway collapse can be partly prevented by reducing the force and/or increasing the lung volume at which the huff is performed. This will place the EPP in the more central rigid airways and thus limit collapse. By using less forceful expirations during huffing at low lung

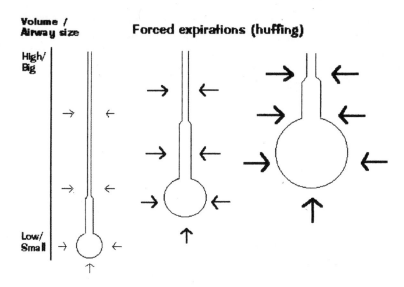

Figure 3 Forced expirations at low lung volumes, and thus small airways, should be performed with less force as compared with forced expirations at high lung volumes. The size of the arrows indicates the amount of muscle power put into each forced expiration.

volumes, airway collapse can be avoided to a great extent. Using optimal expiratory force, the positive effects of dynamic compression are achieved in the more peripheral airways. With proper instructions, most patients learn how to balance the initial lung volume, the lung volume at which the maneuver should be ended, and the amount of muscle force put into each huff. A patient can learn to huff effectively from a small lung volume, which theoretically will mobilize secretions in small airways, and then by huffing from gradually bigger lung volumes effectively transport the mucus to bigger airways from where it easily can be expectorated. These huffing series at different lung volume levels are started repeatedly, allowing adequate time for rest, until lungs are cleared.

Despite proper premedication with bronchodilators in some patients with very hyper-reactive airways, huffs may cause bronchospasms, which leads to tickling cough and increased dyspnea. To avoid this, forced expirations are mixed with relaxed breathing at a comfortable rate, so-called "breathing control." The more hyperreactive the airways, the more time these patients need to spend on relaxation and breathing control between the huffs, to reduce the bronchospasm, and to make each huff as effective as possible.

When treating paretic, weak, or severely ill patients who have overloaded or weak muscles or patients who cannot follow instructions, thoracic compressions can be used to replace or support forced expirations. Thoracic compression must be carried out following the patient's breathing pattern and the physiological movement of the ribs during expiration. Abdominal compression or stabilization is necessary when the abdominal muscles are too poorly activated or too weak to support the expiratory flow. It is important that compressions be gently and fluently applied, because patients who have the opportunity will defend themselves by closing their glottis if the thoracic compression is uncomfortable or painful. This will certainly not lead to an increased expiratory flow.

Forced expirations with an open glottis combined with breathing control is known as the forced expiration technique (FET) or the active cycle of breathing technique (ACBT) (34). In this technique, a cycle consisting of one or more huffs is followed by relaxation and breathing control at a rate comfortable for the patient. The breathing control can consist of ordinary tidal volume breaths or, if needed, pursed-lips breathing. The time needed for this part of the FET is dependent on the patient's pulmonary status and needs to be individually tailored (35). Sutton et al. (36) compared the effects of FET alone, FET with postural drainage, and directed coughing. In this study it was found that the amount of expectorated mucus was higher during FET with postural drainage than during directed coughing alone. However, in more recent studies, using more reliable outcome variables like radioactive tracer clearance, no clear difference in effect was found between coughing and FET (22,23,26). Huffing and FET were developed and first used as adjuncts to postural drainage. Today FET is a part of other airway-clearance techniques as well, such as positive expiratory pressure (PEP), oscillating PEP, and physical exercise (discussed later in this chapter).

ACBT is a cycle consisting of different components (34): thoracic expansion exercises, relaxed breathing control, and huffing. Cycles of this technique are carried out with thoracic expansion exercises, and breathing control is combined with one or two huffs followed by relaxation and breathing control. ACBT/FET is performed either in postural drainage positions, in specific or modified gravity-assisted positions, or in a sitting position. It is usually but not necessarily accompanied by chest clapping during thoracic expansion exercises and vibrations (shaking) during huffs. Thoracic expansion exercises may not be essential to achieve the ACBT effect. White et al. (37) found that there is no difference in spirometry, amount of expectorated mucus, and oxygenation during ACBT with thoracic expansion exercises as compared with ACBT without thoracic expansion exercises. ACBT is repeated in each position until the lungs have cleared.

IV. Breathing Techniques

Different kinds of breathing techniques are frequently used as a part of chest physical therapy, but the aims of using these components are many: to reduce dyspnea, to improve ventilation distribution, to reduce bronchospasm, to reduce the cost of breathing, or to support airway clearance.

Pursed-lips breathing is one of the best-known breathing techniques in chest physical therapy, and it can be used in several different ways and situations. In this technique the patient breathes relaxed against an expiratory resistance (almost closed lips), which results in a positive mouth pressure during expiration of about 5 cm H_2O (38). It is thought that this resistance and the resulting pressure will limit the initial peak flow and increase the intrabronchial pressure and thereby delay airway collapse during expiration. This may give a patient with severe airway obstruction the opportunity to breathe at a lower lung volume. Breathing against an expiratory resistance also leads to increased expiratory and inspiratory muscle activity (39,40) and thereby to an increased tidal volume and reduced dead space ventilation (41). At rest, this type of breathing results in increased tidal volume due to increased inspiratory muscle activity and thereby to improved blood gasses (42–45). During exercise, ventilation is more efficient due to a higher tidal volume and lower breathing frequency, but this is accompanied by increased dyspnea sensations (41).

Pursed-lips breathing is also used to reduce bronchoconstriction (46) during airway-clearance techniques. The use of pursed-lips breathing to reduce airway obstruction is mainly based on clinical experience of patients and caregivers. Wardlaw et al. (46) found that after hyperventilation-induced bronchoconstriction, the fall in FEV_1 was significantly less when patients used pursed-lips breathing than open mouth breathing. The explanation of this effect is not clear, but it supports the spontaneous use of pursed-lips breathing by patients in case of (increased) airway obstruction.

Deep inspirations, also called thoracic expansion exercises, sometimes combined with a breath hold, may open clogged or collapsed airways. Slow, sometimes deep inspirations are meant to distribute inspired air to a larger extent also to obstructed parts of the lungs, to bring air behind secretions. The effect of these exercises on mucus clearance is limited (37).

V. Postural Drainage

Originally the aim of postural drainage was to increase transport of mucus in the airways by the help of gravity (34). Many different specific drainage positions are used to promote clearance from all different lobes and segments. The object is to hold each position long enough to allow mucus to "slide down the airway walls." The duration for which the position is held ranges from the recommended minimum of 10 minutes to the patient's staying all night in a gravity-assisted position. Some studies found that postural drainage improves mucus transport in the airways (47,48), although in a study of Oldenburg (21) no effect was seen. It is important to realize that some positions might affect ventilation perfusion, cardiac output, and saturation in a negative way (49). Postural drainage can also cause reflux (50,51) and increase intracranial pressure.

Another aspect of some postural drainage positions is that the physiological effects of gravity influence regional distribution of ventilation and the regional FRC levels. Postural drainage in this sense may function as an adjunct therapy when other techniques alone are not sufficient. This mainly concerns right and left side lying. In the dependent (lowest) part of the lungs, FRC is decreased, which influences the emptying of that part of the lung toward a regional RV level. This situation may improve secretion mobilization in an otherwise hyperinflated obstructed patient and is consistent with the finding that postural drainage may increase mucus transport in the dependent lung (52). In the independent (highest) part of the lung, FRC will increase. Increased FRC might help to open clogged or collapsed airways, to get air behind secretions before trying to mobilize and transport it to the central airways using another (opposite) position.

VI. Percussion/Clapping: Vibration/Shaking

Percussion can be applied manually on the thorax with a frequency of 3–6 Hz or mechanically with higher frequencies up to 40 Hz. The aim of these techniques is to loosen secretion by applying forces to the chest wall supposed to be transferred to the airway wall, of varying frequency and amplitude. These external forces may induce small coughs superimposed on tidal breathing (53). Another possible explanation for the effect of these techniques is that a reduction of the mucus viscosity may arise. App et al. (54) found a reduction of sputum viscoelasticity after flutter breathing (see Chapter 17). Using these kinds of techniques the patient is usually passive and dependent on an assistant or device. Patients may learn to carry out the clapping and shaking themselves, which is possible on some parts of the thorax, but they will always be dependent on somebody else who can carry out the treatment on the back.

Several studies have failed to show any effects of percussion/vibration. Campbell et al. (55) and Wollmer et al. (56) found that bronchoconstriction induced by percussion was responsible for a decrease in the FEV_1 when used on patients with an exacerbation of chronic bronchitis. In an animal study, the application of vibration and percussion was associated with the development of atelectasis (57). Mechanical clapping has been compared with manual chest percussion, and no significant difference was found between the two (58). In patients with COPD manual percussion had a small effect on mucus transport but did not add to the effectiveness of coughing (59). In a mixed group of patients with hypersecretion, percussion did not affect mucus transport (60). A frequency of about 10–15 Hz, which is outside the range of manual techniques but lower than most commercial vibrators, seems to have the best effect on mucus transport. This is consistent with the finding that in CF patients the intra-thoracic pressures induced by vibration and thus the vibration-induced expiratory flows appeared to be frequency dependent (61). The direction of the induced flow is also important. Based on the results of experimental studies it can be concluded that the oscillation/vibration should lead to an expiratory bi-ased flow, i.e., a higher expiratory than inspiratory flow (62–65), particularly when there is increased mucus rigidity (62). Studies have not demonstrated any additional increase in mucus transport when vibration was added to percussion in patients with COPD or CF (58–60,66), although one study found an improvement in the "rate of expectoration of mucus" when vibration was added to chest physical therapy (67).

There are insufficient data to justify the routine use of percussion, vibration, or oscillation techniques added to chest physical therapy. The experimental results of high-frequency oscillation are quite promising. Nevertheless, controlled clinical studies are needed to investigate the effect on mucus transport and to clarify under which circumstances or in which type of patient this technique would be most effective or which patients are at risk for adverse effects from these interventions.

VII. Autogenic Drainage

Autogenic drainage is another technique used to loosen and mobilize secretions (68). This technique was developed years ago, and its use is gradually increasing as the knowledge is spreading. Without any device patients move mucus in a relaxed sighing manner, simply by regulating airflow and velocity with their expiratory muscles. They must avoid applying an expiratory resistance in their upper airways and avoid using pursed-lips breathing. Instead they learn a breathing technique as follows: 1) slow diaphragmatic inspiration through the nose; 2) an inspiratory pause, 2–3 seconds; and 3) expiring with completely open upper airways in a relaxed sighing manner. The slow inspiration and the inspiratory pause also allow the obstructed airways to be part of the ventilation to a larger extent. The completely open upper airways during expirations are important to achieve an optimal expiratory flow and velocity, great enough to transport mucus. The optimal airflow is achieved without forcing the expiration, trying to avoid airway collapse (69). Patients are instructed to "breath through the secretions" and to "push the secretions up the airways" with the help of the air expired. The optimal airflow varies with the lung volume level at which autogenic drainage is carried out. Autogenic drainage is performed at different lung volume levels, starting at a low lung volume to mobilize mucus from small

.airways, continuing at gradually larger volumes to transport it to gradually bigger airways. If the expiratory force is too high when working at a low lung level, the small airways will collapse. The typical soft sound of mucus moving tells the patient whether the maneuver was optimal. Autogenic drainage is performed in a sitting position mostly but can be used during relaxation in supine and in other (modified) gravity-assisted positions as well. It is sometimes also used during nebulization therapy. Autogenic drainage can be difficult to learn, but once patients know how to carry it out and have learned how to control it, it is a gentle and independent way to carry out the treatment. They need neither assistants nor devices. For patients with unstable or hyperreactive airways where forceful expirations and coughs more easily cause obstruction and create airway closure, autogenic drainage may be an efficient alternative.

Giles et al. (70) compared autogenic drainage with conventional physical therapy in patients with cystic fibrosis. In this study no differences were found in the amount of expectorated mucus or pulmonary function. Miller et al. (71) found no differences in pulmonary function or amount of expectorated mucus between ACBT and autogenic drainage. Pfleger et al. found that autogenic drainage cleared less mucus than positive expiratory pressure breathing in patients with cystic fibrosis (72).

VIII. Physical Exercise and Sports

General physical activity may have a beneficial effect on exercise capacity and well-being as well as on clearing mucus. Improved working capacity, increased muscle strength, and retained mobility in shoulders and thoracic joints are examples of positive effects that can be gained at the same time as clearing mucus. Good mobility in the chest is a prerequisite for effective airway-clearance maneuvers no matter what technique is chosen, and good muscle strength and body knowledge is necessary for effective huffing/coughing. Self-confidence and the feeling of well-being that often comes along with good physical status are important for many reasons.

Physical exercise can be used to loosen secretions, especially if organized as somewhat modified interval or circuit training. The type of activity carried out naturally depends on age, physical status, surroundings, and other factors. Using physical exercise as a part of airway clearance is based on different mechanisms, such as getting air behind and loosening secretions and increasing ventilation and expiratory flow. Physical exercise carried out in this context is often followed by a short period of rest that might include pursed-lips breathing. Then either FET or autogenic drainage may be added. The cycle of exercise, period of rest, and FET or autogenic drainage are repeated until the lungs are sufficiently cleared or the agreed-upon program has been carried out.

Some adolescent and adult patients prefer using physical exercise (especially jogging) to loosen secretions, combined with FET or autogenic drainage. It takes little time, has positive side effects, and looks more like something people usually do.

As the minute ventilation is increased, tidal volume and expiratory flow will increase in patients with no or very little obstruction. In patients with pulmonary obstruction, the FRC will increase during physical activity since the expiratory flow in the peripheral airways is limited; otherwise the peripheral airways tend to collapse. The effect of physical exercise on mobilizing mucus can be due to either of the above, depending on the clinical status of the patient. Some patients may experience some bronchospasm during physical exercise even if optimally treated with bronchodilators beforehand. Others may get an increased instability in the small airways. These patients experience thoracic "stiffness" after having carried out physical activities. This makes physical exercise to loosen secretions an inefficient technique for these patients, since much time throughout the treatment needs to be spent on relaxation and breathing control before huffing or autogenic drainage is possible to carry out.

Many patients are nowadays advised to perform some sort of physical activity either as a part of or added to their chest physical therapy. The use of exercise as a mucus-clearance technique is often based on the study of Wolff et al. (73), in which it was found that exercise increased mucus transport in healthy subjects. However this could not be confirmed in a more recent study of Olséni et al. (74). In patients with pulmonary disease, physical activity alone is usually not sufficient as a clearance technique. Bilton et al. (75) compared four different mucus-clearance protocols in a group of patients with cystic fibrosis: physical therapy for 20 minutes, cycling (at 60% of the VO_2max) for 20 minutes, cycling for 10 minutes followed by physical therapy for 10 minutes, and physical therapy for 10 minutes followed by cycling for 10 minutes. The amount of mucus expectorated was highest during the 20 minutes of physical therapy and lowest during the 20 minutes of cycling. Lannefors et al. (52) found no difference in mucus transport between FET combined with postural drainage, FET combined with positive expiratory pressure breathing, and FET combined with cycling in patients with cystic fibrosis. Olséni and coworkers (76) found no effect of exercise on mucus transport in a mixed group of patients with bronchial hypersecretion. On the other hand, Thomas et al. (5) found in a meta-analysis that in patients with cystic fibrosis the combination of chest physical therapy and exercise clears more mucus from the airways than chest physical therapy alone.

The amount and intensity of physical activity can (in some cases should) be worked out together with a physical therapist. It is very important that the activity level be adapted to the individual patient's capacity for the moment. If necessary, the correct amount of supplemental oxygen should be given and the intensity adjusted so that the individual does not go below 90% oxygen saturation during activity. Inhalation of bronchodilating drugs should precede physical activities if necessary.

Nutritional status is also important to consider. Without a good nutritional base, neither endurance nor muscle strength can be improved or maintained. Patients can consult nutritional experts before beginning therapy so that the physical activities can be of maximum benefit (77–79).

IX. Final Remarks

Many attempts have been made to evaluate the efficacy of different airway-clearance techniques. Different groups have produced different results. One technique may suit one individual or one culture better than another. In general, the various airway-clearance techniques seem to be equally effective when it comes to clearing pulmonary secretions, but they can result in more or less fatigue, discomfort, and good or bad side effects.

It is important that clinicians know what they want to achieve with the chest physical therapy recommended, that they come up with an individual strategy, and that they offer techniques that are regularly and thoroughly assessed in each patient.

We must continue to evaluate the treatments available, developing new, even better techniques for the future, taking evidence-based medicine into consideration. To be able to understand what we actually can do, to produce a strategy for each patient, and to assess the results of the treatment, we have to know respiratory physiology and pathophysiology well.

References

1. Clarke SW. Management of mucus hypersecretion. Eur J Respir Dis Suppl 1987; 153:136–144.
2. Rosenberg W, Donald A. Evidence based medicine: an approach to clinical problem-solving. BMJ 1995; 310:1122–1126.
3. van der Schans CP, Postma DS, Koeter GH, Rubin BK. Physiotherapy and bronchial mucus transport. Eur Respir J 1999; 13:1477–1486.
4. Jones AP, Rowe BH. Bronchopulmonary hygiene physical therapy in chronic obstructive pulmonary disease and bronchiectasis. The Cochrane Libraray 1999. www.cochranelibrary.net.
5. Thomas J, Cook DJ, Brooks D. Chest physical therapy management of patients with cystic fibrosis. A meta-analysis. Am J Respir Crit Care Med 1995; 151:846–850.
6. Seemungal TA, Donaldson GC, Paul EA, Bestall JC, Jeffries DJ, Wedzicha JA. Effect of exacerbation on quality of life in patients with chronic obstructive pulmonary disease. Am J Respir Crit Care Med 1998; 157:1418–1422.

7. Vestbo J, Prescott E, Lange P. Association of chronic mucus hypersecretion with FEV1 decline and chronic obstructive pulmonary disease morbidity. Copenhagen City Heart Study Group. Am J Respir Crit Care Med 1996; 153:1530–1535.

8. Lange P, Vestbo J, Nyboe J. Risk factors for death and hospitalization from pneumonia. A prospective study of a general population. Eur Respir J 1995; 8:1694–1698.

9. Passero MA, Remor B, Salomon J. Patient-reported compliance with cystic fibrosis therapy. Clin Pediatr (Phila) 1981; 20:264–268.

10. Patterson JM, Budd J, Goetz D, Warwick WJ. Family correlates of a 10-year pulmonary health trend in cystic fibrosis. Pediatrics 1993; 91:383–389.

11. Abbott J, Dodd M, Bilton D, Webb AK. Treatment compliance in adults with cystic fibrosis. Thorax 1994; 49:115–120.

12. Abbott J, Dodd M, Webb AK. Health perceptions and treatment adherence in adults with cystic fibrosis. Thorax 1996; 51:1233–1238.

13. Currie DC, Munro C, Gaskell D, Cole PJ. Practice, problems and compliance with postural drainage: a survey of chronic sputum producers. Br J Dis Chest 1986; 80:249–253.

14. Blomquist M, Freyschuss U, Wiman LG, Strandvik B. Physical activity and self treatment in cystic fibrosis. Arch Dis Child 1986; 61:362–367.

15. Masserey M. Manual breathing and coughing aids. In: Bach JR, Haas F, eds. Pulmonary Rehabilitation. Philadelphia: W. B. Saunders, 1996:407–422.

16. Holland N, Williams MT, Parsons D, Hall B, Martin AJ. Clinical technical note. The effect of directed vigorous coughing on energy expenditure and pulmonary function in normal subjects. Physiother Theory Pract 1998; 14:55–61.

17. Wijma J, Tinga DJ, Visser GH. Perineal ultrasonography in women with stress incontinence and controls: the role of the pelvic floor muscles. Gynecol Obstet Invest 1991; 32:176–179.

18. Miller JM, Ashton Miller JA, DeLancey JO. A pelvic muscle precontraction can reduce cough-related urine loss in selected women with mild SUI. J Am Geriatr Soc 1998; 46:870–874.

19. Miller JM, Ashton Miller JA, DeLancey JO. Quantification of cough-related urine loss using the paper towel test. Obstet Gynecol 1998; 91:705–709.

20. Kirilloff LH, Owens GR, Rogers RM, Mazzocco MC. Does chest physical therapy work? Chest 1985; 88:436–444.

21. Oldenburg FA Jr, Dolovich MB, Montgomery JM, Newhouse MT. Effects of postural drainage, exercise, and cough on mucus clearance in chronic bronchitis. Am Rev Respir Dis 1979; 120:739–745.

22. Hasani A, Pavia D, Agnew JE, Clarke SW. Regional lung clearance during cough and forced expiration technique (FET): effects of flow and viscoelasticity. Thorax 1994; 49:557–561.

23. Hasani A, Pavia D, Agnew JE, Clarke SW. Regional mucus transport following unproductive cough and forced expiration technique in patients with airways obstruction. Chest 1994; 105:1420–1425.

24. de Boeck C, Zinman R. Cough versus chest physiotherapy. A comparison of the acute effects on pulmonary function in patients with cystic fibrosis. Am Rev Respir Dis 1984; 129:182–184.

25. Rossman CM, Waldes R, Sampson D, Newhouse MT. Effect of chest physiotherapy on the removal of mucus in patients with cystic fibrosis. Am Rev Respir Dis 1982; 126:131–135.

26. Hasani A, Pavia D, Agnew JE, Clarke SW. The effect of unproductive coughing/FET on regional mucus movement in the human lungs. Respir Med 1991; 85(suppl A):23–26.

27. Scherer PW. Mucus transport by cough. Chest 1981; 80:830–833.

28. Bateman JR, Newman SP, Daunt KM, Sheahan NF, Pavia D, Clarke SW. Is cough as effective as chest physiotherapy in the removal of excessive tracheobronchial secretions? Thorax 1981; 36:683–687.

29. Mead J, Turner JM, Macklem PT, Little JB. Significance of the relationship between lung recoil and maximum expiratory flow. J Appl Physiol 1967; 22:95–108.

30. van der Schans CP, Ramirez OE, Postma DS, Koeter GH, Rubin BK. Effect of airway constriction on the cough transportability of mucus [abstr]. Am J Respir Crit Care Med 1994; 149:A1023.

31. Young S, Abdul Sattar N, Caric D. Glottic closure and high flows are not essential for productive cough. Bull Eur Physiopathol Respir 1987; 23(suppl 10):11s-17s.

32. Zahm JM, King M, Duvivier C, Pierrot D, Girod S, Puchelle E. Role of simulated repetitive coughing in mucus clearance. Eur Respir J 1991; 4:311–315.

33. van der Schans CP, Piers DA, Beekhuis H, Koeter GH, van der Mark TW, Postma DS. Effect of forced expirations on mucus clearance in patients with chronic airflow obstruction: effect of lung recoil pressure. Thorax 1990; 45:623–627.

34. Webber BA, Pryor JA. Physiotherapy skills: techniques and adjuncts. In: Webber BA, Pryor JA, eds. Physiotherapy for Respiratory and Cardiac Problems. London: Churchill Livingstone, 1993.

35. Pryor JA, Webber BA, Hodson ME, Batten JC. Evaluation of the forced expiration technique as an adjunct to postural drainage in treatment of cystic fibrosis. BMJ 1979; 2:417–418.

36. Sutton PP, Parker RA, Webber BA, Newman SP, Garland N, Lopez Vidriero MT, et al. Assessment of the forced expiration technique, postural drainage and directed coughing in chest physiotherapy. Eur J Respir Dis 1983; 64:62–68.

37. White D, Stiller K, Willson K. The role of thoracic expansion exercises during the active cycle of breathing techniques. Physiother Theory Pract 1997; 13:155–162.

38. van der Schans CP, de Jong W, Kort E, Wijkstra PJ, Postma DS, van der Mark TW. Mouth pressures during pursed lip breathing. Physiother Theory Pract 1995; 11:29–34.

39. van der Schans CP, de Jong W, de Vries G, Postma DS, Koeter GH, van der Mark TW. Respiratory muscle activity and pulmonary function during acutely induced airways obstruction. Physiother Res Int 1997; 2:167–177.

40. van der Schans CP, de Jong W, de Vries G, Postma DS, Koeter GH, van der Mark TW. Effect of positive expiratory pressure on breathing pattern in healthy subjects. Eur Respir J 1993; 6:60–66.

41. van der Schans CP, de Jong W, de Vries G, Kaan WA, Postma DS, Koeter GH, et al. Effects of positive expiratory pressure breathing during exercise in patients with COPD. Chest 1994; 105:782–789.

42. Mueller RE, Petty TL, Filley GF. Ventilation and arterial blood gas changes induced by pursed lips breathing. J Appl Physiol 1970; 28:784–789.
43. Tiep BL, Burns M, Kao D, Madison R, Herrera J. Pursed lips breathing training using ear oximetry. Chest 1986; 90:218–221.
44. Thoman RL, Stoker GL, Ross JC. The efficacy of pursed-lips breathing in patients with chronic obstructive pulmonary disease. Am Rev Respir Dis 1966; 93:100–106.
45. Breslin EH. The pattern of respiratory muscle recruitment during pursed-lip breathing. Chest 1992; 101:75–78.
46. Wardlaw JM, Fergusson RJ, Tweeddale PM, McHardy GJ. Pursed-lip breathing reduces hyperventilation-induced bronchoconstriction [letter]. Lancet 1987; 1:1483–1484.
47. Chopra SK, Taplin GV, Simmons DH, Robinson GD Jr, Elam D, Coulson A. Effects of hydration and physical therapy on tracheal transport velocity. Am Rev Respir Dis 1977; 115:1009–1014.
48. Wong JW, Keens TG, Wannamaker EM, Douglas PT, Crozier N, Levison H, et al. Effects of gravity on tracheal mucus transport rates in normal subjects and in patients with cystic fibrosis. Pediatrics 1977; 60:146–152.
49. Ross J, Dean E, Abboud RT. The effect of postural drainage positioning on ventilation homogeneity in healthy subjects. Phys Ther 1992; 72:794–799.
50. Button BM, Heine RG, Catto Smith AG, Phelan PD, Olinsky A. Postural drainage and gastro-oesophageal reflux in infants with cystic fibrosis. Arch Dis Child 1997; 76:148–150.
51. Button BM, Heine RG, Catto-Smith AG, Phelan PD. Postural drainage in cystic fibrosis: is there a link with gastro-oesophageal reflux? J Paediatr Child Health 1998; 34:330–334.
52. Lannefors L, Wollmer P. Mucus clearance with three chest physiotherapy regimes in cystic fibrosis: a comparison between postural drainage, PEP and physical exercise. Eur Respir J 1992; 5:748–753.
53. Hansen LG, Warwick WJ, Hansen KL. Mucus transport mechanisms in relation to the effect of high frequency chest compression (HFCC) on mucus clearance. Pediatr Pulmonol 1994; 17:113–118.
54. App EM, Kieselmann R, Reinhardt D, Lindemann H, Dasgupta B, King M, et al. Sputum rheology changes in cystic fibrosis lung disease following two different types of physiotherapy: flutter versus autogenic drainage. Chest 1998; 114:171–177.
55. Campbell AH, O'Connell JM, Wilson F. The effect of chest physiotherapy upon the FEV1 in chronic bronchitis. Med J Aust 1975; 1:33–35.
56. Wollmer P, Ursing K, Midgren B, Eriksson L. Inefficiency of chest percussion in the physical therapy of chronic bronchitis. Eur J Respir Dis 1985; 66:233–239.
57. Zidulka A, Chrome JF, Wight DW, Burnett S, Bonnier L, Fraser R. Clapping or percussion causes atelectasis in dogs and influences gas exchange. J Appl Physiol 1989; 66:2833–2838.
58. Pryor JA, Parker RA, Webber BA. A comparison of mechanical and manual percussion as adjuncts to postural drainage in the treatment of cystic fibrosis in adolescents and adults. Physiotherapy 1981; 67:140–141.
59. van der Schans CP, Piers DA, Postma DS. Effect of manual percussion on tracheo-

bronchial clearance in patients with chronic airflow obstruction and excessive tracheobronchial secretion. Thorax 1986; 41:448–452.

60. Sutton PP, Lopez Vidriero MT, Pavia D, Newman SP, Clay MM, Webber B, et al. Assessment of percussion, vibratory-shaking and breathing exercises in chest physiotherapy. Eur J Respir Dis 1985; 66:147–152.

61. Flower KA, Eden RI, Lomax L, Mann NM, Burgess J. New mechanical aid to physiotherapy in cystic fibrosis. BMJ 1979; 2:630–631.

62. Chang HK, Weber ME, King M. Mucus transport by high-frequency nonsymmetrical oscillatory airflow. J Appl Physiol 1988; 65:1203–1209.

63. King M, Phillips DM, Zidulka A, Chang HK. Tracheal mucus clearance in high-frequency oscillation. II: Chest wall versus mouth oscillation. Am Rev Respir Dis 1984; 130:703–706.

64. King M, Zidulka A, Phillips DM, Wight D, Gross D, Chang HK. Tracheal mucus clearance in high-frequency oscillation: effect of peak flow rate bias. Eur Respir J 1990; 3:6–13.

65. Freitag L, Long WM, Kim CS, Wanner A. Removal of excessive bronchial secretions by asymmetric high- frequency oscillations. J Appl Physiol 1989; 67:614–619.

66. van Hengstum M, Festen J, Beurskens C, Hankel M, van den Broek W, Corstens F. No effect of oral high frequency oscillation combined with forced expiration manoeuvres on tracheobronchial clearance in chronic bronchitis. Eur Respir J 1990; 3:14–18.

67. Gallon A. Evaluation of chest percussion in the treatment of patients with copious sputum production. Respir Med 1991; 85:45–51.

68. Schoni MH. Autogenic drainage: a modern approach to physiotherapy in cystic fibrosis. J R Soc Med 1989; 82(suppl 16):32–37.

69. Dab I, Alexander F. The mechanism of autogenic drainage studied with flow volume curves. Monogr Paediatr 1979; 10:50–53.

70. Giles DR, Wagener JS, Accurso FJ, Butler Simon N. Short-term effects of postural drainage with clapping versus autogenic drainage on oxygen saturation and sputum recovery in patients with cystic fibrosis. Chest 1995; 108:952–954.

71. Miller S, Hall DO, Clayton CB, Nelson R. Chest physiotherapy in cystic fibrosis: a comparative study of autogenic drainage and the active cycle of breathing techniques with postural drainage. Thorax 1995; 50:165–169.

72. Pfleger A, Theissl B, Oberwaldner B, Zach MS. Self-administered chest physiotherapy in cystic fibrosis: a comparative study of high-pressure PEP and autogenic drainage. Lung 1992; 170:323–330.

73. Wolff RK, Dolovich MB, Obminski G, Newhouse MT. Effects of exercise and eucapnic hyperventilation on bronchial clearance in man. J Appl Physiol 1977; 43: 46–50.

74. Olséni L, Wollmer P. Mucociliary clearance in healthy men at rest and during exercise. Clin Physiol 1990; 10:381–387.

75. Bilton D, Dodd ME, Abbot JV, Webb AK. The benefits of exercise combined with physiotherapy in the treatment of adults with cystic fibrosis. Respir Med 1992; 86: 507–511.

76. Olseni L, Midgren B, Wollmer P. Mucus clearance at rest and during exercise in patients with bronchial hypersecretion. Scand J Rehabil Med 1992; 24:61–64.

77. Palange P, Forte S, Onorati P, Paravati V, Manfredi F, Serra P, et al. Effect of reduced body weight on muscle aerobic capacity in patients with COPD. Chest 1998; 114:12–18.

78. Palange P, Forte S, Felli A, Galassetti P, Serra P, Carlone S. Nutritional state and exercise tolerance in patients with COPD. Chest 1995; 107:1206–1212.

79. Schols AM, Soeters PB, Dingemans AM, Mostert R, Frantzen PJ, Wouters EF. Prevalence and characteristics of nutritional depletion in patients with stable COPD eligible for pulmonary rehabilitation. Am Rev Respir Dis 1993; 147:1151–1156.

17

High-Frequency Oscillation, PEP, and Flutter

JAMES B. FINK

Aerogen, Inc.
Mountain View, California, U.S.A.

MALCOLM KING

University of Alberta
Edmonton, Alberta, Canada

I. Introduction

In the normal lung, mucociliary activity and coughing are the primary mechanisms of removing secretions from the lung. In disease, changes in viscosity, elasticity and volume of secretions, dyskinesia of the cilia, and instability of the airway reduce the ability to clear secretions from the airway, increasing the risk of exacerbation and infection. A variety of breathing maneuvers and mechanical devices have been used to assist patients in mobilizing secretions from the lower respiratory tract, often designed to augment normal mucus transport mechanisms. Breathing maneuvers such as active-cycle breathing (ACB), forced expiratory technique (FET), huff coughing, and autogenic drainage (AD) have been used alone or with devices providing positive airway pressure (PAP) and high-frequency oscillation of the airway (HFOA) and of the chest wall. The purpose of this chapter is to explore how these maneuvers and devices function, their theoretical benefit, and their clinical benefit in the treatment of patients with cystic fibrosis and other chronic obstructive lung disease.

II. Positive Airway Pressure

PAP, as defined in the AARC Clinical Practice Guideline (1), includes continuous positive airway pressure (CPAP), positive expiratory pressure (PEP), and expiratory positive airway pressure (EPAP), used to mobilize secretions and treat atelectasis. PAP bronchial hygiene techniques have proven to provide effective alternatives to chest physical therapy in expanding the lungs and mobilizing secretions. Evidence suggests that PAP therapy is more effective than incentive spirometry and intermittent positive-pressure breathing (IPPB) in the management of postoperative atelectasis (2,3) and as an adjunct to enhance the benefits of aerosol bronchodilator delivery (4,5). Cough and other airway-clearance techniques are essential components of PAP therapy.

A. Definitions (1)

Continuous positive airway pressure (*CPAP*) is the application of a positive airway pressure to the spontaneously breathing patient during both inspiration and expiration. The patient breathes from a pressurized circuit with a threshold resistor on the expiratory limb of the breathing. CPAP maintains a consistent airway pressure (from 5 to 20 cmH$_2$O) throughout the respiratory cycle. CPAP requires that a relatively high gas flow be available to the patient's airway, sufficient to maintain the desired positive airway pressure.

Expiratory positive airway pressure (*EPAP*) applies positive pressure to the airway, much like CPAP, but only during expiration. Unlike CPAP, patients generate subatmospheric pressures on inspiration to take a breath. During EPAP therapy the patient exhales against a threshold resistor, generating preset pressures of 5 to 20 cmH$_2$O.

Positive expiratory pressure (*PEP*) consists of positive pressure generated as a patient exhales through a fixed-orifice resistor generating pressures ranging from 10 to 20 cmH$_2$O (although pressures up to 60 cmH$_2$O have been reported). The fixed-orifice resistor, which differentiates PEP from EPAP, generates pressure only when expired flows are high enough to generate backpressure through the small orifice. EPAP, utilizing a threshold resistor, does not produce the same mechanical or physiological effects that PEP does with a fixed orifice. Further study is required to determine how these differences affect clinical outcome.

Threshold resistors, in theory, exert a predictable, quantifiable, and constant force at the expiratory limb of a circuit. When the force is applied over a unit area, a constant threshold pressure is established. A pressure exceeding threshold opens the valve and allows expiration, while pressures below threshold allow the valve to close, sealing the circuit and stopping the flow of gas. A true threshold resistor will maintain constant pressure in the circuit, independent of changing flow rates. Relatively few CPAP devices are *true* threshold resistors, in that they offer flow-dependent resistance once the valve is open so that pressure varies secondary to changes in flow rates, resulting in increased resistance and work of breathing.

B. Types of Resistors (6)

Underwater seal: The expiratory limb of the circuit is submerged under water. The height of the water above the terminal end of the expiratory limb (cmH_2O) corresponds to the threshold pressure generated (Figure 1a). A variant of the underwater seal is the water column, in which the threshold pressure is generated from a column of water above a diaphragm directly above the expiratory limb of the circuit. The pressure in the circuit must be greater than the pressure of the water to raise the diaphragm and allow gas to exit. In this device, threshold pressure is a product of water-column height and the surface area of the diaphragm.

Weighted ball: A precision ground ball of a specific weight is set above a calibrated orifice immediately above the expiratory limb of the circuit, in a housing with expiratory ports. If the diameter of the orifice is not the narrowest point in the expiratory limb of the circuit, the weight of the ball determines the threshold pressure. Weighted-ball systems require meticulous attention to vertical orientation to maintain consistent pressures (Figure 1b).

Spring-loaded valve: A spring holds a disk or diaphragm down over the end of the expiratory limb of the circuit. The force of the spring must be overcome for gas to leave the circuit. The function of the spring-loaded valve is independent of position (Figure 1c).

Magnetic valve: A bar magnet attracts a ferromagnetic disk to seat on the outlet orifice. As pressure exceeds the attraction of the magnet, the disk is displaced, allowing gas to exit the circuit. The greater the distance between the magnet and the disk, the lower the pressure required for gas to leave the circuit.

Fixed-orifice resistor: A restricted opening of a fixed size is placed at the end of the expiratory limb of a breathing circuit. As gas reaches the restricted orifice, turbulence and airway resistance result in increased pressure within the circuit. For any given gas flow, the smaller the orifice, the higher the pressure generated. Expiratory pressure is flow-dependent, so as flow decreases, pressure decreases. With this device there is no "threshold" pressure to be overcome before gas can exit the system. In fact, no pressure is generated until expiratory flow is high enough to create turbulence upon exiting through the orifice (Figure 1d).

The fixed-orifice resistor was in large part abandoned by the critical care community more than 20 years ago because of concerns that high pressures could be generated with changing flows (i.e., coughing). However, the pressure generated with the fixed-orifice resistor during a cough has not been shown to

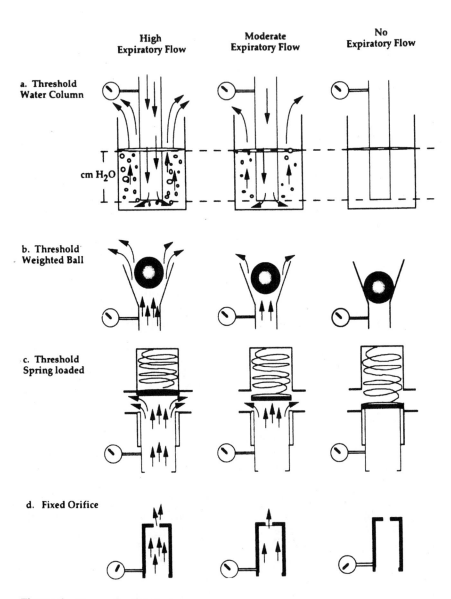

Figure 1 Types of resistors.

be greater than that of a normal cough against a closed glottis, and no adverse effects have been associated with its use.

B.   Rationale (7)

Pursed-lips breathing is a simple procedure that many patients with chronic obstructive lung disease have taught themselves to relieve air-trapping caused by collapse of unstable airways during expiration (Figure 2). It is believed that the resistance at the mouth during a pursed-lips exhalation transmits backpressure to splint open the airways, preventing compression and premature closure

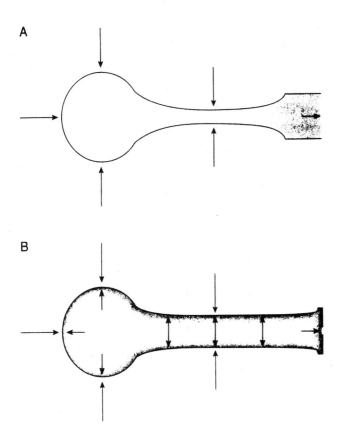

Figure 2   (A) Forces that compress and close unstable airways during forced expiration. (B) The use of positive airway pressure to splint open the airway during expiration. (From Ref. 7.)

(much like the fixed-orifice resistor) (8,9). As an instinctive adaptation to disease, pursed-lips breathing represents a functional predecessor to many of our modern strategies of applying PEP to the airway.

In 1936, Poulton and Odon (10) described the use of the positive-pressure mask for the treatment of congestive heart failure and cardiogenic pulmonary edema. One year later, Barach et al. (11) reported the use of "continuous positive pressure breathing" (CPPB) by mask in patients suffering from respiratory obstruction and pulmonary edema. At that time, the positive-pressure mask did not find application for the treatment or prophylaxis of postoperative pulmonary complications. Thirty years later, Cheney et al. (12) described improvements in PaO_2 following the application of expiratory resistance in anesthetized patients on mechanical ventilation and speculated that this was caused by reversing alveolar collapse. In the late 1960s, articles by Ashbaugh and colleagues (13) established the concept of positive end-expiratory pressure (PEEP) as a technique to improve oxygenation in acute respiratory failure (ARF) and adult respiratory distress syndrome (ARDS). In 1971, Gregory et al. (14) reported a significant reduction in mortality when CPAP was used to treat respiratory distress syndrome of the neonate, leading to its widespread application in the newborn population.

Further research (15–17) established that PEEP and CPAP can be effective in reducing the alveolar-arterial oxygen difference ($A\text{-}aDO_2$) and right-to-left intrapulmonary shunt, increasing functional residual capacity (FRC) in the intubated patient with ARF with or without mechanical ventilation. In 1979 Andersen et al. (18) showed that reinflation of collapsed excised human lungs could be accomplished with CPAP by mechanisms involving collateral ventilation and noted that CPAP "has a potential secretion clearing effect in that pressure is built distal to an obstruction." The following year Andersen and Jespersen (19) made castings of human lungs, identified communications between intersegmental respiratory bronchioles, and concluded that collateral ventilation might be of importance in normal lung function.

The prophylactic and therapeutic use of CPAP and PEEP in nonintubated patients did not receive much attention until the early 1980s (20,21). In 1980, Andersen et al. (22) conducted a prospective, randomized, controlled clinical trial using a sequential-analysis design to determine the effect of conventional therapy versus conventional therapy plus periodic CPAP by mask in the treatment of 24 surgical patients with atelectasis. CPAP was given each hour for 25–35 breaths, with a pressure averaging 15 cmH_2O. At 12 hours, patients in the CPAP group exhibited significantly greater improvement (PaO_2 and radiographic findings) than the control group. This study prompted Pontoppidan (23) to consider periodic CPAP as a tool for treatment of postoperative pulmonary complications. Several studies during the early 1980s explored the application of PEEP and CPAP in different fashions to nonintubated patients with varying results (24–29), including comparisons of mask CPAP with incentive spirometry, deep breathing and coughing (DBC), and IPPB. As more effective strategies were developed, Stock et al. (28,29) concluded that intermittent mask CPAP was as effective as incentive spirometry or DBC in return of pulmonary function following thoracic or upper-abdominal surgery. Additionally, the authors suggested that mask CPAP might be preferable, as it represented a more effortless, painless type of postoperative respiratory care.

Ricksten et al. (3) performed a randomized comparative study that looked at postoperative complications in 43 upper-abdominal-surgery patients. A-aDO$_2$, PEF, and forced vital capacity (FVC) in patients using either CPAP or PEP were compared with measurements in a control group using incentive spirometry. All three groups took 30 breaths each hour while awake for 3 days postoperatively. Although peak flow did not change between groups, FVC was greater in the CPAP and PEP groups. A-aDO$_2$ increased uniformly for all groups for the first 24 hours, but then decreased in the CPAP and PEP groups (being insignificantly lower in the PEP group). Atelectatasis was observed in 6/15 patients in the control group, 1/13 in the CPAP group, and 0/15 in the PEP group. The authors concluded that periodic PEP and CPAP are superior to deep-breathing exercises with respect to gas exchange, preservation of lung volumes, and prevention of postoperative atelectasis following upper-abdominal surgery. They also concluded that "the simple and commercially available PEP mask is as effective as the more complicated CPAP system." A simple PEP system as described earlier certainly represents a cost savings over the use of a more complex CPAP system, which requires a gas flow that will not change FIO$_2$ in response to backpressure, pressure monitor, and oxygen analyzer.

Lindner et al. (30), in a randomized study of 34 upper-abdominal-surgery patients, compared postoperative physiotherapy with postoperative physiotherapy plus mask CPAP. Their findings indicated that the group treated with physiotherapy plus CPAP had a more rapid recovery of vital capacity and FRC with fewer pulmonary complications. Campbell et al. (31) randomized 71 abdominal-surgery patients into group 1 (breathing exercises and huff coughing) and group 2 (same as group 1 plus PAP using a water-column threshold resistor adjusted to produce pressures of 5–15 cmH$_2$O with the patient exhaling through a mouthpiece). There were no differences in pulmonary function between the two groups, and the difference in respiratory complications—31% in group 1, 22% in group 2—was not statistically significant. The authors concluded that PEP could serve as an adjunct to routine chest physiotherapy, particularly with postoperative smokers, in that 43% of the smokers in their study developed respiratory complications, compared with none of the nonsmokers ($p < 0.01$).

By preventing expiratory collapse, PEP is thought to facilitate a more homogeneous distribution of ventilation throughout the lung, via these collateral interbronchiolar channels (86). Groth et al. (32), measuring lung function from the expiratory port of the PEP mask in 12 cystic fibrosis patients, found a significant change in FRC ($p < 0.02$), decrease in volume of trapped gas ($p < 0.05$), and decrease of washout volume ($p < 0.05$), as compared with pretreatment measurements. They concluded that the changes were attributed to an improvement in the distribution of ventilation (more evenly within the lung) and the opening up of airways otherwise closed off during normal ventilation. In contrast, van der Schans and colleagues (33) reported that use of a 5- and 15-cmH_2O threshold resistor for 2 minutes increased FRC from 2.6 to 3.6 and 4.4 L, respectively, and total lung capacity from 5.1 to 5.9 and 6.9 L (Figure 3). These lung volumes returned to baseline immediately. They also found that use of threshold resistor did not influence mucus clearance.

Because a patient must breathe down to subatmospheric pressures on inspiration, both EPAP and PEP are believed to require higher work of breathing than CPAP. Van der Schans et al. (34) examined the effect of EPAP with 5 cmH_2O using a threshold resistor (Vital Signs) in eight COPD patients measuring work of breathing and myoelectrical activity of the scalene, parasternal, and abdominal muscles. During EPAP breathing at rest, mean W_{sp} increased from 0.54 to 1.08 J/L. Expired minute volume decreased from 12.4 to 10.5 L/min and V_d/V_T decreased from 0.39 to 0.34. Increased phasic respiratory muscle activity was increased with EPAP. Dyspnea sensation during exercise test was higher than during the test with undisturbed breathing. It is unclear whether the fixed-orifice resistor, more commonly associated with PEP, would have the same effect.

McIlwaine and associates (35) randomly assigned 40 patients, ages 6 to 17 years, to perform CPT or PEP therapy for a 1-year period. CPT consisted of five or six postural drainage positions, with percussion for 3 to 5 minutes each, followed by deep-breathing exercises combined with vibration on expiration, forced expirations, and vigorous coughing. These 30-minute sessions were repeated twice daily. PEP, as described by Falk, was performed with a fixed-orifice resistor (Astra Meditec); with the patient in a sitting position, 15 tidal breaths with slightly active expiration were taken through the device (approximately 2 minutes). The patient then performed two or three forced expiratory maneuvers, followed by cough, and a 1–2-minute period of relaxed controlled breathing. This sequence was repeated six times in a 20-minute session. In the CPT group, all parameters of pulmonary function declined, similar to the rate of decline reported by Reisman et al. (36) for CPT (FEV_1 −1.9% predicted per year). In contrast, the PEP group had positive changes in FEV_1 ($p = 0.02$) and FVC ($p = 0.02$), improving from baseline in all parameters (FVC, +6.57%; FEV_1, +5.98%; FEF_{25-75}, +3.3%). This has been the most convincing study to date that PEP may be superior to standard CPT.

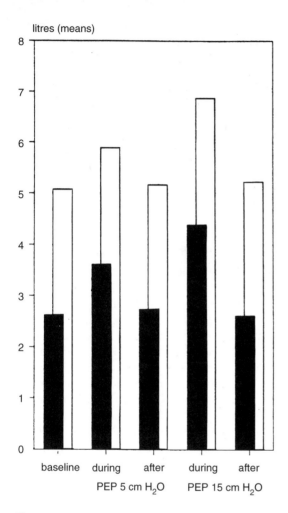

Figure 3 Thoracic gas volume at functional residual capacity (solid bars) and at total lung capacity (hatched bars) during baseline, during, and after 2 minutes of PEP 5 cmH_2O, and during and after 2 minutes of PEP 15 cmH_2O. PEP = positive expiratory pressure breathing. (From Ref. 33.)

C. PEP Administration Techniques (7)

PEP therapy is performed with the subject seated comfortably, elbows resting on a table. Equipment consists of a soft, transparent hand ventilation mask or mouthpiece, T-assembly with a one-way valve, a variety of fixed-orifice resistors (or adjustable expiratory resistor), and a manometer. The mask is applied tightly but comfortably over the mouth and nose. The subject is instructed to relax while performing diaphragmatic breathing, inspiring a volume of air larger than normal tidal volume but not to total lung capacity, through the one-way valve. Exhalation to FRC is active but not forced, through the resistor chosen to achieve a positive airway pressure between 10 and 20 cmH$_2$O (0.98–1.96 kPa) during exhalation.

A series of 10–20 breaths are performed with the mask or mouthpiece in place. The mask or mouthpiece is then removed, and the individual performs several coughs to raise secretions. This sequence of 10–20 PAP breaths followed by huff coughing is repeated four to six times per PEP therapy session. Each session for bronchial hygiene takes from 10 to 20 minutes, and may be performed one to four times a day as needed. For lung expansion, patients should be encouraged to take 10–20 breaths every hour while awake.

D. PEP Administration Considerations

Selection of a resistor with an appropriate orifice size is critical to proper technique. The therapeutic goal of exhalation is to achieve a PEP between 10 and 20 cmH$_2$O, with an inspiratory-to-expiratory ratio (I:E) of 1:3 to 1:4. When using a fixed orifice, most adults achieve this pressure range utilizing a flow-restricting orifice 2.5–4.0 mm in diameter. Selection of the proper resistor also produces the desired of 1:3 to 1:4. A manometer is placed in-line to measure the expiratory pressure while selecting the appropriate size of orifice. Once the proper resistor orifice has been determined, the manometer can be removed from the system. Selection of a resistor with too large an orifice produces a short exhalation, with failure to achieve the proper expiratory pressure. Too small an orifice prolongs the expiratory phase, elevates the pressure above 20 cmH$_2$O, and increases the work of breathing. Performing a PEP session for more than 20 minutes may lead to fatigue. During periods of exacerbation, individuals are encouraged to increase the frequency with which PEP is performed, rather than extending the length of individual sessions.

E. Aerosol Administration with PAP

Aerosol therapy may be done simultaneously with or just prior to a PEP session, either by hand-held nebulizer or metered-dose inhaler (MDI) (Table 1). Andersen and Klausen (4) applied facemask PEEP while administering nebulized bronchodilators to eight patients with severe bronchospasm. A randomized crossover design was used, with each patient subjected to two PEEP treatments and two control treatments with zero end-expiratory pressure (ZEEP), at intervals of 3 hours between each treatment. FEV$_1$, FVC, and peak flow improved significantly following PEEP treatments ($p < 0.05$). They concluded that PEEP

Table 1 Procedures for PAP Administration

1. Explain that PAP therapy is used to re-expand lung tissue and help mobilize secretions. Patients should also be taught to perform the "huff"-directed cough procedure.
2. Instruct the patient to:
   a. Sit comfortably
   b. If using a mask, apply it tightly but comfortably over the nose and mouth. If mouthpiece is used, place lips firmly around it and breathe through mouth.
   c. Take in a breath that is larger than normal, but don't fill lungs completely.
   d. Exhale actively, but not forcefully, creating a positive airway pressure of 10–20 cmH$_2$O during exhalation (determined with manometer during initial therapy sessions). Length of inhalation should be approximately 1/3 of the total breathing cycle (I:E ratio of 1:3).
   e. Perform 10–20 breaths.
   f. Remove the mask or mouthpiece and perform two to three Huff coughs, and rest as needed.
   g. Repeat above cycle four to eight times, not to exceed 20 minutes.
   h. When patients are also receiving bronchodilator aerosol, administer in conjunction with PAP therapy by placing a holding chamber/MDI or nebulizer at the inspiratory port of the PAP device.

improved the efficacy of bronchodilator administration, probably mediated through a better distribution to the peripheral airways.

Frischknecht-Christensen et al. (5) examined the effect of PEP mask applied in conjunction with beta$_2$-agonists administered via MDI with spacer. In a randomized crossover study, eight patients alternately received treatments of two puffs of terbutaline MDI without PEP, terbutaline MDI with PEP, and placebo MDI with PEP. Results showed statistically significant ($p < 0.0001$) improvement in PEF when terbutaline was taken in conjunction with facemask PEP of 10–15 cmH$_2$O. Mahlmeister et al. (7) described the use of an MDI and chamber-style adapter with the Resistex system (Mercury Medical, Clearwater, FL), which accepts a spacer device on the distal inspiratory limb of the PEP assembly.

Although no absolute contraindications to the use of PAP therapies have been reported, common sense dictates that patients with acute sinusitis, ear infection, epistaxis, or recent facial, oral, or skull injury or surgery should be carefully evaluated before a decision is made to initiate PEP mask therapy. Patients who are experiencing active hemoptysis or those with unresolved pneumothorax should avoid using PAP therapy until these acute pulmonary problems have resolved. Complications such as barotrauma or hemodynamic compromise are intuitive with the use of positive pressure; no complications have been reported when PEP mask therapy has been used for lung expansion or secretion clearance, in large part due to the techniques involved in the therapy and the patient population.

In that some authors have used different terms to describe PAP options, Figure 4 shows the difference in pressure patterns generated with CPAP, EPAP (threshold resistors), Flutter, and PEP with fixed-orifice resistor. Further studies are required to better understand the differences in effect of these three types of modalities.

III. High-Frequency Oscillation

High-frequency oscillation (HFO) of the air column in the conducting airways is employed in a variety of techniques designed to enhance clearance of secretions. HFO can be generated by devices providing the oscillations at the airway opening or on the chest wall. The oscillations can administered to the patient, or can be self-generated by expiration through an oscillatory device. HFOs can influence mucus clearance through a variety of mechanisms, including alteration of mucus rheology, enhanced mucus–airflow interaction, and reflex mechanisms.

Pavia and associates (37) studied the effect of an electrically driven vibrating pad at frequencies of 29 to 49 Hz in patients with chronic bronchitis in a reclining body position, and found only a nonsignificant trend to greater clearance and sputum production. King and associates (38) examined the effects of high-frequency chest-wall oscillation applied by means of a pneumatic cuff system driven by a piston pump at frequencies from 3 to 17 Hz. In nine anesthetized dogs, they found that the tracheal mucus clearance rate (TMCR) was acutely increased at all frequencies except 3 Hz. The enhancement of TMCR was most pronounced between 11 and 15 Hz, reaching a peak of 340% of control at 13 Hz. In 1984, King et al. (39) reported a comparison of tracheal mucus clearance rate in eight anesthetized dogs during spontaneous breathing, HFO via the airway opening (AO), and HFO via the chest wall (CW). TMCR was increased to 240% of control with HFO/CW, while with HFO/AO, TMCR was less than or equal to control. In a separate experiment (40), HFO/CW enhanced both peripheral and central mucus clearance in dogs, as determined by radioaerosol clearance, and was found to be safe when moderate pressures were applied. These early experiments on chest-wall oscillation established the basis for the development of the Advanced Respiratory Vest® for mucus-clearance physiotherapy in cystic fibrosis.

Rubin et al. (41) found that a commercial percussor at 40 Hz produced a mean maximum expiratory flow rate of 0.25 L/s in dogs, with no measurable

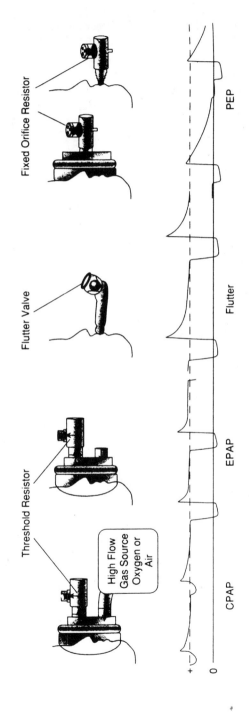

Figure 4 Comparison of pressure waveforms, continuous positive airway pressure (CPAP), expiratory positive airway pressure (EPAP), positive expiratory pressure (PEP), and Flutter.

effect on tracheal mucus velocity (TMV). An experimental oscillator using an unbiased sine wave at 13 Hz increased TMV to 204% of control ($p < 0.003$) when the power level was sufficient to produce flows of 2–3 L/s.

Freitag et al. (42) studied the effects of expiratory bias, inspiratory bias, and posture on the rate of mucus clearance on anesthetized sheep. Applying HFO at 14 Hz with asymmetrical waveforms (e.g., PEF 3.8 L/s, peak inspiratory flow 1.3 L/s), they found that mucus clearance in the horizontal position with expiratory biased HFO was 3.5 mL/10 min, in the head-down tilt position without HFO it was 3.1 mL/10 min, and in combination was 11.0 mL/10 min. No clearance occurred with inspiratory bias, even in the head-down position.

The role of orally applied airflow oscillations on secretion clearance remains less clear. George and colleagues (43) found an increase in mucociliary clearance in normal man induced by HFO, with the time required for 90% clearance of a radiolabeled aerosol decreasing from 4 hr 50 min to 3 hr 43 min during HFO ($p < 0.05$). In contrast, van Hengstum et al. (44) reported no effect of oral HFO combined with forced expiration maneuvers on tracheobronchial clearance in eight patients with chronic bronchitis. Comparing 30-minute sessions of FET with huff, CPT in six positions, and breathing exercises with HFOA at 9.25 to 25 Hz, and control with huff only, they found that FET was more effective for radioaerosol clearance than HFOA or control. Further studies need to be carried out.

Shearing at the air–mucus interface could be a significant factor in the enhanced tracheal mucus clearance during HFO (45). HFO has been found to reduce the apparent viscosity of sputum in vitro (46), and it has been demonstrated that a decrease in mechanical impedance (the vectorial sum of elasticity and viscosity) of mucus has a positive effect on clearance induced by in vitro simulated cough. Dasgupta and colleagues (47) demonstrated that airflow oscillations applied to CF sputum at frequencies similar to those used in physiotherapy reduced viscoelasticity with increasing oscillation time. This was also true for mucus gel simulants exposed to airflow oscillations at 0, 12, and 22 Hz; the higher the applied frequency, the greater the reduction in viscoelasticity (48). Although the mechanism for the reduction in viscoelasticity is unknown, likely possibilities involve the cooperative unfolding of the physical entanglements between the primary network of mucus glycoproteins and other structural macromolecules, the rupture of cross-linking bonds such as disulfide bridges, or the fragmentation of larger molecules such as DNA of F-actin, which are present as a byproduct of infection and can increase mucus viscoelasticity owing to their interactions with glycoproteins (49).

A variety of devices utilize HFO to mobilize secretions. In the case of the commercially available devices that apply HFOs to the airway, application of positive airway pressure appears to be a common attribute. In evaluating the benefit of these devices it is difficult to isolate the role of HFO and PAP.

IV. Flutter Valve

Developed in Switzerland by VarioRaw SA, the Flutter® mucus clearance device combines the techniques of PAP with high-frequency oscillations at the airway opening (HFao). A pipe-shaped device with a steel ball in the "bowl" is loosely covered by a perforated cap (Figure 4). The weight of the ball serves as an EPAP device (at approximately 10 cmH$_2$O) while the internal shape of the bowl allows the ball to flutter, generating oscillations of about 15 Hz (2–32 Hz), varying with the position of the device. The proposed mechanism of effect includes shearing of mucus from the airway wall by oscillatory action, stabilization of airways preventing early airway closure, facilitation of cephalad flow of mucus, and changes in mucus rheology.

Although the Flutter has been available in Europe for many years, little has been published on its efficacy (50,51). In 1994, Konstan and coworkers (52) reported that the amount of sputum expectorated by 18 patients with cystic fibrosis was more than three times the amount expectorated with either voluntary cough (described as vigorous cough every 2 minutes for 15 minutes) or postural drainage (up to 10 positions in 15 minutes). These findings merit additional scrutiny in that patients in the study continued to receive their regular chest physiotherapy throughout the 2-week period, so the study only looked at measured sputum from an extra therapy session each day (53). Patients with CF (and other COPD) tend to have their airways close prematurely during vigorous cough (rather than FET, Huff, or ACB), resulting in trapped gas and secretions. National guidelines suggest that effective postural drainage requires somewhere between 3 and 10 minutes per position (54), so those 10 drainage positions would require between 30 and 100 minutes to provide effective results. It appears that neither the cough nor the postural-drainage legs of the protocol were designed in light of available research to provide optimal results.

Later in 1994, Pryor et al. (55), studying 24 CF patients who averaged >11.9 g of sputum per day using ACB as their standard bronchial hygiene, reported that ACB alone resulted in significantly more sputum production than 10 minutes of Flutter followed by ACB. The authors expressed concern about the possibility of increased sputum retention when the Flutter was used.

Homnick et al. (56) studied 24 CF patients (age 8 to 44 years) during hospitalization for acute exacerbation, assigned to receive standard CPT or supervised Flutter four times a day. Significant improvements were noted from admission to discharge within each group. No significant differences were found in clinical score or pulmonary function tests between CPT and Flutter from hospital admission to discharge. Similarly, Padman et al. (57) compared Flutter, EPAP, and CPT in CF patients. In 6 of 15 patients who completed the study, they found no significant differences in PFT or assessment parameters, but reported a patient preference for Flutter.

Oscillations are capable of decreasing mucus viscoelasticity at frequencies and amplitudes achievable with the Flutter device. App et al. (58) evaluated AD and Flutter in 14 CF patients using a crossover design, with a separate 4-week course of therapy with either AD or Flutter. Overall, significant changes in FVC, FEV_1, or sputum volume were noted. At the end of the study, both groups showed a 6% improvement in FVC (nonsignificant), and there was a nonsignificant increase in sputum production during Flutter use. Sputum viscoelasticity was significantly lower ($p < 0.01$) with Flutter therapy than with AD. The mucus rheology changes are shown in Figure 5. App et al. also reported in vitro results that the elasticity of CF sputum samples, as measured by a filancemeter, was decreased by 19-Hz oscillations, generated by a Flutter device for 15 and 30 minutes, with a mean airflow velocity of 1.5 L/s.

Weiner and coworkers (59) compared use of Flutter with sham treatment in a comparative study of 20 COPD patients. After 3 months, FVC, FEV_1, and 12-minute walk increased in the treatment group and was unchanged in the sham group. The authors reported an improvement in COPD symptoms in the Flutter group compared with baseline ($p < 0.05$). Nakamura and Kawakami (60) reported similar findings in a group of COPD patients. Girard and Terki (61) studied patients suffering from hyperproductive asthma with a hypersensitivity to Ascaris as a major allergen; using Flutter for 5×5 min daily for 30–45 days, they reported objective and subjective improvement in 18 of 20 patients.

To better understand how this device compares to other PAP devices, Fink (62) compared the Flutter valve with both threshold resistors and fixed-orifice resistors to determine effects on the airway in vitro. Pressure patterns, peak expiratory flows (PEFR, L/min), peak expiratory pressure (P_{exp}, cmH_2O), mean airway pressures (MAP, cmH_2O), work of breathing (W_{pt}, Joule/L), and changes in residual volume (RV, mL above baseline) during passive exhalation (V_T 500 mL, PIF 40 L/min) were measured using a test lung with a compliance of 0.02 cmH_2O/L. The results with the Flutter valve, two levels of threshold resistor, and two sizes of fixed-orifice resistor are shown in Table 2.

FACING PAGE

Figure 5 A Mucus rheology changes for sputum samples collected after autogenic drainage (AD) and Flutter therapy after an acute session at the beginning and end of 4 weeks of therapy, followed by a crossover period to the opposite therapy. The rheological measurements were made using a magnetic microrheometer at a measuring frequency of 1 or 100 rad/s. Sputum viscoelasticity is reported as log G*, an index of rigidity. (From Ref. 58.) B Mucus-clearability indices for sputum samples collected after AD and Flutter therapy, as in Figure 5A, The clearance indices (MCI-mucociliary clearability index; CCI-cough clearability index) were calculated from the sputum viscoelastic data. (From Ref. 58.)

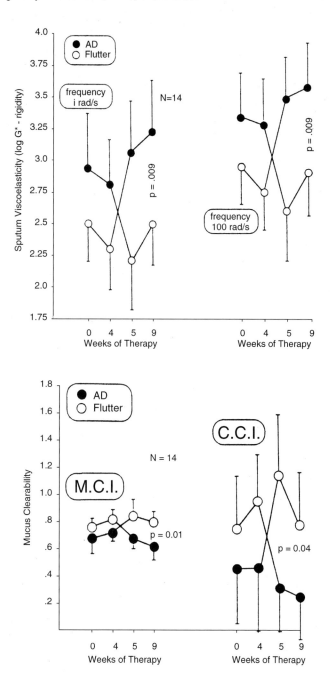

Table 2 Comparison of Devices' Effects on the Airway In Vitro

	PEFR	P_{exp}	EPAP	W(pt)	MAP	RV
Flutter	27.1	18.8	8.4	1.406	7.5	450
Threshold resistor						
10 cmH$_2$O	39	15.5	7.5	1.255	6.6	450
15 cmH$_2$O	40	20.6	12.5	1.694	9.9	700
Fixed-orifice resistor						
4.0 mm	23.7	9.5	00.3	0.738	0.8	0
3.0 mm	13.4	10.2	0.3	0.714	1.6	0

The Flutter developed lower PEFR than the threshold resistor but higher flows than the fixed-orifice resistor. In all other respects the Flutter resembled the threshold resistor (Figure 4). The fixed-orifice resistor developed lower peak flows, peak and mean airway pressures, work of breathing, and residual volume than either of the threshold resistors or the Flutter ($p < 0.001$).

EPAP requires greater work of breathing than CPAP (63) (Table 3). In this laboratory study, both the Flutter and threshold resistors produced a greater measured work of breathing than the fixed-orifice resistor. It is unclear what the effect of this increased patient work may be in the severely obstructed COPD patient. Clearly CPAP has a role in reducing dyspnea (64,65) while EPAP may not achieve this purpose (at least during exercise) (34). Further, large-scale studies are required to determine the benefits of the Flutter relative to those of the less expensive PAP and breathing-maneuver therapies.

V. Percussionaire

Intermittent percussive ventilation (IPV) of the lungs as a therapeutic form of chest physical therapy has been advanced by Dr. Forrest Bird as a treatment for patients with COPD utilizing a pneumatic device called a Percussionator®. IPV was designed to treat diffuse patchy atelectasis, enhance the mobilization and clearance of retained secretions, and deliver nebulized medications and wetting agents to the distal airways (66). With IPV, the patient breathes through a mouthpiece that delivers high-flow-rate "mini-bursts" at rates of over 200 cycles/minute (Figure 6). During these percussive bursts of gas into the airway, a continuous airway pressure is maintained while the "pulsatile percussive intra-airway pressure" rises progressively. Each percussive cycle is programmed by the patient or clinician, by holding down a thumb button for 5–10 seconds for percussive inspiratory cycle and releasing the button for exhalation. Treatments of approximately 20 minutes are recommended by the manufacturer. Impaction

Table 3 Procedures for Flutter Administration

1. Practitioner will assess whether Flutter therapy is indicated and design a treatment program designed to accomplish treatment objectives.
    a. Practitioner will bring equipment to bedside and provide initial therapy to patient, adjusting pressure settings to meet patient need.
    b. After initial patient treatment and/or training, practitioner will communicate treatment plan to physician and nurse, and provide instruction to nursing staff if required.
2. Explain that Flutter therapy is used to re-expand lung tissue and help mobilize secretions. Patients should also be taught to perform the "Huff" directed cough procedure.
3. Instruct the patient to:
    a. Sit comfortably.
    b. Take in a breath that is larger than normal, but don't fill lungs completely.
    c. Place Flutter mouthpiece in mouth, lips sealed firmly, and exhale actively but not forcefully, holding the flutter valve at an angle that produces maximum oscillation.
    d. Perform 10–20 breaths.
    e. Remove the Flutter mouthpiece and perform two or three huff coughs, and rest as needed.
    f. Repeat above cycle four to eight times, not to exceed 20 minutes.
3. Evaluate the patient for his or her ability to self-administer.
4. When appropriate, teach patient to self-administer. Observations on several occasions of proper technique uncoached should precede allowing the patient to self-administer without supervision.
5. When patients are also receiving bronchodilator aerosol, administer in conjunction with Flutter by administering bronchodilator immediately preceding the Flutter breaths.
6. When visibly soiled, rinse Flutter device with sterile water and shake/air-dry; leave within reach at patient's bedside.
7. Send the Flutter device home with the patient.
8. Document in the patient's medical record procedures performed (including device, number of breaths per treatment, and frequency), response to therapy, patient teaching provided, and ability to self-administer.

pressures of 25 to 40 psig are delivered with a frequency from <100 to 225 percussive cycles/minute at 40 psig. The IPV-2 includes nonoscillatory-demand CPAP and/or oscillatory-demand CPAP with IMV. Clinicians have prescribed the use of IPV through both inspiratory and expiratory cycles.

Natale et al. (67) reported that a single IPV treatment was as effective as standard chest physiotherapy in improving acute pulmonary function and enhancing sputum expectoration in nine cystic fibrosis patients. Homnick et al.

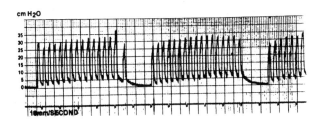

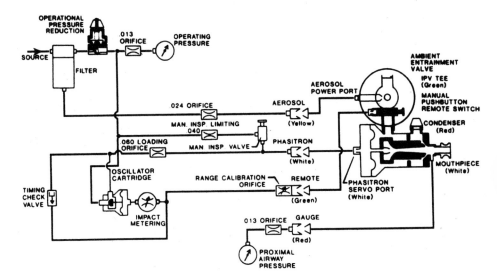

Figure 6 Percussionator (bottom) and waveform (top). (Courtesy of Percussionaire, Sandpoint, ID.)

(68) later undertook a 6-month parallel comparative trial comparing IPV with standard manual chest physiotherapy in accordance with Cystic Fibrosis Foundation guidelines in 16 cystic fibrosis patients (children and adults). They found no significant differences between treatment groups, and concluded that the two methods were comparable. One IPV patient had light hemoptysis during the study.

Newhouse and coworkers (69) compared IPV and Flutter with standard CPT in children and adults with CF. No difference in sputum quantity was found between methods, but transient lower oxygen saturation was found with CPT. Trends to lower lung volumes at 1 and 4 hours postadministration were noted with all three therapies.

Further studies would be valuable in determining the relative merit of IPV in comparison with other lung-expansion/secretion-clearance techniques. With so little published on the use of IPV (70–72), one might assume that contraindications and hazards are similar to those associated with other forms of mechanical ventilation. The manufacturer lists potential side effects as including sore ribs, fatigue, stress, and irritation.

VI. High-Frequency External Chest-Wall Compression

High-frequency chest-wall compression (HFCWC or HFCC) has been shown to increase tracheal mucus-clearance rates and to correlate with improved ventilation in both animal and clinical studies (38–46). HFCWC was originally developed as a means of providing ventilatory support for patients for whom conventional mechanical ventilation was inadequate (73). Because HFCWC was observed to mobilize secretions in anesthetized dogs, its effect on tracheal mucus clearance was studied. King and coworkers (38) reported in 1983 that HFCWC in healthy anesthetized dogs increased the clearance rate of tracheal mucus marker particles by as much as threefold compared with quiet breathing. The enhancement of clearance was also seen in peripheral airways, using inhaled radioaerosols (41). Orally applied high-frequency airflow oscillations had no significant effect on tracheal mucus clearance in the canine model (39).

HFCWC is believed to act via a combination of three possible mechanisms. According to the findings of in vitro experiments (38,47,48), high-frequency airflow oscillations of amplitude comparable to those achieved in vivo are capable of reducing the viscoelastic and cohesive properties of mucus, thus making it more easily clearable by the air–liquid interactions associated with cephalad airflow velocity bias. Second, the high-frequency oscillations may reinforce the interaction with the cilia or the natural harmonics of the cheat wall. Evidence for this comes from the fact that optimal frequencies for clearance by HFCWC are in the range of 13–15 Hz (38). Third, HFCWC may stimulate the release of fresh secretions by a vagal reflex mechanism, the fresh secretions being more easily mobilized by airflow interactions (45).

VII. The Vest

The Vest (Advanced Respiratory, St. Paul, MN) was developed by Warwick and colleagues at the University of Minnesota. The Vest device, designed for self-therapy, consists of a large-volume variable-frequency airpulse delivery system attached to a nonstretchable inflatable vest, which is worn by the patient extending over the entire torso down to the iliac crest. Pressure pulses that fill the vest and vibrate the chest wall are controlled by the patient (with a foot pedal) and applied during expiration or the entire respiratory cycle. Pulse frequency is adjustable from 5 to 25 Hz, with pressure in the vest varying from 28 mmHg at 5 Hz to 39 mmHg at 25 Hz.

In theory, these vibrations to the chest wall cause transient increases in airflow in the lungs, to improve gas–liquid interactions and the movement of mucus. Animal and clinical studies demonstrated that the frequency of oscillations (cycles/second) and flow bias (inspiratory vs. expiratory) are important in determining effectiveness. Flow bias determines whether secretions move upstream or downstream (45). Conjecture that this device has a role in lung expansion for patients other than those with cystic fibrosis in the acute care settings has not been empirically established.

The Vest has been purported to be more effective than postural drainage in secretion clearance on the basis of a limited study in cystic fibrosis patients (74). Kluft and associates (75) studied HFCWC vs. CPT/PD in a crossover trial of 29 cystic fibrosis patients, randomly alternated on a daily basis. Each day consisted of three 30-minute sessions of therapy. Sputum was collected during and 15 minutes post session. For HFCWC, six frequencies (6, 8, 14, 15, 18, and 19 Hz) were applied for 5 minutes each in order of increasing frequency. Each frequency application was followed by a deep breath with huff, with the device turned off, and the patient actively coughed. Patients received nebulized normal saline via a small-volume nebulizer during treatment. CPT/PD included chest percussion with postural drainage of five sites for 2–3 minutes per position, followed by vibration and forced cough. The five positions rotated during each of three session to cover all lobes in 24 hours. The CPT sessions did not include huff and there was no mention of nebulization of saline. Sputum wet and dry weights were determined for each type of therapy. There was significantly more sputum production with HFCWC than with CPT.

Arens et al. (76) studied 50 cystic fibrosis patients randomly assigned to t.i.d. therapy during admission for acute exacerbation. CPT was performed with six positions over 30 minutes (four lying and two sitting, with 4 minutes of percussion with each position). HFCC treatments consisted of six frequencies for 4–5 minutes each. All patients were administered aerosol with albuterol prior (CPT) or during therapy. The 1-hour wet weight of sputum with HFCC was greater than with CPT (14.6 ± 2.9 g vs. 6.0 ± 1.8 g; $p < 0.035$). The authors concluded that HFCC and CPT were equally safe and effective when used during acute exacerbation.

VIII. The Hayek Oscillator

The Hayek Oscillator is an electrically powered, microprocessor-controlled noninvasive oscillator ventilator that utilizes an external flexible chest enclosure (cuirass) to apply negative and positive pressure to the chest wall to deliver noninvasive oscillation to the lungs. The negative pressure generated in the cuirass causes the chest wall to expand for inspiration, while positive pressure compresses the chest to produce a forced expiration. Both inspiratory and expiratory phases may be active and not reliant on passive recoil of the chest. Expiratory pressure can be positive, atmospheric, or negative, allowing ventilation to occur above, at, or below the patient's normal FRC. Several groups have reported success in using this device as a method of ventilatory support (78,79). Four adjustable parameters with the Hayek include frequency range (to 999 oscillations/minute), I:E ratio (6:1–1:6), inspiratory, and pressure (−70 to +70 cmH_2O).

Clinicians' anecdotal observations of "spontaneous expulsion of secretions" (80,81) during high-frequency ventilation has led to development of several discrete secretion-management-program recommendations in which the chest is oscillated through two sets of cycles: several minutes at a high frequency of up to 999 (usually 600/720) cycles per minute at an I:E ratio of 1:1 followed a 60/90 cycles/minute at an I:E ratio of 5:1. Setting can be changed according to the patient's "need." Reports of efficacy of this or similar protocols for secretion management with the Hayek have yet to be published.

Scherer and colleagues (82) reported that HFO applied via the airway or via the chest wall and CPT have comparable augmenting effects on expectorated sputum weight without changing PFTs or oxygen saturation. According to earlier experiments, prerequisites for optimal transport of mucus by air–liquid interaction in a cephalad direction include airflow with an expiratory bias, which needs to be in the range of 1 to 3 L/s, and for airway oscillation an oscillation frequency between 8 and 15 Hz. This was confirmed in the experiment, and high-frequency chest-wall oscillation was found to improve oxygenation and ventilation in patients with normal lungs, patients with respiratory failure, and patients with COPD (Figure 7).

IX. Comparison of Flow, Airway, and Esophageal Pressures

To better understand the relative effects of these devices, a normal volunteer, with an esophageal balloon in place, was asked to breathe in accordance with manufacturers' instructions with a variety of devices. Airway pressures and flow rates were determined with a pneumotachometer placed at the airway using a VenTrak monitor (Novametrix, CT). In Figures 8–14, the upper panel represents flow (L/min) and the lower panel shows airway and esophageal pressures.

Normal tidal breathing (Figure 8): expiratory flow rates up to 40 L/min, esophageal pressures between −6 and −12 cmH_2O. Airway pressure fluctuation

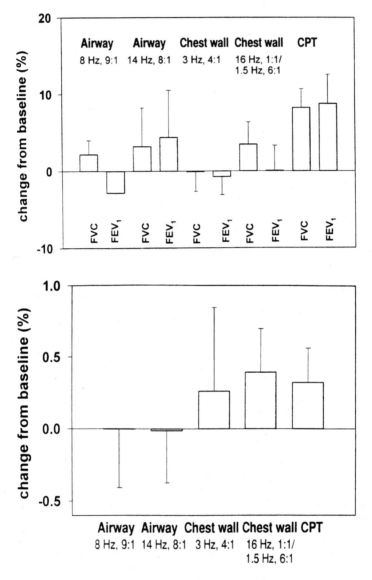

Figure 7 A Effect of airway and chest wall treatments on pulmonary function parameters. Mean changes (±SEM) expressed as percent of baseline. None of the parameters was significantly altered in the treatments. (From Ref. 159.) B Effect of airway and chest wall treatments on oxygen saturation. There were no significant differences among the treatments. (From Ref. 159.)

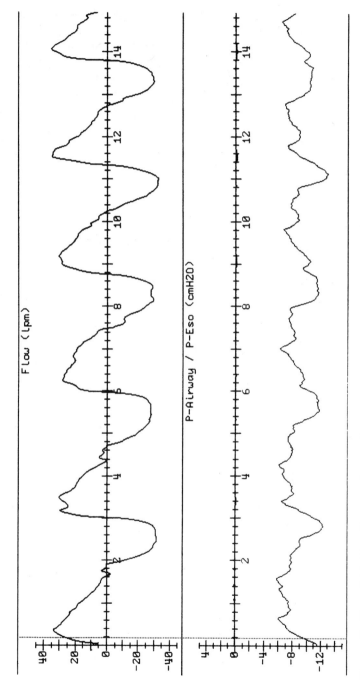

Figure 8 Normal tidal breathing—expiratory flow rates up to 40 L/min, esophageal pressures between −6 and −12 cmH$_2$O. Airway pressure fluctuation less than 1 cmH$_2$O at atmospheric baseline. Esophageal pressures are subatmospheric, with tidal changes between −6 and −12 cmH$_2$O; minor rhythmic fluctuations 0.5 to 2.0 cmH$_2$O occur at a rate of 64/minute and correlate with heart rate.

less than 1 cmH$_2$O at atmospheric baseline. Esophageal pressures are subatmospheric, with tidal changes between −6 and −12 cmH$_2$O; minor rhythmic fluctuations 0.5 to 2.0 cmH$_2$O occur at a rate of 64/minute and correlate with heart rate.

Fixed-orifice resistor (TheraPEP®) (Figure 9): Expiratory flow is restricted to <20 L/min, airway pressure peaks at 10 cmH$_2$O, returning to 0. Esophageal pressure normal on inspiration, increases to positive during expiration, reducing with reduced flow. On prolonged active inspiration, esophageal pressure steadily increases with time and may exceed airway pressure.

Spring-loaded threshold resistor (vital signs valve—10 cmH$_2$O): Expiratory flow appears unrestricted at 40 L/min with square wave pattern; airway pressure peaks and maintains a plateau until exhalation begins (square wave); esophageal pressure equalizes with airway pressure early in expiratory phase. As active exhalation continues past midpoint (1.5 to 2.0 seconds), esophageal pressure increases above airway pressure by 8–10 cmH$_2$O. (Figure 10).

Weighted-ball threshold resistor (Flutter): Fluctuations of flow and airway pressure similar during expiration, with less than 0.5 cmH$_2$O fluctuation in esophageal pressure. Expiratory flow >40 L/min appears to be unrestricted, decreasing gradually toward end of expiration. Airway pressure and esophageal pressure equalize early in expiratory phase, and as exhalation continues past midpoint, esophageal pressure exceeds airway pressure by as much as 10 cmH$_2$O (Figure 11).

High-frequency oral oscillation—IPV: Large fluctuations in flow rate, greater on expiration than inspiration. Airway pressure fluctuations of 4–8 cmH$_2$O, esophageal fluctuations 1–2 cmH$_2$O. Airway pressure on expiration is square wave (increases to peak and plateaus until expiration); esophageal pressure increases to match airway in approximately 2 seconds (Figure 12).

HFCWC—Vest: Flow of 40 L/min appears unrestricted; as flow decreases, the fluctuations increased. Airway pressure remained at baseline with tidal breathing, with fluctuations of 0.5 to 0.75 cmH$_2$O, and esophageal pressures had normal subatmospheric pattern with fluctuation of 0.25. to 1.0 cmH$_2$O (Figure 13).

HFCWC—Hayek: Expiratory flow appears unrestricted, airway pressure fluctuations greater on expiration, with esophageal pressure fluctuations from 0.5 to 2.0 cmH$_2$O (Figure 14).

It appears that the HFCWC devices create similar airflow and pressure patterns, with differences in frequency. Both threshold resistors demonstrate a square-wave pattern of flow and airway pressure. The fixed-orifice device effectively reduces expiratory flow, with both flow and airway pressure decreasing in a ramp pattern. With both the threshold and fixed-orifice resistors, the esophageal pressures become positive early in expiration, and during the course of active inspiration can exceed the airway pressure. While we found this pattern

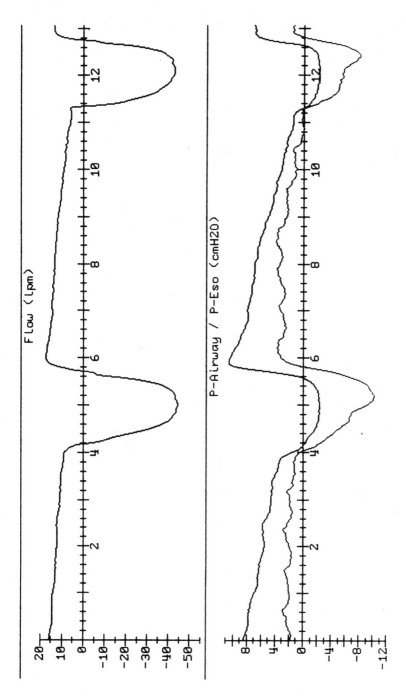

Figure 9 Fixed-orifice resistor (TheraPEP)—expiratory flow is restricted to <20 L/min; airway pressure peaks at 10 cmH$_2$O, returning to zero. Esophageal pressure normal on inspiration, increases to positive during expiration, decreasing with reduced flow. On prolonged active inspiration, esophageal pressure steadily increases with time and may exceed airway pressure.

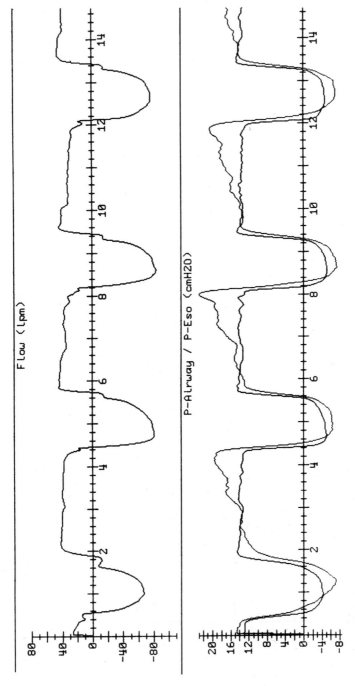

Figure 10 Spring-loaded threshold resistor (vital signs valve 10 cmH₂O). Expiratory flow appears unrestricted at 40 L/min with square-wave pattern; airway pressure peaks and maintains a plateau until exhalation begins (square wave); esophageal pressure equalizes with airway pressure early in expiratory phase. As active exhalation continues past midpoint (1.5 to 2.0 seconds), esophageal pressure increases above airway pressure by 8–10 cmH₂O.

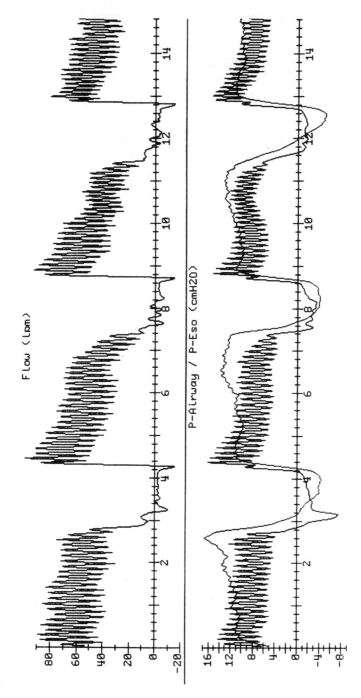

Figure 11 Weighted-ball threshold resistor (Flutter)—fluctuations of flow and airway pressure similar during expiration, with less than 0.5 cmH₂O fluctuation in esophageal pressure. Expiratory flow >40 L/min appears to be unrestricted, decreasing gradually toward end of expiration. Airway pressure and esophageal pressure equalize early in expiratory phase, and as exhalation continues past midpoint, esophageal pressure exceeds airway pressure by as much as 10 cmH₂O.

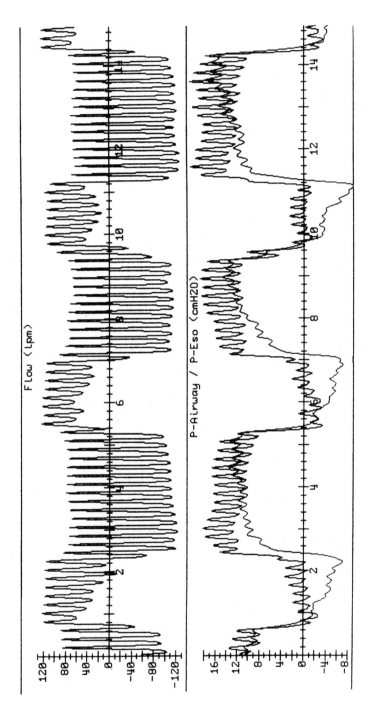

Figure 12 High-frequency oral oscillation—IPV: large fluctuations in flow rate, greater on expiration than inspiration. Airway pressure fluctuations of 4–8 cmH₂O, esophageal fluctuations 1–2 cmH₂O. Airway pressure on expiration is square wave (increases to peak and plateaus until expiration); esophageal pressure increases to match airway in approximately 2 seconds.

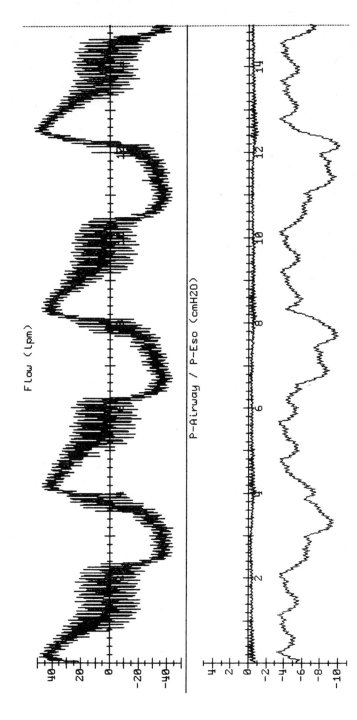

Figure 13 High-frequency chest-wall oscillation—Vest: flow of 40 L/min appears unrestricted; as flow decreases, the fluctuations increased. Airway pressure remained at baseline with tidal breathing, with fluctuations of 0.5 to 0.75 cmH$_2$O, and esophageal pressures had normal pattern subatmospheric pattern with fluctuation of 0.25 to 1.0 cmH$_2$O.

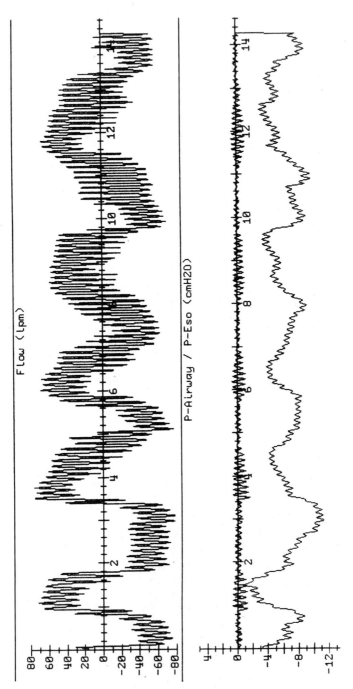

Figure 14 High-frequency chest-wall oscillation—Hayek: expiratory flow appears unrestricted, airway pressure fluctuations greater on expiration, with esophageal pressure fluctuations from 0.5 to 2.0 cmH$_2$O.

routinely with the threshold resistor, it rarely happened with the fixed-orifice resistor unless T_{exp} >10 seconds, secondary to using too small an orifice for the patient.

X. Summary

It would appear that many of these maneuvers and devices have a place in promoting bronchial hygiene in patients with cystic fibrosis, and perhaps in other lung diseases. As we learn more about the normal mechanisms of mucociliary clearance, it becomes apparent that maneuvers that reinforce or complement these mechanisms provide improved secretion clearance with considerably less effort and inconvenience than postural drainage. While the research to date has not identified one "superior" therapy, we have identified a substantial number of viable alternatives that appear to be as good or better than postural drainage. Over the course of several decades of life, cystic fibrosis patients may have the need or opportunity to utilize any number of these techniques. The ultimate key to their success may be how comfortable and convenient any particular device may prove to be for the individual patient.

References

1. Hilling L, Bakow E, Fink J, Kelly C, Sobush D, Southorn PA. AARC Clinical Practice Guideline: use of positive airway pressure adjuncts to bronchial hygiene therapy. Respir Care 1993; 38:516–521.
2. Paul WL, Downs JB. Postoperative atelectasis: intermittent positive pressure breathing, incentive spirometry, and face-mask positive end-expiratory pressure. Arch Surg 1981; 116:861–863.
3. Ricksten SE, Bengtsson A, Soderberg C, Thorden M, Kvist H. Effects of periodic positive airway pressure by mask on postoperative pulmonary function. Chest 1986; 89:774–781.
4. Andersen JB, Klausen NO. A new mode of administration of nebulized bronchodilator in severe bronchospasm. Eur J Respir Dis 1982; 63(suppl 119):97–100.
5. Frischknecht-Christensen E, Norregaard O, Dahl R. Treatment of bronchial asthma with terbutaline inhaled by conespacer combined with positive expiratory pressure mask. Chest 1991; 100:317–321.
6. Kacmarek RM, Dimas S, Reynolds J, Shapiro B. Technical aspects of positive end expiratory pressure (PEEP): Part I. Physics of PEEP devices. Respir Care 1982; 27:1478–1489.
7. Mahlmeister MJ, Fink JB, Hoffman GL, Fifer LF. Positive-expiratory-pressure mask therapy: theoretical and practical considerations and a review of the literature. Respir Care 1991; 36:1218–1230.
8. Thoman RL, Stoker GL, Ross JC. The efficacy of pursed-lips breathing in patients with chronic obstructive pulmonary disease. Am Rev Respir Dis 1968; 93:100–106.

9. Petty TL, ed. Chronic Obstructive Pulmonary Disease. New York: Marcel Dekker, 1978.
10. Poulton EP, Odon DM. Left-sided heart failure with pulmonary oedema: its treatment with the "pulmonary plus pressure machine." Lancet 1936; 231:981–983.
11. Barach AL, Martin J, Eckman L. Positive pressure respiration and its application to the treatment of acute pulmonary edema and respiratory obstruction. Proc Am Soc Clin Invest 1937; 16:664–680.
12. Cheney FW, Hornbein TF, Crawford EW. The effect of expiratory resistance on the blood gas tensions of anesthetized patients. Anesthesiology 1967; 28:670–676.
13. Ashbaugh DG, Petty TL, Bigelow DB, Harris TM. Continuous positive pressure breathing (CPPB) in adult respiratory distress syndrome. J Thorac Cardiovasc Surg 1969; 57:31–41.
14. Gregory GA, Kitterman JA, Phibbs RH. Treatment of the idiopathic respiratory distress syndrome with continuous positive airway pressure. N Engl J Med 1971; 284:1333–1340.
15. Pontoppidan H, Wilson RS, Rie MA, Schneider RC. Respiratory intensive care. Anesthesiology 1977; 47:96–116.
16. Katz JA. PEEP and CPAP in perioperative respiratory care. Respir Care 1984; 29:6:614–623.
17. Garrard CS, Shah M. The effects of expiratory positive airway pressure on function residual capacity in normal subjects. Crit Care Med 1978; 6:320–332.
18. Andersen JB, Qvist H, Kann T. Recruiting collapsed lung through collateral channels with positive end-expiratory pressure. Scand J Respir Dis 1979; 60:260–266.
19. Andersen JB, Jespersen W. Demonstration of intersegmental respiratory bronchioles in normal lungs. Eur J Respir Dis 1980; 61:337–341.
20. Branson RD, Hurst JM, DeHaven CB. Mask CPAP: state of the art. Respir Care 1985; 30:846–857.
21. Branson RD. PEEP without endotracheal intubation. Respir Care 1988; 33:598–610.
22. Andersen JB, Olesen KP, Eikard E, Jansen E, Qvist J. Periodic continuous positive airway pressure, CPAP, by mask in the treatment of atelectasis: a sequential analysis. Eur J Respir Dis 1980; 61:20–25.
23. Pontoppidan H. Mechanical aids to lung expansion in nonintubated surgical patients. Am Rev Respir Dis 1980; 122:109–119.
24. Carlsson C, Sonden B, Thylen U. Can postoperative continuous positive airway pressure (CPAP) prevent pulmonary complications after abdominal surgery? Intensive Care Med 1981; 7:225–229.
25. Martin JG, Shore S, Engel LA. Effect of continuous positive pressure on respiratory mechanics and pattern of breathing in induced asthma. Am Rev Respir Dis 1982; 126:812–817.
26. Stock MC, Downs JB. Administration of continuous positive airway pressure by mask. Acute Care 1983/84; 10:184–188.
27. Stock MC, Downs JB, Corkran ML. Pulmonary function before and after prolonged positive airway pressure by mask. Crit Care Med 1984; 12:973–974.
28. Stock MC, Downs JB, Cooper RB, et al. Comparison of continuous positive airway

pressure, incentive spirometry, and conservative therapy after cardiac operations. Crit Care Med 1984; 12:969–972.

29. Stock MC, Downs JB, Gauer PK, Alster JM, Imrey PB. Prevention of postoperative pulmonary complication with CPAP, incentive spirometry and conservative therapy. Chest 1985; 87:151–157.

30. Lindner KH, Lotz P, Ahnefeld FW. Continuous positive airway pressure effect on functional residual capacity, vital capacity and its subdivisions. Chest 1987; 92: 66–70.

31. Campbell T, Ferguson N, McKinlay RGC. The use of a simple self-administered method of positive expiratory pressure (PEP) in chest physiotherapy after abdominal surgery. Physiotherapy 1986; 72:498–500.

32. Groth S, Stafanger G, Dirksen H, Andersen JB, Falk M, Kelstrup M. Positive expiratory pressure (PEP mask) physiotherapy improves ventilation and reduces volume of trapped gas in cystic fibrosis. Bull Eur Physiopathol Respir 1985; 21:339–343.

33. van der Schans CP, van der Mark TW, de Vries G, et al. Effect of positive expiratory pressure breathing in patients with cystic fibrosis. Thorax 1991; 46:252–256.

34. van der Schans CP, de Jong W, de Vries G, et al. Effects of positive expiratory pressure breathing during exercise in patients with COPD. Chest 1994; 105:782–789.

35. McIlwaine PM, Wong LT, Peacock D, Davidson GF. Long-term comparative trial of conventional postural drainage and percussion versus positive expiratory pressure physiotherapy in the treatment of cystic fibrosis. J Pediatr 1997; 131:570–574.

36. Reisman JJ, Rivington-Law B, Corey M, et al. Role of conventional physiotherapy in cystic fibrosis. J Pediatr 1988; 113:632–636.

37. Pavia D, Thomson ML, Phillipakos D. A preliminary study of the effect of a vibrating pad on bronchial clearance. Am Rev Respir Dis 1976; 113:92–96.

38. King M, Phillips DM, Gross D, Vartian V, Chang HK, Zidulka A. Enhanced tracheal mucus clearance with high frequency chest wall compression. Am Rev Respir Dis 1983; 128:511–515.

39. King M, Phillips DM, Zidulka A, Chang HK. Tracheal mucus clearance in high frequency oscillation II: chest wall versus mouth oscillation. Am Rev Respir Dis 1984; 130:703–706.

40. Gross D, Zidulka A, O'Brien C, Wight D, Fraser R, Rosenthal L, King M. Peripheral mucocilliary clearance with high-frequency chest wall compression. J Appl Physiol 1985; 58:1157–1163.

41. Rubin E, Scantlen GE, Chapman GA, Eldridge M, Menendez R, Wanner A. Effect of chest wall oscillation on mucus clearance: comparison of two vibrators. Pediatr Pulmonol 1989; 6:122–126.

42. Freitag L, Long WM, Kim CS, Wanner A. Removal of excessive bronchial secretions by asymmetrical high-frequency oscillations. J Appl Physiol 1989; 67:614–619.

43. George RJ, Johnson MA, Pavia D, Agnew JE, Clarke SE, Geddes DM. Increase in mucocilliary clearance in normal man induced by oral high frequency oscillation. Thorax 1985; 40:433–437.

44. van Hengstum M, Festen J, Beurskens C, Hankel M, van den Broek W, Corstens

F. No effect of oral high frequency oscillation combined with forced expiration manoeuvres on tracheobronchial clearance in chronic bronchitis. Eur Respir J 1990; 3:14–18.

45. King M, Zidulka A, Phillips DM, Wight D, Gross D, Chang HK. Tracheal mucus clearance in high-frequency oscillation: effect of peak flow rate bias. Eur Respir J 1990; 3:6–13.

46. Chang HK, Weber ME, King M. Mucus transport by high-frequency nonsymmetrical oscillatory airflow. J Appl Physiol 1988; 65:1203–1209.

47. Dasgupta B, Tomkiewicz RP, Boyd WA, Brown NE, King M. Effects of combined treatment with rhDNase and airflow oscillations on spinnability of cystic fibrosis sputum *in vitro*. Pediatr Pulmonol 1995; 20:78–82.

48. Tomkiewicz RP, Biviji AA, King M. Effects of oscillating air on the rheological properties and clearability for mucus gel simulant. Biorheology 1994; 124:689–93.

49. King M, Rubin BK. Mucus-controlling agents: past and present. Respir Care Clin N Am 1999; 5(4):575–594.

50. Lindemann H. [The value of physical therapy with VRP 1—Desitin ("Flutter").] Pneumologie 1992; 46:626–630.

51. Huls G, Boldt A, Kieselmann R, Lindemann H. Child physiotherapy in cases of chronic retention of mucus. Der Kinderarzt 1992; 23:2004–2011.

52. Konstan MW, Stern RC, Doershuk CF. Efficacy of the Flutter device for airway mucus clearance in patients with cystic fibrosis. J Pediatr 1994; 124:689–693.

53. Mahesh VK, McDougal JA, Haluszka L. Efficacy of the Flutter device for airway mcus clearance in patients with cystic fibrosis [letter]. J Pediatr 1996; 128:165–166.

54. Hilling L, Bakow E, Fink J, Kelly C, Sobush D, Southorn PA. AARC Clinical Practice Guideline: Postural Drainage Therapy. Respiratory Care 1993; 36:1418–1426.

55. Pryor JA, Webber BA, Hodson, ME, Warner JO. The Flutter VRP1 as an adjunct to chest physiotherapy in cystic fibrosis. Respir Med 1994; 88:677–681.

56. Homnick DN, Anderson K, Marks JH. Comparison of the flutter device to standard chest physiotherapy in hospitalized patients with cystic fibrosis: a pilot study. Chest 1998; 114:993–997.

57. Padman R, Geouque DM, Englehardt MT. Effects of the flutter device on pulmonary function studies among pediatric cystic fibrosis patients. Del Med J 1999; 71:13–18.

58. App EM, Kieselman R, Reinhardt D, et al. Sputum rheology changes in cystic fibrosis lung disease following two different types of physiotherapy: flutter *vs* autogenic drainage. Chest 1998; 114:171–177.

59. Weiner P, Zamir D, Waizman J, Weiner M. Physiotherapy in chronic obstructive pulmonary disease: oscillatory breathing with Flutter VRP1. Harefuah 1996. 131:14–17.

60. Nakamura S, Kawakami M. Acute effect of use of the Flutter on expectoration of sputum in patients with chronic respiratory diseases. Jpn J Thorac Dis 1996; 34:180.

61. Girard JP, Terki N. The Flutter VRP1: a new personal pocket therapeutic device

used as an adjunct to drug therapy in the management of bronchial hygiene. J Invest Allergol Clin Immunol 1994; 4:23–27.

62. Fink J. A comparison of Flutter to other airway clearance valves: a laboratory study [abstr]. Chest 1995; 108:147S.

63. Schlobohm, RM, Fallrick RT, Quan SF, Katz JA. Lung volumes, mechanics and oxygenation during spontaneous positive pressure ventilation: the advantage of CPAP over EPAP. Anesthesiology 1981; 55:426–422.

64. Petrof BJ, Calderini E, Gottfried SB. Effect of CPAP on respiratory effort and dyspnea during exercise in severe COPD. J Appl Physiol 1990; 69:179–188.

65. Petrof BJ, Legare M, Godberg P, Milic-Emili J, Gottfried SB. Continuous positive airway pressure reduces work of breathing and dyspnea during weaning from mechanical ventilation in severe chronic obstructive pulmonary disease. Am Rev Respir Dis 1990; 141:281–289.

66. McInturff SL, Shaw LI. Intrapulmonary percussive ventilation. Resp Care 1985; 30:884–885.

67. Natale JE, Pfeifle J, Homnick DN. Comparison of intramulmonary percussive ventilation and chest physiotherapy. Chest 1994; 105:1789–1793.

68. Homnick DN, White F, de Castro C. Comparison of effects of an intrapulmonary percussive ventilator to standard aerosol and chest physiotherapy in treatment of cystic fibrosis. Pediatr Pulmonol 1995; 20:50–55.

69. Newhouse PA, White F, Marks JH, Homnick DN. Clin Pediatr 1998; 37:427–432.

70. Davis KJ, Hurst JM, et al. High frequency percussive ventilation. Respir Care 1989; 34:39–47.

71. Hurst JM, Branson, RD. High-frequency percussive ventilation in the management of elevated intracranial pressure. J Trauma 1988; 28:1363–1367.

72. Cioffi WG, Major MC. High frequency percussive ventilation in patients with inhalation injury. J Trauma 1989; 29:350–354.

73. Zidulka A, Gross D, Minami H, Vartian V, Chang HK. Ventilation by high-frequency chest wall compression in dogs with normal lungs. Am Rev Respir Dis 1983; 127:709–713.

74. Hansen L, Warwick W. High frequency chest compression system to aid in clearance of mucus from the lung. Biomed Instrum Tech 1990; 24:289–294.

75. Kluft, J, Beker L, Castagnino M, Gaiser J, Chaney H, Fink RJ. A comparison of bronchial drainage treatments in cystic fibrosis. Pediatr Pulmonol 1996; 22:271–274.

76. Arens R, Gozal D, Omlin KJ, et al. Comparison of high frequency chest compression and conventional chest physiotherapy in hospitalized patients with cystic fibrosis. Am J Respir Crit Care Med 1994; 150:1154–1157

77. Spitzer SA, Fink G, Mittelman M. External high-frequency ventilation in severe chronic obstructive pulmonary disease. Chest 1993; 104:1698–1701.

78. Soo Hoo GW, Ellison MJ, Zhang C, Williams AJ, Belman MJ. Effects of external chest wall oscillation in stable COPD patients. Am J Respir Crit Care Med 1994; 149:A637.

79. Smithline HA, Rivers EP, Rady MY, Blake HC, Nowak RM. Biphasic extrathoracic pressure CPR: a human pilot study. Chest 1994; 105:842–846.

80. Segawa J, Nakashima Y, Kuroiwa A, et al. The efficacy of external high frequency oscillation: experience in a quadriplegic patient with alveolar hypoventilation. Kokyu To Junkan 1993; 41:271–275.

81. Gaitini L, Krimerman S, Smorgik J, Gruber A, Werczberger A. External high frequency ventilation for weaning from the mechanical ventilation. Recent Adv Anaesth Pain Int Care Emerg 1990; 5:137–138.

82. Scherer TA, Barandun J, Martinez E, Wanner A, Rubin EM. Effect of high-frequency oral airway and chest wall oscillation and conventional chest physical therapy on expectoration in patients with stable cystic fibrosis. Chest 1998; 113: 1019–1027.

18

Pediatric Mucus Clearance by Chest Physiotherapy

Principles and Practice

MAXIMILIAN S. ZACH and BEATRICE OBERWALDNER

University of Graz
Graz, Austria

I. Introduction

Chest physiotherapy (CPT) for mucus clearance is an established therapeutic component in the management of various acute and chronic respiratory disorders and complications in pediatric patients (1). Its application is based on the concept of thereby treating or preventing the mechanical consequences of obstructing secretions, such as local hyperinflation, atelectasis, increased work of breathing, and maldistribution of ventilation. In addition, CPT can remove infectious material and proteolytic activity from the airways, thereby effectively reducing inflammatory tissue damage (2). Furthermore, microbiological and other investigations of recovered secretions can aid the diagnostic work-up, and mucus clearance of airways will facilitate the aerosol treatment of respiratory disorders.

The application of CPT for mucus clearance is traditionally based on the clinical impression of a therapeutic effectiveness in various airway disorders that are complicated by abundant intrabronchial secretions. Over the last two decades, a slowly increasing number of relevant studies commenced to provide a body of scientific evidence for the effectiveness of CPT. Some studies of therapeutic effects, however, have remained negative, and some of these discouraging results might be explained by faulty technique and/or application of mucus clearance techniques in disorders and situations that provide no clear rationale for CPT (3). In addition, some of these CPT studies are flawed by a poor scientific approach, lack of controls, and insufficient sample size and power. So far, there are no studies of methodological details that might assist the therapist in tailoring her or his approach to the prevailing pathophysiology. Moreover, some of the CPT literature has been motivated by an ongoing search for the "best" technique; unfortunately, such publications tend to contribute parochialism and bias rather than sound scientific data to an already prevailing confusion. Some authors consider such comparative studies in patient groups with some pathophysiological inhomogeneity as a scientific misconception and have advocated an individualized approach in which different techniques are used to provide a quiver of therapeutic details for fine-tuning CPT to the prevailing disease situation of the patient (1,4). Pediatric chest physiotherapists increasingly adhere to this principle, but so far they are only guided by accumulated bedside experience and by trial and error.

Because CPT for mucus clearance consists of mechanical interventions applied to the patient's respiratory tract, it might be considered as a therapeutic application of respiratory physiology. It follows that respiratory physiology constitutes a body of knowledge that extends into clinical practice via a diagnostic (lung function testing) and a therapeutic (CPT) arm. This concept provides an additional approach to the prescription and practice of CPT, i.e., a physiology-based analysis of the prevailing respiratory disease, which is then translated into a spectrum of matching techniques and methodological details for maximal effectiveness.

Such an approach, however, will be particularly complex in pediatric patients, as they present numerous age-specific physiological peculiarities that not only differ substantially from the adult situation, but also change continuously with growth and development. In addition, there are disease-inflicted changes that further modify this developmentally defined baseline; moreover, the psychological basis for the therapist-patient interaction also changes substantially with age.

This chapter outlines a physiologically and developmentally oriented approach to CPT for mucus clearance by looking at the pediatric patient from a physiological, clinical, psychological, and pathophysiological perspective, and then scrutinizing the available techniques for best fit. For obvious reasons of length and volume, this chapter does not aim at being comprehensive; by reviewing and discussing specific examples and details, it rather tries to illustrate a newly emerging strategy of decision making which might help to optimize the practice of pediatric CPT. Methodological characteristics of available CPT techniques are only discussed to the extent of their physiological relevance; for more detailed information, the reader is referred to current textbook articles (1,5,6).

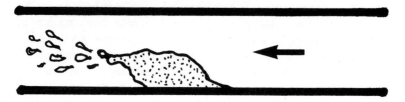

Figure 1   Shearing forces; the expiration carries mucus downstream.

II. Physiological Perspectives

A. Therapeutic Principles

Mobilization and transport of secretions is achieved by a few basic mechanisms, namely the effects of shearing forces on the air/liquid interface, the mechanics of a forced expiration, and gas-liquid pumping (1).

Shearing forces (Fig. 1) are effected by a high-velocity expiratory airstream that carries mucus downstream towards the pharynx. With the rapid increase in the summarized bronchial cross-sectional area, expiratory airstream velocity progressively decreases towards the periphery. It follows that, even with forced expirations, this simple mechanism will only be effective in the most central airways, namely, the trachea and larynx. However, as secretions will cause a local stenosis in the airway, airstream velocity will increase locally, and this might occasionally support a more peripheral effectiveness of the shearing mechanism.

From the more central part of the tracheobronchial tree, secretions are cleared by a different albeit related mechanism (Fig. 2), namely the dynamic compression of airways, which occurs with any forced expiration (7,8). The

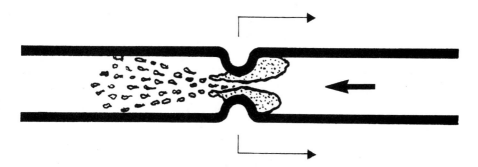

Figure 2   Dynamic compression of the airway in a forced expiration; secretions are caught in an upstream moving choke point and are ejected downstream.

mechanics of a forced expiratory maneuver are characterized by a progressive upstream movement of the equal pressure points. Dynamic compression of the airway occurs immediately downstream of each equal pressure point; with an ongoing forced expiration, this results in a wave of choke points that run towards the periphery. Any mucus plug, once reached and caught by such a choke point, will be ejected downstream through this stenosis by the expiratory airflow. The most important prerequisite for this mechanism to be effective is a sufficient degree of bronchial stability. An overly stiff airway will not narrow enough to form an effective stenosis; this, however, will rarely be of clinical relevance. More important is complete airway closure, occurring with exaggerated bronchial compressibility and effectively interrupting airflow and mucus transport (9). Furthermore, the mechanics of a forced expiration will depend on expiratory airflow velocity; thus, as shown by radioaerosol studies of coughing, they will progressively lose effectiveness towards the bronchial periphery (10).

The third, poorly understood mechanism for mobilizing abundant intrabronchial secretions is gas-liquid pumping (Fig. 3). In contrast to the two previously discussed therapeutic principles, it does not depend on expiratory airflow velocity and thus might be the only mechanism with some effectiveness in the periphery. Air inspired through secretions will mix with the latter, and the

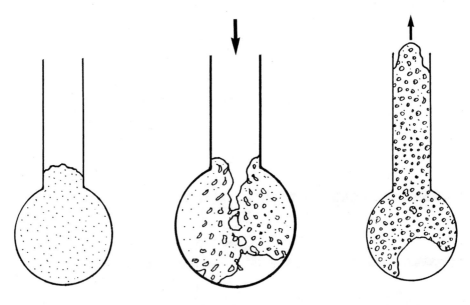

Figure 3 Gas-liquid pumping: (left) secretions in the periphery; (center) inspiration—airspaces are dilated and inspired air mixes with secretions; (right) expiration—airspaces decrease in size and air-liquid mixture moves downstream.

resulting foam will occupy more space than any pool of airless secretions. This should effect expansion, and with the alveolar side of the system being a dead end, one can speculate that such expansion will result in a net movement of secretions towards more central parts of the tracheobronchial tree. Prerequisites for this mechanism becoming effective should be viscoelastic properties of the secretions that allow for mixing with air and large rhythmic volume changes of airways and alveoli as occur with hyperventilation (exercise).

Properly mobilized and transported mucus ultimately arrives in the pharynx, from which it is expectorated. To this end, the above-discussed mechanisms have to interact effectively, i.e., one mechanism will have to guide secretions to the next. Most likely, the intrathoracic trachea is the transitional zone where dynamic compression of airways transitions to the shearing forces of the high-velocity expiratory airstream. It is less clear in which bronchial generation the forced expiratory mechanics take over from gas-liquid pumping, and it is this transition where occasionally one mechanism might fail to link with the other, resulting in an inability to clear secretions from the periphery.

All these therapeutic principles are equally important for pediatric CPT as they are for mucus clearance in adults. However, substantial differences in respiratory structure and function between the adult and the pediatric patient set the physiological stage for their varied applications.

B. Lung Volume

All CPT techniques for clearance of intrabronchial secretions aim at initially bringing air behind obstructing mucus, thus facilitating gas-liquid pumping and expiratory mobilization and transport of secretions (6). This is achieved by increasing the lung volume. Bronchodilation enhances inspiration beyond mucus plugs, and the alveolar space behind the occluded airways can be inflated via collateral ventilation channels; furthermore, the phenomenon of interdependence, i.e., expanding forces exerted between adjacent alveoli, is more effective in the reexpansion of lung tissue at a higher lung volume (11).

This therapeutic principle pertains to patients of all ages and thus constitutes an important physiological basis for mucus clearance in both adult and pediatric patients. Where the newborn and the infant differs substantially from the older patient, however, is in its age-specific weakness in maintaining lung volume at a level high enough for airway patency. This stems from an unstable chest wall; its compliance is two to six times that of the lung in preterm and full-term infants (12–14). This ratio decreases gradually towards young adulthood, when chest roughly equals lung compliance (15,16). As a consequence, the elastic equilibrium volume of the respiratory system, i.e., that volume where the inward recoil of the lungs and the outward recoil of the chest are balanced, occurs at a lower percentage of total lung capacity (TLC) in newborns and

infants than in older subjects (17). It follows that some airways would close at
end expiration if tidal breathing occurred at this low level of lung volume and
static-elastic recoil pressure. This is prevented by a spectrum of strategies to
dynamically elevate functional residual capacity (FRC), the most important being shortened expiratory time, postinspiratory diaphragmatic activity, and expiratory laryngeal braking (18). The relative importance of shortened expiratory
time is unclear, but it might be a mechanism that increases in effectiveness with
increased respiratory rate in disease. The two other mechanisms (i.e., diaphragmatic activity extending into expiration and braking of expiratory airflow by
adducted vocal cords) change in effectiveness with time. During rapid eye
movement (REM) sleep, postinspiratory diaphragmatic activity was found to be
decreased in newborns (19,20), and expiratory vocal cord adduction was shown
to be reduced in animal experiments (21,22). In addition, there is some evidence
that chest wall stability is further reduced during REM sleep via decreased intercostal muscle activity (23). Once FRC has decreased critically in preterm infants, sighs are used as a reserve mechanism for restoring lung volume (24). In
summary, the newborn and the young infant have a special problem maintaining
a lung volume sufficient for airway patency, and this age-specific situation, in
combination with an underdeveloped collateral ventilation, renders these very
young patients especially prone to respiratory complications that may be caused
by abundant intrabronchial secretions. This not only explains the phenomenon
of chest physiotherapists having to treat atelectasis more often in this age group
than in any other, but also suggests that lung volume management is more important in early childhood than at any later age.

There is a spectrum of therapeutic approaches with which this special
demand of the newborn and young infant can be met. Continuous positive airway pressure (CPAP) will effectively support any small patient who is unable
to sufficiently elevate his or her FRC by physiological means for alveolar filling
and airways patency. CPAP will thus be beneficial when other mechanisms for
dynamic elevation of FRC are hampered. Laryngeal expiratory breaking is ren-
dered ineffective by any artificial airway (endotracheal tube, tracheostomy cannula). The clinically noted accumulation of mucus problems in small children
with artificial airways is readily explained by this handicap in combination with
an interrupted mucociliary escalator and a mechanically neutralized cough
mechanism. Thus, CPAP should be applied liberally to children with an artificial
airway, especially during respiratory infections, when airway patency is further
compromised by inflammatory edema of the bronchial mucosa and excessive
mucus production.

Other strategies of lung volume management are required in cases where
CPAP is not available. Manual bagging, monitored by a manometer in small
children to avoid excessive pressures, raises lung volume for mobilization of
secretions by a slow long insufflation with end-inspiratory hold and positive

end-expiratory pressure (PEEP). Many experienced chest physiotherapists bring the infant's chest manually into a position mimicking a deep inspiration prior to any expiratory maneuver for mucus clearance.

The problem in newborns and infants of maintaining lung volume and airway patency is of particular relevance when suctioning secretions from the bronchial tree through an artificial airway. Negative suction pressure will further tilt the already compromised mechanical balance between lungs and thoracic cage towards decreased lung volume and occluded airways. Consequently, high negative pressures and deep suctioning were found to be risk factors for the development of right upper lobe collapse in intubated children (25). Suctioning was observed to produce a marked fall in the pulmonary compliance of intubated infants, and this effect increased when suction was prolonged and a larger catheter was used (26). The same study showed that compliance could be restored by applying positive pressure to the respiratory system; if the lungs were not inflated after suctioning, however, they remained partially collapsed. Thus, it seems of particular importance in this age group to routinely reinflate the system by manual bagging or mechanical insufflation after each suction procedure.

In schoolchildren, like in adults, lung volume can be raised by training the patient to inspire deeply with breathholding at end inspiration. In preschool children a deep inspiration might be achieved by blowing games, where lengthy expirations are usually followed by deep inspirations. In addition, there are therapeutic games in which different semipermeable articles have to be sucked against the opening of a thin tube and held there for as long as possible.

With an unstable and highly compliant chest, a deep inspiration per se is mechanically a much more difficult task for the newborn and infant than for any older patient. The muscular contribution to such an inspiration changes with body position. While the chest is passively driven by the diaphragm in the upright body position, an active contraction of the intercostal muscles is required for rib cage expansion in the supine subject (27). For the predominantly supine infant, a REM-associated decrease in intercostal muscle activity (23) thus results not only in a less stable chest but also in a less effective inspiration in this sleep stage, thereby providing for increased paradoxical rib cage motion (28).

It follows that, with this problem of the breathing pump, all other mechanisms that decrease inspiratory resistance have to be maximally utilized. The importance of reducing inspiratory resistance is illustrated by a spectrum of strategies that the newborn applies for increasing upper airway patency. Preterm infants show pronounced nasal flaring in periods of increased demands on respiration (29). Alae nasi activation and the thereby effected reduction in nasal resistance may help to stabilize the upper airway by preventing the development of large negative pharyngeal pressures. While being dedicated nose breathers, preterm infants switch to oral breathing with nasal occlusion, but this change of inspiratory route is preceded by a decrease in oxygen saturation and respiratory frequency (30). In healthy newborns, blocking of a nostril effects a reduction in respiratory rate and a fall in minute ventilation (31). Children with congenital upper airway stenosis try to reduce upper airway resistance by dilating the pharynx (32,33).

Thus, the therapist's practical approach to patients of this age group will be to support inspiration whenever possible. This means that additional obstacles that further elevate inspiratory work have to be recognized and, if possible, treated, removed, or avoided. One prominent example is the increased nasal resistance to inspiratory airflow that occurs in the course of a viral infection. Decongestant nose drops might have a more important preventive and therapeutic role in this age group than in any older patient, and clearing of the nasal air passages by suction is to be seen from the same perspective. In addition, therapeutic interventions that compromise upper airway patency should be minimized or avoided altogether. As one would expect, a nasogastric tube significantly increases nasal and total airway resistance in newborns and thus will result in a markedly increased work of breathing (34). Removal of nasogastric feeding tubes was observed to reduce apnea rate in newborn infants (35). It follows that this particular route of tube feeding, albeit often favored by nursing staff because of its practical advantages in the passing and fixation of the tube, should be seen critically from the chest physiotherapist's perspective, especially in spontaneously breathing infants with respiratory compromise and in those patients with marginal muscular resources for the work of breathing. In these patients the first therapeutic step is to protect the airway and not to block it (36).

In summary, obtaining high lung volume is a much more difficult task for newborns and infants, and a spectrum of chest wall stability and inspiration problems favors the occurrence of respiratory complications caused by mucus plugging. Reduced lung volume results in decreased static elastic recoil pressure, and the thereby lowered radial traction effects a reduction of airway patency. In combination with intrabronchial secretions, this leads to atelectasis and hyperinflating valve mechanisms. Hence, lung volume management is of particular importance for mucus clearance in this age group.

The other side of this coin is that a properly applied therapeutic increase in lung volume appears to be of particular effectiveness for mucus clearance in newborns and infants. This might explain an age-specific success rate of pediatric CPT in the treatment of mucus-effected respiratory complications of >90% (37). Furthermore, the unstable and highly compliant chest of the very young patient, while being the main cause of the aforementioned difficulties in maintaining lung volume, offers itself as a highly accessible therapeutic interface, which renders mucus clearance maneuvers like chest compression, shaking, clapping, and vibration much more effective than the stiff, big, and noncompliant chest of the older patient.

C. Body Position

One of the more traditional concepts in CPT is "postural drainage," i.e., placing the patient's body in a position that allows mucus to flow from the uppermost diseased lung units down towards the more central airways, from where it can be expectorated (6). Some have speculated that thereby effected mobilization of secretions is not so much due to gravitational forces, but rather to redistribution of ventilation occurring with changes of body position (38,39). Locally enhanced ventilation, i.e., lung volume changes, will result in more effective gas-liquid pumping; deeper inspirations will support patency of airways. Positioning of the patient offers an approach to locally modify or maximize these mechanisms.

Normally, the weight of lung tissue causes distension of the uppermost segments; there, an increased static-elastic recoil will not only effect dilation of the alveolar space, but also a higher degree of airway patency. In the adult, however, the increased negative transthoracic pressure of an inspiration brings more air to the dependent lung units, which then will exhale a larger volume in the subsequent expiration (40). It follows that breathing-associated changes in airway caliber, airflow, and lung volume in the adult are more pronounced in those dependent regions with less airway patency. One might speculate that this creates a dilemma as to positioning for mucus clearance, as there should be more gas-liquid pumping in the dependent lung units that at the same time appear at a disadvantage, both in terms of airway patency and gravitational forces.

Evidence indicates that regional ventilation, at least in lateral decubitus positions, differs between pediatric and adult patients. Radionuclide ventilation scans comparing the left decubitus position (right lung uppermost) and right decubitus position (left lung uppermost) have shown reduced ventilation of the dependent and enhanced ventilation of the uppermost lung in children, while adults display the reverse pattern (41). The reasons for this striking difference might be found in the much more compliant chest of the child, a less rigid mediastinum, and a narrow abdomen, resulting in less difference in the preload of the two hemidiaphragms (42). As one might expect, there is no difference between adults and children in the distribution of perfusion, which favors the dependent lung irrespective of age (43). Consequently, the ventilation/perfusion ratio decreases in the dependent lung, when children are moved into the lateral decubitus position (43). These findings have important implications for positioning in unilateral lung disease. In this situation, the preferential distribution of ventilation to the dependent lung regions was found to be of clinical relevance in adult patients (44). When the good lung is positioned uppermost, however, gas exchange generally worsens in adults, but improves in children (45).

Extrapolating these findings to mucus clearance, the child appears at an advantage when compared to the adult. With more ventilation, the uppermost lung regions should be more effective in gas-liquid pumping while, at the same time, having the advantage of both increased bronchial patency and cooperating gravitational forces. Thus, paradoxically, the concept of postural drainage, while originally developed in adults and only extrapolated to children, appears physiologically more sound in pediatric than in adult patients.

D. Airway Stability

Considering the effectiveness of forced expiration for mucus clearance, it is no surprise that most CPT techniques employ and modify forced expiration mechanics. However, a prerequisite for the effectiveness of coughing and forced expiration is adequate bronchial stability, which, in combination with positive transthoracic pressure, should provide for a stenosis, but must avoid complete occlusion of the airway. Furthermore, there should be a hierarchy of decreasing bronchial wall stability from the intrathoracic trachea towards the periphery, thus optimally matching the changing pressure situation that occurs with ongoing forced expiration. Such a hierarchy, in fact, appears nicely illustrated by a changing bronchial wall anatomy, with decreasing and finally disappearing cartilage components towards the higher bronchial generations.

Sufficient bronchial stability for effective mucus clearance is not fully present in the premature baby, the newborn, and the young infant. Several studies have documented a markedly increased bronchial compliance for this age group (46–48). These findings are in agreement with the observation of a reduced bronchial muscle mass in neonates, which only slowly increases with age (49), and with the finding of extremely compliant tracheal cartilage in preterm animals, which subsequently increase in stiffness with age (50). One consequence of enhanced bronchial compressibility in early postnatal life should be a mechanically less effective cough mechanism, but this has not been evaluated in relevant clinical studies. It is, however, interesting to consider the frequent occurrence of staccato cough with respiratory disorders in early infancy (51) from this perspective. It seems reasonable to interrupt expiratory airflow by glottic closure as soon as positive transthoracic pressure threatens to occlude extremely compliant airways. Fortunately, the healthy infant will grow out of this developmentally reduced bronchial wall stability in the second half of the first year.

What are the practical consequences for pediatric CPT? Obviously, high externally applied transthoracic pressures have to be avoided when performing chest compressions in this age group. Rather, such therapist-effected maneuvers have to aim at achieving sufficiently enhanced but still uninterrupted expiratory flows. This requires an individualized and highly sensitive approach to the patient, backed up by substantial professional routine and manual skill in working with these small chests. Thoracic compression maneuvers can be slightly enhanced if the child is on CPAP, as the positive airway pressure will support bronchial patency. Some therapists have adopted the routine of using small PEP masks in combination with thoracic compression maneuvers, as the backpressure from the expiratory resistor will again support airway patency.

An issue to be considered in this context is the use of bronchodilators prior to the administration of CPT. This is a widely established routine, based on the concept that patients with airway hyperresponsiveness tend to react with bronchospasm to the applied spectrum of mechanical interventions (52). Furthermore, bronchodilation prior to CPT promises to provide sufficiently patent airways for effective transport of secretions. Bronchodilators, however, are airway smooth muscle relaxants, and airway smooth muscle tone is a major determinant of airway wall stability (53–55). Consequently, small infants with bronchiolitis, who expire actively against the resistance of their obstructed intrathoracic airways, might react paradoxically to a medication with $ß_2$-stimulants (56), indicating that bronchial smooth muscle relaxation had further reduced an age-specific low bronchial wall stability. From this aspect, the above-mentioned routine of bronchodilator medication before CPT should be seen critically for the newborn period and for early infancy. In cases where a carefully tailored individualized approach, probably backed up by infant lung function testing (rapid thoracic compression technique), is not possible, a general policy of abstention from bronchodilators appears advisable.

In summary, careful consideration of bronchial stability problems is an essential basis for application of any mucus clearance technique that includes forced expirations in patients with developmentally high airway compressibility, i.e., newborns and young infants.

III. Clinical Perspectives

A. Size

Pediatric CPT encounters massive differences in the size of its patients. The weight of the treated subjects ranges from less than 1 kg for the extremely premature baby to occasionally well over 70 kg for adolescents, thus spanning a body mass spectrum of more than 100-fold.

From a practical perspective, small size and low weight is frequently an advantage in pediatric CPT. While it takes considerable effort and strength plus the availability of mechanical support (tilting boards, special beds) to position an adolescent who is unable to cooperate actively, the "handful of human life" of a premature baby is easily positioned with a single hand. The infant rides on the palm and forearm and is stabilized by the grip of the same hand; this leaves the therapist's other hand free to administer interventions to the chest.

B. Vulnerability

The wide size and age range encountered in pediatric CPT illustrates enormous developmental differences, from the highly immature organ systems of the prematurely born to the adult end of growth and development. This spectrum of size, age, and vulnerability is faced by the same individual (i.e., chest physiotherapist), who is thus challenged to adapt the dose of the mechanical intervention to an extreme extent. This situation carries the risk of undertreating the upper end of the size spectrum, while administering interventions that are too aggressive at its lower end.

One example would be the therapist's physical interaction with the patient's chest in conventional CPT (postural drainage, chest clapping, shaking, vibration, compression, assisted coughing). There is little documentation on the effectiveness of these interventions in the relevant literature (1); moreover, no study has ever evaluated effectiveness in relation to size and age. From clinical experience, most chest physiotherapists claim that these interventions are hardly effective on the big, stiff, and uncompliant chest of the adolescent and adult. In contrast, the highly compliant, soft, and small chest of the newborn and infant seems to provide for a high effectiveness of conventional CPT, albeit with a concomitant risk of damage. The latter possibility is suggested by reports of physiotherapy-inflicted rib fractures in premature and newborn infants (57).

Another CPT technique for mucus clearance to be considered from the perspective of age-related differences in vulnerability is suctioning in the intubated patient. For adults, the effects of catheter insertion and tracheal stimulation on systemic vascular and cerebrovascular status have been studied mainly in mechanically ventilated patients with brain injury. Generally, these patients respond with an increase of mean arterial and intracranial pressure (58), and transmission of cough-induced increases in intrathoracic pressure to the cerebral venous system were found to be instrumental for these changes (59). The effects of consecutive suction passes on mean arterial and intracranial pressure seem to be cumulative (60). Suctioning causes similar changes of systemic and cerebral hemodynamics in mechanically ventilated preterm infants, who also respond by marked increases in intracranial pressure (61,62). These changes were found to be effected by a suction-induced stimulation of sympathoexcitatory receptors that are localized in the large airways (63). Due to an age-specific special cerebrovascular vulnerability, each preterm infant is at risk for the occurence of intraventricular hemorrhage. This means that a special hazard in a special adult patient group turns into a much more general one in preterm babies. In practice, the necessity to restrict suction frequency to an absolute minimum, in combination with the avoidance of any time-based routine, therefore pertains not only to adult patients with brain injury, but also to each mechanically ventilated preterm infant.

A somewhat related issue has been raised by a publication that suggests a causal relationship between frequent CPT in the first weeks of life and the occurrence of a characteristic form of brain damage (encephaloclastic porencephaly) in very low birthweight babies (64). As these lesions resemble those seen in older infants with nonaccidental shaking injury, these authors speculate that it might be mechanical interventions occurring in the course of CPT that are responsible for cerebral damage; as a practical consequence of their findings, they have stopped administering CPT in very low birthweight infants altogether. The practical consequence, however, remains debatable, as witholding CPT in these patients, who frequently do have problems with intrabronchial secretions, will result in a different spectrum of problems and complications. One could also react to these disturbing findings with other less radical measures. One of these would be to reduce the frequency of CPT sessions by avoiding any time-based routine and replacing it by targeted interventions that are exclusively based on clinical findings suggestive of mucus-related complications. Another is to modify the methodological details of CPT in the direction of avoiding any shaking or similar mechanical interventions and paying meticulous attention to proper stabilization of the baby's head. Whatever the clinical conclusions drawn, this problem once again dramatically illustrates the special vulnerability of those found at the bottom end of the pediatric size and age spectrum.

Suction trauma, i.e., mucosal damage by tracheobronchial suctioning, has been described in pediatric and adult patients with artificial airways (65–67). Mucosal hemorrhage and erosion are produced when a catheter is inserted too deeply and negative pressure pulls the mucosa into its end and side holes. If this insult is repetitive, it can lead to the formation of granulation tissue and scarring, and these repair processes can eventually result in bronchial obstruction and thereby effected atelectasis. Such severe and permanent damage, usually localized in the basal segments of the right lower lobe, has mostly been observed in mechanically ventilated infants (67,68). This suggests that suction trauma, while occuring in both pediatric and adult patients, might have more severe sequelae in intubated neonates and small children than in any other age group, again highlighting the special vulnerability of the very young pediatric patient. This is further underlined by reports of pneumothoraces in neonates, secondary to perforation of segmental bronchi (again most often occuring in the basal segments of the right lower lobe) by suction catheters (69,70). Imperfect technique applied in the most fragile infants with the most severe lung disease is believed to be responsible for this complication (67). The small size of the newborn makes the distance from the lower end of the endotracheal tube to the entrances of the lower lobe's segmental bronchi particularly short; thus, relatively small errors in the depth of catheter insertion carry a high risk of mucosal damage in this age group.

There is an increased prevalence of gastroesophageal reflux in children with chronic respiratory disease, especially cystic fibrosis, and the predominant reflux mechanism is a transient inappropriate lower esophageal sphincter relaxation (71). Reflux was observed to occur more often in children when CPT was administered (72). Recent studies suggest that the number of reflux episodes is only increased in infants with cystic fibrosis when CPT is performed with a head-down tilt; it might be that this form of postural drainage, rather than other mechanical interventions, is responsible for enhancing reflux (73,74). The clinical relevance of these findings is as yet unclear, as it is not the frequency of reflux episodes, but rather the duration of these episodes and the speed with which the acid is cleared, that matters (75). However, any association of gastroesophageal reflux and CPT in this patient group remains a serious concern, as reflux might occasionally lead to microaspiration and reflex bronchospasm, thus further complicating chronic respiratory disease (76). In older children and adults, gastroesophageal reflux is also recognized as an aggravating factor that can cause or worsen chronic lung disease, but so far there is only one report of an assocation between CPT and reflux (77). This raises the question as to whether gastroesophageal reflux might be an age-specific complication of CPT that occurs predominantly in infancy and early childhood.

IV. Psychological Perspectives

A. Cooperation

Clearly, the psychology of the therapist-patient interaction in pediatric CPT is complex. So far no studies have attempted to systematically explore this area, but clinical experience strongly supports the feasibility of an age-specific approach. No matter their age, all children should always be handled with a maximum of care and respect.

Newborns and infants usually cooperate passively with CPT, i.e., they tolerate the treatment without any sign of discomfort. Most children in this age group seem to like the manipulations of a skillful therapist and rapidly familiarize themselves with the concomitant sensations like the therapist's touch and voice. Schoolchildren usually become actively cooperating partners, and a treatment session will provide them with both a therapeutic and a learning experience. The most difficult patient is certainly the toddler and preschool child who will no longer cooperate passively with CPT yet cannot be persuaded into active cooperation. Experienced pediatric chest physiotherapists collect a quiver full of strategies and tricks to interact productively with children of this age group. Cooperation might be obtained by distraction or persuasion; little gifts and tokens as rewards for good behavior and courage are helpful. As a general rule, severity of disease often correlates with the extent of a small child's cooperation. In the face of serious respiratory compromise, children tend to react to CPT as if they know that these interventions have the potential to make them better and their breathing easier.

B. Teaching

While CPT for clearance of secretions still consists of postural drainage, chest clapping, shaking, vibration, compression, and coughing for the infant and toddler, there is now a spectrum of self-administered techniques for schoolchildren, adolescents, and adults with chronic respiratory disorders (1,78). It follows that the chest physiotherapist is the person who actively administers treatment to the newborn, infant, and preschool child and, occasionally, teaches techniques to parents. In the older patient, the therapist's role is changed into that of an instructor, monitor, and assistant. This situation confronts the pediatric chest physiotherapist with a spectrum of different challenges, and applied clinical psychology is as important a prerequisite as physiological knowledge and manual skills (79,80). The special problem of interacting constructively with younger children is illustrated by studies in patients with cystic fibrosis that report significantly more treatment-related behavioral difficulties and adjustment problems to new aspects of therapy for younger pediatric patients (81).

Adults learn self-administered CPT techniques by accumulating knowledge about the subject. Group teaching that uses strategies of participation and interaction—preferably coordinated and not led—plus offering the additional experience of a friendly and supportive environment is particularly effective. Written information material will often be helpful; the therapist can expect an attention span of 30 minutes or more. While children with chronic respiratory disorders like cystic fibrosis can and will learn the same self-administered techniques for mucus clearance, the approach to teaching and training must be adapted to the age of the patient.

Education in these techniques should commence in the preschool-age child who is able to understand basic concepts. As responsibilities are generally deferred to adults, teaching this age group should include the adult caregivers, and an overly ambitious focus on the patient alone is not yet particularly helpful. Simple, boldly colored pictures and objects, plus a spectrum of easy-to-understand "blowing games," are routinely included in the psychological armentarium of any chest physiotherapist teaching children of this age group. The environment for training should not be perceived as threatening by the small patient; ideally, the entire learning process is experienced as fun, i.e., enjoyable and stimulating. Teaching concepts should take the short attention span of young children (about 5–10 minutes) into account.

School-age children start to benefit from slightly more complex teaching strategies. Verbal explanations begin to be effective as adjuncts to pictures, playful exercises, and demonstrations. Imitation is a key principle to be utilized in the early school age; thus, games and plays based on imitation will be particularly effective. Beyond primary school, both the complexity of such games and the dimension of concomitant verbal explanations should expand. Attention span gradually increases from 10 to 20 minutes or more. Ability and motivation to learn peak in preadolescence, when children are intense and interested. More sophisticated learning resources like books, videos, films, and computer programs can safely be included in educational concepts for preadolescents.

Adolescents are a very difficult and challenging group to educate, and approaches that are highly effective in preadolescence rapidly lose their impact in this developmental stage. Formal education is often ineffective, and interest as a key to successful teaching is both essential and hard to recruit. Any educational environment that is felt to be dominated by adults is usually rejected, but response to messages from peers and peer idols is often enthusiastic. A learning situation in which the patient has ample opportunity to give her or his opinion and to interact intensively with the therapist is essential for recruiting cooperation; involving personalities from the realms of sports, music, fashion, and film for raising and maintaining interest is a successful approach to education in this age group. Attention span, if supported by interest, can range up to or beyond 30 minutes.

In summary, teaching a self-administered CPT technique to pediatric patients with chronic respiratory disorders must utilize age-specific approaches. Ideally, the therapist is already familiar with the patient and his or her family, life, and disease situation, and thus will be able to employ teaching strategies that are not only age-specific but also tailored to the psychological profile of the individual patient.

V. Pathophysiological Perspectives

A. Airway Hyperresponsiveness

Clinical observation and lung function data suggest that CPT can induce bronchospasm in both pediatric and adult patients with airway hyperresponsiveness (6,52,82,83). Airway hyperresponsiveness is a pathophysiological hallmark of bronchial asthma, but can episodically complicate many other acute and chronic respiratory disorders in childhood. Consequently, the therapist should have a high level of awareness of the clinical symptoms of bronchospasm; in case of doubt, lung function testing will help to identify patients who tend to develop this complication. The mechanisms by which CPT triggers a bronchospastic response have never been explored in detail, but it seems reasonable to assume that mechanical irritation per se has a causal role.

Physiotherapy-induced bronchospasm will not only make the patient breathless, but will also hamper mobilization and transport of secretions via a compromise of bronchial lumen, thus rendering the entire treatment session ineffective. The pediatric chest physiotherapist has basically two options to prevent this complication in patients at risk. One is premedication with bronchodilator drugs, usually inhaled β_2-sympathomimetics. This is the most frequently chosen approach, but there remain some reservations against adopting such a bronchodilator-CPT sequence as a fixed therapeutic routine. These reservations pertain to the influence of bronchial smooth muscle relaxants on bronchial wall stability. The other strategy to avoid physiotherapy-induced bronchospasm in patients with airway hyperresponsiveness is the choice of a therapeutic technique that largely avoids mechanical irritation of the tracheobronchial tree. Last but not least, other therapeutic interventions that might cause bronchospasm should either be avoided altogether or timed in a way so as not to jeopardize mucus clearance. One example of such an intervention is the inhalation of aerosolized antibiotics (84); such potentially irritating medication is best administered after mucus clearance has been accomplished successfully.

B. Airway Instability

As discussed previously, the effectiveness of cough and forced expiration for mucus clearance depends on a delicate balance between the magnitude of positive expiratory transthoracic pressure on one side and evenly distributed airway stability that gradually tapers off towards the periphery on the other. This balance is disturbed not only by the developmentally increased airway compressibility of early infancy, but also and more so by localized instability lesions, which occur as congenital airway malformations or as the acquired result of inflammatory tissue destruction.

Some patients suffer from localized instability lesions in the central intrathorac airways throughout their first decade of life and sometimes even into adulthood. These children suffer from tracheo- and/or bronchomalacia, a type of congenital malformation increasingly recognized with the more liberal diagnostic use of flexible fiberoptic bronchoscopy (85,86). These instability lesions are seen in association with tracheoesophageal fistula, vascular rings, more complex cardiac malformations, and generalized disorders of cartilage development; however, they also occur as acquired defects in the context of bronchopulmonary dysplasia (87). Whatever the cause, these lesions predispose the central airways to complete closure with positive transthoracic pressure, thereby effectively interrupting expiratory airflow and clearance of mucus.

Instability lesions will present a special mechanical disadvantage when coexisting with abundant intrabronchial secretions that have to be cleared by CPT. This is the case in generalized or localized bronchiectasis, especially in cystic fibrosis. Advanced stages of this disorder present with countless bronchiectatic lesions, which increase the bronchial volume proportion of the lung from a normal of around 4% to 20% or more (88,89). Lesions start to develop as bronchiectatic ulcers and abscesses, which show histological evidence for active elastolysis (90); in combination with the finding of significantly increased urinary excretion of elastin cross-links and markedly elevated proteolytic activity in the sputum of patients (91), this indicates that the progression of bronchiectasis is effected by ongoing proteolytic damage of bronchial tissue. Proteolytic activity mainly stems from lysosomal enzymes of hyperstimulated neutrophils; in combination with the release of oxygen radicals, this hyperstimulated immune response overwhelms antiprotease defenses and, as a net result, perpetuates bronchial wall damage (92). Physiologically, this ongoing inflammation and tissue destruction results in a combination of more peripherally located airway obstruction (inflammatory mucosal edema and mucus plugging) and more centrally located instability lesions (bronchiectatic ulcers) (Fig. 4); an understanding of lung function alterations in cystic fibrosis via this airway instability concept explains several observed peculiarities like paradoxical responses to pharmacological bronchodilation and bronchial challenges (92–96).

From the chest physiotherapist's perspective, this pathophysiology amounts to an additional rationale for mucus clearance, but also to a substantial mechanical problem. Effective clearance of secretions in cystic fibrosis, as well as in other disorders with generalized or localized bronchiectasis, should not only prevent the mechanical consequences of obstructing mucus and pus like atelectasis or regional hyperinflation, but should also reduce the ongoing damage of the airway walls by removing proteolytic and oxidative activity (2). Disseminated bronchial instability lesions, on the other hand, will predispose to airway collapse when subjected to positive transthoracic pressure, thereby preventing airflow and mucus clearance by cough and forced expirations (1,9). CPT has met this challenge by mucus clearance techniques that modify the physiology of a forced expiration towards preventing such bronchial collapse; these techniques will be discussed subsequently.

As already addressed above, bronchodilators, i.e., bronchial smooth muscle relexants, will further enhance airway compressibility. It follows that abstention from bronchodilator medication appears advisable for any child with tracheo- or bronchomalacia (97). In bronchiectasis, the clinical decision for or against medication with a β_2-stimulant is more complex and should be individualized. A therapeutic trial with an inhaled bronchodilator, monitored by recording of a maximum expiratory flow–volume curve, can be helpful for clinical decision making. An observed increase in end-expiratory flow suggests a thera-

---

FACING PAGE

Figure 4 Advanced airway damage in CF as a combination of central bronchiectasis and more peripheral obstruction: (top) inspiration—air is inhaled into alveoli but also into dilating instable airways; (center) early forced expiration—high flow from alveoli and previously dilated bronchi; (bottom) late forced expiration—severely compromised flow due to airway obstruction and compression; (right) corresponding typical flow-volume loop. $\dot{V}_E$ = expiratory flow; $\dot{V}_I$ = inspiratory flow; V = volume; TLC = total lung capacity; RV = residual volume. (From Ref. 96.)

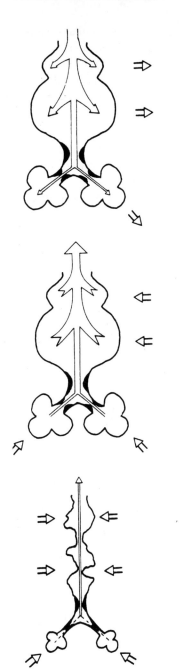
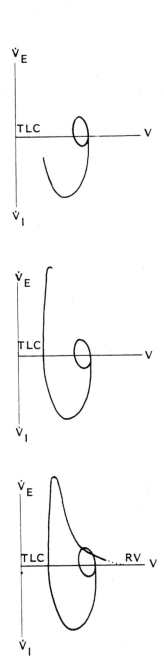

peutically effected reduction of bronchospasm, while a bronchodilator-induced further decrease of end-expiratory flow should be interpreted as indicating a potentially harmful compromise of bronchial wall stability (94). Bronchodilator premedication can be used more liberally when the therapist plans to apply a CPT technique that mechanically compensates for bronchial compression.

C. Lung Volume Derangement

Most respiratory diseases in childhood effect alterations of lung volume; thus, the chest physiotherapist is more often than not treating a patient whose volume level of breathing has been shifted away from normal.

By far the most frequent type of lung volume alteration in pediatric patients is hyperinflation secondary to obstruction of intrathoracic airways (51). The mechanisms effecting an increase of FRC and residual volume during acute and chronic airway obstruction are complex (98). In most cases, this obstruction, whether inflammatory mucosal edema, accumulated secretions, or bronchospastic narrowing of airways, will be disseminated, and hyperinflation will be distributed somewhat inhomogeneously throughout the lungs. As evident from a markedly elevated FRC, tidal breathing is shifted into a higher percentage of TLC, thus providing for the necessary minimum of bronchial patency by an increased static-elastic recoil with more radial traction on airways.

Advanced chronic interstitial lung disease is rare in pediatric patients. When compared to normal, these patients show a restrictive pattern of lung function changes (99,100); they breathe at a lower lung volume, but the level of tidal breathing has not shifted massively in terms of percentage of TLC. Rather, TLC and FRC have decreased proportionally. Airways, if not directly involved in the disease process, are patent.

A somewhat different type of restrictive lung volume derangement prevails in infants and children with progressive neuromuscular disease (100,101). Comparable to the situation in the premature baby, a chest that lacks sufficient muscular support for stability suspends lungs with a normal recoil; consequently, the elastic equilibrium of the system and tidal breathing are shifted to an abnormally low lung volume. Airway patency is compromised via a low static-elastic recoil pressure. This abnormally high chest wall complicance, and the thereby effected lung volume changes, however, are only typical for pediatric patients (102); adults with neuromuscular disease have decreased chest wall compliance, which is speculatively attributed to years of low tidal volume breathing leading to contractures of joints and increased stiffness of the soft chest wall tissues (101,103). Often the situation is further complicated by the development of scoliosis that contributes to lung volume restriction in these patients (104).

It follows that the pediatric chest physiotherapist might be confronted by both developmental and disease-inflicted lung volume problems or a combination of both. This raises the question as to whether different lung volume alterations require a different approach to mucus clearance. Most likely, the answer is that the essentials of the technique should remain unchanged, while therapeutic details require some modifications.

Mucus clearance from a markedly hyperinflated lung will nevertheless have to commence with further raising the lung volume, as the treatment will have to target those lung units that are already underventilated because of compromised bronchial patency. Once secretions have been mobilized, however, their transport through the airways towards expectoration is subject to a delicate interaction of patent lumen, stability, airstream velocity, and compression waves. Unobstructed airways that are widely distended by the increased parenchymal recoil of elevated lung volume might occasionally disturb this mechanical interaction by being overly patent. Experienced pediatric chest physiotherapists will tend to emphasize volume reduction (chest compression, voluntary expirations to low lung volume) when transport of mobilized secretions is required in children with hyperinflated lungs. This routine is based on the clinical observation of more effective mucus clearance with lung volume reduction.

CPT for mucus clearance will rarely be required in pediatric interstitial lung disease. The therapist can train the patient in breathing patterns that save energy. Distension techniques (deep inspirations, inspiratory muscle training) will have no significant effect on the fibrotic lungs.

More often CPT will be required for mucus clearance in patients with neuromuscular disease. A weak cough, a low tidal volume, and reduced bronchial patency all combine to produce a high likelihood of mucus-effected respiratory complications. In addition, muscle weakness will result in a decreased incidence of body position changes; consequently, redistribution of ventilation will occur less often than required for homogeneous alveolar inflation. Here, the chest physiotherapist will not only raise lung volume for initial mobilization of secretions, but will continue to emphasize lung volume management in order to provide sufficient bronchial patency for transport of secretions. In the preterm and newborn infant, CPAP appears to be an effective strategy to prevent or treat complications from intrabronchial secretions in children with neuromuscular disease, especially during respiratory infections. In combination with CPT, CPAP provides a well-inflated alveolar region and sufficiently dilated airways as a basis for any attempt at mucus clearance.

VI. Practical Perspectives

A. Techniques

A spectrum of CPT techniques has been developed for mucus clearance in pediatric patients; for more detailed information on history of technique, practical details, and clinical studies, the reader is referred to relevant articles (1,5,6,

78,105). In order to tailor CPT to the individual needs of a pediatric patient, one has to analyze the patient and disease situation from a developmental, physiological, pathophysiological, psychological, and clinical perspective and then scrutinize the quiver of available techniques for the one that best satisfies the therapeutic needs.

Conventional CPT (postural drainage, lung volume management, chest percussion, shaking, vibration, compression, and assisted coughing or suctioning) is a traditional technique that is therapist-administered, requires little cooperation, and thus remains the only method available for premature babies, newborns, infants, and toddlers as well as for unconscious and immobilized (artificially ventilated) patients (5,6). Change of body position and all applied strategies of lung volume management aim at getting air behind obstructing mucus plugs; chest percussion, shaking, and vibration are based on a concept of pressure waves that shake secretions from the airway wall (moblization); coughing, either induced by mobilized mucus or stimulated by the therapist, moves secretions (transport) via the mechanisms of a forced expiration. Because this technique, when applied in nonintubated patients, uses coughing for transport of secretions, it can be hampered by airway instability lesions that allow for bronchial closure under positive transthoracic pressure. The chest is a therapeutic interface that reduces its initially supportive role with growth. A soft and compliant chest wall will sufficiently transmit externally applied mechanical interventions to the lungs; thus, mobilization of secretions by conventional CPT will be more effective in the very young than in the older patient. Mechanical forces acting on the airways may suffice for inducing bronchospasm in the presence of airway hyperresponsiveness.

In contrast to conventional CPT, all self-administered techniques require the active cooperation of the patient. When scrutinized from the perspective of respiratory physiology, all these methods basically employ the airflow and airway mechanics of a forced expiration. As discussed previously, any localized instability lesion will result in complete airway collapse, once incorporated in the compressed downstream segment, thereby effectively terminating expiratory airflow and mucus transport from these lung units. All the subsequently described CPT techniques have in common the attempt to circumnavigate these untoward effects of airway instability lesions by various modifications of forced expiration mechanics.

The active cycle of breathing techniques consists of thoracic expansion exercises for raising lung volume plus the forced expiration technique for mobilizing and transporting secretions (106). The technique is relatively easy to learn, given a dedicated chest physiotherapist as teacher; nevertheless, it takes some time to develop the required skills, and thus the technique is usually taught to patients with chronic disorders like cystic fibrosis. The "huff," i.e., the forced expiratory maneuver for mucus clearance, works by the above-described physiology of a forced expiration. The lung volume at which a huff is initiated can be adjusted to the momentary location of intrabronchial secretions, and more peripherally deposited mucus is targeted by huffing at a low lung volume. As the forced expiration technique allows for adapting applied positive transthoracic pressure to existing instability lesions, huffing with carefully titrated effort might be more effective than coughing for mucus clearance in the presence of bronchiectasis; it has been observed that transpulmonary pressures developed with coughing are in excess of those occuring in a forced expiratory maneuver (107). Forced expirations might occasionally induce bronchospasm in patients with hyperresponsive airways. This complication can be prevented by alternating forced expirations with breathing control (6); in addition, a bronchodilator can be inhaled before commencing CPT. Bronchodilator premedication, however, carries the risk of further reducing bronchial stability and thereby enhancing bronchial collapse.

Positive expiratory pressure (PEP) mask therapy utilizes expirations against a stenosis for mobilizing secretions. There are two distinctly different techniques of PEP mask therapy: the conventional (or low pressure) one, which avoids higher expiratory efforts and pressures (108), and the high-pressure technique, which incorporates forced expirations into the treatment cycle (109). The high-pressure technique has the advantage of being very effective in a short period of time and the occasionally relevant disadvantage of being energy consuming.

PEP-mask breathing (low-pressure technique) effects a marked attenuation of dynamic expiratory airway compression (110) and complex changes of lung functions like increased tidal and decreased residual volume (111,112). The physiological consequences of exhaling forcefully against a resistive load (high-pressure technique) are even more complex; they are discussed in some detail elsewhere (109). Briefly, the entire tracheobronchial tree remains dilated upstream segment for a large portion of the forced expiration; however, an upstream movement of the equal pressure point, although also subject to the equalizing effect of the external expiratory resistor, occurs at the end of a properly performed maneuver. Backpressure and thereby effected airway dilation will enhance filling of underventilated lung regions; the terminal upstream movement of choke points will mobilize and transport secretions. The resistor's equalizing effect on the expiratory behavior of different lung units is paid for by a substantially increased expiratory muscle effort and by a decreased airstream velocity. In comparison to a normal forced expiratory maneuver, however, the latter will only be a disadvantage for the first few bronchial generations, as expiratory flow decreases rapidly towards the periphery in any case.

While basically developed for self-administered CPT in chronic disorders, PEP mask therapy is easy enough to learn for therapeutic application against acute complications like atelectasis. Even in the presence of advanced airway instability lesions, bronchial collapse is prevented by the backpressure of the expiratory resistor. Bronchospasm will complicate the high-pressure technique, but bronchodilator premedication can be used liberally as the effected further reduction of bronchial wall stability will be compensated for by the inherent mechanical effects of the technique.

Autogenic drainage is a special breathing technique that avoids higher transthoracic pressures and thereby effected bronchial compression and tries to adapt the lung volume to the perceived location of intrabronchial secretions (113). Physiologically, autogenic drainage can be seen as a modification of the forced expiration technique that applies comparable mechanical principles. It aims to achieve an individually determined ideal expiratory flow rate that suffices for mobilizing and transporting secretions but, at the same time, avoids the application of transthoracic pressures of sufficient magnitude to occlude destabilized airways. This type of compromise will be determined by the most collapsible parts of the system; thus, the technique is focused on treating those lung regions with more advanced bronchiectatic airway wall damage.

It takes considerable time to learn to perform the technique properly and to develop the required proprioceptive abilities; consequently, autogenic drainage will mainly be taught to older patients with chronic disoders. Unlike the high-pressure PEP mask technique, autogenic drainage is more time and less energy consuming; thus, it is particularly suited for exhausted and weak patients. As it avoids forced expiratory maneuvers, autogenic drainage is one of the techniques that offer themselves for application in patients with airway instability lesions. For the same reason, bronchospasm will rarely be a handicap when using this technique.

There are other techniques for mucus clearance in pediatric patients, such as high-frequency chest compression (114) or oscillating PEP (flutter) therapy (115), but more data are required to determine whether these newer developments are of equal effectiveness or even offer advantages when compared to the aforementioned methods. So far, comparative studies have failed to demonstrate a superiority of flutter CPT over other techniques in the treatment of cystic fibrosis (116,117). Physical exercise and sports can also facilitate mucus clearance in patients with chronic suppurative lung disease (118,119); one can assume that hyperventilation with physical activity and sports effects enhanced gas-liquid pumping.

B. Knowledge

In addition to practical experience in administering and teaching the above techniques to patients, a pediatric chest physiotherapist must have detailed knowledge of the respiratory physiology of newborns, infants, children, and adolescents. Such knowledge is acquired in relevant courses, from textbooks and other teaching material, and, most importantly, by integrating the CPT service into the organizational framework of a pediatric respiratory center with a busy lung function laboratory. Besides gaining visual experience in the interpretation of chest radiographs and endoscopies, a pediatric chest physiotherapist should have easy access to lung function testing for monitoring mucus clearance interventions (1). Still more important will be a physiologically oriented approach to the clinical assessment of the individual patient; a keen recognition of signs and symptoms, complemented by their physiological interpretation, will usually provide the therapist with enough information for optimally matching disease situation and therapeutic technique on an individual basis.

VII. Conclusions

In pediatric patients, recognition of developmental peculiarities, in combination with an analysis of the prevailing pathophysiology, will be essential for choosing the appropriate technique and fine-tuning the therapeutic details.

The patient's age will define type and extent of cooperation. Passively cooperating newborns, infants, and toddlers can only be treated by conventional CPT. Given enough time for instruction and training, the active cycle of breathing techniques and PEP mask therapy can be taught to children from an age of about 4 years. Autogenic drainage is better suited for older children and adolescents. Teaching methods will vary with age.

Age also defines an individual respiratory tract's structural and functional stage of development and thereby the necessary methodological modifications. Lung volume management and consideration of bronchial stability issues will be of special relevance for mucus clearance in premature babies, newborns, and young infants. Children in this age group also demand special consideration of their increased vulnerability in order to avoid any negative side effects of CPT. Positioning will have different physiological effects in the first decade of life than later in adolescence or adulthood.

Detailed analysis of prevailing disease mechanisms is the other prerequisite for an individualized approach to mucus clearance. This starts with the trivial realization that CPT can only clear mucus that is abundant in the airways. Airway obstruction due to inflammatory mucosal edema or bronchospasm has to be differentiated carefully by clinical, radiological, and physiological means from the signs and consequences of accumulated intrabronchial secretions before commencing CPT. Airway hyperresponsiveness calls for less irritating mechanical interventions or bronchodilator premedication. The presence of airway instability lesions requires techniques that mechanically compensate for the increased risk of bronchial collapse. Lung volume derangement calls for modification of the applied technique. Exhausted patients will have to use those techniques that are least energy consuming.

Acute disease and mucus-effected complications like atelectasis demand a CPT technique that does not require a time-consuming learning process on the side of the patient; this suggests conventional CPT as the technique of choice in such situations. CPAP will effectively support conventional CPT in the reinflation of atelectatic lung units. PEP mask therapy is also learned quickly by older patients and thus is a realistic alternative. Chronic disorders remain the most important indication for training in self-administered techniques.

It follows that a developmentally oriented approach to the prescription and administration of CPT will help to guide the therapist through the conundrum of physiological and psychological peculiarities that characterize the pediatric patient. By no means can such an approach substitute for the urgently required results of studies that further explore the potential and the limitations of pediatric CPT. Such studies, however, will also benefit in focus and clinical relevance when guided by developmentally oriented concepts on the interaction of CPT techniques with disease mechanisms.

References

1. Zach MS, Oberwaldner B. Chest physiotherapy. In: Taussig L, Landau L, eds. Textbook of Pediatric Respiratory Medicine. St. Louis: Mosby, 1999:299–311.
2. Zach MS, Oberwaldner B. Chest physiotherapy—the mechanical approach to antiinfective therapy in cystic fibrosis. Infection 1987; 5:381–384.
3. Webber BA. Evaluation and inflation in respiratory care. Physiotherapy 1991; 77:801–804.
4. Williams MT. Chest physiotherapy and cystic fibrosis: why is the most effective form of treatment still unclear? Chest 1994; 106:1872–1882.
5. Parker A, Prasad A. Paediatrics. In: Pryor JA, Webber BA, eds. Physiotherapy for Respiratory and Cardiac Problems. Edinburgh: Churchill-Livingstone, 1998:329–369.
6. Webber BA, Pryor JA, Bethune DD, Potter HM, McKenzie D. Physiotherapy techniques. In: Pryor JA, Webber BA, eds. Physiotherapy for Respiratory and Cardiac Problems. Edinburgh: Churchill-Livingstone, 1998:137–209.
7. Mead J, Turner JM, Macklem PT, Little JB. Significance of the relationship between lung recoil and maximum expiratory flow. J Appl Physiol 1967; 22:95–108.
8. Macklem PT, Mead J. The physiological basis of common pulmonary function tests. Arch Environ Health 1967; 14:5–9.
9. Smaldone GC, Itoh H, Swift DL, Wagner HN. Effect of flow-limiting segments and cough on particle deposition and mucociliary clearance in the lung. Am Rev Respir Dis 1979; 120:747–758.
10. Hasani A, Pavia D, Agnew JE, Clarke SW. Regional lung clearance during cough and forced expiration technique (FET): effects of flow and viscoelasticity. Thorax 1994; 49:557–561.
11. Mead J, Takishima T, Leith D. Stress distribution in lungs: a model of pulmonary elasticity. J Appl Physiol 1970; 28:596–608.
12. Richard CC, Bachman L. Lung and chest wall compliance in apneic paralyzed infants. J Clin Invest 1961; 40:273–278.

13. Gerhard T, Bancalari E. Chest wall compliance in full-term and premature infants. Acta Paediatr Scand 1980; 69:359–364.
14. Davis GM, Coates AL, Papageorgiou A, Bureau MA. Direct measurement of static chest wall compliance in animal and human neonates. J Appl Physiol 1988; 65:1093–1098.
15. Sharp JT, Druz WS, Balagot RC, Bandelin VR, Danon J. Total respiratory compliance in infants and children. J Appl Physiol 1970; 29:775–779.
16. Papastamelos C, Panitch H, England S, Allen J. Developmental changes in chest wall compliance in infancy and early childhood. J Appl Physiol 1995; 78:179–184.
17. Polgar G, Weng TR. The functional development of the respiratory system. From the period of gestation to adulthood. Am Rev Respir Dis 1979; 120:625–695.
18. Bryan AC, England SJ. Maintenance of an elevated FRC in the newborn. Paradox of REM sleep. Am Rev Respir Dis 1984; 129:209–210.
19. Lopes J, Muller NL, Bryan MH, Bryan AC. Importance of inspiratory muscle tone in maintenance of FRC in the newborn. J Appl Physiol 1981; 51:830–834.
20. Stark AR, Cohlan BA, Waggener TB, Frantz JD, Kosch PC. Regulation of end expiratory lung volume during sleep in premature infants. J Appl Physiol Respir Environ Exercise Physiol 1987; 62:1117–1123.
21. Harding R, Johnson P, MacLelland ME. The expiratory role of the larynx during development and the influence of behavioural state. In: von Euler C, Lagercrantz H, eds. Central Nervous Control Mechanisms of Breathing. Oxford, UK: Pergamon Press, 1979:353–359.
22. England SJ, Kent G, Stogryn HAF. Laryngeal muscle and diaphragm activities in conscious dog pups. Respir Physiol 1985; 60:95–108.
23. Hagan R, Bryan AC, Bryan HM, Gulston G. The effect of sleep state on intercostal muscle activity and rib cage motion. Physiologist 1976; 19:214.
24. Poets CF, Rau GA, Neuber K, Gappa M, Seidenberg J. Determinants of lung volume in spontaneously breathing preterm infants. Am J Respir Crit Care Med 1997; 155:649–653.
25. Boothroyd AE, Murthy BV, Darbyshire A, Petros AJ. Endotracheal suctioning causes right upper lobe collapse in intubated children. Acta Paediatr 1996; 85:1422–1425.
26. Brandstater B, Muallem M. Atelectasis following tracheal suctioning in infants. Anaesthesiology 1969; 31:468–473.
27. Tusiewicz K, Moldofsky H, Bryan AC, Bryan MH. Mechanics of the rib cage and diaphragm during sleep. J Appl Physiol Respir Environ Exercise Physiol 1977; 43:600–602.
28. Knill R, Andrews W, Bryan AC, Bryan HM. Respiratory load compensation in infants. J Appl Physiol 1976; 40:357–361.
29. Carlo WA, Martin RJ, Bruce EN, Strohl KP, Fanaroff AA. Alae nasi activation (nasal flaring) decreases nasal resistance in preterm infants. Pediatrics 1983; 72:338–343.
30. De Almeida VL, Alvaro RA, Haider Z, Rehan V, Nowaczyk B, Cates D, Kwiatkowski K, Rigatto H. The effect of nasal occlusion on the initiation of oral breathing in preterm infants. Pediatr Pulmonol 1994; 18:374–378.

31. Purcell M. Response in the newborn to raised upper airway resistance. Arch Dis Child 1976; 51:602–606.

32. Dunbar JS. Upper respiratory tract obstruction in infants and children. Am J Roentgen 1970; 109:227–246.

33. Meine FJ, Lorenzo RL, Lynch PF, Capitanio MA, Kirkpatrick JA. Pharyngeal distension associated with upper airway obstruction. Radiology 1974; 111:395–398.

34. Stocks J. Effect of nasogastric tubes on nasal resistance during infancy. Arch Dis Child 1980; 55:17–21.

35. Van Someren V, Linnett SJ, Stothers JK, Sullivan PG. An investigation into the benefits of resisting nasoenteric feeding tubes. Pediatrics 1984; 74:379–383.

36. Sporik R. Why block a small hole? The adverse effects of nasogastric tubes. Arch Dis Child 1994; 71:393–394.

37. Zach M, Oberwaldner B, Purrer B, Schober P, Grubbauer HM. Thoraxphysiotherapeutische Behandlung bronchopulmonaler Erkrankungen des Kindesalters [Chest physiotherapy in childhood respiratory disorders]. Monatsschr Kinderheilkd 1981; 129:633–636.

38. Mellins RS. Pulmonary physiotherapy in the pediatric age group. Am Rev Respir Dis 1974; 110:137–142.

39. Menkes H, Britt J. Rationale for physical therapy. Am Rev Respir Dis 1980; 122(suppl. 2):127–131.

40. West JB. Pulmonary Pathophysiology. 4th ed. Baltimore: Williams & Wilkins, 1992.

41. Davies H, Helms P, Gordon J. Effect of posture on regional ventilation in children. Pediatr Pulmonol 1992; 12:227–232.

42. Davies H, Kitchman R, Gordon J, Helms P. Regional ventilation in infancy. Reversal of adult pattern. N Engl J Med 1985; 313:1626–1628.

43. Bhuyan U, Peters AM, Gordon J, Davies H, Helms P. Effects of posture on the distribution of pulmonary ventilation and perfusion in children and adults. Thorax 1989; 44:480–484.

44. Remolina C, Khan AU, Santiago TV, Edelman NH. Positional hypoxaemia in unilateral lung disease. N Engl J Med 1981; 304:523–525.

45. Heaf DP, Helms P, Gordon J, Turner HM. Postural effects on gas exchange in infants. N Engl J Med 1983; 308:1505–1508.

46. Croteau JR, Cook CD. Volume-pressure and length-tension measurements in human tracheal and bronchial segments. J Appl Physiol 1961; 16:170–172.

47. Matsuba K, Thurlbeck WM. A morphometric study of bronchial and bronchiolar walls in children. Am Rev Respir Dis 1972; 105:908–913.

48. Shaffer TH, Bhutani VK, Wolfson MR, Penn RB, Tran NN. In vivo mechanical properties of the developing airway. Pediatr Res 1989; 25:143–146.

49. Hislop AA, Haworth SG. Airway size and structure in the normal fetal and infant lung and the effect of premature delivery and artificial ventilation. Am Rev Respir Dis 1989; 140:1717–1726.

50. Penn RB, Wolfson MR, Shaffer TH. Developmental differences in tracheal cartilage mechanics. Pediatr Res 1989; 26:429–433.

51. Phelan PD, Olinsky A, Robertson CF. Respiratory Illness in Children. 4th ed. Oxford, UK: Blackwell Scientific Publications, 1994.
52. Rochester DF, Goldberg SK. Techniques of respiratory physical therapy. Am Rev Respir Dis 1980; 122:133–146.
53. Olsen CR, Stevens AE, McIlroy MB. Rigidity of trachea and bronchi during muscular constriction. J Appl Physiol 1967; 23:27–34.
54. Olsen CR, Stevens AE, Pride NB, Staub NC. Structural basis for decreased compressibility of constricted trachea and bronchi. J Appl Physiol 1967; 23:35–39.
55. Bouhuys A, van de Woestijne KP. Mechanical consequences of airway smooth muscle relaxation. J Appl Physiol 1971; 30:670–676.
56. Prendiville A, Green S, Silverman M. Paradoxical response to nebulised salbutamol in wheezy infants, assessed by partial expiratory flow-volume curves. Thorax 1987; 42:86–91.
57. Purchit DM, Caldwell C, Levkoff AH. Multiple rib fractures due to physiotherapy in a neonate with hyaline membrane disease. Am J Dis Child 1975; 129:1103–1104.
58. Brucia J, Rudy E. The effect of suction catheter insertion and tracheal stimulation in adults with severe brain injury. Heart Lung 1996; 25:295–303.
59. Werba A, Weinstabl C, Petricek W, Plainer B, Spiss CK. Bedarfsgerechte Muskelrelaxation mit Vecuronium zur Tracheobronchialtoilette bei neurochirurgischen Intensivpatienten. Anaesthesist 1991; 40:328–331.
60. Rudy EB, Turner BS, Baun M, Stone KS, Brucia J. Endotracheal suctioning in adults with head injury. Heart Lung 1991; 20:667–674.
61. Perlman JM, Volpe JJ. Suctioning in the preterm infant: effects on cerebral blood—flow velocity, intracranial pressure, and arterial blood pressure. Pediatrics 1983; 72:329–334.
62. Evans JC. Reducing the hypoxemia, bradycardia, and apnea associated with suctioning in low birthweight infants. J Perinatol 1992; 12:137–142.
63. Segar JL, Merrill DC, Chapleau MW, Robillard JE. Hemodynamic changes during endotracheal suctioning are mediated by increased autonomic activity. Pediatr Res 1993; 33:649–652.
64. Harding JE, Miles FK, Becroft DMO, Allen BC, Knight DB. Chest physiotherapy may be associated with brain damage in extremely premature infants. J Pediatr 1998; 132:440–444.
65. Plum F, Dunning MF. Techniques for minimising trauma to the tracheobronchial tree after tracheostomy. N Engl J Med 1956; 254:193–200.
66. Sackner MA, Landa J, Greeneltch N, Robinson J. Pathogenesis and prevention of tracheobronchial damage with suction procedures. Chest 1973; 64:284–290.
67. Young CS. A review of the adverse effects of airway suction. Physiotherapy 1984; 70:104–106.
68. Nagaraj HS, Fellows R, Shott R, Yacoub U. Recurrent lobar atelectasis due to acquired stenosis in neonates. J Pediatr Surg 1980; 15:411–415.
69. Anderson K, Chandra K. Pneumothorax secondary to perforation of sequential bronchi by suction catheters. J Paediatr Surg 1976; 11:687–693.
70. Vaughan RS, Menke JA Giacoia GP. Pneumothorax: a complication of endotracheal tube suctioning. J Paediatr 1978; 92:633–634.

71. Cucchiara S, Santamaria F, Andreotti MR, Minella R, Ercolini P, Oggero V, de-Ritis G. Mechanisms of gastroesophageal reflux in cystic fibrosis. Arch Dis Child 1991; 66:617–622.

72. Vandenplas Y, Diericx A, Blecker U, Lanciers S, Deneyer M. Esophageal pH monitoring data during chest physiotherapy. J Pediatr Gastroenterol Nutr 1991; 13:23–26.

73. Button BM, Heine RG, Catto-Smith AG, Phelan PD. Postural drainage exacerbates gastroesophageal reflux in patients with lung disease: is positive expiratory pressure a better alternative? Pediatr Res 1994; 36:47A.

74. Button BM, Heine RG, Catto-Smith AG, Phelan PD, Olinsky A. Postural drainage and gastro-oesophageal reflux in infants with cystic fibrosis. Arch Dis Child 1997; 76:148–150.

75. Taylor CJ, Threlfall D. Postural drainage techniques and gastro-oesophageal reflux in cystic fibrosis. Lancet 1997; 349:1567–1568.

76. Orenstein SR, Orenstein DM. Gastroesophageal reflux and respiratory disease in children. J Pediatr 1980; 97:224–249.

77. Foster AC, Voyles JB, Murphy SA. Twenty-four hour pH monitoring in children with cystic fibrosis: association of chest physical therapy to gastroesophageal reflux. Pediatr Res 1983; 17:118A.

78. Hardy KA. A review of airway clearance: new techniques, indications, and recommendations. Respir Care 1994; 39:440–452.

79. Nickel H. Entwicklungspsychologie des Kindes- und Jugendalters. Band 1. [Developmental Psychology of Childhood and Adolescence. Volume 1.] Bern: Hans Huber Verlag, 1976.

80. Nickel H. Entwicklungspsychologie des Kindes- und Jugendalters. Band 2. [Developmental Psychology of Childhood and Adolescence. Volume 2.] Bern: Hans Huber Verlag, 1976.

81. Sanders MR, Gravestock FM, Wanstall K, Dunne M. The relationship between children's treatment-related behaviour problems, age and clinical status in cystic fibrosis. J Paediatr Child Health 1991; 27:290–294.

82. Campbell AH, O'Connell JM, Wilson F. The effect of chest physiotherapy on the FEV_1 in chronic bronchitis. Med J Aust 1975; 1:33–35.

83. Feldman J, Traver GA, Taussig LM. Maximal expiratory flows after postural drainage. Am Rev Respir Dis 1979; 119:239–245.

84. Chua HL, Collis GG, LeSouef PN. Bronchial response to nebulized antibiotics in children with cystic fibrosis. Eur Respir J 1990; 3:1114–1116.

85. Wood RE. Spelunking in the pediatric airways: explorations with the flexible fiberoptic bronchoscope. Pediatr Clin North Am 1984; 31:785–799.

86. Eber E, Zach M. Flexible fiberoptische Bronchoskopie in der Pädiatrie—eine Analyse von 420 Untersuchungen (pediatric flexible fiberoptic bronchoscopy—an analysis of 420 investigations). Wien Klin Wochenschr 1995; 107:246–251.

87. Sotomayor JL, Godinez RI, Borden S, Wilmott RW. Large airway collapse due to acquired tracheobronchomalacia in infancy. Am J Dis Child 1986; 140:367–371.

88. Bedrossian CMW, Greenberg SD, Singer DB, Hansen JJ, Rosenberg HS. The lung in cystic fibrosis. A quantitative study including prevalence of pathologic findings among different age groups. Hum Pathol 1976; 7:195–204.

89. Tomashefski JF, Bruce M, Goldberg HJ, Dearborn DG. Regional distribution of macroscopic lung disease in cystic fibrosis. Am Rev Respir Dis 1986; 133:535–540.

90. Bruce MC, Poncz L, Klinger JD, Stern RC, Tomashefski JF, Dearborn DG. Biochemical and pathologic evidence for proteolytic destruction of lung connective tissue in cystic fibrosis. Am Rev Respir Dis 1985; 132:529–535.

91. Suter S, Schaad UB, Roux L, Nydegger UE, Waldvogel FA. Granulocyte neutral proteases and *Pseudomonas elastase* as possible causes of airway damage in patients with cystic fibrosis. J Infect Dis 1984; 149:523–531.

92. Zach MS. Lung disease in cystic fibrosis—an updated concept. Pediatr Pulmonol 1990; 8:188–202.

93. Landau LJ, Phelan PD. The variable effect of a bronchodilating agent on pulmonary function in cystic fibrosis. J Pediatr 1973; 83:863–868.

94. Zach MS, Oberwaldner B, Forche G, Polgar G. Bronchodilators increase airway instability in cystic fibrosis. Am Rev Respir Dis 1985; 131:537–543.

95. Darga LL, Eason LA, Zach MS, Polgar G. Cold air provocation of airway hyperreactivity in patients with cystic fibrosis. Pediatr Pulmonol 1986; 2:82–88.

96. Eber E, Oberwaldner B, Zach MS. Airway obstruction and airway wall instability in cystic fibrosis: the isolated and combined effect of theophylline and sympathomimetics. Pediatr Pulmonol 1988; 4:205–212.

97. Panitch HB, Keklikian EN, Motley RA, Wolfson MR, Schidlow DV. Effect of altering smooth muscle tone on maximal expiratory flows in patients with tracheomalacia. Pediatr Pulmonol 1990; 9:170–176.

98. Pellegrino R, Brusasco V. On the causes of lung hyperinflation during bronchoconstriction. Eur Respir J 1997; 10:468–475.

99. Thurlbeck WM, Fleetham JA. Usual interstitial pneumonia (cryptogenic or idiopathic fibrosing alveolitis). In: Chernick V, Kendig EL, eds. Disorders of the Respiratory Tract in Children. 5th ed. Philadelphia: W. B. Saunders, 1990:480–485.

100. Bancalari E, Clausen J. Pathophysiology of changes in absolute lung volume. Eur Respir J 1998; 12:248–258.

101. Allen JL. Respiratory function in children with neuromuscular disease. Monaldi Arch Chest Dis 1996; 51:230–235.

102. Papastamelos C, Panitch H, Allen J. Chest wall compliance in very young children with neuromuscular disease. Am J Respir Crit Care Med 1994; 149:A693.

103. Estenne M, Heilporn A, Delhez L, Yernault JC, DeTroyer A. Chest wall stiffness in patients with chronic respiratory muscle weakness. Am Rev Respir Dis 1983; 128:1002–1007.

104. Jenkins JG, Bohn D, Edmonds JF, Levison H, Barker GA. Evaluation of pulmonary function in muscular dystrophy patients requiring spinal surgery. Crit Care Med 1982; 10:645–649.

105. Mahlmeister MJ, Fink JB, Hoffman GL, Fifer LF. Positive-expiratory pressure mask therapy: theoretical and practical considerations and a review of the literature. Respir Care 1991; 36:1218–1229.

106. Pryor JA, Webber BA, Hodson ME, Batten JC. Evaluation of the forced expiration technique as an adjunct to postural drainage in treatment of cystic fibrosis. BMJ 1979; 2:417–418.

107. Langlands J. The dynamics of cough in health and in chronic bronchitis. Thorax 1967; 22:88–96.
108. Falk M, Kelstrup M, Andersen JB, Kinoshita T, Falk P, Stovring S, Gothgen J. Improving the ketchup bottle method with positive expiratory pressure, PEP, in cystic fibrosis. Eur J Respir Dis 1984; 65:423–432.
109. Oberwaldner B, Evans JC, Zach MS. Forced expirations against a variable resistance: a new chest physiotherapy method in cystic fibrosis. Pediatr Pulmonol 1986; 2:358–367.
110. Al-Nahhas A, Hoffmeyer B, Takis C, Obeid E, Pichurko B. Dynamic airway compression limited forced vital capacity is attenuated by positive airway pressure in severe cystic fibrosis. Am J Respir Crit Care Med 1994; 65(4 part 2):A675.
111. Groth S, Stafanger G, Dirksen H, Andersen JB, Falk M, Kelstrup M. Positive expiratory pressure (PEP-mask) physiotherapy improves ventilation and reduces volume of trapped gas in cystic fibrosis. Bull Eur Physiopathol Respir 1985; 21: 339–343.
112. Van der Schans CP, deJong W, deVries G, Postma DS, Koeter GH, van der Mark TW. Effect of positive expiratory pressure on breathing pattern in healthy subjects. Eur Respir J 1993; 6:60–66.
113. Chevallier J. Autogenic drainage. In: Lawson D, ed. Cystic Fibrosis: Horizons. Chichester, UK: John Wiley and Sons, 1984:235.
114. Warwick WJ, Hansen LG. The long-term effect of high-frequency chest compression therapy on pulmonary complications of cystic fibrosis. Pediatr Pulmonol 1991; 11:265–271.
115. Konstan MW, Stern RC, Doershuk CF. Efficacy of the flutter device for airway mucus clearance in patients with cystic fibrosis. J Pediatr 1994; 124:689–693.
116. Pryor JA, Webber BA, Hodson ME, Warner JO. The flutter VRP1 as an adjunct to chest physiotherapy in cystic fibrosis. Respir Med 1994; 88:677–681.
117. Van Winden CMQ, Visser A, Hop W, Sterk PJ, Beckers S, deJongste JC. Effects of flutter and PEP mask physiotherapy on symptoms and lung function in children with cystic fibrosis. Eur Respir J 1998; 12:143–147.
118. Zach MS, Purrer B, Oberwaldner B. Effect of swimming on forced expiration and sputum clearance in cystic fibrosis. Lancet 1981; 2:1201–1203.
119. Zach M, Oberwaldner B, Häusler F. Cystic fibrosis: physical exercise versus chest physiotherapy. Arch Dis Child 1982; 57:587–589.

19

Postoperative Mucus Clearance

LINDA DENEHY

The University of Melbourne
Parkville, Victoria, Australia

J. P. VAN DE LEUR

University Hospital Groningen
Groningen, The Netherlands

I. Introduction

Following upper-abdominal and cardiothoracic surgery, patients are at risk of developing postoperative pulmonary complications, such as atelectasis and pneumonia. Several studies have been performed to determine which category of patient is highrisk. Results from the literature suggest that multiple factors may be involved in the development of complications. These may include reduced lung volumes and changes
in the properties of mucus and mucus transport, all of which may lead to mucus plugging and hypoventilation (1–4).

II. Postoperative Pulmonary Complications

Postoperative pulmonary abnormality was identified as early as 1910 by Pasteur (5) who thought it was due to a failure of respiratory power. In 1914 Eliot et al. and Dingley (6) proposed that postoperative lung collapse was the result of occlusion of the airways by mucus. Subsequent work by Haldane et al. (7), Beecher et al. (8), and Dripps et al. (9) reported the findings of lung collapse after laparotomy. These authors hypothesized that shallow breathing was the major cause of postoperative hypoxia and lung collapse. Notwithstanding subsequent advances in surgery and supportive medications, the morbidity resulting from postoperative pulmonary abnormalities remains a significant problem.

Despite a significant volume of research, the precise definition of pulmonary complications, the causative factors, and the incidence in surgical populations remain unclear. Pulmonary complications documented in the literature include atelectasis, hypoxemia, and pneumonia (10–12). Less commonly, pulmonary embolus, pleural effusion, and pneumothorax are reported (13). Of these, pulmonary atelectasis is the most commonly reported respiratory complication (14).

Atelectasis and collapse are terms used synonymously to mean closure or collapse of alveoli and may be described in relation to radiological appearance, clinical signs and symptoms, or mechanism of occurrence (15). Changes resulting from atelectasis may vary from microatelectasis which is undetectable on chest radiograph, to macroatelectasis, which is accompanied by overt clinical signs and symptoms (16). The common clinical signs and symptoms of atelectasis in the postoperative period include reduced breath sounds on auscultation, tachypnea, tachycardia, hypoxemia, and fever. Although fever is commonly attributed to the presence of atelectasis, there is no direct evidence to support this view (3).

The three major consequences of macroatelectasis are an increased work of breathing, impairment of gas exchange, and a predisposition to infection (3). Atelectasis and pneumonia are terms often included together in the literature to denote a postoperative pulmonary complication. In fact, these problems describe a continuum from atelectasis, which is noninfectious (and may be subclinical), to proven bacterial pneumonia (12). Although the fact that patients with atelectasis may also have a fever make this explanation too simplistic. Given the broad range of possible clinical sequelae resulting from this definition of postoperative pulmonary complication, it is easy to understand the difficulty in interpreting comparative literature in this area.

III. Pathogenesis of Complications

The proposed mechanisms for pathogenesis of postoperative pulmonary abnormalities have altered little since early in the 20th century. There are still two basic theories to explain their occurrence: blockage of airways by mucus and regional hypoventilation. Advocates of the mucus-blockade theory contend that the primary cause of atelectasis is the absorption of alveolar air distal to a mucus plug in the proximal airway, causing eventual collapse unless fresh air enters through collateral channels (3). A high inspired oxygen concentration may facilitate this absorption of air.

In support for this theory, Gamsu et al. (17) measured clearance of tantalum powder, which adheres to airway mucus, in 18 patients following abdominal surgery and seven patients undergoing orthopedic surgery. Patients experienced delayed clearance of the tantalum after abdominal but not orthopedic surgery, atelectasis in areas of retained powder, and clearance of tantalum once the atelectasis had resolved. Pooling of tantalum powder always occurred in the region of the lung where volume loss was evident. The authors used serial chest radiographs and an ordinal scoring system for atelectasis. They concluded that impaired mucociliary function and mucus transport are implicated in postoperative atelectasis and that lung volume is important in mucociliary clearance (17). This paper had several limitations. After the second chest radiograph measurement, patients were managed using different forms of respiratory care that may have included positioning, intermittent positive pressure breathing, nasotracheal suction, or ultrasonic humidification. These treatments may have affected outcomes between patients. These authors, and others, suggest that the cumulative effects of the perioperative process present a significant insult to mucus clearance. These factors are presented in Table 1. In a study of 127 patients undergoing elective upper-abdominal surgery, Dilworth and White (20) found an overall incidence of postoperative pulmonary complications of 20.5%, but in patients with pre-existing respiratory disease characterized by chronic sputum production and airflow obstruction on spirometry, and those who were current smokers, the incidence of postoperative pulmonary complications increased to between 50 and 84%. These authors concluded that mucus hypersecretion is one of the essential determinants of postoperative pulmonary complications (20). Patients are at increased risk of postoperative pulmonary complications due to pre-existing increased mucus production combined with a reduction in clearance of secretions as a result of the operative process.

The second basic process thought to cause atelectasis is regional hypoventilation. There are several physiological factors that may contribute to promote alveolar closure; these relate to reductions in functional residual capacity and

Table 1 Factors Promoting Postoperative Mucociliary Dysfunction

Anesthetic agents
Endotracheal intubation with cuffed tube
Pain medication
Higher inspired oxygen concentrations and airway humidification
Altered breathing pattern, loss of sigh
Decreased alveolar size and stability
Reduced lung volumes and reduced cough efficiency
Decreased, altered mucociliary activity
Increased and/or dry secretions

Source: Refs. 2, 7, and 172.

an altered relationship between functional residual capacity and closing volume. Following upper-abdominal surgery, the functional residual capacity has been shown to decrease to approximately 70% of preoperative value (10,11). As functional residual capacity falls below closing volume, closure of dependent small airways may occur, leading to arterial hypoxemia as perfusion of airless lung units persists (2,10). This altered relationship may exist regionally in the lung, even when overall functional residual capacity exceeds overall closing volume (10,11). The reductions in functional residual capacity have been shown to be closely associated with the degree of arterial hypoxemia after surgery (10). The consequences of the reduction in functional residual capacity are reduced lung compliance, altered surfactant properties (10), impaired gas exchange, retention of lung secretions, and atelectasis (2).

The precise sequence and relative contributions of each of the above mechanisms are still unclear. It is possible that they vary between patients and that both alveolar hypoventilation and secretion plugging coexist to contribute to postoperative lung changes (3).

Clinically, the definition of postoperative pulmonary complications varies significantly; some common definitions cited in the literature are given in Table 2. These definitions usually include new signs and symptoms, including auscultation and sputum production, tests including chest radiograph and sputum results, and administration of antibiotics. Generally the definition includes more than one of these criteria, with many authors combining clinical and radiographic evidence in their definition. More recent papers attempt to define a postoperative pulmonary complication with reference to the clinical significance of the problem, which includes consideration of both hospital and patient costs. In 1992 O'Donohue (18) defined a postoperative pulmonary complication as "a pulmonary abnormality that produces identifiable disease or dysfunction that is clinically significant and adversely affects the clinical course."

The natural history of postoperative atelectasis may vary but generally is one of spontaneous improvement, requiring no specific therapy (14,15). A significant complication is one that may be defined as an unexpected progression of the postoperative recovery to a second disease entity (19). This definition is useful as it allows clinicians to discern between self-limiting clinical sequelae and those that may result in an increased use of resources and increased length of postoperative hospital stay. Unfortunately, specific outcome criteria that accurately describe clinically relevant complications remain elusive. Studies using a combination of multiple-outcome measures rather than single variables may more accurately define a clinically significant postoperative pulmonary complication.

The incidence of postoperative pulmonary complications is a function of the diagnostic criteria used. As a result of the differing criteria used to define a postoperative pulmonary complication and failure to further identify a clinically

Table 2 Criteria Used to Define Postoperative Pulmonary Complication
in the Literature, Following Abdominal or Cardiac Surgery Presented Chronologically

Author (year)	Definition of postoperative pulmonary complication
Wightman (1968)	Productive cough, fever >38, new physical signs
Stein and Cassara (1970)	Any 1 or more of the following: graded from 1^+ to 4^+ by severity, exacerbation of bronchitis with airway obstruction, fever, purulent sputum, atelectasis, pneumonia, pulmonary failure, severe dyspnea
Laszlo et al. (1973)	Classified as type 0 to type 3: 0 = no complication, 1 = deterioration of sputum by 2 or more grades of purulence (bronchitis), 2 = deterioration of cxr to minimal or subsegmental lesions or worse, not accompanied by a change in sputum grading, 3 = deterioration of both cxr and sputum (pneumonia)
Ali et al. (1974)	All of the following: temperature >38°, productive cough, cxr changes of consolidation or atelectasis
Wheatley et al. (1977)	All of the following: productive cough with increase in sputum volume compared with preop, temperature >37.1°, development of new lung signs *or* cxr signs of collapse or consolidation
Morran et al. (1983)	Classified as either atelectasis of chest infection; atelectasis defined as pyrexia, purulent sputum, cxr and clinical evidence of collapse; chest infection defined as pyrexia, purulent sputum, cxr and clinical evidence of collapse, persisting >72 hours
Stock et al. (1985)	Pneumonia diagnosed when two of the following present: change in color or quantity of sputum, oral temperature >38.5° for at least 2 days, infiltrate on cxr; sputum culture then performed
Jenkins et al. (1989)	Temperature >38.5°, cxr signs of consolidation or pronounced lung collapse
Dilworth and White (1992)	(Scored criteria) chest infection = 4 or more, temperature >38 >24 hours (1), cough-increased or developed (1), sputum, increased >2 grades of purulence (3), crackles (1), cxr change c/w infection (1), WCC >11 × 109 (1)
Williams-Russo et al. (1992)	Classed as clinical or cxr complications. Clinical defined as fever >38° and localized adventitious sounds, without cxr evidence; cxr complications defined as evidence of infiltrates or atelectasis
Lawrence et al. (1996)	Pneumonia; cxr evidence and antibiotics, possible pneumonia; cxr changes and no antibiotics or antibiotics but normal cxr
Hall et al. (1996)	Presence of clinical features consistent with collapse or consolidation *plus* temperature >38°, and either positive cxr findings or positive sputum microbiology
Brooks-Bunn (1997)	Minimum of two criteria present for >2 consecutive days anytime in first 6 postop days, criteria: new cough/sputum production, abnormal breath sounds, temperature >38°, cxr signs of new infiltrate or atelectasis, physician documentation of atelectasis or pneumonia

significant postoperative pulmonary complication, the incidence reported in the literature varies considerably. It has been reported to be between 5 and 75% (20). A higher incidence is found for upper-abdominal and cardiothoracic surgical procedures, and a lower incidence for surgery of the lower abdomen and extremities (16). In fact, the incidence of atelectasis measured using chest radiography has been reported to be approximately 70%; however, clinically significant postoperative pulmonary complications develop in few of these patients (14,21). Bourn and Jenkins (22) describe postoperative atelectasis as "the rule rather than the exception," and this view is supported in other literature (23). In more recent studies in which a multicriteria outcome has been used, the reported incidence of postoperative pulmonary complications was as low as 5–20% (24–29). These differences in incidence reflect not only the variation in outcome measures used to assess postoperative pulmonary complications but also the obscurity of the link between subclinical atelectasis and clinically relevant postoperative pulmonary complications. Individual patient risk factors and differences in postoperative management (physiotherapy, pain control) may somehow combine to produce these varied outcomes between patients having similar surgery.

IV. Risk Factors for Developing Postoperative Pulmonary Complications

Problems in mucus clearance may be a result of changes in the cardiorespiratory physiology during the postoperative period. A multifactorial approach (Figure 1) may be used to explain the rationale for the prevention of postoperative pulmonary complications by characterizing patient categories and type of surgery. This approach may be used for setting up treatment hypotheses of postoperative pulmonary complications.

Postoperative pulmonary complications remain a significant cause of morbidity following major surgery, despite advances in perioperative care (12). Many studies have been performed in an attempt to elucidate risk factors for developing postoperative pulmonary complications. These predominately involve patient having cardiothoracic or abdominal surgery.

Identification of patient risk factors or risk factor models helps the health care professional to target certain patient groups and provide respiratory care or treatment that may modify some of the preoperative risk factors, for example, smoking and weight reduction. This risk assessment may then have an effect on patient outcome postoperatively by focusing on prevention (12,30). The importance of the role of preoperative education in modifying outcomes postoperatively has been well documented in the literature (31–34). Preoperative assessment and treatment of patients by physiotherapists are discussed in more detail later in this chapter.

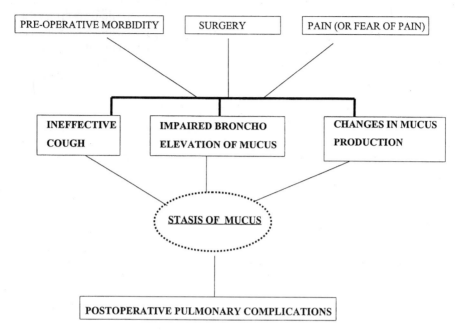

Figure 1 Schematic diagram demonstrating the multifactorial relationships contributing to impaired mucus clearance and postoperative pulmonary complications.

A. Methodology Issues

Several issues arise from a study of the literature related to postoperative pulmonary complications and risk factors. The most important relate to the definition of these variables. Although many studies have been published, there are numerous differences in the operational definitions of both a postoperative pulmonary complication and risk factors. This design limitation between papers limits a valid comparison and produces varied outcomes from the literature (24). In addition, many risk factors are cited in isolation rather than in the context of the multifactorial perioperative process. Whether a single risk factor may be independently responsible for the development of a postoperative pulmonary complication or whether it occurs in combination is critical to the identification of individual patients at risk (12). Univariate analysis examines each risk factor independently and correlates it to the incidence of postoperative pulmonary complication. This technique is useful to establish the main contributing factors and eliminate those with no association to the outcome, thereby increasing the strength of the analysis (35). However, reliance on univariate analysis alone may lead to inaccurate conclusions (24). More recent studies in abdominal surgery focus on multivariate approaches to risk factor identification, ensuring that their importance is considered in the context of other risk factors. Other limitations of existing literature are that older papers may not accurately reflect the perioperative management conditions of the 1990s, sample sizes are too small given the type of statistical analyses necessary, older papers may not meet today's exacting scientific and statistical standards, data have often been collected retrospectively, some of the putative risk factors studied are not routinely assessed before cardiothoracic or abdominal surgery, and a heterogeneous mix of surgical cases is included in studies (24,33,36–39). However, the single most important limitation relates to the definition of a postoperative pulmonary complication. This is the endpoint with which risks are correlated. Obviously, if great variation between studies exists in this definition, then valid conclusions and comparisons in the literature are difficult.

B. Specific Risk Factors

Several patient characteristics have been associated with an increased incidence of postoperative pulmonary complications, these have been classified as pulmonary and nonpulmonary (30). These risk factors are discussed in the subsequent section, which also includes a description of the pathophysiological reasons for the effects of the putative risk factors on the respiratory system.

C. Preoperative Morbidity

Preoperative morbidity can be classified using the American Society of Anesthetists (ASA) score. The ASA score (numbered 1–5) divides patients into five groups and collectively rates patient risk of anesthesia. It was developed as a standardized way for anesthetists to convey information about patients' overall health status and allow outcomes to be stratified by a global assessment of their severity of illness. In practice, the ASA score may be the only overall documentation of preoperative condition that is used widely. Because of this, it is frequently recorded in studies to estimate operative risk (40). The classification of physical status recommended by the House of Delegates of the American Society of Anesthesiologists (41) are: 1) a normal healthy patient, 2) a patient with mild to moderate systemic disease, 3) a patient with a severe systemic disease that limits activity but is not incapacitating, 4) a patient with an incapacitating systemic disease that is a constant threat to life, and 5) a moribund patient not expected to survive 24 hours with or without operation. The attending anesthetist ascribes a score to each patient upon preoperative assessment.

There is some controversy in the literature as to the predictive ability of the ASA score. Hall et al. (42), in their prospective study of 1000 patients undergoing abdominal surgery, identified the ASA score as the most powerful indicator of surgical risk in both uni- and multivariate analyses. They report that the combination of ASA score >1 and age >59 years identified 88% of the patients who developed a postoperative pulmonary complication. These results are supported in other studies (40,43,44). However, Brooks-Bunn (24) and Lawrence et al. (38), in large studies of patients having abdominal surgery, report significance of ASA in univariate analysis but not when subjected to multivariate analysis. In a prospective study of 151 vascular surgical patients, Vodinh et al. (45) found that ASA classification was not associated with increased risks. In a more recent examination of risk factors using a multicenter trial of 276 patients, Brookes-Bunn (46) identified different patient risk factors when assessing the validity of her previously developed six-risk model. These included a higher ASA classification. Because the ASA score considers comorbidities, extremes of age and weight, and emergency operations, it is not surprising that it has been found to be a significant indicator of risk in much of the literature (43). Indeed, it may be that the identification of significant comorbidity is the most powerful determinant of operative outcome (47). The strengths of ASA class are that it is a common, well-defined, and valid (48) assessment tool used by anesthetists and as such can be compared across different patient populations and countries.

Increasing age is considered in most of the surgical literature to be a risk factor for developing postoperative pulmonary complications. However, the definition of the critical age varies between studies. Many papers report that an age over 60 years increases risk after surgery (24,42,49), while others found that age greater than 70 (43,47) or 75 years (40,50) was a significant risk factor. Not all studies analyzing risk factors found age to be important (20,39,51,52). Where age has been identified as a risk factor, the findings have been attributed to the normal changes of aging, specifically relating to alterations in lung volumes and P_aO_2. The closing capacity of the lungs increases with age (53) and as it rises above functional residual capacity, closure of small airways can occur. In fact, after the age of approximately 65 years, this occurs in normal adult lungs during quiet breathing in a seated position (53,54). Although changes with aging are normal, a distinction can be made between chronological and physiological age (55). Patients with poor physical status rather than advanced age may be the ones at higher risk. Greenburg et al. (56) concur with this view and suggest that age may be a minor factor in surgical risk. Based on a retrospective study of 468 patients, the authors suggested that if the vital organs, especially heart and lungs, were physiologically intact there were no differences in mortality between patients over 70 years and younger patients. However, patients who are older tend to have more comorbid disease (40), which may be the factor influencing patient risk rather than chronological age. Wightman (52) suggested that there may be a higher incidence of respiratory disease in older patients, which may account for the apparent effects of age as a risk factor.

Obesity and malnutrition are frequently studied as clinical risk factors for postoperative pulmonary complications. Obesity has been studied using a comparison to ideal weight or body mass index (BMI), which is a calculated measure found by dividing a person's weight (in kilograms) by his or her height (in meters) squared. The normal range for BMI is 20–25 (24) while the definition of obesity may vary between studies. The literature provides conflicting evidence for this risk factor; however, there is a general view that weight is important, but only when patients are morbidly obese (20,51,55). Weight greater than 30% of ideal has been linked to increased risk of postoperative pulmonary complications. Calligaro et al. (43) found that in a population of 181 patients undergoing abdominal aortic aneurysm repair, obesity did not reach statistical significance until greater than 50% above ideal weight. This is in contrast to some studies in which excess weight of only 10% was significant (57). More recent research defined a BMI of greater than 25 (42) or 27 (24) as a preoperative risk factor. In these two studies BMI was found to be a significant preoperative risk factor for postoperative pulmonary complications when analyzed using multivariate statistics. Brookes-Bunn (24) reported that a BMI greater than 27 increased patients' risk of developing postoperative pulmonary complications by a factor of 2.8.

The physiological changes associated with obesity that may account for increased postoperative risks are a reduction in FRC, produced mainly as a result of decreased chest wall compliance, and a lower than normal P_aO_2 (54). The reduction in FRC postoperatively is aggravated by the supine position (13).

Malnutrition has been recognized as a risk factor for more than 50 years (58), but has not been widely addressed in recent literature. Preoperative protein depletion may contribute to respiratory muscle weakness, including a reduction in diaphragmatic muscle mass (59), loss of periodic sighing (60), hypoventilation, and impaired immune-system function (55), thus increasing the potential for an ineffective cough and an increased risk of postoperative pulmonary complications. Windsor and Hill (58) advocate dynamic preoperative assessment of nutritional status and intravenous feeding if this can be found to be cost-effective in reducing the incidence of postoperative pulmonary complications in patients with protein depletion.

The components of cigarette smoke have major adverse effects on cardiovascular and respiratory function (61). The reader is referred to a detailed review by Pearce and Jones (61). The effect of smoking history on the development of postoperative pulmonary complications, however, remains somewhat uncertain. A large body of literature supports the inclusion of cigarette smoking as a preoperative risk factor (12,20,52,62). Bluman et al. (63) reported a fourfold increase in postoperative pulmonary complications, in current compared with never-smokers following elective noncardiac surgery. This difference was obtained after controlling for possible confounding factors such as type of surgery, age, pulmonary disease, and BMI. However, the difference was evident only for minor postoperative pulmonary complication (atelectasis or worsening of atelectasis on chest x-ray), not for major complication (infection, reintubation). In contrast, some studies report no association between smoking and increased risk of postoperative pulmonary complications (30,43,58). In addition, there is considerable disagreement about the effects and timing of preoperative smoking abstinence. The smoking pack-year threshold necessary for significant adverse effects of smoking has been reported to be 20 pack-years (one pack-year may be defined as smoking 20 cigarettes per day for one year). Dilworth and White (20) also report significant increased risk for postoperative pulmonary complications in heavy smokers (>20 pack-years) compared with lighter smokers (<20 pack-years).

In addition there is considerable disagreement about the effects and timing of preoperative smoking abstinence. Recommendations for cessation of smoking 48 hours to 1 or 2 weeks before surgery have been reported; these were based on several physiological factors: the time for the carboxyhemoglobin levels of smokers to return to nonsmoking levels and thus produce a rise in oxygen content and availability, improvement in ciliary activity, and reduced mucus hypersecretion (61). In a retrospective analysis of patients undergoing coronary artery bypass grafting, Warner et al. (64) found a statistically significant decrease in the incidence of postoperative pulmonary complications for patients who quit smoking at least 8 weeks prior to surgery. These results are supported in a recent prospective study of 400 patients in which the authors found that an age >60 years, history of cancer, abdominal incision, and smoking within 8 weeks of surgery was associated with twice the risk of postoperative pulmonary complication compared with others (24). This time period may be required to improve small airway function, closing volumes, and tracheobronchial clearance and reduce sputum production (49).

It may be argued that smoking per se is less important as an independent risk factor than as a coexisting variable in patients who have lung disease and reduced forced expiratory volume in 1 second (FEV$_1$). Many smokers exhibit the signs and symptoms of respiratory disease, such as cough, increased secretion volume, and airflow limitation; as a result, the importance of smoking as an independent preoperative risk factor is uncertain, as it may identify a high-risk population of patients with respiratory disease.

Pre-existing chronic obstructive pulmonary disease (COPD) is often considered an important risk factor for postoperative pulmonary complications (39, 47,51,52,65). It has been suggested that mucus hypersecretion is the important factor that increases risk in these patients (52,66). Other predictive markers studied extensively in COPD have been pulmonary-function test indices. It appears from a review of the literature that no specific spirometric test has been consistently used, but that tests measuring expiratory flow such as forced expiratory flow 25% to 75% (FEF$_{25-75\%}$) and maximal expiratory flow–volume curves may be useful (49,66). In addition, the degree of abnormality in pulmonary-function tests indices necessary to increase risks has not been well defined. Preoperative hypercapnia ($P_aCO_2 > 50$ mm Hg) has also been identified as a factor that may increase risk of serious postoperative pulmonary complications (67).

In a study comparing risk between patients with varying degrees of COPD and those without the disease, Kroenke et al. (47) reported that those with severe COPD experienced higher rates of serious postoperative pulmonary complication and mortality compared with the other group. The higher incidence of mortality in this study occurred in patients having coronary artery surgery rather than abdominal surgery, and the authors concluded that COPD should be regarded as an independent indicator of risk in the coronary artery surgery population. This view is supported in other studies of postoperative risk following coronary artery surgery (68,69). In contrast, several authors report that a history of COPD was not associated with increased risk following abdominal surgery (24,38,42,43).

Patients with suppurative lung diseases presenting for cardiac, thoracic, transplant, or abdominal surgery have increased risks for pulmonary complications. There are few published data examining this patient population in isolation (Table 1); however, given the perioperative changes to mucus and mucus clearance, lung volumes, and effective coughing, it would seem plausible physiologically that these patients experience significantly increased risks of sputum plugging, atelectasis, and postoperative pulmonary infection (Fig. 1).

The use of spirometry for assessment of risk prior to surgery was supported in several early studies, the most often cited being those by Stein et al. (70). More recent literature suggests that physical examination and clinical assessment may be equally useful in predicting postoperative pulmonary complications (67). There may be subgroups of patients who may still benefit from preoperative spirometry, including patients with extensive smoking histories and evidence of severe pulmonary disease (71). In a systematic review of current literature Lawrence et al. (72) found the predictive value of preoperative spirometry to be unproven. Despite this, preoperative spirometry may still be overutilized and thus incur unnecessary increased costs in patient management (71).

Several other potential factors have been reported that may contribute to postoperative morbidity and mortality. In cardiac surgical patients Spivack et al. (73) found that left ventricular ejection fraction was a good predictor of an uncomplicated postoperative course. The combination of this with pre-existing comorbid conditions such as diabetes, angina, current smoking, and congestive cardiac failure served as a modest risk factor for prolonged ventilation after coronary artery surgery. There has been more research into risks before cardiac surgery than other types of surgery. Most literature in this field reports risk factors associated with the type of cardiac surgery being performed, the functional status of the heart at the time of surgery, and associated cardiac risk factors (68,69,73).

Other preoperative risk factors reported to be significant but less commonly cited include a history of cancer (24), tumor stage (74), emergency surgery (75), male gender, prolonged preoperative hospital stay, impaired cognitive function (24), presence of a nasogastric tube (65), and reduced preoperative P_aO_2 (45,76). Intraoperative factors such as residual intraperitoneal sepsis (36), excessive blood loss, and incision length larger than 30 centimeters (46) have also been reported.

D. Anesthesia

General anesthesia, irrespective of the anesthetic agents used, results in a reduction in functional residual capacity of the magnitude of 20% (11,77). Juno et al. (78) found a decrease in functional residual capacity and closing capacity in patients during anesthesia. Alterations in the chest wall and reduced lung volumes seem to be most important in the etiology of functional abnormalities following anesthesia. Carryover of these changes may occur postoperatively, when several factors conspire to further reduce lung volumes and affect gas exchange and mucociliary clearance (16). However, there is no evidence that general anesthesia per se causes postoperative pulmonary complications (55). Patient risk factors are thought to potentiate this deterioration in pulmonary function following abdominal and cardiothoracic surgery (12).

It is generally agreed in the literature that operations of longer duration carry increased risks of postoperative pulmonary complications. Windsor and Hill (58) report that an anesthetic lasting longer than 2 hours is significantly associated with increased morbidity, and Garibaldi et al. (51), using univariate analysis, identified a duration of surgery greater than 4 hours as being associated with a significant risk of postoperative pneumonia in patients following upper-abominal surgery. Although Williams-Russo et al. (39) also report an increased incidence of postoperative pulmonary complications with longer duration of surgery, this did not reach significance when subjected to multivariate risk analysis. Others also report a lack of significance for duration of surgery as an independent risk factor (20,52). The risk associated with duration of surgery may reflect the complexity of the surgical procedure itself rather than the length of anesthesia administration (30). This argument is supported by Kotani et al. (79), who also proposed that longer or more complex surgery may cause death of alveolar macrophages in humans. However, the relevance of this finding to the development of postoperative pulmonary complications needs further investigation.

E. Site of Surgery

The site of surgery has been identified as having a major influence on risk of postoperative pulmonary complications (16,80). Patients undergoing upper-abdominal or thoracic surgery are at a higher risk of developing respiratory problems compared with patients who have surgery on the lower abdomen or the extremities (10,16,25,51,67,81). In recent comparative reviews the site of surgery has been identified as a significant risk factor (24,42). Furthermore, Celli (30) states that the site of the surgery may be the single most important risk factor.

The wide variation that exists after surgery in spirometry may be explained by different incision sites (10,11,82,83) and operation techniques. For instance, Johnson (83) investigated the reduction in spirometry after surgery and found a 25% reduction of the preoperative values of vital capacity in subcostal thoracotomy and 39% for lower midline incisions. However, Ali et al. (10) found that a thoracotomy incision led to a 40% reduction in preoperative vital capacity, lower abdominal surgery resulted in a 42% reduction, and an upper-abdominal incision a 37% reduction. In the study by Johnson (83), the type of surgery performed was not clearly described. The difference in postoperative reduction of pulmonary function between Johnson's groups and Ali's groups may be explained by the type and extent of surgery. Garcia-Valdecasas et al. (84) demonstrated significant differences between groups of patients having subcostal abdominal versus midline abdominal incisions. They found lower vital capacity values in midline incisions compared with subcostal incisions. On the other hand, Tsui et al. (85) found no differences in pulmonary function in patients after esophageal surgery comparing two different incision sites, abdominal and thoraco-abdominal, and Frazee et al. (86) described reduced pulmonary function following open cholecystectomy compared with patients following laparoscopic surgery. These results demonstrate that a decline in pulmonary function is at least partly dependent on the surgical procedure.

The influence of site of surgery as a significant risk factor is explained predominantly by alterations in diaphragmatic function caused by surgery performed in close proximity to the diaphragm (30,57). Ford et al. (82) demonstrated that the diaphragmatic contribution to tidal ventilation was reduced following upper-abdominal surgery in 15 subjects who underwent open cholecystectomy. Blaney and Sawyer (142) measured diaphragm displacement before and after upper-abdominal surgery in 18 subjects, using ultrasonography, and found that mean diaphragm displacement was reduced by 57% on the first day after surgery (142). Dureuil et al. (87) reported significantly less diaphragm dysfunction in lower- compared with upper-abdominal surgery. These authors postulated that a decrease in diaphragmatic motion following upper-abdominal surgery may result in diminished ventilation and expansion of the dependent lung zones. Pansard et al. (88) found diaphragm inhibition in patients after upper-abdominal surgery as measured by changes in diaphragmatic pressure and excursion of the chest and abdomen. These authors suggested that this inhibition of the phrenic nerve was mainly a result of postoperative analgesia. The loss of diaphragm function also occurs in minimally invasive surgery. Erice et al. (89) described changes in maximum transdiaphragmatic pressure after laparoscopic abdominal surgery. The authors therefore posed a second hypothesis of loss of diaphragmatic function through stimulation of the mesenteric plexus. This hypothesis was originally discussed by Reeve et al. (90).

However, the primary cause of postoperative dysfunction appears to be the chest as the site of surgery, which causes reflex inhibition of the diaphragm and intercostal muscles (87,91,92). Another possible explanation may be increased intra-abdominal pressure as a result of abdominal distension, which may limit normal diaphragmatic function (3).

Pulmonary complications following thoracic surgery relate to both the site of incision and the removal of previously healthy lung tissue (55). A vertical laparotomy has been reported to increase morbidity compared with subcostal or transverse incisions (93). Although median sternotomy for cardiac surgery has been reported to have less impact on respiratory function than thoracotomy or abdominal incisions, the effects of the cardiac surgical process (median sternotomy, cardiopulmonary bypass, and topical cardioplegia) may increase the risk of developing postoperative pulmonary complications (92,94,95). Left-lower-lobe abnormality is a frequent finding after cardiac surgery (94,96). The reasons are unclear, but factors that may influence this are: diaphragmatic dysfunction, lung trauma due to retraction, compression of the left lower lobe by the heart during surgery, and pleurotomy (94).

Numerous pathophysiological factors may be responsible for the alterations in respiratory mechanics following abdominal surgery. Although the precise reasons for the development of postoperative pulmonary complications in individual patients may be a complex interaction of events, there is strong support in the literature that the site of surgery is an important nonpulmonary risk factor influencing their development.

F. Postoperative Pain

Surgery is associated with varying degrees of acute postoperative pain, brought about by tissue injury, which reduces with the natural healing process (97). The severity of the pain may depend on the type and site of surgery, the age of the patient, and the individual's response to the stress of the operation. Several other factors influence pain severity, including a patient's personality, previous pain experience, cultural background, and conditioning. As an acute pain, postoperative pain is often accompanied by changes in autonomic activity that are largely sympathetic and may consist of hypertension, tachycardia, sweating, and decreased gut motility.

Pain is difficult to define because it is a purely sensory experience; as such, it is also very difficult to measure. To date, there appears to be no single reliable objective measure of pain (97). Stress responses, as an objective measurement of pain, are nonspecific, and pulmonary function is influenced by factors other than pain. Most research measures patients' estimate of the severity of their pain. Literature measuring the perioperative incidence of postoperative pulmonary complications and methods used in its reduction often report on patient pain by using verbal rating scales (VRS) or visual analog scales (VAS). Of these, the VAS is the best established; the patient is asked to place a mark on a 100-mm line between two verbal anchors such as "no pain" and "worst possible pain." In addition to difficulties in choosing a measurement tool for pain, controversy exists as to whether pain should be measured at rest or with activity to provide the most meaningful outcomes (98). With respect to postoperative pulmonary complications and their prophylaxis, movement pain is more significant. However, not all studies examining postoperative pulmonary complications measure patient pain scores. Differences in pain intensity and pain management between populations studied introduce a potential confounding variable that may render comparisons between these studies less reliable.

Reduction in postoperative pain intensity is essential for patient comfort but also to reduce the incidence of severe or life-threatening postoperative pulmonary complications. It is widely assumed that if patients are relatively pain-free, their recovery from surgery will be quicker and uneventful (98). Sabanathan et al. (99) suggest that pain in the early postoperative period may be the factor most responsible for ineffective ventilation.

Many methods of pain relief are available to patients in the new millennum. Much comparative research exists that examines the efficacy of one method of analgesia over another. More recent developments in pain management include the introduction of postoperative pain services led by anesthetists or nurses, recognition of the possible value of pre-emptive analgesia (analgesics given immediately prior to surgical incision to prevent nerve impulses arising from intraoperative events from sensitizing central neural structures) (100,101), use of multimodal analgesic techniques rather than single-drug administration, more sophisticated drug administration techniques such as patient-controlled analgesia (PCA), and use of the epidural route on surgical wards. These developments evolved in an attempt to improve patient comfort and outcome by reducing pain levels, preventing significant central sensitization of pain, reducing the incidence of analgesic side effects, and improving patient mobility and well-being (102).

Opioid analgesics remain the most commonly used method of postoperative pain relief (97,98), and morphine remains the benchmark drug (102). However, some authors disagree and recommend that opiates not be used for patients following thoracotomy because of their respiratory-depression effects (99). The introduction of multimodal methods has seen an increase in the use of nonsteroidal anti-inflammatory drugs (NSAIDs) given in addition to narcotics delivered using PCA or epidural local anesthetics and opioids for postoperative pain. NSAIDs are used as opioid-sparing agents, but have also been shown to improve analgesia (102). Paracetamol may also be added to these treatment regimens (102).

In an extensive review and meta-analysis, Ballantyne et al. (98) report on the comparative benefits of one method of analgesia over another for preventing pulmonary morbidity after surgery. They conclude that the incidence of postoperative pulmonary complications is significantly lower when patients receive epidural opioid and/or epidural local anesthetic treatments in comparison with systemic opioids. This is not a view shared by all authors (103).

G. Stasis of Mucus

Mucociliary transport, a first-line nonimmunological defense mechanism of the respiratory tract, is influenced by many factors. The factors that determine the normal clearance of airway secretion include mucus production, a mucociliary elevator, and an effective cough. All these factors may be altered by changes of respiratory physiology in the responsible structure during the perioperative period. The cause-and-effect relationships of the three factors are discussed in the following section.

Impaired Mucociliary Transport

Mucociliary clearance is a major function of the airway epithelium. This important function depends both on the physicochemical properties of the airway mucus and on the activity of the cilia, and is dependent mainly on the quality and quantity of mucus glycoproteins or mucins. Many factors can impair mucociliary function. The respiratory epithelium consists of cilia, which contribute to the normal elevation of mucus, bacteria, and debris. During the perioperative phase, many events such as medical interventions or disease can have an effect on the cilia and their bronchial elevatory system, for example, structural loss of cilia and changes in size and beating frequency. Intubation and ventilation of the patient during and after surgery will influence the internal milieu, by providing a bypass of the vocal cord and introducing foreign substances such as anesthetic gasses. By bypassing the normal barrier, the lower airway is opened for an intrusion of bacteria, viruses, yeasts, and other foreign substances. Several postoperative factors may contribute to the development of lower-airway infection. In order to colonize the epithelium, some bacteria or viruses delay expectoration by adhering to the mucus layer. Certain pathogens penetrate the mucociliary barrier to reach the epithelial surface, where disruption of the tight junction in the epithelium and the endothelium can take place (104). For instance, *Pseudomonas aeruginosa* will result in a ciliary disorientation as well as delay in mucociliary transport. This might be a result of changes in the ionic content in and around the periciliary fluid. In the presence of host-derived infection, such as human leukocyte elastase, neutral protienase and bacteria-derived products can adversely affect ciliary function. Impaired mucociliary transport in intubated patients is associated with a loss of cilia rather than ultrastructural abnormalities of cilia (105). An increase in ciliary beat frequency with different concentrations of oxygen at normobaric pressures has been observed in vitro by Stanek et al. (106). This effect might influence the efficacy of ciliary beat and therefore impair the mucus transport. In the perioperative phase, there might be a combination of effects on the ciliary beat. The ciliary beat frequency reduces after anesthesia with isoflurane but not with propofol (107). These data suggest that different anesthetic agents may impair respiratory defense mechanisms to differing degrees. In neonates, decreased mucociliary clearance following halothane anesthesia is due, at least in part, to a directly depressant effect of halothane on ciliated cells (108). The previous authors might have found a contradiction, as in one study the beat frequency increases and in the other it decreases. A clinical view regarding the overall effect of the total treatment in the perioperative phase is not yet known.

An animal study (109) shows that reduced humidity produces longer cilia and altered function. Alterations in tracheobronchial structure and function result from exposure to dry gases and are amplified by the duration of exposure. Because of all the medical interventions during surgery, the bronchociliary elevator can be impaired for a period ranging from 2 to 6 days postoperatively (17).

Changes in Mucus Production

Respiratory mucus represents the products derived from secretion of the submucosal glands and the goblet cells. The relationship between the humidity and temperature of inspired gas and the function of the airway mucosa suggests that there is an optimal temperature and humidity above and below which there is impaired mucosal function. This optimal level of temperature and humidity is core temperature and 100% relative humidity. However, existing data are sufficient to test this model only for gas conditions below core temperature and 100% relative humidity. The data concur with the model in that region. No studies have yet looked at this relationship beyond 24 hours.

The main factors contributing to abnormalities in mucus clearance during the postoperative phase are flow reduction and decreased relative humidity. This could lead to changes in the mucus viscosity and accumulation of mucus. If this progresses, in theory this might lead to obstruction of airways, plugging, atelectasis, and gas-exchange abnormalities.

Impaired Cough

A cough has been defined by Leith (110) as a brief rapid inspiration of a volume of air larger than the normal resting tidal volume (V_t). The glottis is then closed for about 0.2 second. During that time the pressure in abdominal, pleural, and alveolar spaces is raised to 50–100 mm Hg or more by an expiratory effort that includes agonist–antagonist interaction between inspiratory and expiratory muscles, of both ribcage and diaphragm. Abdominal pressure thus exceeds intrathoracic pressure. Circulatory and cerebrospinal fluid systems are affected in this rise of pressure, as might be expected, during this brief violent Valsalva maneuver. Intraocular pressures also rise. The glottis suddenly opens actively as subglottic pressure continues to rise. Expiratory flow at the mouth accelerates rapidly; within 30–50 msec, flow reaches a peak that may exceed 12 L/sec. Oscillations of tissue and gas cause a characteristic explosive sound and may play a role in suspending secretion in the moving gas stream. During this time, the lower trachea and other intrathoracic airways collapse, contributing a transient spike of flow on top of the more sustained expiratory flow through the airway from lung parachyma. About half a second later, after a liter or less of gas has been expired, flow is stopped by one of two methods: either the glottis closes with a characteristic second sound or expiratory-muscle agonist–antagonist activity is adjusted so that alveolar pressure falls to zero. The sequence may be repeated rapidly several times, sweeping down through lung volume toward residual volume and progressively collapsing more and more of the airways.

This normal cough has many variations. Initial inspiration may not occur. Starting volume, volume expired, and flow rates are quite variable, as are the pressures developed. Expiratory effort often starts just before the glottis closes, causing a characteristic voiced "huh" sound. A similar sound may occur one or several times during such a series (111).

An effective cough is important for transport and expectoration of lung mucus. Several elements contribute to the efficiency of the cough (112). Primarily it is believed to be a function of peak airflow velocities in the airways. Several elements may participate in producing the initial transient supramaximal flows (113) that are characteristic of a cough: initial high lung volume, muscle-generated pulmonary pressures, coordinated glottis participation, and airway compression resulting in adequate expiratory flow.

Initial High Lung Volume

The initial high lung volumes during cough have several effects. Greater expiratory-muscle pressure and higher expiratory flow are achievable. The effects of gravity on the lung are minimized, so inflation of lung regions is more uniform, and the number of closed lung units is minimized.

Muscle-Generated Pulmonary Pressures

Adequate musculoskeletal function and pulmonary compliance must be present for an efficient cough. Pressures generated are variable and limited by age, gender, and physical condition (114). In the perioperative phase these pressures may be reduced (89). Two limiting factors for the production of pulmonary pressures must be considered in the perioperative phase. First, the velocity of shortening of expiratory muscles can be regarded as depending on the rate of change of thoracic gas volume. Second, peak pressures are reached after a substantial volume has been expired and by the closure of the glottis or mouth. Higher lung volumes have an advantage in production of peak pressures due to better muscle force–length relationship and geometry. In the perioperative phase these two factors are relevant, but their effect is limited. The abdominal muscles are more active during anesthesia in a nonparalyzed patient; however, this activity has no significant effect on the functional residual capacity postsurgery (115). In curarized patients Arora and Gal (59) found a progressive decline in functional residual capacity. Some of the diaphragm muscle function may be regained by administration of medication, such as aminophylline (116,117).

High expiratory flow is generated through the interaction of respiratory muscle function and gravitational forces acting on the skeletal system. In the postoperative phase the diaphragmatic pressures were decreased by $22 \pm 16\%$ in a study by Pansard et al. (88). In the postoperative situation expiratory flow may therefore be limited.

Coordinated Glottis Participation

Among the most interesting aspects of expiratory flow during a cough are those associated with the extremely rapid collapse of intrathoracic airways when the glottis opens. As the equal pressure point migrates upstream in intrathoracic airways, negative transmural pressures are applied to airways downstream from it. The resulting dynamic compression accounts for most of the airway volume change. In contrast, flow from the parenchyma is sustained over time, falling relatively slowly as lung volume decreases. The timing of the rise of flow from the parenchyma is uncertain.

Effective lung clearance is not entirely dependent on glottis closure. Clearing lower airways by sharp forced expiration without glottis closure is common—for example, use of the forced expiration technique, which will be discussed later in this chapter. Airway compression results in adequate expiratory flow during breathing, airways narrow during coughing, and dynamic compression and contraction of smooth muscle occur in airway walls. This dynamic collapse of airways contributes to increased flow velocities. Persistent coughing, however, can precipitate wheezing and reduce expiratory flow, and may provoke asthma in susceptible patients.

As a result of anesthesia, the airway caliber is reduced, The airway may therefore have a further increase in resistance and related obstruction.

Dynamic compression (118) of the intrathoracic airway is undoubtedly an essential part of an effective cough, as the compression makes it possible for the high kinetic energy of the expiratory flow to shift material at the airway wall. The potential kinetic energy of flowing gas may not change, except in coronary artery surgery, when the force–velocity behavior of expiratory muscle is involved. After abdominal surgery a decrease in maximum flow might occur. The reduction of, for instance, peak expiratory flow could also be explained by an impairment in the voluntary contraction of the abdominal muscles or reduced motivation due to fear of pain. Cotes (119) and Nunn (120) describe peak expiratory flow as having an effort-dependent factor due to many inhibiting factors, including motivation and muscular force. As a result, during the postoperative phase patients might be restrained in producing maximal flows, which are needed to cough. A change in muscle force–length relationships may also be involved.

A cough is a tool to prevent particles from entering further into the respiratory tract. To trigger this reaction the sensory system of the trachea and the first generations of bronchi must be alert. In the postoperative phase the sensory system is reduced and cough threshold is therefore increased on the first postoperative day (121). Thus the efferent information needs more stimuli to produce an evacuating cough. In this situation the intruders, bacteria and debris, may attack the epithelium and lay a foundation for postoperative pulmonary complications (104).

H. Summary

Given the conflicting nature of the results from review of current literature pertaining to preoperative risk-factor assessment, more research is obviously necessary. This research should be performed with the aim of developing and validating risk profiles or models that will allow clinicians to more accurately identify individual patients at risk. Risk models do exist; the cardiopulmonary risk index (CPRI) developed by Epstein et al. (122) has undergone the most rigorous testing. Higgins et al. (68) developed a weighted severity score for morbidity and mortality in a coronary artery surgery population, but report that the model may overestimate morbidity in high-risk patients. The Acute Physiological and Chronic Health Evaluation (APACHE) models II and III is a predictive outcome score used upon admission to critical care units and is used in many units across the world. Brooks-Bunn (24,46) has attempted to validate a six-factor risk model for abdominal surgery; others have advocated development of models (62,72), but as yet no valid model exists. Acceptance by authors of standardized criteria for definition of postoperative pulmonary complications would help this process; until this occurs no model will be applicable across the different patient populations throughout the world. The other factor that has contributed to failure of model validation is the differing methods for selection of the population (123). A risk index or model that included thoracic, cardiac, and abdominal surgery would be most useful in clinical practice but more difficult to validate

(46). Furthermore, the ability of clinicians to reliably use a risk model must also be tested. Different members of the health care team may perform this task in different countries; these may include doctors, nurses, or physiotherapists. Ability to reliably assess patients most at risk of developing postoperative pulmonary complications would allow more effective and cost-efficient management by targeting patients at high risk, both pre- and postoperatively.

At present, given the literature available, the factors that clinicians should note in preoperative assessment are: site of surgery (upper-abdominal, thoracic), age, nutritional status (obese or undernourished), smoking history, and presence of comorbid disease (55). Significant postoperative factors to note, in addition to a physical examination, are duration of anesthesia, effectiveness of pain control, and ability to mobilize secretions.

Examination of literature pertaining to risk factors for development of postoperative pulmonary complications has been extensively reported. The interplay of pre-, intra-, and postoperative factors in the development of postoperative pulmonary complications are extremely complex, and no valid model for predicting outcome has been developed. Research in this field is hindered by the diverse patient groups studied and the plethora of definitions for outcome variables. Future research should aim to define consistent outcome criteria for use as endpoints and to validate a risk score or model against these variables.

V.   Effect of Physiotherapy on Perioperative Respiratory Function

A.   Rationale for Physiotherapy

In 1910, Pasteur (5) described in elegant detail several types of postoperative pulmonary complications. Although pulmonary treatment regimens were not defined, Pasteur stated in his concluding words that the deficiency of inspiratory power will occupy an important position in the search and determination of causes of postoperative lung complications. In this respect, breathing exercises, concentrating on inspiratory volume and expiratory techniques, could be key issues in prevention and treatment of problems of mucus clearance. One of the earliest publications regarding increasing inspiratory effort through breathing exercises and manual control during expiratory maneuvers such as coughing was described by MacMahon in 1933 (124).

A review of the well-recognized physiological changes of the postoperative period provides empirical support for the role of physiotherapy treatment to prevent or minimize hypoventilation and secretion plugging. Supporting evidence for this role was provided almost 50 years ago (34). Since then, several randomized controlled trials have reported beneficial effects of prophylactic physiotherapy in reducing the incidence of postoperative pulmonary complications following major surgery (25,32,33,125–127). In contrast, several other studies report no additional benefit of prophylactic physiotherapy (29,96,128). Respiratory physiotherapy may include preoperative assessment and education and postoperative prophylactic management. Many physiotherapy techniques may be used in the treatment of patients after surgery, with the primary aims of improving lung ventilation, clearing excess secretions, and minimizing risk of postoperative pulmonary complications. These may include deep-breathing strategies, forced expiratory maneuvers, mobilization, airway-clearance techniques, and positive-pressure devices. O'Donohue (18) cites three important factors that should be considered in postoperative management: the need for and effectiveness of therapy, the importance of treatment to recovery, and the cost vs. benefit of the chosen form of prophylaxis. The comparative efficacy of these techniques, specifically in clearing pulmonary secretions, and the rationale for their use forms the basis of the following section of this chapter. An extensive search of the MEDLINE, CINAHL, Cochrane, and PedRO databases for published literature on postoperative care and physiotherapy was undertaken in preparation of the material in this section.

The use of specific airway-clearance techniques such as postural drainage, percussion, and vibration may be necessary pre- and postoperatively, especially when patients have underlying respiratory diseases involving excessive pulmonary secretions (bronchiectasis, chronic bronchitis, cystic fibrosis). These techniques are described elsewhere in this book. Their use in the perioperative period may need modification, especially percussion and vibration, because postoperative pain and incision site may limit their performance. Patients with suppurative lung disease are at high risk of developing postoperative pulmonary complications. These patients should be assessed and treated by a physiotherapist in the immediate preoperative period, with the aim of reducing secretion volume. In these patients, it may be necessary to delay surgical intervention to mid-morning in order to allow clearance of secretions prior to anesthesia (129). Close postoperative monitoring is essential and effective analgesia is vital (even after minor procedures) to enable patients to perform airway-clearance techniques (129). The addition of humidified supplemental oxygen may also be of benefit in this patient group, both intra- and postoperatively (129,130), because reduced humidification alters ciliary function (109). Nebulized saline, and in some cases brochodilators, following surgery may also be helpful in improving secretion clearance (130). In general, however, the use of such airway-clearance techniques is less common following surgery for patients without suppurative lung disease.

B. Methodology Issues

In reviewing the research into the efficacy and relative contributions of various physiotherapy treatment techniques used in the management of postoperative patients, a number of factors must be considered.

The natural history of postoperative pulmonary complications is one of spontaneous recovery (17). For this reason, studies need to be adequately controlled; inclusion of a control (no-treatment) group is the optimal research design. The literature reviewing physiotherapy practice often fails to control and/ or measure variables such as patient mobilization, body position, and pain levels that may confound results. These factors may be considered active treatment components in their own right (131). Unfortunately, few studies include a true control group—several control groups actually received some form of treatment (132). The frequency of performance of treatment techniques may be insufficient (18) and/or not documented. In addition, equivalence between frequency for all techniques being compared is not always achieved (18). Patient adherence to practice of techniques is difficult to assess, but this may confound the effectiveness of results obtained (132). Lack of complete descriptions of methodology render between-study comparisons and generalizability of results difficult. Furthermore, the inclusion of mixed surgical procedures (lower- and upper-abdominal surgery) and patients with varying preoperative risk factors also hinders accurate comparisons between studies. Finally, the small subject numbers studied in many of the papers reviewed often did not allow clear conclusions to be made from the data.

C. Preoperative Education

In recent years, considerable attention has been focused on preoperative intervention. Preoperative explanation including information regarding the effects of the surgical process on respiratory function, location of the wound, and drips and drains may help to reduce pain and hasten postoperative recovery (133). A decrease in postsurgical complications and length of stay was reported by Healy (134) in patients receiving preoperative intervention prior to abdominal surgery. Preoperative education may also reduce the anxiety levels of patients (135). However, there is some controversy over this finding, as other studies have reported no differences in patient anxiety levels despite preoperative education (205). In addition to general education, the physiotherapist may explain the advantages of regular maximal inspirations, wound support during forced expiratory techniques, especially if the patient has excess secretion production preoperatively (13), and the benefits of early ambulation after surgery. Many physiotherapists also provide written instructions (206), although the value of these has not been studied in upper-abdominal surgery or cardiothoracic surgical patients. Physiotherapists, through the preoperative assessment, can identify any risk factors that may predispose to increased risk of postoperative respiratory complication (54). A number of other preventive measures may be worthwhile prior to surgery, including cessation of smoking, loss of weight, and regular physiotherapy if excessive secretions are a problem (54).

Several studies have assessed the role of preoperative physiotherapy. The work of Thoren (34) paved the way for prophylactic pre- and postoperative physiotherapy. In a nonrandomized trial, the author found a reduced incidence of postoperative pulmonary complications in patients receiving both pre- and postoperative physiotherapy (12%) compared with postoperative (27%) or no therapy (42%). Preoperative instruction alone was as effective as pre- and postoperative physiotherapy in minimizing the incidence of postoperative pulmonary complications in 48 patients following cholecystectomy (136). These results have recently been supported in a study of 368 elective abdominal surgical patients (33). The incidence of postoperative pulmonary complications was found to be 6% in the group who received preoperative instruction in deep breathing, coughing, and the benefits of early mobilization, compared with 27% in the control (no-treatment) group, and this difference was found to be statistically significant. However, it was clear from the description of the methodology that patients in the treatment group did receive postoperative physiotherapy. More accurate conclusions from this research are that prophylactic pre- and postoperative physiotherapy (not preoperative physiotherapy as stated) are significantly more effective than no treatment in reducing the incidence of postoperative pulmonary complications.

D. Breathing Strategies

As previously outlined, the pulmonary complications occurring perioperatively are thought to be due to a multifactorial process involving either or both of two main pathophysiological factors: hypoventilation and secretion plugging. In the available literature describing breathing strategies (exercises) there is use of inconsistent terminology. Traditionally, deep-breathing strategies (thoracic expansion exercises, diaphragmatic breathing, sustained maximal inspiration) to increase lung volume, redistribute ventilation, improve gas exchange, increase thoracic mobility, and aid in secretion mobilization (137) have been the mainstay of physiotherapy for this patient group. Evidence supporting their efficacy in achieving these aims is scant (131,138,139) and often conflicting. However, O'Donohue (18) and Celli (30) both stress the importance of regular maximal inspirations in a prophylactic perioperative treatment regimen, whereas others question the need to include breathing exercises at all (96,27,131). The effects of breathing exercises, in isolation, in aiding secretion clearance have not been studied.

Most deep-breathing exercises that aim to improve lung volume are performed from functional residual capacity to total lung capacity (TLC). As a result of the effect of body position on lung volume, they are often performed in an erect sitting position but may also be used in combination with gravity-assisted drainage and forced expiratory maneuvers. Variations in inspiratory flow are thought to alter the distribution of ventilation (137). To improve ventilation to dependent lung regions, which are the most affected following major surgery, a slow inspiratory flow is recommended. As lung volume increases, the influence of flow on distribution of ventilation is reduced (137). The importance of periodic deep breaths in people with normal lungs was evaluated, and results showed that regular large breaths to TLC were essential to maintain inflation. Furthermore, it was reported that five consecutive breaths to TLC were needed for effective inflation of alveoli (140). Based on this research, the number of maximal sequential breaths needed for physiological effects is thought to be five, performed once every waking hour (140). The time spent on breathing exercises and respiratory maneuvers described as being most beneficial is reported to be approximately 20 minutes (126).

No recent research examines the effects of altering duration and frequency of breathing exercises on outcomes. In clinical practice, physiotherapists may chose to perform deep-breathing exercises by using tactile stimulation over a patient's lower ribs laterally or anteriorly over the costal margin. The addition of resistance through the hands and application of a quick stretch is thought to encourage a maximal inspiration (141). Figure 2 illustrates a patient receiving breathing exercises while sitting out of bed. The physiotherapist is using a

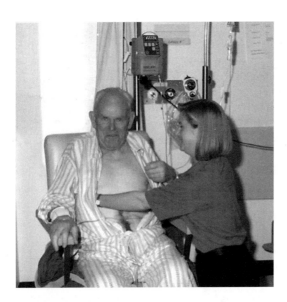

Figure 2 A patient, 1 day following upper-abdominal surgery, receiving breathing exercises from a physiotherapist.

"hands-on" approach. Blaney and Sawyer (142) studied diaphragmatic motion using ultrasonography in 18 patients following upper-abdominal surgery. The authors compared three breathing strategies with the patients sitting, receiving verbal instruction to take only deep breaths, and coached in diaphragmatic breathing and thoracic expansion exercises pre- and postoperatively. Results showed a significant increase in diaphragmatic excursion following surgery when the two tactile, or hands-on, breathing techniques were compared with verbal instruction alone (142).

A convincing body of literature supports the view that reflex inhibition of the diaphragm occurs following upper-abdominal surgery (87,144,143) and the ribcage contribution to respiration increases at the expense of abdominal-compartment movement (82,145). These alterations in diaphragmatic function may be responsible for atelectasis, reduced lung volumes, and hypoxemia in postoperative patients (82). There is a paucity of literature that seeks to evaluate the role of different methods of applying breathing strategies by physiotherapists. It is unclear whether it is more effective to teach deep-breathing exercises by encouraging greater abdominal excursion or facilitating bilateral costal (bucket-handle) movement, or whether just asking the patient for a maximal inspiration is sufficient. The results of Blaney and Sawyer (142) are in favor of a hands-on approach to breathing exercises, but the small sample size of the study limits the generalizability of results. This area requires further research.

The addition of a 3-second breath hold at TLC has been recommended (146,147). A sustained maximal inspiration mimics a sigh or yawn and aims to increase transpulmonary pressure (147). It may also allow time for alveoli with slow time constants to fill. Redistribution of gas into areas of low lung compliance utilizing collateral ventilation pathways and lung interdependence may re-expand collapsed alveoli (18,146,148). If regional ventilation is reduced as a result of secretion plugging, the re-expansion of collapsed alveoli may allow air to move behind the secretions and assist their removal using forced expiration techniques (148,149).

Lung volume is important in mucus clearance, as demonstrated by Gamsu et al. (17). The postoperative clearance of tantalum powder (adhered to airway mucus) was measured in 18 patients following abdominal surgery. These patients experienced delayed clearance of the tantulum, atelectasis in areas of retained powder, and clearance of tantulum once the atelectasis had resolved. Restoration of lung volumes following surgery using breathing strategies may therefore be important in promoting more effective mucus clearance. Improved lung volumes will enhance the effectiveness of a cough and thus also promote more efficient mucus clearance.

Incentive spirometry was developed to stimulate patients to perform deep-breathing exercises under supervision or independently. The additional effects of incentive spirometry compared with deep-breathing exercises have been widely discussed in the literature. Incentive spirometry is a simple tool in the clinical setting to facilitate deep breathing. Many conflicting articles have been written about its physiological effects (28,145,150–153) or absence of them (154–156). Other benefits, such as cost-effectiveness, have been described by Hall et al. (42) and refuted by Denehy et al. (157) and others (158,159). The use of incentive spirometry has been evaluated in different patient categories such as those undergoing cardiac surgery and a pediatric population (160,161). Many questions regarding its effectiveness remain unanswered. The patient category most likely to benefit from this tool are high-risk patients after thoracic or upper-abdominal surgery (154,162). In a recent well-designed study it was reported that the addition of incentive spirometry to physiotherapy, including deep-breathing exercises and early mobilization, in 67 patients did not significantly alter the incidence of postoperative pulmonary complications following thoracic and esophageal surgery (207). The fact that the incentive spirometer could be used as a pre- and postoperative screening device has been described (163,164). Bastin et al. (165), although describing a postlobectomy population, found a moderate correlation with outcome. Their conclusion that incentive spirometry was a simple means to follow up pulmonary function is debatable, because the gap between the real maximum inspiratory capacity and forced vital capacity is larger than the difference between the incentive spirometry and forced vital capacity. Incentive spirometry therefore underestimates the maximum inspiratory capacity.

The efficacy of deep-breathing strategies in clinical practice (deep-breathing exercises, sustained maximal inspiration, and incentive spirometry) for reducing postoperative morbidity has been studied by several authors. Different methods of postoperative prophylaxis have been compared; the results of these studies are given in Tables 3 and 4. It seems apparent from these studies that different breathing strategies (independent deep breathing, incentive spirometry, positive expiratory pressure) may be equally effective and that some form of deep breathing is better than no intervention in minimizing the incidence of postoperative pulmonary complications.

E. Forced Expiratory Manuevers

With respect to expiratory techniques, little research exits that compares the efficacy of mucus-mobilizing techniques in the postoperative phase. Forced expiration is one technique used for mobilizing and expectorating excess bronchial secretions (149). The technique incorporates one or two forced expirations (huffs) and breathing control. Extensive information outlining the definition and efficacy of this technique has been published (149,166). Much of this research was performed in medical patients with copious secretions. The specific role of the forced expiratory technique in the management of patients after surgery has not

Table 3 Description and Results of Comparative Physiotherapy Research in Patients Following Abdominal Surgery

Author (year)	Intervention	Patient category and sample size	Outcome variable	Conclusion
Jung (1980)	IS vs. IPPB	AS (126)	PPC, CXR	n.s.
Stock (1984)	CPAP vs. IS vs. DBEX	AS (63)	PPC, CXR, PFT	CPAP > IS = DBEX
Morran (1983)	No physio treatment vs. DBEX	AS (102)	PPC, CXR, ABG,	DBEX > no treatment
Celli (1984)	No treatment vs. IPPB vs. IS vs. DBEX	AS (172)	PPC, CXR	IPPB = IS = DBEX > no treatment
Hallbrook (1984)	Advice DBEX, cough DBEX, cough, PD DBEX, cough, PD, bronchodilator	AS (137)	ABG, CXR	n.s.
Ricksten (1986)	IS vs. CPAP vs. PEP	AS (45)	[A-a] 02 diff, FVC	PEP = CPAP > IS
Schwieger (1986)	No physio treatment vs. IS	AS, low risk (40)	CXR, ABG, PFT	n.s.
Roukema (1988)	No physio treatment vs. IS	AS nonsmokers (153)	CXR, ABG	DBEX > no treatment
Hall (1991)	IS, mob vs. DBEX, cough mob	AS (876)	PPC, CXR, PaO$_2$, LOS	n.s.
Christensen (1991)	DBEX vs. DBEX + PEP vs. DBEX + IR-PEP	AS (365)	PPC, PFT, LOS	n.s.
Condie (1993)	DBEX cough, mob preop DBEX, cough, mob pre- and postop	AS nonsmokers (330)	PPC	n.s.

Table 3 (Continued)

Author (year)	Intervention	Patient category and sample size	Outcome variable	Conclusion
Denehy (1996)	DBEX, FET, mob DBEX, FET, mob and CPAP 15 min DBEX, FET, mob and CPAP 30 min	AS (50)	PPC, FRC, VC, SaO$_2$, CXR	n.s.
Hall (1996)	Low-risk group: IS vs. DBEX, cough High-risk group: IS vs. IS + maximal inspiration	AS (456)	PPC, CXR, ABG	Low risk: DBEX and cough > IS High risk: IS > IS + maximal inspiration
Chumillas (1998)	No physio treatment DBEX, SMI, FET, mob	AS (81)	PPC, CXR, ABG, FVC	DBEX > no treatment in PPC, n.s. others
Olsen (1997)	No physio treatment Preop physio (DBEX, cough ± PE)	AS (368)	PPC, SaO$_2$, FVC	Preop physio > no treatment in PPC and SaO$_2$

CABG: coronary arterial bypass graft; AS: abdominal surgery; ABG: arterial blood gases; PPC: postoperative pulmonary complications; BDEX: deep-breathing exercises; FET: forced expiration technique; SMI: sustained maximal inspiration; mob: mobilization; physio: physiotherapy; preop: preoperative; IS: incentive spirometry; IPPB: intermittent positive-pressure breathing; PEP: positive expiratory pressure; IR-PEP: inspiratory resistance positive expiratory pressure; CPAP: continuous positive airway pressure; PFT: pulmonary function tests; VC: vital capacity; SaO$_2$: arterial saturation; FVC: forced vital capacity; PEFR: peak expiratory flow rate; CXR: chest x-ray; LOS: length of postoperative hospital stay; BD: twice daily; QID: four times daily; n.s.: nonsignificant.

Table 4 Description and Results of Comparative Physiotherapy Research in Patients Following Cardiac Surgery

Author (year)	Interventions	Patient category and sample size	Outcome variables	Conclusion
Gale (1980)	IS vs. IPPB	CABG/valve (109)	VC, PaO$_2$, CXR	n.s.
Dull (1983)	Mob, cough, and IS Mob, cough, DBEX Mob, cough	CABG/valve (49)	Fever, mucus, auscultation	n.s.
Stock (1984)	CPAP vs. IS vs. DBEX	CABG/valve (38)	FRC, PaO$_2$, CXR, PPC	n.s.
Jenkins (1989)	Mob cough Mob, cough, DBEX Mob, cough, DBEX, IS	CABG (110)	VC, FRC, PaO$_2$, PPC	n.s.
Oikkonen (1991)	IS, cough, DBEX IPPB, cough, DBEX	CABG (52)	VC, PEFR, PaO$_2$, CXR	n.s.
Ingwerson (1993)	DBEX, huff, and CPAP DBEX, huff, and PEP DBEX, huff, and IR-PEP	Cardiothoracic (120)	CXR	n.s.
Stiller (1994)	No physio treatment DBEX, cough (BD) Intensive DBEX, cough (QID)	CABG (120)	PPC	n.s.
Johnson (1995)	Minimal atelectasis at extubation Mob, DBEX Mob, DBEX, SMI Marked atelectasis at extubation Mob, DBEX, SMI Mob, DBEX, SMI, manual percussion	CABG (228)	PPC, CXR, LOS	n.s.
Stiller (1995) Stiller (1994)	No pre- or postop physio treatment Mob (nurses)	CABG (127)	PPC	n.s. compared
Crowe (1997)	DBEX, huff, mob DBEX, huff, mob, and IS	CABG (185)	PPC, CXR	n.s.

Abbreviations as in Table 3.

been studied. Many studies support its efficacy in clearing excess secretions. However, teaching the correct performance of the huff from mid- to low lung volume with the glottis open may be best done preoperatively. It is our experience that drowsy patients who are taking nothing by mouth and experiencing pain find that the forced expiration technique is difficult to perform effectively immediately after surgery unless they have been instructed in its use prior to surgery. The use of wound support during the technique is recommended in a way similar to that of teaching a patient to cough. The role of coughing in secretion clearance is discussed in Section IV. Coughing with wound support should be encouraged as part of any prophylactic treatment regimen following major surgery.

Because of the increased metabolic demand in the postoperative phase, respiratory manuevers or exercises may be tiring for patients. Schulze and Thorup (167) described fatigue after laparoscopic cholesystectomy. Directed vigorous coughing (168) was shown to increase oxygen expenditure in young healthy adults. This might suggest that vigorous coughing results in a high increase in expenditure in patients, either surgical or nonsurgical. For this reason it is far better to teach patients to perform one or two effective coughs than numerous less effective maneuvers.

Routine pulmonary-function testing in the postoperative period is uncommon, and it may provide an additional strain for the patient. Using equipment that allows a combination of deep-breathing exercises and measurement of vital capacity may be beneficial for the patient and clinician in providing an objective means to evaluate the patient's recovery process.

F. Mobilization

The cardiovascular and respiratory effects of immobility and bed rest have been well documented (131,169–171). These include reduced lung volumes and capacities, especially functional residual capacity; reduced PaO_2; decreased $VO_{2\,max}$, cardiac output, and stroke volume; increased heart rate; and orthostatic intolerance (169). The goal of mobilization of postoperative patients is exercise at a level sufficient to increase minute ventilation and cardiac output—within safe physiological limits (170). Given the previously described physiological changes associated with major surgery, a technique that can increase ventilation may improve outcome in this patient group. Effective analgesia is necessary in order to actively mobilize patients (99). It has long been recognized that body position affects respiratory function (172,173). Adoption of the upright position and increased tidal volumes may aid in recruitment of alveoli in dependent lung zones, improve ventilation/perfusion (V/Q) matching, and promote secretion mobilization (170,174).

Several studies have examined the efficacy of this technique in isolation. Dull and Dull (175) and Jenkins et al. (176) advocate early mobilization in the respiratory prophylaxis of patients following coronary artery surgery. No additional benefits of breathing exercises or incentive spirometry were found in either study. Hallböök et al. (177) reported similar results in patients following cholecystectomy. Wolff et al. (178) studied the effects of exercise hyperventilation compared with eucapnic hyperventilation using radioactive isotopes in normal subjects. The authors reported a significant improvement in secretion mobilization with exercise hyperventilation.

Close monitoring is essential during and immediately following mobilization, but specific exercise guidelines must relate to individual patients and assessment and reassessment by the physiotherapist. Figure 3 illustrates a patient being ambulated with assistance 2 days after surgery. Early mobilization of patients following major surgery is common physiotherapy and nursing practice. Previously, although patients were mobilized during physiotherapy treatment, improving mobility was not recognized as an important short-term goal by physiotherapists. Further research is necessary to identify the optimal distance, speed, and frequency of mobilization necessary to gain maximum benefit (54). With more research and a greater emphasis on a pathophysiological basis for treat-

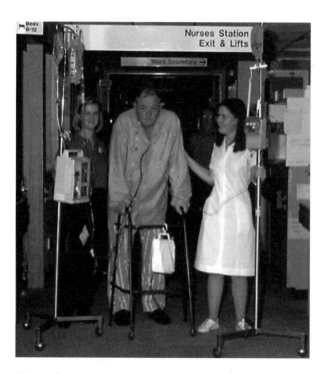

Figure 3 Ambulation following upper-abdominal surgery often requires two assistants to help manage drips and drains.

ment, early mobilization has become increasingly important as a technique in its own right (131).

G. Positive-Pressure Techniques

Physiotherapists have used positive-pressure devices since intermittent positive-pressure breathing (IPPB) was first introduced to clinical management (179). Apart from IPPB, some physiotherapists may use positive expiratory pressure (PEP) and continuous positive airway pressure (CPAP) in the management of patients following major surgery. Several studies have compared the efficacy of PEP with that of other techniques in the postoperative period; these are reviewed in Tables 3 and 4.

Intermittent Positive-Pressure Breathing

There is a large body of literature examining the physiological effects and efficacy of IPPB in different patient populations. The results of this literature were both inconsistent and controversial (180). IPPB has been used in clinical practice primarily to improve lung volumes and decrease the work of breathing (181–183). In postoperative patients the efficacy of IPPB was compared with IS, breathing strategies, and respiratory physiotherapy. The results of this extensive research were equivocal, with IPPB conferring no added benefit when compared with other methods of postoperative prophylaxis (25,155,158,184–186). This literature is plagued by methodological problems, especially related to frequency, dosage, and application of IPPB, as discussed in Section V.B.

Few studies have investigated the efficacy of IPPB in mobilizing secretions. Pavia et al. (187) found no differences in tracheobronchial clearance between conventional physiotherapy, IPPB, and combined treatment in eight patients with excessive secretion production. IPPB may be a useful tool in the management of postoperative patients who cannot or will not inspire maximally (18). For patients with reduced lung volumes, improvement in vital capacity may provide the patient with a more effective cough, thereby improving secretion clearance. Because the aims of IPPB need to be directed toward improving volumes, the pressure and flow rate settings must be set accordingly for individual patients and will depend on their body position and underlying lung pathology (18,25). However, because of cost-benefit considerations, IPPB should never be used as a prophylactic treatment technique.

Positive Expiratory Pressure

Physiotherapy treatment with the PEP mask was pioneered in Denmark (208). Research evidence reporting the clinical efficacy of PEP-mask physiotherapy is conflicting, and most research was performed in patients with chronic sputum production. Thomas and colleagues (209), in a systematic review, identified eight clinical trials involving a total of 228 patients that compared PEP with traditional airway-clearance modalities. The pooled results showed equivalence of efficacy for the outcome measures, which were sputum weight and lung function. Although three of these studies reported significant results for PEP over traditional therapy (210–212), conclusions from this research are hampered by use of different PEP treatment regimens and the lack of equivalence in frequency of the other physiotherapy techniques with which PEP was compared. In the treatment of patients undergoing upper-abdominal surgery, PEP has been compared with CPAP, incentive spirometry, and conventional pre- and postoperative physiotherapy. The effect of adding PEP to conventional physiotherapy was measured in 71 patients after elective abdominal surgery, and the incidence of postoperative pulmonary complications was found to be 31% after conventional physiotherapy and 22% after physiotherapy plus PEP (213). The PEP device used in this study is now commonly known as "bubble" PEP because the end expiratory pressure is maintained by the height of a column of water in a plastic bottle. In this study no manometer was added to the circuit so accurate PEP pressure was not maintained.

In a comparison of PEP-mask physiotherapy with CPAP and incentive spirometry, Ricksten et al. (202) found that PEP and CPAP were significantly more effective than incentive spirometry in maintaining gas exchange and lung volumes postoperatively and lowering the incidence of atelectasis in 43 patients undergoing elective upper-abdominal surgery. All patients performed 30 breaths every waking hour for 3 days after surgery. The PEP and CPAP pressures were set at 10–15 cm H_2O and monitored using a manometer. A record was kept of the number of treatment occasions, which were not significantly different between groups. The results from this well-controlled study suggest that both CPAP and PEP may be equally effective in prophylaxis postoperatively. The physiological mechanisms for the effectiveness of PEP are thought to be through recruitment of lung through collateral channels; however, few studies have investigated the effects of PEP on physiological parameters (214).

While the use of PEP in the management of patients undergoing upper-abdominal surgery has been supported in two studies (33,213), the extent of its use in clinical practice has not been studied. Further research is necessary to establish whether PEP-mask physiotherapy administered postoperatively is more effective than simpler treatment regimens. The advances in pain management since these studies were performed may influence the results of future studies.

Continuous Positive Airway Pressure

CPAP may be defined as the maintenance of positive airway pressure throughout the whole respiratory cycle (188). Because CPAP has been shown to increase functional residual capacity, it was adopted as a therapeutic tool for management of reduced lung volumes following surgery (30).

Its clinical use as a noninvasive technique was pioneered by Gregory et al. (189) in 1971 for newborn infants with respiratory distress. Its use by physiotherapists involves intermittent—otherwise known as periodic—application. Use of intermittent CPAP application developed from cadaver studies that demonstrated recruitment of atelectasis with a single CPAP application (190). The physiological mechanisms by which CPAP increases functional residual capacity are thought to be through a progressively increasing alveolar volume with increases in applied positive end expiratory pressure (191,192), a time-dependent increase in lung volume somewhat like pressure–volume hysteresis (191), and increased transpulmonary pressure at end expiration favoring recruitment of collapsed alveoli (193), possibly through collateral channels (190).

Following upper-abdominal surgery, functional residual capacity can decrease to 70% of preoperative levels, the greatest reductions occurring 16–24 hours postoperatively (11). This reduction alters the relationship between functional residual capacity and closing volume, which may lead to closure of dependent small airways and arterial hypoxemia (194). Application of CPAP following upper-abdominal surgery has been shown to improve functional residual capacity compared with other forms of prophylaxis (195,196). However, no significant benefits were reported by Carlsson et al. (215), studying the same patient group. In patients following coronary artery surgery, results of administration of intermittent CPAP are also conflicting (196,197). There is support for the improvement of atelectasis with CPAP application after abdominal surgery (196,198–200). However, the effects of CPAP on the incidence of significant postoperative pulmonary complications are unclear (196). Denehy et al. (201) studied the effects of two different CPAP application times and physiotherapy treatment on postoperative pulmonary complications in 50 patients following upper-abdominal surgery. The authors found a trend toward a reduction in the incidence of clinically relevent postoperative pulmonary complications in patients receiving 30 minutes of CPAP four times daily compared with 10 minutes, and with physiotherapy-only groups. The incidence of postoperative pulmonary complications was low in all groups. On reviewing the evidence, it appears CPAP may be effective in improving lung volumes more quickly than voluntary inspiratory maneuvers but that this does not necessarily have important clinical benefits (18).

A review of the literature failed to identify any research that measures sputum clearance as a primary outcome of treatment with CPAP in postoperative patients. If atelectasis was associated with sputum plugging or sputum retention, it is conceivable that improving functional residual capacity and thereby collateral ventilation may allow airflow behind secretions and enhance their movement up the bronchial tree (198).

An optimal treatment regimen has not yet been established for the use of CPAP. Application patterns vary between and within countries. There are differences in the level of positive pressure used and the length of time and method of application, for example, 30 breaths hourly compared with 15 minutes every 4 hours (196,202). As a result, comparisons in the literature must be drawn with caution. Most studies examine the prophylactic use of CPAP postoperatively but not its efficacy in patients who have developed a significant postoperative complication. This research is still necessary. The introduction of intermittent CPAP to clinical management of patients following surgery may not be the decision of the physiotherapist. In some centers, it may be that of the referring doctor or a joint decision between the physiotherapist and doctor. Prescription of CPAP for respiratory failure, acute pulmonary edema, or obstructive sleep apnea is generally a medical decision.

H. Physiotherapy Intervention

The previous discussion illustrates that research into the use of different techniques for postoperative prophylaxis has been extensive, often poorly controlled, and somewhat contradictory. Tables 3 and 4 present a summary of studies performed in upper-abdominal surgery and coronary artery surgery using different methods of perioperative prophylaxis. Outcome measures used to test the efficacy of such techniques vary considerably, as does the definition for the same outcome across numerous studies. Research that uses radiological evidence of atelectasis as the main outcome variable may provide spurious results since most patients develop some degree of atelectasis following upper-abdominal or coronary artery surgery (22). Measuring clinically relevant complications that, by definition, may adversely affect the postoperative course of the patient (18) is critical to providing relevant answers as we move further into the new millennium.

The type, dosage, and frequency of physiotherapy techniques utilized in different countries (and within the same country) also vary significan tly. Given all this information regarding the most appropriate outcome measure, patient risk assessment, and pre- and postoperative prophylaxis, two main questions arise: do patients need routine prophylaxis after major surgery, and, if so, what are the most effective and cost-efficient methods of providing it?

Results from the literature to date suggest that high-risk patients should be targeted (increasing age, history of respiratory disease, morbid obesity, cardiothoracic or upper-abdominal surgery). These patients may be taught a prophylactic postoperative treatment regimen including some form of maximal inspiratory maneuver (deep-breathing strategies, incentive spirometry, PEP). Reassessment after surgery may be required to assess postoperative risk factors (pain levels, mobility). Ambulation should be encouraged as soon as possible following surgery. Patients may need respiratory physiotherapy management for only 1 or 2 days after surgery. Indeed, they may only require postoperative assessment and reinforcement of their practice routine by the physiotherapist.

There is mounting evidence that following coronary artery surgery early ambulation alone is sufficient to minimize postoperative pulmonary complications in uncomplicated patients (175,176). Stiller et al. (96) report that the provision of routine prophylactic physiotherapy needs to be reviewed in coronary artery surgery patients. Patients with excess secretions perioperatively are at very high risk for developing postoperative pulmonary complications and may benefit from specific airway-clearance techniques preoperatively.

It seems that many methods of treatment may be effective for prophylaxis, and the specific method used will ultimately depend on individual patients' needs, available resources (30), and, to some extent, the training of the physiotherapist.

The role of physiotherapy in the management of routine (low-risk) patients is less clear. Advances in the surgical process (pain management, minimally invasive surgery) have meant that the incidence of postoperative pulmonary complications in this population is decreasing. Several studies suggest that preoperative education alone may be sufficient for patients having upper-abdominal surgery. In patients who have developed refractory atelectasis or infection postoperatively, the role and effectiveness of physiotherapy have not been adequately studied. Another change in patient management in many centers is the use of preadmission clinics. Patients visit the hospital as outpatients for admission details and information up to 1 to 3 weeks before their surgery. They are then admitted as inpatients on the day of surgery. If patients undergoing upper-abdominal surgery or cardiothoracic surgery benefit from preoperative physiotherapy, then the physiotherapist needs to be involved in the preadmission of these patients. Research, particularly in cardiac surgical patients, has shown positive perioperative benefits from preadmission education (203,204).

More comparative research, including the use of no-treatment control groups, is necessary to evaluate the specific continuing role of physiotherapy for patients following major surgery. Furthemore, the comparative efficacy of physiotherapy interventions, especially in relation to mucus clearance, needs to be evaluated. Measurement of treatment efficacy remains a significant problem because the wet or dry weight of sputum produced may not necessarily measure mucus clearance validly.

Resources for surgical units occupy a prominent part of physiotherapy department staffing budgets, and the cost of perioperative respiratory physiotherapy is substantial (54). It is essential that more research be performed to add to the current body of knowledge regarding treatment of surgical patients, in order that physiotherapists can provide evidence-based practice. This research should be aimed at identifying preoperative risk factors, developing a risk-factor model for clinical use, and examining the efficacy of postoperative physiotherapy in specific patient populations (especially thoracic and esophageal surgery) using a no-treatment control group and multicenter research if possible.

To conclude, the statement by O'Donohue (18) is one that may be reflected on by clinical physiotherapists: "treating a spontaneously reversible pulmonary condition that is a normal consequence of surgery may have little relevance or benefit to recovery."

References

1. Bartlett RH. Pulmonary pathophysiology in surgical patients. Surg Clin North Am 1980; 60:1323–1338.
2. Fairshter RD, Williams JH Jr. Pulmonary physiology in the postoperative period. Crit Care Clin 1987; 3:287–306.
3. Marini JJ. Post-operative atelctasis: pathophysiology, clinical importance and principle of management. Respir Care 1984; 29:516–528.
4. Pierce AK, Robertson J. Pulmonary complications of general surgery. Annu Rev Med 1977; 28:211–221.
5. Pasteur W. Active lobar collapse of the lung. Lancet 1910; 1080–1083.
6. Elliot TR, Dingley LA. Massive collapse of the lungs following abdominal operations. Lancet 1914; 1305–1309.
7. Haldane J, Meakins J, Priestly J. The effects of shallow breathing. J Physiol 1919; 52:433–453.
8. Beecher H. The measured effect of laparotomy on the respiration. J Clin Invest 1933; 12:639–658.
9. Dripps R. Post-operative atelectasis and pneumonia. Ann Surg 1946; 124:94–110.
10. Ali J, Weisel RD, Layug AB, Kripke BJ, Hechtman HB. Consequences of postoperative alterations in respiratory mechanics. Am J Surg 1974; 128:376–382.
11. Craig DB. Postoperative recovery of pulmonary function. Anesth Analg 1981; 60: 46–52.
12. Brooks-Brunn J. Postoperative atelectasis and pneumonia. Heart Lung 1995; 24: 94–115.
13. Ridley S. Surgery for adults. In: Pryor J, Webber B, eds. Physiotherapy for Respiratory and Cardiac Problems. London: Churchill Livingstone, 1998:295–327.
14. O'Donohue WJ Jr. Prevention and treatment of postoperative atelectasis: can it and will it be adequately studied? [editorial]. Chest 1985; 87:1–2.
15. Johnson N, Pierson D. The spectrum of pulmonary atelectasis: pathophysiology, diagnosis and therapy. Respir Care 1999; 31:1107–1120.
16. Tisi GM. Preoperative evaluation of pulmonary function: validity, indications, and benefits. Am Rev Respir Dis 1979; 119:293–310.
17. Gamsu G, Singer MM, Vincent HH, Berry S, Nadel JA. Postoperative impairment of mucous transport in the lung. Am Rev Respir Dis 1976; 114:673–679.
18. O'Donohue WJ Jr. Postoperative pulmonary complications: when are preventive and therapeutic measures necessary? Postgrad Med 1992; 91:167–5.
19. Brooks D, Thomas J. Interrater reliability of auscultation of breath sounds among physical therapists. Phys Ther 1995; 75:1082–1088.
20. Dilworth JP, White RJ. Postoperative chest infection after upper abdominal surgery: an important problem for smokers. Respir Med 1992; 86:205–210.

21. Jenkins S, Soutar SA, Loukota JM, Johnson LC, Moxham J. A comparison of breathing exercises, incentive spirometry and mobilization after coronary bypass surgery. Physiother Theory Pract 1990; 6:117–126.
22. Bourn J, Jenkins S. Post-operative respiratory physiotherapy. Physiotherapy 1992; 78:80–85.
23. Platell C, Hall JC. Atelectasis after abdominal surgery. J Am Coll Surg 1997; 185:584–592.
24. Brooks-Brunn J. Predictors of postoperative pulmonary complications following abdominal surgery. Chest 1997; 111:564–571.
25. Celli BR, Rodriguez KS, Snider GL. A controlled trial of intermittent positive pressure breathing, incentive spirometry, and deep breathing exercises in preventing pulmonary complications after abdominal surgery. Am Rev Respir Dis 1984; 130:12–15.
26. Craven JL, Evans GA, Davenport PJ, Williams RH. The evaluation of the incentive spirometer in the management of postoperative pulmonary complications. Br J Surg 1974; 61:793–797.
27. Jenkins SC, Soutar SA, Forsyth A, Keates JR, Moxham J. Lung function after coronary artery surgery using the internal mammary artery and the saphenous vein. Thorax 1989; 44:209–211.
28. Hall JC, Tarala RA, Tapper J, Hall JL. Prevention of respiratory complications after abdominal surgery: a randomised clinical trial [comments]. Br Med J 1996; 312:148–152.
29. Stiller K, Crawford R, McInnes M, Montarello J, Hall B. The incidence of pulmonary complications in patients not receiving phrophylactic chest physiotherapy after cardiac surgery: a randomized clinical trial. Physiother Theory Pract 1995; 11:205–208.
30. Celli BR. Perioperative respiratory care of the patient undergoing upper abdominal surgery. Clin Chest Med 1993; 14:253–261.
31. Castillo R, Haas A. Chest physical therapy: comparative efficacy of preoperative and postoperative in the elderly. Arch Phys Med Rehabil 1985; 66:376–379.
32. Chumillas S, Ponce JL, Delgado F, Viciano V, Mateu M. Prevention of postoperative pulmonary complications through respiratory rehabilitation: a controlled clinical study. Arch Phys Med Rehabil 1998; 79:5–9.
33. Fagevik O, Hahn I, Nordgren S, Lönroth H, Lundholm K. Randomized controlled trial of prophylactic chest physiotherapy in major abdominal surgery. Br J Surg 1997; 84:1535–1538.
34. Thoren L. Post-operative pulmonary complication: observation on their prevention by means of physiotherapy. Acta Chir Scandinav 1954; CVII:193–205.
35. Norman G, Streiner D. Biostatistics: the bare essentials. St. Louis: Mosby Yearbook, 1994.
36. Hall JC, Tarala R, Harris J, Tapper J, Christiansen K. Incentive spirometry versus routine chest physiotherapy for prevention of pulmonary complications after abdominal surgery [comments]. Lancet 1991; 337:953–956.
37. Hayhurst MD. Preoperative pulmonary function testing [editorial; comments]. Respir Med 1993; 87:161–163.

38. Lawrence VA, Dhanda R, Hilsenbeck SG, Page CP. Risk of pulmonary complications after elective abdominal surgery [comments]. Chest 1996; 110:744–750.

39. Williams-Russo P, Charlson ME, MacKenzie CR, Gold JP, Shires GT. Predicting postoperative pulmonary complications: is it a real problem? Arch Intern Med 1992; 152:1209–1213.

40. Cullen DJ, Apolone G, Greenfield S, Guadagnoli E, Cleary P. ASA physical status and age predict morbidity after three surgical procedures [comments]. Ann Surg 1994; 220:3–9.

41. Owens WD, Felts JA, Spitznagel-EL J. ASA physical status classifications: a study of consistency of ratings. Anesthesiology 1978; 49:239–243.

42. Hall JC, Tarala RA, Hall JL, Mander J. A multivariate analysis of the risk of pulmonary complications after laparotomy. Chest 1991; 99:923–927.

43. Calligaro KD, Azurin DJ, Dougherty MJ, Dandora R, Bajgier SM, Simper S, et al. Pulmonary risk factors of elective abdominal aortic surgery. J Vasc Surg 1993; 18:914–920.

44. Cohen D, Horiuchi K, Kemper M, Weissman C. Modulating effects of propofol on metabolic and cardiopulmonary responses to stressful intensive care unit procedures. Crit Care Med 1996; 24:612–617.

45. Vodinh J, Bonnet F, Touboul C, Lefloch JP, Becquemin JP, Harf A. Risk factors of postoperative pulmonary complications after vascular surgery. Surgery 1989; 105:360–365.

46. Brooks-Brunn J. Validation of a predictive model for postoperative pulmonary complications. Heart Lung 1998; 27:151–158.

47. Kroenke K, Lawrence VA, Theroux JF, Tuley MR, Hilsenbeck S. Postoperative complications after thoracic and major abdominal surgery in patients with and without obstructive lung disease. Chest 1993; 104:1445–1451.

48. Brown D. Risk and Outcome in Anesthesia. Philadephia: Lippincott, 1988.

49. Jackson CV. Preoperative pulmonary evaluation [comments]. Arch Intern Med 1988; 148:2120–2127.

50. Mendes-da CP, Lurquin P. Gastrointestinal surgery in the aged. Br J Surg 1993; 80:329

51. Garibaldi RA, Britt MR, Coleman ML, Reading JC, Pace NL. Risk factors for postoperative pneumonia. Am J Med 1981; 70:677–680.

52. Wightman JA. A prospective survey of the incidence of postoperative pulmonary complications. Br J Surg 1968; 55:85–91.

53. Leblanc P, Ruff F, Milic EJ. Effects of age and body position on "airway closure" in man. J Appl Physiol 1970; 28:448–451.

54. Jenkins S. Pre-operative and post-operative physiotherapy: are they necessary? In: Pryor J, ed. Respiratory Care. 7th ed. London: Longman Group, 1991:147–168.

55. Luce JM. Clinical risk factors for post-operative pulmonary complications. Respir Care 1984; 29:484–491.

56. Greenburg AG, Saik RP, Pridham D. Influence of age on mortality of colon surgery. Am J Surg 1985; 150:65–70.

57. Latimer RG, Dickman M, Day WC, Gunn ML, Schmidt CD. Ventilatory patterns and pulmonary complications after upper abdominal surgery determined by preop-

erative and postoperative computerized spirometry and blood gas analysis. Am J Surg 1971; 122:622–632.

58. Windsor JA, Hill GL. Risk factors for postoperative pneumonia: the importance of protein depletion. Ann Surg 1988; 208:209–214.

59. Arora NS, Gal TJ. Cough dynamics during progressive expiratory muscle weakness in healthy curarized subjects. J Appl Physiol 1981; 51:494–498.

60. Rosenbaum S, Askanazi J, Hyman A, Silverberg P, Milic-Emili J, Kinney JM. Respiratory patterns in profound nutritional depletion. Anesthesiology 1982; 51S: 36.

61. Pearce AC, Jones RM. Smoking and anesthesia: preoperative abstinence and perioperative morbidity. Anesthesiology 1984; 61:576–584.

62. Kocabas A, Kara K, Ozgur G, Sonmez H, Burgut R. Value of preoperative spirometry to predict postoperative pulmonary complications. Respir Med 1996; 90: 25–33.

63. Bluman LG, Mosca L, Newman N, Simon DG. Preoperative smoking habits and postoperative pulmonary complications [comments]. Chest 1998; 113:883–889.

64. Warner MA, Offord KP, Warner ME, Lennon RL, Conover MA, Jansson-Schumacher U. Role of preoperative cessation of smoking and other factors in postoperative pulmonary complications: a blinded prospective study of coronary artery bypass patients. Mayo Clin Proc 1989; 64:609–616.

65. Ephgrave KS, Kleiman WR, Pfaller M, Booth B, Werkmeister L, Young S. Postoperative pneumonia: a prospective study of risk factors and morbidity. Surgery 1993; 114:815–819.

66. Gracey DR, Divertie MB, Didier EP. Preoperative pulmonary preparation of patients with chronic obstructive pulmonary disease: a prospective study. Chest 1979; 76:123–129.

67. Cain HD, Stevens PM, Adaniya R. Preoperative pulmonary function and complications after cardiovascular surgery. Chest 1979; 76:130–135.

68. Higgins TL, Estafanous FG, Loop FD, Beck GJ, Blum JM, Paranandi L. Stratification of morbidity and mortality outcome by preoperative risk factors in coronary artery bypass patients: a clinical severity score [published erratum appears in JAMA 1992; 268(14):1860] [comments]. JAMA 1992; 267:2344–2348.

69. Grover FL, Hammermeister KE, Burchfiel C. Initial report of the Veterans Administration Preoperative Risk Assessment Study for Cardiac Surgery. Ann Thorac Surg 1990; 50:12–26.

70. Stein M, Cassara EL. Preoperative pulmonary evaluation and therapy for surgery patients. JAMA 1970; 211:787–790.

71. De Nino LA, Lawrence VA, Averyt EC, Hilsenbeck SG, Dhanda R, Page CP. Preoperative spirometry and laparotomy: blowing away dollars. Chest 1997; 111: 1536–1541.

72. Lawrence VA, Page CP, Harris GD. Preoperative spirometry before abdominal operations: a critical appraisal of its predictive value. Arch Intern Med 1989; 149:280–285.

73. Spivack SD, Shinozaki T, Albertini JJ, Deane R. Preoperative prediction of postoperative respiratory outcome: coronary artery bypass grafting. Chest 1996; 109: 1222–1230.

74. Nagawa H, Kobori O, Muto T. Prediction of pulmonary complications after transthoracic oesophagectomy. Br J Surg 1994; 81:860–862.

75. Linn BS, Linn MW, Wallen N. Evaluation of results of surgical procedures in the elderly. Ann Surg 1982; 195:90–96.

76. Fan ST, Lau WY, Yip WC, Poon GP, Yeung C, Lam WK, et al. Prediction of postoperative pulmonary complications in oesophagogastric cancer surgery. Br J Surg 1987; 74:408–410.

77. Richardson J, Sabanathan S. Prevention of respiratory complications after abdominal surgery. Thorax 1997; 52(suppl)3:S35–S40.

78. Juno J, Marsh HM, Knopp TJ, Rehder K. Closing capacity in awake and anesthetized-paralyzed man. J Appl Physiol 1978; 44:238–244.

79. Kotani N, Lin CY, Wang JS, Gurley JM, Tolin FP, Michelassi F, et al. Loss of alveolar macrophages during anesthesia and operation in humans. Anesth Analg 1995; 81:1255–1262.

80. McKeague H, Cunningham AJ. Postoperative respiratory dysfunction: is the site of surgery crucial? [editorial; comment]. Br J Anaesth 1997; 79:415–416.

81. Seymour DG, Pringle R. Post-operative complications in the elderly surgical patient. Gerontology 1983; 29:262–270.

82. Ford GT, Rosenal TW, Clergue F, Whitelaw WA. Respiratory physiology in upper abdominal surgery. Clin Chest Med 1993; 14:237–252.

83. Johnson WC. Postoperative ventilatory performance: dependence upon surgical incision. Am Surg 1975; 41:615–619.

84. Garcia-Valdecasas J, Almenara R, Cabrer C, de-Lacy AM, Sust M, Taura P, et al. Subcostal incision versus midline laparotomy in gallstone surgery: a prospective and randomized trial. Br J Surg 1988; 75:473–475.

85. Tsui SL, Chan CS, Chan AS, Wong SJ, Lam CS, Jones RD. Postoperative analgesia for oesophageal surgery: a comparison of three analgesic regimens. Anaesth Intensive Care 1991; 19:329–337.

86. Frazee RC, Roberts JW, Symmonds RE, Snyder SK, Hendricks JC, Smith RW, et al. A prospective randomized trial comparing open versus laparoscopic appendectomy. Ann Surg 1994; 219:725–731.

87. Dureuil B, Cantineau JP, Desmonts JM. Effects of upper or lower abdominal surgery on diaphragmatic function. Br J Anaesth 1987; 59:1230–1235.

88. Pansard JL, Mankikian B, Bertrand M, Kieffer E, Clergue F, Viars P. Effects of thoracic extradural block on diaphragmatic electrical activity and contractility after upper abdominal surgery. Anesthesiology 1993; 78:63–71.

89. Erice F, Fox GS, Salib YM, Romano E, Meakins JL, Magder SA. Diaphragmatic function before and after laparoscopic cholecystectomy. Anesthesiology 1993; 79:966–975.

90. Reeve EB, Nanson EM, Rundle FF. Observation on inhibitory reflexes during abdominal surgery. Clin Sci 1951; 10:65–87.

91. Estenne M, Yernault JC, De-Smet JM, De-Troyer A. Phrenic and diaphragm function after coronary artery bypass grafting. Thorax 1985; 40:293–299.

92. Locke TJ, Griffiths TL, Mould H, Gibson GJ. Rib cage mechanics after median sternotomy. Thorax 1990; 45:465–468.

93. Vaughan RW, Wise L. Choice of abdominal operative incision in the obese patient: a study using blood gas measurements. Ann Surg 1975; 181:829–835.

94. Matthay MA, Wiener KJ. Respiratory management after cardiac surgery. Chest 1989; 95:424–434.

95. Vargas FS, Cukier A, Terra FM, Hueb W, Teixeira LR, Light RW. Influence of atelectasis on pulmonary function after coronary artery bypass grafting. Chest 1993; 104:434–437.

96. Stiller K, Montarello J, Wallace M, Daff M, Grant R, Jenkins S, et al. Efficacy of breathing and coughing exercises in the prevention of pulmonary complications after coronary artery surgery [comments]. Chest 1994; 105:741–747.

97. Dodson M. The management of post-operative pain. In: Dodson M, ed. Current Topics in Anaesthesia. 8th ed. London: Edward Arnold, 1985.

98. Ballantyne JC, Carr DB, deFerranti S, Suarez T, Lau J, Chalmers TC, et al. The comparative effects of postoperative analgesic therapies on pulmonary outcome: cumulative meta-analyses of randomized, controlled trials. Anesth Analg 1998; 86:598–612.

99. Sabanathan S, Shah R, Tsiamis A, Richardson J. Oesophagogastrectomy in the elderly high risk patients: role of effective regional analgesia and early mobilisation. J Cardiovasc Surg Torino 1999; 40:153–156.

100. Katz J. Preop analgesia for postop pain [comment]. Lancet 1993; 342:65–66.

101. Richmond CE, Bromley LM, Woolf CJ. Preoperative morphine pre-empts postoperative pain [comments]. Lancet 1993; 342:73–75.

102. Barrat S. Advances in acute pain management. Int Anaesthesiol Clin 1997; 35: 27–33.

103. Jayr C, Matthay MA, Goldstone J, Gold WM, Wiener KJ. Preoperative and intraoperative factors associated with prolonged mechanical ventilation: a study in patients following major abdominal vascular surgery. Chest 1993; 103:1231–1236.

104. Wilson R, Dowling RB, Jackson AD. The biology of bacterial colonization and invasion of the respiratory mucosa [comments]. Eur Respir J 1996; 9:1523–1530.

105. Konrad F, Schiener R, Marx T, Georgieff M. Ultrastructure and mucociliary transport of bronchial respiratory epithelium in intubated patients. Intensive Care Med 1995; 21:482–489.

106. Stanek A, Brambrink AM, Latorre F, Bender B, Kleemann PP. Effects of normobaric oxygen on ciliary beat frequency of human respiratory epithelium. Br J Anaesth 1998; 80:660–664.

107. Raphael JH, Butt MW. Comparison of isoflurane with propofol on respiratory cilia. Br J Anaesth 1997; 79:473–475.

108. O'Callaghan C, Atherton M, Karim K, Gyi A, Langton JA, Zamudio I, et al. The effect of halothane on neonatal ciliary beat frequency. J Paediatr Child Health 1994; 30:429–431.

109. Branson RD, Campbell RS, Davis K, Porembka DT. Anaesthesia circuits, humidity output, and mucociliary structure and function. Anaesth Intensive Care 1998; 26:178–183.

110. Leith DE. The development of cough. Am Rev Respir Dis 1985; 131:S39–S42

111. Bennett WD, Foster WM, Chapman WF. Cough-enhanced mucus clearance in the normal lung. J Appl Physiol 1990; 69:1670–1675.

112. Bouros D, Siafakas NM, Green M. Cough. In: Roussos C, ed. The Thorax, Part B: Applied Physiology. 2nd ed. New York: Marcel Dekker, 1995:1335–1354.

113. Knudson RJ, Mead J, Knudson DE. Contribution of airway collapse to supramaximal expiratory flows. J Appl Physiol 1974; 36:653–667.

114. Enright PL, Kronmal RA, Manolio TA, Schenker MB, Hyatt RE. Respiratory muscle strength in the elderly: correlates and reference values. Cardiovascular Health Study Research Group. Am J Respir Crit Care Med 1994; 149:430–438.

115. Hewlett AM, Hulands GH, Nunn JF, Heath JR. Functional residual capacity during anaesthesia. II. Spontaneous respiration. Br J Anaesth 1974; 46:486–494.

116. Siafakas NM, Stoubou A, Stathopoulou M, Haviaras V, Tzanakis N, Bouros D. Effect of aminophylline on respiratory muscle strength after upper abdominal surgery: a double blind study [comments]. Thorax 1993; 48:693–697.

117. Celli B. Respiratory muscle strength after upper abdominal surgery [editorial; comment]. Thorax 1993; 48:683–684.

118. Macklem PT. Airway obstruction and collateral ventilation. Physiol Rev 1971; 51:368–436.

119. Cotes JE. Maximal flow rates. In: Cotes JE, ed. Lung Function: Assessment and Application in Medicine. 5th ed. London: Blackwell, 1993:114–121.

120. Nunn JF. Measurement of ventilatory capacity. In: Nunn JF, ed. Applied Respiratory Physiology. 4th ed. London: Butterworth, 1993:

121. Dilworth JP, Pounsford JC. Cough following general anaesthesia and abdominal surgery. Respir Med 1991; 85(suppl A):13–16.

122. Epstein SK, Faling LJ, Daly BD, Celli BR. Predicting complications after pulmonary resection: preoperative exercise testing vs a multifactorial cardiopulmonary risk index. Chest 1993; 104:694–700.

123. Charlson ME, Ales KL, Simon R, MacKenzie CR. Why predictive indexes perform less well in validation studies: is it magic or methods? Arch Intern Med 1987; 147:2155–2161.

124. MacMahon C. Breathing and physical exercises for use in wounds in the pleura, lung and diaphragm. Lancet 1915; 2:769–770.

125. Bartlett RH, Gazzaniga AB, Geraghty TR. Respiratory maneuvers to prevent postoperative pulmonary complications: a critical review. JAMA 1973;224:1017–1021.

126. Morran CG, Finlay IG, Mathieson M, McKay AJ, Wilson N, McArdle CS. Randomized controlled trial of physiotherapy for postoperative pulmonary complications. Br J Anaesth 1983; 55:1113–1117.

127. Roukema JA, Carol EJ, Prins JG. The prevention of pulmonary complications after upper abdominal surgery in patients with noncompromised pulmonary status. Arch Surg 1988; 123:30–34.

128. Laszlo G, Archer GG, Darrell JH, Dawson JM, Fletcher CM. The diagnosis and prophylaxis of pulmonary complications of surgical operation. Br J Surg 1973; 60:129–134.

129. Weeks AM, Buckland MR. Anaesthesia for adults with cystic fibrosis. Anaesth Intensive Care 1995; 23:332–338.

130. Walsh TS, Young CH. Anaesthesia and cystic fibrosis. Anaesthesia 1995; 50:614–622.

131. Dean E, Ross J. Discordance between cardiopulmonary physiology and physical therapy: toward a rational basis for practice [comments]. Chest 1992; 101:1694–1698.
132. Thomas JA, McIntosh JM. Are incentive spirometry, intermittent positive pressure breathing, and deep breathing exercises effective in the prevention of postoperative pulmonary complications after upper abdominal surgery? A systematic overview and meta-analysis. Phys Ther 1994; 74:3–10.
133. Auerbach S, Kilman P. Crisis intervention: a review of outcome. Psychol Bull 1974; 84:1189–1217.
134. Healy K. Does pre-operative instruction make a difference? Am J Nursing 1968; 68:62–67.
135. Meeker B. Pre-operative patient education: evaluating post-operative patient outcomes. Patient Educ Couns 1994; 23:41–47.
136. Bourn JEA, Conway JH, Holgate ST. The effect of ost-operative physiotherapy on pulmonary complications and lung function after abdominal surgery. Eur Respir J 1991; 4S:325.
137. Tucker B, Jenkins S. The effect of breathing exercises with body positioning on regional ventilation. Aust J Physiother 1996; 42:219–227.
138. Sampson MG, Smaldone GC. Voluntary induced alterations in regional ventilation in normal humans. J Appl Physiol 1984; 56:196–201.
139. Roussos CS, Fixley M, Genest J, Cosio M, Kelly S, Martin RR, et al. Voluntary factors influencing the distribution of inspired gas. Am Rev Respir Dis 1977; 116:457–467.
140. Ferris B, Pollard D. Effect of deep and quiet breathing on pulmonary compliance in man. J Clin Invest 1960; 39:143–149.
141. Levenson CR. Breathing exercises. In: Zadii CC, ed. Pulmonary Management in Physical Therapy. New York: Churchill-Livingstone, 1992:135–154.
142. Blaney F, Sawyer T. Sonographic measurement of diaphragmatic motion after upper abdominal surgery: a comparion of three breathing manoeuvres. Physiother Theory Pract 1997; 13:207–2115.
143. Simonneau G, Vivien A, Sartene R, Kunstlinger F, Samii K, Noviant Y, et al. Diaphragm dysfunction induced by upper abdominal surgery: role of postoperative pain. Am Rev Respir Dis 1983; 128:899–903.
144. Katagiri H, Katagiri M, Kieser TM, Easton PA. Diaphragm function during sighs in awake dogs after laparotomy. Am J Respir Crit Care Med 1998; 157:1085–1092.
145. Chuter TA, Weissman C, Starker PM, Gump FE. Effect of incentive spirometry on diaphragmatic function after surgery. Surgery 1989; 105:488–493.
146. Terry PB, Traystman RJ, Newball HH, Batra G, Menkes HA. Collateral ventilation in man. N Engl J Med 1978; 298:10–15.
147. Bakow ED. Sustained maximal inspiration: a rationale for its use. Respir Care 1977; 22:379–382.
148. Menkes HA, Traystman RJ. Collateral ventilation. Am Rev Respir Dis 1977; 116:287–309.
149. Pryor J. The forced expiration technique. In: Pryor J., ed. Respiratory Care. London: Churchill Livingstone, 1991:79–99.

150. Weiner P, Man A, Weiner M, Rabner M, Waizman J, Magadle R, et al. The effect of incentive spirometry and inspiratory muscle training on pulmonary function after lung resection. J Thorac Cardiovasc Surg 1997; 113:552–557.

151. Melendez JA, Alagesan R, Reinsel R, Weissman C, Burt M. Postthoracotomy respiratory muscle mechanics during incentive spirometry using respiratory inductance plethysmography. Chest 1992; 101:432–436.

152. Minschaert M, Vincent JL, Ros AM, Kahn RJ. Influence of incentive spirometry on pulmonary volumes after laparotomy. Acta Anaesthesiol Belg 1982; 33:203–209.

153. Parker A, Verne S. Incentive spirometry versus routine chest physiotherapy [letter; comment]. Lancet 1991; 337:1350.

154. Crowe JM, Bradley CA. The effectiveness of incentive spirometry with physical therapy for high-risk patients after coronary artery bypass surgery. Phys Ther 1997; 77:260–268.

155. Oikkonen M, Karjalainen K, Kahara V, Kuosa R, Schavikin L. Comparison of incentive spirometry and intermittent positive pressure breathing after coronary artery bypass graft. Chest 1991; 99:60–65.

156. Schwieger I, Gamulin Z, Forster A, Meyer P, Gemperle M, Suter PM. Absence of benefit of incentive spirometry in low-risk patients undergoing elective cholecystectomy: a controlled randomized study. Chest 1986; 89:652–656.

157. Denehy L, Ntoumenopoulos G, Maclellan DG. The cost-efficiency of incentive spirometry after abdominal surgery [letter; comment]. Aust NZ J Surg 1994; 64:637–639.

158. Ayres SM. Magnitude of use and costs of in-hospital respiratory therapy. Am Rev Respir Dis 1980; 122:11–13.

159. Kester L, Stoller JK. Ordering respiratory care services for hospitalized patients: practices of overuse and underuse. Cleve Clin J Med 1992; 59:581–585.

160. Krastins I, Corey ML, McLeod A, Edmonds J, Levison H, Moes F. An evaluation of incentive spirometry in the management of pulmonary complications after cardiac surgery in a pediatric population. Crit Care Med 1982; 10:525–528.

161. Gale GD, Sanders DE. Incentive spirometry: its value after cardiac surgery. Can Anaesth Soc J 1980; 27:475–480.

162. Hall JC, Tapper J, Tarala R. The cost-efficiency of incentive spirometry after abdominal surgery [comments]. Aust NZ J Surg 1993; 63:356–359.

163. Dewan AK, Rao N, Kumar S. Incentive spirometry as screening pulmonary test. J Surg Oncol 1996; 63:209

164. Kips JC. Preoperative pulmonary evaluation. Acta Clin Belg 1997; 52:301–305.

165. Bastin R, Moraine JJ, Bardocsky G, Kahn RJ, Melot C. Incentive spirometry performance: a reliable indicator of pulmonary function in the early postoperative period after lobectomy? Chest 1997; 111:559–563.

166. Webber B, Pryor J. Physiotherapy techniques. In: Pryor J, Webber B, eds. Physiotherapy for Respiratory and Cardiac Problems. London: Churchill-Livingstone, 1998:138–145.

167. Schulze S, Thorup J. Pulmonary function, pain, and fatigue after laparoscopic cholecystectomy. Eur J Surg 1993; 159:361–364.

168. Holland N, Williams MT, Parsons D, Hall B, Martin AJ. The effect of directed

vigour coughing on energy expenditure and pulmonary function in normal subjects. Physiother Theory Pract 1998; 14:55–61.

169. Dean E. Mobilization and exercise. In: Frownfelter D, Dean E, eds. Principles and Practice of Cardiopulmonary Physical Therapy. New York: Mosby, 1987: 265–296.
170. Ross J, Dean E. Integrating physiological principles into the comprehensive management of cardiopulmonary dysfunction. Phys Ther 1989; 69:255–259.
171. Winslow EH. Cardiovascular consequences of bed rest. Heart Lung 1985; 14: 236–246.
172. Wahba RW. Perioperative functional residual capacity [comments]. Can J Anaesth 1991; 38:384–400.
173. Crosbie W, Sim D. The effect of postural modification on some aspects of pulmonary function following surgery of the abdomen. Physiotherapy 1986; 72:487–492.
174. Jenkins S, Soutar SA, Gray B, Evans J, Moxham J. The acute effects of respiratory manoeuvers in post-operative patients. Physiother Pract 1988; 4:63–68.
175. Dull JL, Dull WL. Are maximal inspiratory breathing exercises or incentive spirometry better than early mobilization after cardiopulmonary bypass? Phys Ther 1983; 63:655–659.
176. Jenkins SC, Soutar SA, Loukota JM, Johnson LC, Moxham J. Physiotherapy after coronary artery surgery: are breathing exercises necessary? Thorax 1989; 44:634–639.
177. Hallböök T, Lindblad B, Lindroth B, Wolff T. Prophylaxis against pulmonary complications in patients undergoing gall-bladder surgery: a comparison between early mobilization, physiotherapy with and without bronchodilatation. Ann Chir Gynaecol 1984; 73:55–58.
178. Wolff RK, Dolovich MB, Obminski G, Newhouse MT. Effects of exercise and eucapnic hyperventilation on bronchial clearance in man. J Appl Physiol 1977; 43:46–50.
179. Bott J, Keilty S, Brown A, Ward E. Nasal positive pressure ventilation. Physiotherapy 1992; 78:93–96.
180. Bott J, Keilty S, Noone L. Intermittend possitive pressure breathing: a dying art? Physiotherapy 1992; 78:656–660.
181. Emmanuel G, Smith W, Briscoe W. The effect of intermittent positive pressure breathing and voluntary hyperventilation upon the distribution of ventilation and pulmonary blood flow to the lung in chronic obstructed pulmonary disease. J Clin Invest 1966; 45:1221–1223.
182. Sukumalchantra Y, Park S, Williams M. The effect of intermittent positive pressure breating in acute ventilatory failure. Am Rev Respir Dis 1965; 92:885–893.
183. Torres G, Lyons H, Emerson P. The effects of intermittent pressure breathing on the interpulmonary distribution of inspired air. Am J Med 1960; 29:946–954.
184. Baxter WD, Levine RS. An evaluation of intermittent positive pressure breathing in the prevention of postoperative pulmonary complications. Arch Surg 1969; 98: 795–798.
185. Jung R, Wight J, Nusser R, Rosoff L. Comparison of three methods of respiratory care following upper abdominal surgery. Chest 1980; 78:31–35.

186. Iverson LI, Ecker RR, Fox HE, May IA. A comparative study of IPPB, the incentive spirometer, and blow bottles: the prevention of atelectasis following cardiac surgery. Ann Thorac Surg 1978; 25:197–200.

187. Pavia D, Webber B, Agnew J. The role of IPPB in bronchial toilet. Eur Respir J 1988; 1S:250

188. Oh TE. Mechanical ventilatory support. In: Oh TE, ed. Intensive Care Manual. Oxford: Butterworth Heinmann, 1990:155–161.

189. Gregory GA, Kitterman JA, Phibbs RH, Tooley WH, Hamilton WK. Treatment of the idiopathic respiratory-distress syndrome with continuous positive airway pressure. N Engl J Med 1971; 84:1333–1340.

190. Andersen JB, Qvist J, Kann T. Recruiting collapsed lung through collateral channels with positive end-expiratory pressure. Scand J Respir Dis 1979; 60:260–266.

191. Katz JA, Ozanne GM, Zinn SE, Fairley HB. Time course and mechanisms of lung-volume increase with PEEP in acute pulmonary failure. Anesthesiology 1981; 54:9–16.

192. Peruzzi W. The current status of PEEP. Respir Care 1996; 41:273–279.

193. Lum H, Huang I, Mitzner W. Morphological evidence for alveolar recruitment during inflation at high transpulmonary pressure. J Appl Physiol 1990; 68:2280–2286.

194. Wilson R. Intermittent CPAP to prevent atelectasis in post-operative patients. Respir Care 1983; 28:71–73.

195. Lindner K, Lotz P, Ahnefeld F. Continuous positive airway pressure effect on functional residual capacity, vital capacity and its subdivisions. Chest 1987; 92: 66–70.

196. Stock MC, Downs JB, Gauer PK, Alster JM, Imrey PB. Prevention of postoperative pulmonary complications with CPAP, incentive spirometry, and conservative therapy. Chest 1985; 87:151–157.

197. Pinilla JC, Oleniuk FH, Tan L, Rebeyka I, Tanna N, Wilkinson A, et al. Use of a nasal continuous positive airway pressure mask in the treatment of postoperative atelectasis in aortocoronary bypass surgery [comments]. Crit Care Med 1990; 18: 836–840.

198. Andersen JB, Olesen B, Eikhard B, Jansen E, Qvist J. Periodic continuous positive airway pressure by mask in the treatment of atelectasis. Eur J Resp Dis 1980; 61: 20–25.

199. Duncan SR, Negrin RS, Mihm FG, Guilleminault C, Raffin TA. Nasal continuous positive airway pressure in atelectasis. Chest 1987; 92:621–624.

200. Williamson DC, Modell JH. Intermittent continuous positive airway pressure by mask: its use in the treatment of atelectasis. Arch Surg 1982; 117:970–972.

201. Denehy L, Carroll S, Ntoumneopoulos G, Jenkins S. A randomized contolled trial comparing periodic mask CPAP with physiotherapy after abdominal surgery. Physiother Res Int 2001; 6(4):236–250.

202. Ricksten SE, Bengtsson A, Soderberg C, Thorden M, Kvist H. Effects of periodic positive airway pressure by mask on postoperative pulmonary function. Chest 1986; 89:774–781.

203. Rice VH, Mullin MH, Jarosz P. Preadmission self-instruction effects on postad-

mission and postoperative indicators in CABG patients: partial replication and extension. Res Nurs Health 1992; 15:253–259.

204. Recker D. Patient perception of preoperative cardiac surgical teaching done pre- and postadmission. Crit Care Nurse 1994; 14:52–58.

205. Anderson EA. Preoperative preparation for cardiac surgery facilitates recovery, reduces psychological distress and reduces the incidence of acute postoperative hypertension. J Consult Clin Psychol 1987, 55:513–520.

206. Chase L, Elkins J, Shepard K. Perceptions of physical therapists toward patient education. Physical Therapy 1993, 73:787–796.

207. Gosselink R, Schrever K, Cops P, Witvrouwen H, De Leyn P, Troosters T, Lerut A, Deneffe G, Decramer M Incentive spirometry does not enhance recovery after thoracic surgery. Crit Care Med 2000, 28:679–683.

208. Falk M, Kelstrup M, Andersen J, Falk P, Stovring. Improving the ketchup bottle method with positive expiratory pressure, PEP, in cystic fibrosis. Eur J Respir Dis 1984, 65:423–432.

209. Thomas J, Cook DJ, Brooks D. Chest physical therapy management of patients with cystic fibrosis: a meta-analysis. Am J Respir Crit Care Med 1995, 151:846–850.

210. Tonneson P, Stovring S. Positive expiratory pressure (PEP) as lung physiotherapy in cystic fibrosis: a pilot study. Eur J Resp Dis 1984; 65:419–422.

211. Oberwaldner B, Theissl B, Rucker A, Zach MS. Chest physiotherapy in hospitalized patients with cystic fibrosis: a study of lung function effects and sputum production. Eur Respir J 1991; 4:152–158.

212. Lannefors L, Wollmer P. Mucus clearance with three chest physiotherapy regimens in cystic fibrosis: a comparison between postural drainage, PEP and physical exercise. Eur Respir J 1992; 5:748–753.

213. Campbell T, Ferguson N, McKinlay R. the use of a simple self-administered method of postive expiratory pressure (PEP) in chest pjhysiotherapy after abdominal surgery. Physiotherapy 1986; 72:498–500.

214. Van Hengstrum M, Festen J, Beurskens C, Hankel M, Beekman F, Corstens F. Effect of PEP versus forced expiration technique on regional lung clearance in chronic bronchitis. Eur Respir J 1991; 4:651–654.

215. Carlsson C, Sonden B, Tyhlen U. Can continuous positive airway pressure prevent pulmonary complications after abdominal surgery? Intens Care Med 1981; 7:225–229.

20

Management of Airway Secretions in Patients with Severe Respiratory Muscle Dysfunction

JOHN R. BACH and JODI THOMAS

UMDNJ–The New Jersey Medical School
Newark, New Jersey, U.S.A.

I. Introduction

There is much debate about the indications for instituting nocturnal noninvasive mechanical ventilation for patients with neuromuscular inspiratory muscle dysfunction (1). In reality, the emphasis on when and how to provide nocturnal ventilatory assistance is a little misplaced when one realizes that respiratory failure is caused primarily by expiratory muscle rather than inspiratory muscle dysfunction. Numerous investigators have demonstrated that for most neuromuscular diseases, the expiratory muscles are weaker than the inspiratory muscles (4). The same is true for patients with spinal cord injury as well as for many other conditions. In fact, it has been shown that about 90% of the time acute respiratory failure is caused by airway secretion retention that occurs during otherwise benign chest colds for patients with severe respiratory muscle dysfunction (3).

Adequate expiratory muscle function is critical for clearing airway secretions and bronchial mucus. This may be a constant problem for patients with severe bulbar muscle weakness who essentially continually aspirate upper airway secretions or food. However, most often it becomes a critical problem only during intercurrent chest colds, following general anesthesia, and during other periods of bronchial hypersecretion. Few clinicians, however, are aware of how to assist expiratory muscle function and avert translaryngeal intubation and resort to tracheostomy. In this chapter it will be made clear how noninvasive inspiratory and expiratory muscle aids can be used to prevent respiratory failure indefinitely for the majority of people with progressive or severe respiratory muscle dysfunction and how they can be used to decrease or eliminate the need for hospitalizing these patients.

II. Ventilatory Versus Oxygenation Impairment

Before discussing the respiratory muscle aids, it is important to distinguish between patients who have processes that cause primarily oxygenation impairment from those who have primarily impairment of alveolar ventilation. Although episodes of respiratory failure can often not be averted for the former, they often can be averted for the latter. Noninvasive ventilation and physical methods to facilitate the mobilization of airway secretions have been explored for patients with primarily oxygenation impairment, but use of these methods is controversial, and evidence of their efficacy is essentially lacking (5). On the other hand, despite the fact that the use of inspiratory and expiratory muscle aids by patients with primarily lung ventilation impairment can prevent respiratory complications and the need for hospitalizations (5–7), these methods continue to be underutilized (8).

Ventilation impairment can result from any neuromuscular or skeletal disorder that causes respiratory muscle dysfunction. Although the inspiratory muscles of patients with advanced chronic obstructive pulmonary disease (COPD) can also become exhausted, COPD patients have lung disease with essentially irreversible small airways obstruction. Unlike for patients whose respiratory impairment is a direct result of respiratory muscle weakness, since the weakness of respiratory muscles in COPD is not the primary reason for respiratory impairment and the respiratory muscles are not necessarily weak in this condition, the use of inspiratory and expiratory muscle aids may not be expected to markedly affect their clinical courses. For the purposes of this chapter, the terms "ventilatory insufficiency" or "failure" will pertain to patients whose hypoxia is secondary to lung hypoventilation and whose oxyhemoglobin saturation (SpO_2) can be normalized by correcting lung ventilation and increasing cough flows to eliminate airway secretions. The terms "respiratory insufficiency" and "failure" will apply to clinical situations in which hypoxia is due to intrinsic lung or airways disease that is not correctable by normalizing ventilation and for whom cough flows cannot be increased to effectively eliminate airway secretions.

Many clinicians have polysomnography performed on their patients with neuromuscular disease, and when the polysomnogram suggests some combination of "central or obstructive apneas," continuous positive airway pressure (CPAP) or pressure support ventilation with positive end-expiratory pressure delivered by a bilevel positive airway pressure (BiPAP) machine is prescribed. This is often done whether or not the patient has clear symptoms of sleep-disordered breathing and despite the fact that the primary problem is one of respiratory muscle weakness rather than one of central or obstructive apneas. Instead of suggesting CPAP or low-level pressure support ventilation, other clinicians, realizing that the condition is progressive and ventilatory failure is inevitable, recommend "prophylactic tracheostomy." Still other clinicians prescribe supplemental oxygen administration, thinking this will decrease the tendency for central apneas. All three of these approaches are, at best, inappropriate and, at worst, harmful for the majority of patients with respiratory muscle dysfunction on the basis of neuromuscular disease.

CPAP does not assist inspiratory muscle function and does not, therefore, provide any significant clinical benefit for neuromuscular disease patients. Although bilevel positive airway pressure can assist the inspiratory muscles as a function of the inspiratory positive airway pressure (IPAP)/expiratory positive airway pressure (EPAP) difference or span, BiPAP machines are usually used at spans that can assist only the least affected patients, and these machines cannot provide the deep insufflations these patients need to clear airway secretions during intercurrent chest colds. Prophylactic tracheostomy is not warranted because most patients with neuromuscular disease who use respiratory muscle aids never require tracheostomy. Further, patients who have used both tracheostomy for intermittent positive pressure ventilation (IPPV) and noninvasive IPPV almost invariably prefer the latter (2), and they have fewer respiratory complications and require many fewer hospitalizations and hospitalization days when using the latter for even 24-hour ventilatory support (3). Oxygen supplementation is an even poorer substitute for the use of respiratory muscle aids because it not only can result in more severe hypercapnia, it also greatly increases the risk of pulmonary morbidity (3).

Patients with certain diagnoses develop primarily ventilatory impairment and can most benefit from the use of respiratory muscle aids. Many if not most patients with these diagnoses can cooperate with and have sufficient bulbar muscle function to use the required respiratory techniques and equipment and can thereby avoid endotracheal intubation and long-term ventilatory support via indwelling tracheostomy tubes.

III. The Normal Cough

A normal cough requires a precough inspiration or insufflation to about 85–90% of total lung capacity (9). Glottic closure follows for about 0.2 s, and sufficient intrathoracic pressures are generated to obtain peak transient expiratory flows or peak cough flows (PCF) exceeding 6 L/s upon glottic opening (10,11). Total expiratory volume during normal coughing is about 2.3 ± 0.5 L (9). Before the first half of the volume is expired, flow is stopped by glottic closure or airway muscle activity. This may be repeated several times before complete expiration (9). When attempting to cough, patients with severe bulbar muscle dysfunction or inability to close the glottis for any reason deliver peak expiratory rather than PCF. PCF are generally somewhat greater than peak expiratory flows, except for patients with severe bulbar muscle dysfunction.

IV. Why Expiratory Muscle Aids Are Needed

> If the only tool you know is a hammer, the whole world begins to look like a nail.

Patients with primarily lung and airways diseases like COPD collapse their airways during the expiratory phase of coughing. This can reduce PCF to below 160 L/m, the very minimum required to expel airway debris (12). These patients are usually managed with a combination of oxygen therapy, bronchodilators, mucoactive agents, and chest physical therapy. On the other hand, the great majority of patients with primarily respiratory muscle weakness have essentially normal airway physiology and mechanics. Nevertheless, most physicians treat these patients with the same modalities they use for patients with primarily oxygenation impairment. However, modalities like bronchodilators and oxygen therapy do not address the primary problem of muscle weakness and can even hasten the development of respiratory failure and resort to translaryngeal intubation and tracheostomy (11). Beta$_2$-agonists can, in themselves, increase airway secretions, and other commonly used medications such as corticosteroids and aminoglycosides can suppress immune function.

Since acute respiratory failure is most often caused by the airway secretion retention that occurs during chest colds (11), and the greater the PCF, the more effective the cough and the less likely that a patient will develop respiratory failure or other pulmonary complications (7,10), the strategy should be to assist the respiratory muscles to maximize PCF. It is important to understand that it is often necessary to first assist the inspiratory muscles in order to optimally assist the expiratory muscles. This is because normal cough flows involve the passage of over 2 L volumes of air, but patients with weak inspiratory muscles cannot attain adequate volumes because they often have vital capacities (VCs) below 1 L. One must, therefore, first assist the inspiratory muscles to achieve an optimal volume of air before aiding the expiratory muscles in increasing PCF.

The VC, forced vital capacity, and ability to cough or PCF are diminished following general anesthesia as well as during chest colds because of fatigue, temporary weakening of inspiratory and expiratory muscles (13), and bronchial mucus plugging. Concomitant weakness of oropharyngeal muscles exacerbates the problem. The attainment of adequate PCF is an appropriate clinical goal and extremely important for preventing serious pulmonary complications in these patients (14).

V. Respiratory Muscle Aids

The respiratory muscles can be aided by manually or mechanically applying forces to the body or intermittent pressure to the airway. The devices that act on the body include the negative pressure body ventilators and oscillators, which assist respiratory muscles by creating atmospheric pressure changes around the thorax and abdomen, body ventilators and exsufflation devices that apply forces directly to the body to mechanically displace respiratory muscles, and devices that apply intermittent pressure changes directly to the airway. Glossopharyngeal breathing (GPB) is also an inspiratory technique that patients with weak inspiratory muscles, but functional bulbar muscles, can use to autonomously obtain a deep breath and thereby indirectly aid the expiratory muscles (15).

VI. Glossopharyngeal Breathing

Glossopharyngeal breathing was first recognized and described in the early 1950s as an assist for coughing (16). It involves the use of the glottis to project boluses of air into the lungs and to thereby add to an inspiratory effort. The glottis closes with each "gulp." One breath usually consists of six to nine gulps of 60–200 mL each. During the training period the efficiency of GPB can be monitored by spirometrically measuring the milliliters of air per gulp, gulps per breath, and breaths per minute (Fig. 1). An excellent training manual and video are available (17,18).

GPB can also provide an individual with weak inspiratory muscles and little or no measurable VC or ventilator-free breathing ability with normal alveolar ventilation for hours and safety when not using a ventilator or in the event of sudden ventilator failure day or night (15,19). Only severe oropharyngeal muscle weakness can limit the usefulness of GPB. However, Baydur et al. (20) reported two Duchenne muscular dystrophy (DMD) ventilator users, and we have cared for six other DMD ventilator users and many other individuals with progressive neuromuscular diseases and no ventilator-free breathing ability who could use GPB to both dramatically increase PCF and successfully ventilate their lungs for hours of ventilator-free time. Although potentially extremely useful, GPB is rarely taught since few health care professionals are familiar with the technique. GPB is also rarely useful in the presence of an indwelling tracheostomy tube. It cannot be used when the tube is uncapped as it is during trache-

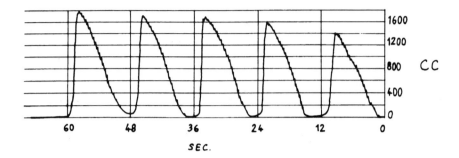

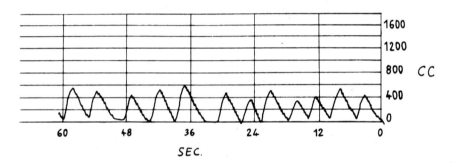

Figure 1   (Top) Maximal GPB minute ventilation 8.39 L/min, GPB inspirations average 1.67 L, 20 gulps, 84 mL/gulp for each breath in a patient with a vital capacity of 0 mL. (Bottom) Same patient regular GPB minute ventilation 4.76 L/min, 12.5 breaths, average 8 gulps per breath, 47.5 mL/gulp performed over a 1-minute period. (With appreciation to the March of Dimes for republication of this illustration.)

ostomy IPPV, and even when capped, the gulped air tends to leak around the outer walls of the tube and out the tracheostomy site as airway volumes and pressures increase during the air stacking process of GPB. The safety and versatility afforded by effective GPB are key reasons to eliminate tracheostomy in favor of noninvasive aids.

VII. Inspiratory Muscle Aids

Inspiratory muscle aids are important to increase precough lung volumes for patients with VCs below 1.5 L and to dramatically increase PCF for patients with

VCs below 1 L (10). Although negative pressure body ventilators can function as inspiratory muscle aids, their use is not practical for providing deep insufflations for assisted coughing, and they will no longer be considered here (6). Likewise, oscillation methods do not assist respiratory muscle function, and although it has been suggested that their application can augment airway secretion mobilization for patients with primarily lung or airways disease, and they may be helpful to mobilize airway secretions for patients with neuromuscular conditions; they are not a substitute for assisted coughing.

The rocking bed and the intermittent abdominal pressure ventilator (IAPV) apply forces directly to the body to assist inspiratory muscle function. The rocking bed (J. H. Emerson Co, Cambridge, MA) rocks the patient an arc of 15–30° during which gravity cyclically displaces the abdominal contents and ventilates the lungs. Since it is not as effective as other noninvasive inspiratory muscle aids, it will no longer be considered here (6). However, the IAPV involves the intermittent inflation of an air sac or bladder that is contained in a corset or belt. The bladder is inflated by a positive pressure ventilator. Bladder action moves the diaphragm upwards causing a forced exsufflation. During bladder deflation the abdominal contents and diaphragm fall to the resting position and inspiration occurs passively. A trunk angle of 30° or more from the horizontal is necessary for its effectiveness. If the patient has any inspiratory capacity or is capable of GPB, he can add his autonomous tidal volume to the mechanically assisted inspiration. Insufflation volumes as high as 1200 ml over patient tidal volumes have been reported (21). Thus, this device can augment cough flows by providing a deeper volume of air to the lungs and by assisting expiratory muscles by applying pressure to the abdominal wall.

VIII. Noninvasive IPPV

> And the Lord God formed man of the dust of the ground and [gave him IPPV via nasal access] the breath of life.
>
> Gen. 2:7

Noninvasive IPPV can be delivered to patients with little or no VC or autonomous ability to breathe via simple mouthpieces kept in or fixed adjacent to the mouth for easy patient access (Fig. 2). Mouthpieces are most commonly fixed near the mouth by a metal clamp attached either to the wheelchair or to the controls that operate the motorized wheelchair (sip and puff, chin control, etc.) (Fig. 2). In this manner over 200 patients have been described to use up to 24-hour ventilatory support without the presence of an indwelling tracheostomy tube (22). Patients usually easily learn how to receive IPPV via a mouthpiece and prevent the insufflation volume from leaking out of the nose. Not only is

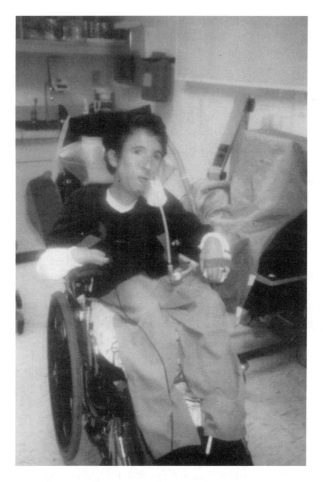

Figure 2 Patient with Duchenne muscular dystrophy who has used 24-hour mouth intermittent positive pressure ventilation for 6 years, now with no ventilator-free breathing ability. The mouthpiece is kept adjacent to his mouth for easy daytime access.

mouthpiece IPPV the most practical and important method of daytime ventilatory support, it is also extremely important for delivering maximal insufflations to increase PCF (10). Mouthpiece IPPV, particularly with lipseal retention (Fig. 3), can also be used as an alternative to nasal IPPV for nocturnal ventilatory support (22). Orthodontic bite plates and custom fabricated shells can be fabri-

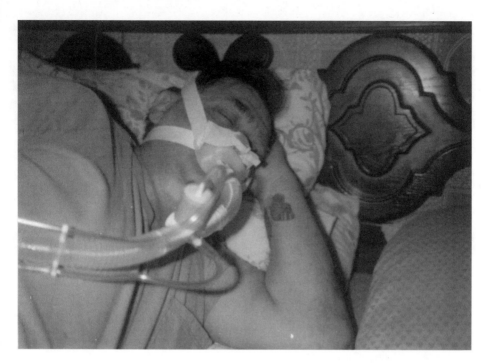

Figure 3 Patient with severe sleep-disordered breathing using mouthpiece intermittent positive pressure ventilation with lipseal (Mallincrodt, Pleasanton, CA) retention and nose plugged with cotton pledgets.

cated to increase comfort and efficacy and eliminate the risk of orthodontic deformity with long-term use.

For patients whose lips or neck are too weak to grab a mouthpiece or whose buccal or bulbar muscles are too weak to direct the insufflation volumes into the lungs, nasal IPPV can also be used both for continuous ventilatory support as well as to deliver the maximal insufflations required for an optimal cough. There are now over 20 commercially available CPAP masks that can be used as nasal interfaces for nasal IPPV. Custom molded nasal interfaces are also available (Fig. 4) (23).

Maximal insufflation, whether via nasal, oral, or oral-nasal interface, can be delivered by manual resuscitator, portable volume-cycled ventilator, or via an In-exsufflator (J. H. Emerson Company, Cambridge, MA). Patients adept at GPB can maximally inflate their lungs without resort to mechanical means.

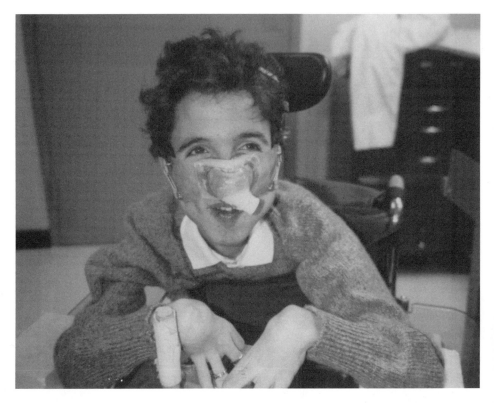

Figure 4 Patient with Duchenne muscular dystrophy and no ventilator-free breathing ability who uses a low-profile custom acrylic nasal interface for nocturnal intermittent positive pressure ventilation.

IX. The Evolution to Tracheostomy IPPV

Trendelenburg was the first to describe the use of a tracheostomy tube with an inflated cuff for assisting ventilation during anesthesia of a human in 1869 (24). The use of transoral intubation during anesthesia was described soon afterward (25). Tracheostomy and the use of a mechanical bellows for ventilatory support were popularized for anesthesia during World War I (26). However, despite this and the fact that tracheostomies were often placed for managing airway secretions in patients ventilated by body ventilators in the 1940s, tracheostomy tubes were not used for ongoing ventilatory support before the inadequate supply of body ventilators made this a necessity during the 1952 poliomyelitis epidemic in Denmark (27).

During the Danish epidemic, the mortality rate was 94% for patients with respiratory paralysis and concomitant bulbar involvement and 28% for those without bulbar involvement (27). Lassen reported that mortality figures for ventilator supported patients decreased from 80% to 41%, or to about 7% for the entire acute paralytic poliomyelitis population overall. This was in part due to more frequent use of tracheostomy, particularly for those with severe bulbar involvement (27). However, specialized centers in the United States also reported equally significant decreases in mortality from 12–15%, depending on the center, in 1948 to 2% in 1952 without resort to tracheostomy for ventilatory support or airway secretion management (28). It was concluded that the previously high fatality rate was not because of inadequacy of body ventilators to ventilate the lungs but because of bulbar insufficiency and ineffective airway secretion management. Better nursing care and attention to managing airway secretions including the use of devices to assist the expiratory muscles in eliminating them were factors in decreasing mortality (30). In 1958 Forbes (31) wrote "Tracheotomy, which is designed to provide a more efficient airway and access to the trachea in certain patients, does not materially assist in ridding the bronchi of secretions which must migrate to the upper bronchi and trachea before they become accessible to suction through the tracheotomy tube. The inaccessibility of these secretions in the lower bronchial tree even to bronchoscopy makes it necessary to provide indirect means for their mechanical expulsion." Forbes noted that the published mortality figures in six studies among acute patients were lower with tank respiration than with tracheostomy IPPV and that with tracheostomy in patients with respiratory paralysis without pharyngeal paralysis, tracheal damage, loss of capability for GPB, and loss of "the routine application of chest compression" and mechanical insufflation-exsufflation (MI-E) made for a worse prognosis by comparison to patients managed by noninvasive methods (31). Despite this, the lack of knowledge of noninvasive IPPV and expiratory muscle aids and the fact that body ventilators restrict patients' activities led to the widespread use of translaryngeal intubation and tracheostomy to clear airway secretions and provide ventilatory support.

As the use of endotracheal methods became widespread, so did complications resulting from their use (6). Mouthpiece IPPV was described in 1969 (32) and was used for large numbers of patients requiring mechanical ventilation in the 1980s (22). Nasal IPPV was described in 1987 (33), and mechanical methods to assist expiratory muscles to eliminate airway secretions became available in 1993 (10).

X. Noninvasive Expiratory Muscle Aids

A. Manually Assisted Coughing

Postural drainage and chest percussion are routinely used to mobilize airway
secretions. However, application of the former can be difficult for patients with
severe musculotendinous contractures or skeletal injury and no independent mobility, and the latter appears to have limited indications and be of questionable
efficacy except for patients with very high quantities of purulent airway secretions (5). In a not well-controlled comparison of cough versus chest physiotherapy on pulmonary function and secretion clearance in patients with cystic fibrosis, the same short-term functional response and sputum yield were seen with
vigorous coughing alone as with complete chest physiotherapy and coughing.
Since suctioning via the mouth or nose is difficult and rarely tolerated or effective, when unassisted coughing is inadequate the only recourse is manually or
mechanically assisted coughing.

   Techniques of manually assisted coughing involve different hand and arm
placements for the expiratory cycle thrusts (Fig. 5) (34). At least nine different

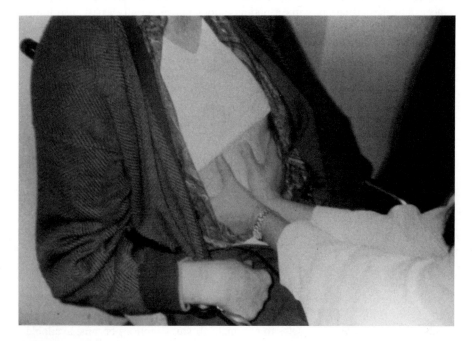

Figure 5 Manually assisted coughing using the abdominal thrust following a maximal
insufflation.

hand placements have been described for manually assisted coughing (35). The two best studied, which probably provide the greatest augmentation in PCF, are the simple abdominal thrust (Fig. 5), in which each hand is placed under the rib cage and the thrusts are delivered in and up, and the use of an epigastric thrust with counterpressure applied across the thorax by the other arm. The counterpressure is used to prevent loss of PCF by air expanding the upper chest rather than being directed out through the upper airway. This technique increases assisted PCF over those achieved by simple abdominal thrusts in about 20% of individuals (10). For patients with less than 1.5 L of VC, efficacy is enhanced by preceding the assisted exsufflation with a deep insufflation, as described in the preceding section.

Manually assisted coughing requires a cooperative patient, good coordination between the patient and caregiver, and adequate physical effort and often frequent application by the caregiver. It is usually ineffective in the presence of significant scoliosis, and certain techniques must be performed with caution in the presence of an osteoporotic rib cage. Unfortunately, since it is no longer widely taught to health care professionals (36), manually assisted coughing is greatly underutilized. When inadequate, the most effective alternative for generating optimal PCF and clearing deep airway secretions is the use of mechanical insufflation-exsufflation (MI-E).

B. Mechanical Insufflation-Exsufflation

> Sir Patrick: Don't misunderstand me, my boy, I'm not belittling your discovery. Most discoveries are made regularly every fifteen years; and it's fully a hundred and fifty since yours was made last. That's something to be proud of . . .
>
> George Bernard Shaw, *The Doctor's Dilemma*

According to Beck and Barach, "the life-saving value of exsufflation with negative pressure was made clear through the relief of obstructive dyspnea as a result of immediate elimination of large amounts of purulent sputum, and, in a second episode, by the substantial clearing of pulmonary atelectasis after 12 hours' treatment" (37).

In the late 1940s Henry Seeler, working for the U.S. Air Force, developed a mechanical insufflator-exsufflator designed to deliver alternating positive and negative pressures to ventilate and exsufflate patients suffering from exposure to "chemical weapons" and "nerve gas" (38). In 1951 Barach et al. (39) described an exsufflator attachment for iron lungs. The device used a vacuum cleaner motor with a 5-inch solenoid valve attachment to an iron lung portal. With the valve closed, the motor developed a negative intratank pressure to -40 mmHg. At peak negative pressure the valve opened, triggering a return to atmospheric pressure in 0.06 s and causing a passive exsufflation. This increased PCF in six ventilator-supported poliomyelitis patients from 1.2 L/s unassisted to 1.6 L/s, or

45%. An additional increase was obtained by timing an abdominal compression with valve opening (40). These techniques were sufficiently effective for the investigators to report that the exsufflation produced by this device "completely replaced bronchoscopy as a means of keeping the airway clear of thick tenacious secretions." Another "patient would have required bronchoscopy or re-opening of the tracheotomy if the exsufflator had not been successful in clearing the airway" (39).

In 1953 various portable devices were manufactured to deliver MI-E directly to the airway via a mouthpiece, mask, or endotracheal tube (41,42). Insufflation and exsufflation pressures were independently adjusted for comfort and efficacy. The best known of these devices was the Cof-Flator (OEM Co, Norwalk, CT) (41). The Cof-Flator consists of a two-stage axial compressor that gradually inflates the lungs with positive pressures of 35–40 mmHg over a 2-s period. The pressure in the upper respiratory passageway is then dropped to 35–40 mmHg below atmosphere in 0.02 s by the swift opening of a solenoid valve connected to a negative-pressure blower. The negative pressure is usually maintained for 1–3 s (30,43).

In February 1993, a mechanical insufflator-exsufflator (In-Exsufflator, J. H. Emerson Co., Cambridge, MA) that operates like the Cof-Flator except that cycling between positive and negative pressure had to be done manually was released on the American market. This manual cycling feature facilitates caregiver-patient coordination of inspiration and expiration with insufflation and exsufflation but requires an additional hand for an abdominal thrust or if one hand is inadequate to affix the mask. In 1994 an automatically cycling In-exsufflator with the option to use a manually cycling mode became available.

One treatment consists of about five cycles of MI-E followed by a period of normal breathing or ventilator use for 20–30 s to avoid hyperventilation. Five or more treatments are given in one sitting, and the treatments are repeated until no further secretions are expulsed. Use can be required as frequently as every 10 minutes during chest colds. An abdominal thrust applied during the exsufflation cycle further increases PCF and airway secretion expulsion (10). Although no medications are usually required for effective MI-E in neuromuscular ventilator users, in the author's experience liquefaction of sputum using heated aerosol treatments or instillation of normal saline drops may, at times, facilitate exsufflation when secretions are inspissated.

The efficacy of MI-E was demonstrated both clinically and on animal models (43). At least for patients without significant obstructive airway disease, flow generation is adequate in both proximal and distal airways to effectively eliminate respiratory tract debris (44,45). Vital capacity, pulmonary flow rates, and Spo2, when abnormal, improve immediately with clearing of secretions by MI-E (22,26). An increase in VC of 15–42% was noted immediately following treatment in 67 patients with "obstructive dyspnea," and a 55% increase in VC was noted following MI-E in patients with neuromuscular conditions (46). We have observed 15–300% improvement in VC and normalization of Spo2 as MI-E eliminates secretions for acutely ill ventilator-assisted neuromuscular patients (Fig. 6) (10).

Significant increases in PCF have been demonstrated by MI-E in patients with poliomyelitis, bronchiectasis, asthma, and pulmonary emphysema (30). Following instillation of a mucin–thorium dioxide suspension into the lungs of anesthetized dogs, bronchograms revealed virtually complete elimination of the suspension after 6 minutes of MI-E (43). The technique was shown to be equally effective in expulsing bronchoscopically inserted foreign bodies (43). The use of MI-E through an indwelling tracheostomy tube was demonstrated to be effective in reversing acute atelectasis associated with productive airway secretions in 1954 (37); however, PCF were noted to be even greater when MI-E was applied via a mask (47). Barach and Beck (46) demonstrated clinical and radiographic improvement in 92 of 103 acutely ill bronchopulmonary and neuromuscular patients with chest colds with the use of MI-E. This included 72 patients with bronchopulmonary disease and 27 with skeletal or neuromuscular conditions including poliomyelitis (37); however, it was more effective for the latter than for the former (46).

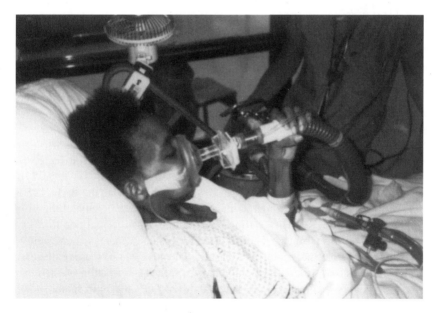

Figure 6 A patient with myasthenia gravis who self-applies mechanical insufflation-exsufflation from the Cough-Assist. (J. H. Emerson Co, Cambridge, MA.)

Colebatch (48) observed that applying negative pressure of 40–50 mmHg is unlikely to have any deleterious effects on pulmonary tissues. He noted that since the negative pressure applied to the airways is analogous to positive pressure on the surface of the lungs during a normal cough, it is improbable that this negative pressure can be more detrimental to the lungs than the normal cough pressure gradient. Bickerman (43) found no evidence of parenchymal damage, hemorrhage, alveolar tears, or emphysematous blebs in the lungs of animals treated with MI-E. Barach and Beck (40) reported no serious complications in the 103 patients they treated with over 2000 courses of MI-E, and for no patient did MI-E have to be discontinued. Many of these patients had COPD. They did not report aggravation of airway obstruction in their patients with hyperdynamic airways. We have also reported that, at least for patients with neuromuscular conditions, FEV_1 has always either increased or remained unchanged following use of MI-E (10). This indicates that no persistent airway collapse is engendered by MI-E, at least for patients without hyperdynamic airways. Barach and Beck also noted that the initial transient appearance of blood-streaked sputum seen in a few patients probably originated from the bronchial wall sites of detachment of mucus plugs. Immediately following the initial elimination of blood-streaked sputum, the profuse outpouring of mucopurulent sputum indicated that "obstruction of the atelectatic area had been relieved." In one study one of 19 patients complained of transient nausea associated with the onset of MI-E. This passed with continued use (49). No reports of damaging side effects have been disclosed in more than 6000 treatments in over 400 patients with MI-E, most of whom had primarily lung disease (48–50). Consistent with this is the fact in over 850 patient-years and many hundreds of applications of MI-E by our neuromuscular ventilator users, no episodes of pneumothorax or aspiration of gastric contents were observed. Blood-streaking of sputum occurs on rare occasions as mucus plugs are torn from the underlying epithelium. Borborygmus and abdominal distention are infrequent and eliminated by decreasing insufflation pressures below the patient's inspiratory reserve volume. As noted below, caution must be observed and insufflation and exsufflation increased gradually when MI-E is used for acute traumatic tetraplegics.

Physiological effects of MI-E were studied in depth in the early 1950s (51). Peripheral venous pressures as measured in the anterior cubital vein are slightly raised, i.e., 5.8 cmH$_2$O, during exsufflation. This is about one-third the increase seen during normal coughing. Blood pressure is increased an average of 8 mmHg in systole and 4 mmHg in diastole. The pulse can increase or decrease during MI-E, and electrocardiographic changes reflect the rotation of the heart at peak inspiratory volumes. For the acute high-level tetraplegic in spinal shock, severe bradyarrhythmias including complete heart block can occur in some patients unless premedication with anticholinergics is used. The increase in intragastric pressure is 26 mmHg during MI-E and 85 mmHg during normal coughing (52).

Dayman (53) found that in patients with emphysema, the production of high intrathoracic pressures during the glottic-closure phase of unassisted coughing and the subsequent pressure drop may result in an even greater pressure difference between the alveoli and lumen of the bronchioles than is normally present. The resulting high alveolar-bronchial pressure gradient may result in closure of bronchioles and obstruction to air exiting the alveoli. Coughing is thus often ineffective for these patients. Part of the benefit of MI-E for COPD patients was explained by the fact that high expiratory flows occur with lower intrathoracic pressures (46). It was suggested that for COPD patients and others with severe intrinsic disease, the patient should practice passive MI-E (50). Further research is required to determine if patients with intrinsic lung or airways disease can derive significant clinical benefits from MI-E.

MI-E has been noted to be effective in the elimination of sputum before and of contrast medium after bronchography in patients with bronchial asthma and bronchiectasis, and it has been suggested that MI-E may improve the results of bronchoscopy in clearing secretions (46). Williams and Holaday (54) reported that MI-E could effectively eliminate airway secretions and ventilate patients in the minutes following generalized anesthesia. They applied MI-E both to cooperative and to unconscious patients and reported normalization of blood gases in all seven patients studied, including two with advanced pulmonary emphysema. In addition, improved breath sounds, increased percussion resonance, reduced respiratory rate, clearing of cyanosis, and reversal of right lower lobe collapse were reported for particular patients as a direct result of MI-E. Patients with wounds of the abdomen or chest reported less wound pain during MI-E than during spontaneous coughing. No incidence of aspiration of gastric contents was found either in this population (54) or in that of anesthetized dogs treated with MI-E (43). The use of MI-E has permitted us to consistently extubate elective surgical neuromuscular patients immediately post–general anesthesia despite their having little or no ventilator-free breathing ability and convert them to the use of noninvasive IPPV when MI-E and mucus elimination alone were not enough to permit them to effectively ventilate their lungs. It has also permitted us to avoid intubation or quickly extubate neuromuscular patients in acute respiratory failure due to intercurrent chest colds with profuse airway secretions.

C. Other Techniques That Assist Respiratory Muscle Effort

For patients with paralyzed abdominal musculature from spinal cord injury, use of a thoracoabdominal corset restricts the descent of the diaphragm and limits the increase in functional residual capacity that otherwise increases when the patient assumes the upright position. Although it does not assist respiratory muscles for the patient when supine, when sitting it assists diaphragm activity by permitting increased excursion. It has no significant effect on PCF in the supine position, but the mildly increased VC when sitting can increase PCF in this position. It can also help to maintain blood pressure and trunk stability for these patients when sitting (55). Use of an abdominal binder has also been reported to decrease the subjective effort of breathing, relieve accessory neck muscle and upper intercostal respiration, decrease the respiratory rate, and increase tidal air with a lowering of the total pulmonary ventilation for patients with neuromuscular disease or pulmonary emphysema (37).

A 4-inch-wide abdominal belt with hand grips or handles has been designed as a postoperative coughing aid (56). When the patient needs to cough, he or she passes one handle through the other and pulls with both hands. This instantaneously applies pressure to the abdomen and facilitates a pain-free cough.

An abdominal binder with functional electrical stimulation electrodes has become available to enhance the cough of spinal cord quadriplegics (Quik Coff Belt Company, Sunnyvale, CA). It has been shown to increase maximum expiratory pressure at the mouth during coughing from 30 cmH_2O for spontaneous coughing to 60 cmH_2O and compares favorably with the 80 cmH_2O obtained during manually assisted coughing. Further studies are needed to determine whether adequate PCF can be achieved using this apparatus (57).

XI. Treatment Protocol

Ideally, patients with neuromuscular conditions need to be evaluated every 2–12 months depending on the rapidity of evolution of the condition. The evaluation includes assessment for symptoms of chronic alveolar hypoventilation and measurement of VC, maximum insufflation capacity (maximum volume of air stacked breaths), assisted and unassisted PCF (Access Peak Flow Meter, HealthScan, Inc., Cedar Grove, NJ), end-tidal carbon dioxide ($EtCO_2$) levels, and SpO_2. An oral-nasal interface or lipseal (Mallincrodt, Pleasanton, CA) can be used for spirometric and PCF measurements when lip muscles are too weak to grab a mouthpiece. For assisted PCF measurements, patients with VCs less than 1500 mL are insufflated to their maximum insufflation capacities then the expiratory muscles are assisted by coordinating an abdominal thrust to glottic opening.

For patients with functional bulbar musculature, unassisted PCF are greater than peak expiratory flows. People with essentially totally dysfunctional bulbar musculature cannot generate cough flows, and their peak expiratory flows are usually inadequate to clear airway secretions. Although peak expiratory flows can be created from the maximum insufflation capacity, they would be suboptimal without the use of an abdominal thrust to maximize them, in which case they become assisted PCF.

Patients are considered to be at risk for chest cold–associated respiratory failure when they have maximum assisted PCF below 270 L/m. Since the VC is also usually below 1000 mL at this point, these patients are trained in air stacking manual resuscitator–delivered volumes to their maximum insufflation capacities. They are also prescribed oximeters and trained in manually assisted coughing and in MI-E. If not already using noninvasive IPPV, they are provided with rapid access (2 h) to a portable volume ventilator, to various mouthpieces and nasal interfaces, and to a mechanical insufflator-exsufflator (In-Exsufflator, J. H. Emerson Co., Cambridge, MA). The patients and care providers are instructed to monitor SpO_2 whenever the patient is fatigued, short of breath, or ill. They are instructed that any decreases in SpO_2 below 95% indicate either hypoventilation or bronchial mucus plugging and that these must be corrected to prevent atelectasis, pneumonia, and respiratory failure. The protocol consists of using noninvasive IPPV and manually and mechanically assisted coughing as needed to maintain normal SpO_2, particularly during intercurrent chest colds. Other than for infants with spinal muscular atrophy who can require acute cardiopulmonary resuscitation at any time, no supplemental oxygen is provided for any patient outside of the hospital (7).

In a recent study of DMD patients who used this protocol, episodes of respiratory failure, tracheostomy, and hospitalizations were consistently averted (7). Averted hospitalizations were defined as acute episodes of respiratory distress relieved by 24-hour noninvasive IPPV along with the use of assisted coughing and MI-E—to expel mucus and to immediately reverse oxyhemoglobin desaturation-associated secretion retention. DMD patients who did not use the physical medicine aid protocol and underwent tracheostomy were hospitalized a mean of 72.2 ± 11.2 days when having their tracheostomy tubes placed, whereas the protocol patients were hospitalized a mean of 6.0 ± 2.4 days ($p < 0.0005$) when beginning lifetime ventilatory assistance. Even when requiring 24-hour noninvasive ventilatory support, the noninvasive aids users had fewer hospitalization days than the patients with indwelling tracheostomy (7). The study demonstrated that, given effective care providers, the use of noninvasive inspiratory and expiratory aids with oximetry feedback can significantly decrease the incidence of respiratory hospitalization and prolong survival for DMD patients without resort to tracheostomy. The study also demonstrated that hospitalization days can be significantly fewer for part-time and for full-time noninvasive IPPV users than for tracheostomy IPPV users long term.

XII. Difficulties in Initiating the Use of Noninvasive Aids

Despite patient and caregiver preferences for noninvasive approaches, the ability of these methods to lower the cost of home mechanical ventilation, to eliminate the need for hospitalization, intubation, and bronchoscopy, particularly for patients with neuromuscular weakness, and their safety and efficacy for long-term ventilatory support and secretion management, there are few centers in the United States that use these techniques. They are not a part of medical or other health professional school curricula, and current invasive approaches are centered around the general tendency to resort to the highest available technology. Physician and hospital reimbursement is procedure oriented and directed towards inpatient management rather than preventive care. One can be remunerated for hospitalizing a patient for respiratory failure, intubating or placing a tracheostomy, and performing bronchoscopy, but outpatient management that prevents hospitalization by using noninvasive IPPV, oximetry, and MI-E is not understood by third-party payors and is likely to require letters of explanation. Such letters need to emphasize that without these preventive measures respiratory failure is an inevitability, frequent and long hospitalizations likely, and tracheostomy or premature death a virtual certainty.

In addition, hospitals are ill prepared to use these noninvasive techniques when they do not own portable ventilators and In-exsufflators and when the staff is inexperienced in their use. The initial use of noninvasive inspiratory aids requires patience on the part of the caregiver and considerable time allocation for evaluating various CPAP masks and possibly other interfaces to optimize comfort and effectiveness. Yet another difficulty is the low volume of patients with neuromuscular hypoventilation seen by pulmonologists and physiatrist pulmonary specialists. Neuromuscular patients are rarely referred before an episode of acute respiratory failure has led to their being intubated. This is in part because less than 1% of the over 220 Muscular Dystrophy Association clinics in the United States have pulmonologists as co-directors and only 18% have physiatrists in this role. The neurologists and other physicians who usually direct these clinics are rarely experienced in the use of noninvasive respiratory muscle aids (8). Our experience with the neuromuscular patient has been consistent with the following statement (48):

> As experience with exsufflation with negative pressure increased, bronchoscopy was performed less frequently for the removal of bronchial secretions. At times bronchoscopic aspiration did relieve acute obstructive anoxia; but it is clear from the case reports that bronchoscopy contributed little to the overall control of bronchial secretions. . . . Had not artificial coughing been available, death might well have followed bronchoscopy in (several cases). The only possible value of bronchoscopy is to relieve obstruction due to secretions in the trachea and main bronchi. This is usually only of transient benefit, and as the relief can be more easily achieved with exsufflation with negative pressure, bronchoscopic aspiration should rarely, if ever, be performed in patients undergoing artificial respiration.

Clearly, for some individuals access to MI-E may be life-saving and pivotal in permitting the long-term use of 24-hour noninvasive ventilatory support. However, instead of noninvasively maintaining lung ventilation and increasing PCF to clear airway secretions, the common practice remains that of providing supplemental oxygen for underventilated or airway secretion–encumbered patients until they arrest, undergo tracheotomy, or die.

References

1. Robert D, Willig TN, Paulus J, Leger P, Bach JR, Barois A, Chevrolet JC, Durocher A, Echenne B, Floret D, Gajdos P, Polu JM, Soudon P. Long-term nasal ventilation in neuromuscular disorders: report of a consensus conference. Eur Respir Rev 1993; 6:599–606.
2. Bach JR. A comparison of long-term ventilatory support alternatives from the perspective of the patient and care giver. Chest 1993; 104:1702–1706.
3. Bach JR, Rajaraman R, Ballanger F, Tzeng AC, Ishikawa Y, Kulessa R, Bansal T. Neuromuscular ventilatory insufficiency: the effect of home mechanical ventilator use vs. oxygen therapy on pneumonia and hospitalization rates. Am J Phys Med Rehabil 1998; 77:8–19.
4. Profiles of neuromuscular diseases. Am J Phys Med Rehabil 1995; 74.
5. Bach JR. Update and perspectives on noninvasive respiratory muscle aids: part 2—the expiratory muscle aids. Chest 1994; 105:1538–1544.
6. Bach JR. Update and perspectives on noninvasive respiratory muscle aids: part 1—the inspiratory muscle aids. Chest 1994; 105:1230–1240.
7. Bach JR, Ishikawa Y, Kim H. Prevention of pulmonary morbidity for patients with Duchenne muscular dystrophy. Chest 1997; 112:1024–1028.
8. Bach JR. Ventilator use by muscular dystrophy association patients: an update. Arch Phys Med Rehabil 1992; 73:179–183.
9. Leith DE. Cough. In: Brain JD, Proctor D, Reid L, eds. Lung Biology in Health and Disease: Respiratory Defense Mechanisms, Part 2. New York: Marcel Dekker, 1977:545–592.
10. Bach JR. Mechanical insufflation-exsufflation: comparison of peak expiratory flows with manually assisted and unassisted coughing techniques. Chest 1993; 104:1553–1562.
11. Fugl-Meyer AR, Grimby G. Ventilatory function in tetraplegic patients. Scand J Rehab Med 1971; 3:151–160.
12. Bach JR, Saporito LR. Criteria for extubation and tracheostomy tube removal for patients with ventilatory failure: a different approach to weaning. Chest 1996; 110:1566–1571.
13. Mier-Jedrzejowicz A, Brophy C, Green M. Respiratory muscle weakness during upper respiratory tract infections. Am Rev Respir Dis 1988; 138:5–7.
14. King M, Brock G, Lundell C. Clearance of mucus by simulated cough. J Appl Physiol 1985; 58:1776–1785.
15. Bach JR, Alba AS, Bodofsky E, Curran FJ, Schultheiss M. Glossopharyngeal

breathing and non-invasive aids in the management of post-polio respiratory insufficiency. Birth Defects 1987; 23:99–113.

16. Feigelson CI, Dickinson DG, Talner NS, Wilson JL. Glossopharyngeal breathing as an aid to the coughing mechanism in the patient with chronic poliomyelitis in a respirator. N Engl J Med 1956; 254:611–613.

17. Dail CW, Affeldt JE. Glossopharyngeal Breathing [video]. Los Angeles: Department of Visual Education, College of Medical Evangelists, 1954.

18. Dail C, Rodgers M, Guess V, Adkins HV. Glossopharyngeal Breathing Manual. Downey, CA: Professional Staff Association of Rancho Los Amigos Hospital, 1979.

19. Bach JR. New approaches in the rehabilitation of the traumatic high level quadriplegic. Am J Phys Med Rehabil 1991; 70:13–20.

20. Baydur A, Gilgoff I, Prentice W, Carlson M, Fischer A. Decline in respiratory function and experience with long-term assisted ventilation in advanced Duchenne's muscular dystrophy. Chest 1990; 97:884–889.

21. Bach JR, Alba AS. Total ventilatory support by the intermittent abdominal pressure ventilator. Chest 1991; 99:630–636.

22. Bach JR, Alba AS, Saporito LR. Intermittent positive pressure ventilation via the mouth as an alternative to tracheostomy for 257 ventilator users. Chest 1993; 103: 174–182.

23. McDermott I, Bach JR, Parker C, Sortor S. Custom-fabricated interfaces for intermittent positive pressure ventilation. Int J Prosthodont 1989; 2:224–233.

24. Trendelenburg F. Beitrage zur den Operationen an den Luftwagen 2. Tamponnade der Trachea. Arch Klin Chir 1871; 12:121–233.

25. MacEwen W. Clinical observations on the introduction of tracheal tubes by the mouth instead of performing tracheotomy or laryngotomy. Br Med J 1880; 2:122–124.

26. Magill IW. Development of endotracheal anesthesia. Proc R Soc Med 1928; 22: 83–88.

27. Lassen HCA. The epidemic of poliomyelitis in Copenhagen, 1952. Proc R Soc Med 1954; 47:67–71.

28. Hodes HL. Treatment of respiratory difficulty in poliomyelitis. In: Poliomyelitis: Papers and Discussions Presented at the Third International Poliomyelitis Conference. Philadelphia: Lippincott, 1955:91–113.

29. Gutierrez M, Beroiza T, Contreras G, Diaz O, Cruz E, Moreno R, Lisboa C. Weekly cuirass ventilation improves blood gases and inspiratory muscle strength in patients with chronic air-flow limitation and hypercarbia. Am Rev Respir Dis 1988; 138:617–623.

30. Barach AL, Beck GJ, Smith RH. Mechanical production of expiratory flow rates surpassing the capacity of human coughing. Am J Med Sci 1953; 226:241–248.

31. Forbes JA. Management of respiratory paralysis using a "mechanical cough" respirator. Br Med J 1958; 1:798–802.

32. Alba A, Solomon M, Trainor FS. Management of respiratory insufficiency in spinal cord lesions. In: Proceedings of the 17th Veteran's Administration Spinal Cord Injury Conference, 1969. 0-436-398. U.S. Government Printing Office, Washington, DC, 1971:101.

33. Bach JR, Alba AS, Mosher R, Delaubier A. Intermittent positive pressure ventila-

tion via nasal access in the management of respiratory insufficiency. Chest 1987; 92:168–170.

34. Sortor S, McKenzie M. Toward Independence: Assisted Cough [video]. Dallas, TX: BioScience Communications of Dallas, 1986.

35. Massery M. Manual breathing and coughing aids. Phys Med Rehabil Clin N Am 1996; 7:407–422.

36. Bach JR, Smith WH, Michaels J, Saporito LS, Alba AS, Dayal R, Pan J. Airway secretion clearance by mechanical exsufflation for post-poliomyelitis ventilator assisted individuals. Arch Phys Med Rehabil 1993; 74:170–177.

37. Beck GJ, Barach AL. Value of mechanical aids in the management of a patient with poliomyelitis. Ann Intern Med 1954; 40:1081–1094.

38. Dempsey CA. 50 Years of Research On Man in Flight. Wright-Patterson Air Force Base, OH: U.S. Air Force, Aerospace Medical Research Laboratory.

39. Barach AL, Beck GJ, Bickerman HA, Seanor HE. Mechanical coughing: studies on physical methods of producing high velocity flow rates during the expiratory cycle. Tr A Am Physicians 1951; 64:360–363.

40. Barach AL, Beck GJ, Bickerman HA, Seanor HE, Smith W. Physical methods simulating mechanisms of the human cough. J Appl Physiol 1952; 5:85–91.

41. The OEM Cof-flator Portable Cough Machine. St. Louis, MO: Shampaine Industries.

42. Segal MS, Salomon A, Herschfus JA. Alternating positive-negative pressures in mechanical respiration (the cycling valve device employing air pressures). Dis Chest 1954; 25:640–648.

43. Bickerman HA. Exsufflation with negative pressure: elimination of radiopaque material and foreign bodies from bronchi of anesthetized dogs. Arch Int Med 1954; 93:698–704.

44. Siebens AA, Kirby NA, Poulos DA. Cough following transection of spinal cord at C-6. Arch Phys Med Rehabil 1964; 45:1–8.

45. Leiner GC, Abramowitz S, Small MJ, Stenby VB, Lewis WA. Expiratory peak flow rate: standard values for normal subjects. Am Rev Resp Dis 1963; 88:644.

46. Barach AL, Beck GJ. Exsufflation with negative pressure: physiologic and clinical studies in poliomyelitis, bronchial asthma, pulmonary emphysema and bronchiectasis. Arch Int Med 1954; 93:825–841.

47. Beck GJ, Graham GC, Barach AL. Effect of physical methods on the mechanics of breathing in poliomyelitis. Ann Intern Med 1955; 43:549–566.

48. Colebatch HJH. Artificial coughing for patients with respiratory paralysis. Australas J Med 1961; 10:201–212.

49. Cherniack RM, Hildes JA, Alcock AJW. The clinical use of the exsufflator attachment for tank respirators in poliomyelitis. Ann Intern Med 1954; 40:540–548.

50. Barach AL. The application of pressure, including exsufflation, in pulmonary emphysema. Am J Surg 1955; 89:372–382.

51. Beck GJ, Scarrone LA. Physiological effects of exsufflation with negative pressure. Dis Chest 1956; 29:1–16.

52. Freitag L, Long WM, Kim CS, Wanner A. Removal of excessive bronchial secretions by asymmetric high-frequency oscillations. J Appl Physiol 1989; 67:614–619.

53. Dayman HG. Mechanics of airflow in health and emphysema. J Clin Investig 1951; 30:1175–1190.

54. Williams EK, Holaday DA. The use of exsufflation with negative pressure in post-operative patients. Am J Surg 1955; 90:637–640.
55. Kirby NA, Barnerias MJ, Siebens AA. An evaluation of assisted cough in quadriparetic patients. Arch Phys Med Rehabil 1966; 47:705–710.
56. Rennie H, Wilson JAC. A coughing-belt. Lancet 1983; 1.1:138–139.
57. Linder SH. Functional electrical stimulation to enhance cough in quadriplegia. Chest 1993; 103:166–169.

Index

[Mucoregulatory agents]
macrolide antibiotics, 140
peptide, peptide antagonists, 331–332
Mucous glycoproteins, viscoelasticity, 381
Mucus clearance. *See under* specific condition
Mucus obstruction. *See under* specific condition
Muscle dysfunction, respiratory, 553–576
abdominal binder, 570
cough, normal, 555–556
expiratory muscle aids, 556–557
glossopharyngeal breathing, 557–558
initiating use of aids, 571–573
inspiratory muscle aids, 558–559
intermittent abdominal pressure ventilator, noninvasive, 559–562
noninvasive expiratory muscle aids, 564–570
manually assisted coughing, 564–565
mechanical insufflation-exsufflation, 565–569
paralyzed abdominal musculature, patients with, 569–570
respiratory muscle dysfunction, noninvasive expiratory muscle aids
thoracoabdominal corset, 569–570
tracheostomy intermittent positive pressure ventilation, 562–563
treatment protocol, 570–571
ventilatory impairment, *vs.* oxygenation impairment, 554–555
Muscle-generated pulmonary pressures, postoperative, 521–522
Mustard, 179
Mycoplasma pneumoniae, bacterial products, effect on mucociliary function, 263
Myristicin, 192

N

N-acetylcysteine, 17, 132, 157, 158–159, 194, 209–210, 382

Nacystelyn, 132, 195
additive effect on viscoelasticity of sputum, 218
NAL. *See* Nacystelyn
NANC agents, regulation of gland secretion by, 61–64
Narcotics, 244
effect on cilia, 253
effect on mucociliary function, 276
Nesosteine, 195
Neurohumoral regulation, surface epithelium, 51–53
Neuropeptide Y, effect on mucociliary function, 270
Neuropeptides, effect on cilia, 249
Neurotransmitters, 362–363
Neutrophil elastase, 62
N-guanylcysteine, 195
Nitric oxide, 363
Non-cystic fibrosis transmembrane regulator
channel activation, 134–135
channel regulation, 133–134
Nondestructive mucolysis, ionic, hydrogen bonds, 212–213
Noninvasive expiratory muscle aids, 564–570
manually assisted coughing, 564–565
mechanical insufflation-exsufflation, 565–569
Nonsteroidal anti-inflammatory drugs
effect on cilia, 253
effect on mucociliary function, 276–277
Norfloxacin, 385–386
Nose, structure of, 373–375

O

Oligosaccharide mucolytic agents, 214–216
Ophiopogonis, 196
Oral mucokinetic agents, mechanisms of action, 179
Oral mucolytics, 209–210